Texas Children's Hospital Handbook of Congenital Heart Disease

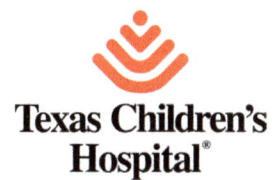

Texas Children's Hospital Handbook of
Congenital Heart Disease

Editors

Carlos M. Mery, MD, MPH
Associate Professor, Surgery and Perioperative Care, and Pediatrics
Associate Chief, Pediatric and Congenital Cardiothoracic Surgery
Director, Health Transformation and Design in Congenital Heart Disease
University of Texas Dell Medical School / Dell Children's Medical Center
Austin, TX

Patricia Bastero, MD
Assistant Professor in Critical Care Medicine
Associate Director of Simulation - Faculty Development
Medical Director of Simulation for Critical Care Medicine
Texas Children's Hospital / Baylor College of Medicine
Houston, TX

Stuart R. Hall, MD, FAAP
Assistant Professor of Anesthesiology, Pediatrics, and Critical Care
Texas Children's Hospital / Baylor College of Medicine
Houston, TX

Antonio G. Cabrera, MD, FAAP, FACC, FAHA
L. George Veasy Presidential Endowed Chair
Chief of Pediatric Cardiology
Co-Director, Primary Children's Heart Center
Associate Professor of Pediatrics
University of Utah Health
Salt Lake City, UT

Senior Editors

Daniel J. Penny, MD, PhD, MHA
Professor of Pediatrics
Baylor College of Medicine
Chief of Cardiology
Texas Children's Hospital
Houston, TX

Lara S. Shekerdemian, MD, MHA
Professor and Chief, Critical Care
Vice Chair for Clinical Affairs, Department of Pediatrics
Baylor College of Medicine, Texas Children's Hospital
Houston, TX

Dean B. Andropoulos, MD, MHCM
Anesthesiologist-in-Chief, Texas Children's Hospital
Department of Anesthesiology, Perioperative and Pain Medicine
Burdett S. Dunbar MD Chair in Pediatric Anesthesiology
Professor, Anesthesiology and Pediatrics
Vice Chair for Clinical Affairs, Department of Anesthesiology
Baylor College of Medicine
Houston, TX

Charles D. Fraser Jr., MD, FACS
Professor of Surgery and Perioperative Care, and Pediatrics
Section Chief for Pediatric and Congenital Cariothoracic Surgery
Director, Texas Center for Pediatric and Congenital Heart Disease
University of Texas Dell Medical School / Dell Children's Medical Center
Austin, TX

Christopher A. Caldarone, MD
Donovan Chair and Chief, Congenital Heart Surgery
Professor of Surgery and Pediatrics
Baylor College of Medicine, Texas Children's Hospital
Houston, TX

Texas Children's Hospital Handbook of Congenital Heart Disease

Digital content editor and contributor (echocardiography): Josh Kailin

Illustrations: Beth Sumner Vuelta, David Aten, Scott Weldon, Carlos Mery

Photography: Phil Steffek

Statistics: Martín Chacón-Portillo, Rodrigo Zea-Vera, Carmen Watrin

Formatting and typesetting: Terrance Johnson, Carlos Mery

Cover: Sheila A. Hall

Project management: Shon Bower, Laura L. Higgins, Carlos Mery

ISBN: 978-1-7342721-1-6 (hardcover)

Library of Congress Control Number: 2019919125

Copyright © 2020 by Texas Children's Hospital

6621 Fannin St
Houston, TX 77030

All rights reserved. This book is protected by copyright. No part of this book may be reproduced in any form or by any means, electronic or mechanical, without permission from the copyright owner.

This book presents generally accepted practices at Texas Children's Hospital, and care has been taken to confirm the accuracy of the information presented. However, the material is only intended as a general guidance for medical professionals. It is the ultimate responsibility of individual providers to review the material, check appropriate medications and dosages, and use their judgement and experience to treat individual patients. The authors, editors, and publisher do not accept any legal responsibility or liability for any errors or omissions made.

Suggested citation: Mery CM, Bastero P, Hall SR, Cabrera AG (eds). Texas Children's Hospital Handbook of Congenital Heart Disease. Houston, TX: Texas Children's Hospital, 2020.

To all children and adults living with congenital heart disease;

To our colleagues who care for them day in and day out;

To our families for allowing us to do so ourselves.

Contributing Authors

Barbara-Jo Achuff, MD, FAAP
Assistant Professor
Department of Pediatrics,
  Cardiac Critical Care
Baylor College of Medicine
Texas Children's Hospital
Houston, TX

Iki Adachi, MD
Director, Mechanical Circulatory Support
Congenital Heart Surgery
Texas Children's Hospital
Associate Professor,
  Michael E. DeBakey Department of Surgery
Baylor College of Medicine
Houston, TX

Natasha Afonso, MD, MPH
Assistant Professor
Section of Critical Care Medicine
Department of Pediatrics
Texas Children's Hospital
Baylor College of Medicine
Houston, TX

Varun Aggarwal, MD
Pediatric Interventional Cardiologist
Assistant Professor of Pediatrics
University of Minnesota Masonic Children's Hospital
Minneapolis, MN

Mubbasheer Ahmed, MD
Assistant Professor
Baylor College of Medicine /
  Texas Children's Hospital
Houston, TX

Ayse Akcan-Arikan, MD
Associate Professor
Department of Pediatrics
Baylor College of Medicine
Sections of Critical Care and Nephrology
Medical Director, Extracorporeal Liver Support
Medical Director, Critical Care Nephrology
Texas Children's Hospital
Houston, TX

Carolyn A. Altman, MD, FACC, FAHA, FASE
Associate Chief, Pediatric Cardiology
Professor of Pediatrics
Texas Children's Hospital
Baylor College of Medicine
Houston, TX

Meghan Anderson, DNP, APRN, CPNP-AC
Nurse Practitioner, Congenital Heart Surgery
Texas Children's Hospital
Houston, TX

Dean B. Andropoulos, MD, MHCM
Anesthesiologist-in-Chief, Texas Children's Hospital
Department of Anesthesiology,
  Perioperative and Pain Medicine
Burdett S. Dunbar MD Chair in
  Pediatric Anesthesiology
Professor, Anesthesiology and Pediatrics
Vice Chair for Clinical Affairs, Department of
  Anesthesiology
Baylor College of Medicine
Houston, TX

Nancy A. Ayres, MD
Director of Non-Invasive Imaging
  and Pediatric Cardiology
Texas Children's Hospital
Assistant Professor of Pediatrics
Baylor College of Medicine
Houston, TX

Patricia Bastero, MD
Assistant Professor in Critical Care Medicine
Associate Director of Simulation -
  Faculty Development
Medical Director of Simulation
  for Critical Care Medicine
Texas Children's Hospital / Baylor College of Medicine
Houston, TX

Aarti Bavare, MD, MPH
Assistant Professor
Section of Critical Care and Cardiology,
  Department of Pediatrics
Baylor College of Medicine
Houston, TX

Judith A. Becker, MD
Associate Professor, Pediatric Cardiology
Baylor College of Medicine
Texas Children's Hospital
Houston, TX

Taylor Beecroft, MS, CGC
Certified Genetic Counselor
Pediatric Cardiology
Baylor College of Medicine
Houston, TX

Ziyad M. Binsalamah, MD, MSc, FRCSC
Assistant Professor in Congenital Heart Surgery
Baylor College of Medicine and
  Texas Children's Hospital
Houston, TX

Claire E. Bocchini, MD, MS
Assistant Professor of Pediatrics – Infectious Disease
Texas Children's Hospital / Baylor College of Medicine
Houston, TX

Ken Brady, MD
Ann & Robert H. Lurie Children's Hospital of Chicago
Northwestern Feinberg School of Medicine
Chicago, IL

Ronald A. Bronicki, MD, FCCM, FACC
Professor with Tenure
Department of Pediatrics
Baylor College of Medicine
Texas Children's Hospital
Section of Critical Care Medicine & Cardiology
Houston, TX

Cole Burgman, CCP
Texas Children's Hospital
Houston, TX

Antonio G. Cabrera, MD, FAAP, FACC, FAHA
L. George Veasy Presidential Endowed Chair
Chief of Pediatric Cardiology
Co-Director, Primary Children's Heart Center
Associate Professor of Pediatrics
University of Utah Health
Salt Lake City, UT

Christopher A. Caldarone, MD
Donovan Chair and Chief, Congenital Heart Surgery
Professor of Surgery and Pediatrics
Baylor College of Medicine
Texas Children's Hospital
Houston, TX

Natalie Cannon, MS, RD, LD, CNSC
Department of Clinical Nutrition
Texas Children's Hospital
Houston, TX

Lisa Caplan, MD
Associate Professor of Anesthesiology
Pediatric Cardiac Anesthesiology
Baylor College of Medicine /
  Texas Children's Hospital
Houston, TX

Corey Chartan, DO, FAAP
Assistant Professor of Pediatrics
Pediatric Critical Care Medicine
  & Pediatric Pulmonary Hypertension
Associate Medical Director -
  Right Ventricular Failure Program
Assistant Medical Director of ECMO - Education
Texas Children's Hospital /
  Baylor College of Medicine
Houston, TX

Paul A. Checchia, MD, FCCM, FACC
Professor of Pediatrics
Associate Section Chief for Cardiac Services and
  Business Operations
Section of Critical Care Medicine
Texas Children's Hospital and
  Baylor College of Medicine
Houston, TX

Ryan D. Coleman, MD, FAAP
Pediatric Critical Care / Pulmonary Hypertension
Medical Director - Right Ventricular Failure Program
Assistant Medical Director - ECMO
Assistant Professor of Pediatrics and Medical Ethics
Texas Children's Hospital / Baylor College of Medicine
Houston, TX

Lisa C.A. D'Alessandro, MD, FRCPC, FAAP
Assistant Professor, Pediatrics, University of Toronto
Pediatric Cardiology, Trillium Health Partners
Mississauga, Ontario, Canada

Caridad M. de la Uz, MD
Assistant Professor
Director of Pediatric Electrophysiology
Johns Hopkins Children's Center
Baltimore, MD

Susan W. Denfield, MD, FAAP, FACC
Associate Professor of Pediatrics
Lillie Frank Abercrombie
  Division of Pediatric Cardiology
Baylor College of Medicine
Texas Children's Hospital
Houston, TX

Heather A. Dickerson, MD
Assistant Professor of Pediatrics
Texas Children's Hospital
Baylor College of Medicine
Houston, TX

William J. Dreyer, MD, FAAP, FACC
Professor of Pediatrics
Baylor College of Medicine
Medical Director, Heart Failure,
  Cardiomyopathy and Cardiac Transplantation
Texas Children's Hospital
Houston, TX

R. Blaine Easley, MD
Professor, Departments of
  Anesthesiology and Pediatrics
Baylor College of Medicine
Associate Anesthesiologist-in-Chief,
  Academic Affairs
Medical Director, Surgical Intensive Care Unit
Texas Children's Hospital
Houston, TX

Justin Elhoff, MD, MSCR, FACC
Assistant Professor,
 Baylor College of Medicine
Department of Pediatrics
Sections of Critical Care Medicine and Cardiology
Texas Children's Hospital
Houston, TX

Barbara A. Elias BSN, RN, CCRN
VAD Coordinator – Congenital Heart Surgery
Texas Children's Hospital
Houston, TX

Peter Ermis, MD, FACC
Medical Director -
 Adult Congenital Heart Disease
Program Director - ACHD Fellowship
Head of Adult Medicine
Texas Children's Hospital
Assistant Professor - Pediatrics
Baylor College of Medicine
Houston, TX

Zhe Amy Fang, MD, FRCPC
Department of Anesthesia and Pain Medicine
Hospital for Sick Children
Toronto, Ontario, Canada

Saul Flores, MD, FAAP, FACC
Cardiac Intensive Care Unit
Section of Critical Care
Texas Children's Hospital
Assistant Professor of Pediatrics
Baylor College of Medicine
Houston, TX

Wayne J. Franklin, MD, FACC
Phoenix Children's Hospital
Co-Director, PCH Heart Center
Chair, Department of Adult Medicine
Director, Adult Congenital Heart Disease
Professor, University of Arizona
Phoenix, AZ

Charles D. Fraser Jr., MD, FACS
Professor of Surgery and Perioperative Care,
 and Pediatrics
Section Chief for Pediatric
 and Congenital Cariothoracic Surgery
Director, Texas Center for Pediatric
 and Congenital Heart Disease
University of Texas Dell Medical School /
 Dell Children's Medical Center
Austin, TX

Nancy S. Ghanayem, MD, MS
Texas Children's Hospital
Baylor College of Medicine
Houston, TX

Jordana Goldman, MD
Assistant Professor
Baylor College of Medicine
Houston, TX

Angela Gooden, MSN, APRN, CPNP-PC/AC
Director, Advanced Practice Providers
Nurse Practitioner, Cardiology
Texas Children's Hospital
Instructor, Baylor College of Medicine
Houston, TX

Erin A. Gottlieb, MD
Associate Professor of Surgery and
 Perioperative Care
The University of Texas at
 Austin Dell Medical School
Chief, Pediatric Cardiac Anesthesiology
Dell Children's Medical Center
Austin, TX

Srinath T. Gowda, MD
Associate Professor of Pediatrics
Pediatric Interventional Cardiology
Texas Children's Hospital
Houston, TX

Stuart R. Hall, MD, FAAP
Assistant Professor of Anesthesiology,
 Pediatrics, and Critical Care
Texas Children's Hospital /
 Baylor College of Medicine
Houston, TX

Lauren Hannigan, MOT, OTR/L
Clinical Specialist
Physical Medicine and Rehabilitation
Texas Children's Hospital
Houston, TX

Amy Hemingway, MSN, CNS, CPNP-AC/PC
Texas Children's Hospital
Clinical Assistant Professor,
 Baylor College of Medicine
Houston, TX

Timothy J. Humlicek, PharmD, BCPS
Clinical Pharmacy Specialist – Cardiology
Texas Children's Hospital
Houston, TX

Siddharth P. Jadhav, MD
Associate Professor
Department of Pediatric Radiology
Division of Cardiovascular, Body and Musculoskeletal
 Imaging
Associate Director, Pediatric Cardiovascular Imaging
 Fellowship Program
Texas Children's Hospital and
Baylor College of Medicine
Houston, TX

Parag Jain, MD, FAAP
Assistant Professor of Pediatrics
Section of Critical Care Medicine
Texas Children's Hospital and Baylor College of
  Medicine
Houston, TX

Henri Justino, MD, CM, FRCPC, FACC, FSCAI, FAAP
Director, Cardiology Innovation
Co-Director, CE Mullins Cardiac
  Catheterization Laboratories,
Texas Children's Hospital
Professor (Tenured) of Pediatrics,
Baylor College of Medicine
Houston, TX

Josh Kailin, MD
Assistant Professor
Baylor College of Medicine
Texas Children's Hospital
Houston, TX

Debra L. Kearney, MD
Pediatric Cardiovascular Pathologist
Medical Director of Autopsy Service
Texas Children's Hospital
Associate Professor of Pathology & Immunology
Baylor College of Medicine
Houston, TX

Asra Khan, MD
Assistant Professor of Pediatrics
Division of Pediatric Cardiology
Baylor College of Medicine / Texas Children's Hospital
Houston, TX

Jeffrey J. Kim, MD
Texas Children's Hospital
Baylor College of Medicine
Houston, TX

Kimberly Krauklis, MSN, APRN, NP-C, PNP-AC
Pediatric Nurse Practitioner
Manager of Advance Practice Providers
Texas Center for Pediatric and
  Congenital Heart Disease
Dell Medical School, University of Texas at Austin
Austin, TX

William Buck Kyle, MD
Associate Professor
Baylor College of Medicine / Texas Children's Hospital
Houston, TX

Wilson Lam, MD
Assistant Professor, Baylor College of Medicine
Departments of Pediatrics and Medicine
Texas Adult Congenital Heart Program
Houston, TX

M. Regina Lantin Hermoso MD, FAAP, FASE, FACC
Associate Professor of Pediatrics
Section of Cardiology
Baylor College of Medicine
Medical Director
Out-Patient Clinics, Main Campus
Texas Children's Heart Center
Houston, TX

Javier J. Lasa, MD, FAAP
Assistant Professor
Department of Pediatrics
Sections of Critical Care Medicine and Cardiology
Texas Children's Hospital
Houston, TX

Aimee Liou MD, FSCAI, FAAP
Assistant Professor of Pediatrics
Division of Pediatric Cardiology
Baylor College of Medicine
Texas Children's Hospital
Houston, TX

Keila N. Lopez, MD, MPH
Assistant Professor, Pediatrics
Director, Transition Medicine,
  Section of Pediatric Cardiology
Baylor College of Medicine /
  Texas Children's Hospital
Houston, TX

Prakash M. Masand, MD
Division Chief, Body & Cardiovascular Imaging
Edward B. Singleton Department of Radiology, Texas
  Children's Hospital
Associate Professor, Baylor College of Medicine
Houston, TX

Estrella Mazarico de Thomas, RN
Clinical Nurse Coordinator
Cardiology Department
Texas Children's Hospital
Houston, TX

Mary Claire McGarry, LP, CCP, FPP
Perfusionist, Congenital Heart Surgery
Texas Children's Hospital
Houston, TX

Carlos M. Mery, MD, MPH
Associate Professor, Surgery and
  Perioperative Care, and Pediatrics
Associate Chief, Pediatric and Congenital
  Cardiothoracic Surgery
Director, Health Transformation and
  Design in Congenital Heart Disease
University of Texas Dell Medical School / Dell
  Children's Medical Center
Austin, TX

Wanda C. Miller-Hance, MD, FACC, FAAP, FASE
Professor of Anesthesiology and Pediatrics
Department of Anesthesiology,
  Perioperative and Pain Medicine
Arthur S. Keats Division of Pediatric
  Cardiovascular Anesthesiology
Department of Pediatrics, Section of Cardiology
Baylor College of Medicine
Texas Children's Hospital
Houston, TX

Christina Y. Miyake, MD, MS
Associate Professor, Department of Pediatrics,
  Texas Children's Hospital
Associate Professor, Department of Molecular
  Physiology and Biophysics,
  Baylor College of Medicine
Houston, TX

Brady S. Moffett, PharmD, MPH, MBA
Assistant Director, Pharmacy
Texas Children's Hospital – The Woodlands
Assistant Professor, Pediatrics
Baylor College of Medicine
Houston, TX

Silvana Molossi, MD, PhD
Associate Chief, Section of Cardiology
Medical Director, Coronary Anomalies Program
Associate Professor, Department of Pediatrics
Texas Children's Hospital
Baylor College of Medicine
Houston, TX

Shaine A. Morris, MD, MPH
Associate Professor of Pediatrics,
  Section of Cardiology
Medical Director, Cardiovascular Genetics
Associate Director,
  Pediatric Cardiology Fellowship Program
Associate Director,
  Fetal Cardiac Intervention Program
Texas Children's Hospital and
  Baylor College of Medicine
Houston, TX

Emad B. Mossad, MD
Associate Anesthesiologist-in-Chief Clinical Affairs
Department of Anesthesiology, Perioperative and
  Pain Medicine
Division Chief, Pediatric Cardiac Anesthesia
Texas Children's Hospital
Houston, TX

Antonio R. Mott, MD
Associate Professor of Pediatrics
Baylor College of Medicine
Medical Director, Inpatient Cardiology Service
The Legacy Tower Heart Center
Texas Children's Hospital
Houston, TX

Pablo Motta, MD, FAAP
Associate Professor of Anesthesiology,
  Perioperative and Pain Medicine
Baylor College of Medicine
Arthur S. Keats Division of Pediatric Cardiovascular
  Anesthesiology
Texas Children's Hospital
Houston, TX

Cory V. Noel, MD
Pediatric Cardiology of Alaska –
  Seattle Children's Hospital
Anchorage, AK

Elena C. Ocampo, MD
Assistant Professor of Pediatrics
Baylor College of Medicine
Texas Children's Hospital
Houston, TX

Katie Persha, CCLS
Certified Life Specialist II
Heart Failure/Heart Transplant
Texas Children's Hospital
Houston, TX

Jack F. Price, MD, FACC, FAAP
Associate Professor of Pediatrics (Cardiology)
Baylor College of Medicine
Texas Children's Hospital
Houston, TX

Zoel A. Quinonez, MD
Assistant Professor
Lucile Packard Children's Hospital
Stanford University
Stanford, CA

Athar M. Qureshi, MD, FSCAI, FAAP
Medical Director of Interventional Cardiology
  (Clinical)
CE Mullins Cardiac Catheterization Laboratories
The Lillie Frank Abercrombie Section of Cardiology,
  Texas Children's Hospital
Associate Professor of Pediatrics, Baylor College of
  Medicine
Attending Physician, Internal Medicine/Cardiology,
  Baylor St. Luke's Medical Center
Houston, TX

Karla V. Resendiz, PharmD, BCPPS
Clinical Pharmacy Specialist
Pediatric Critical Care
Department of Pharmacy Services
Children's Hospital of Philadelphia
Philadelphia, PA

Ashraf Resheidat, MD
Assistant Professor
Department of Anesthesiology
Division of Pediatric Cardiovascular Anesthesiology
Baylor College of Medicine / Texas Children's Hospital
Houston, TX

Guill Reyes, BSN, RN
Cardiovascular ICU
Texas Children's Hospital
Houston, TX

Sara H. Reynolds, CCLS
Certified Child Life Specialist
Cardiac Intensive Care Unit
Texas Children's Hospital
Houston, TX

Christopher J. Rhee, MD, MS
Assistant Professor of Pediatrics
Baylor College of Medicine
Texas Children's Hospital
Houston, TX

Alan F. Riley, MD, FAAP
Assistant Professor
Department of Pediatrics, Pediatric Cardiology
Baylor College of Medicine
Texas Children's Hospital
Houston, TX

D. Jeramy Roddy, MD, FAAP
Assistant Professor of Pediatrics
Baylor College of Medicine
Attending Physician, CICU
Section of Critical Care Medicine
Texas Children's Hospital
Houston, TX

Miranda A. Rodrigues, DNP, RN, CNL, CCRN-K
Clinical Specialist - Nursing
Cardiac Intensive Care Unit
Texas Children's Hospital
Houston, TX

Alexia B. Santos, MD
Assistant Professor, Pediatric Cardiology
Texas Children's Hospital / Baylor College of Medicine
Houston, TX

Fabio Savorgnan, MD, FAAP, FACC
Cardiac Intensive Care Unit
Section of Critical Care
Texas Children's Hospital
Assistant Professor of Pediatrics
Baylor College of Medicine
Houston, TX

Tobias R. Schlingmann, MD, PhD
Assistant Professor, Baylor College of Medicine
Pediatric Cardiologist, Texas Children's Hospital
Houston, TX

Robin Rae Schlosser, PT
Inpatient Specialty Therapy Coordinator
Texas Children's Hospital
Houston, TX

Thomas J. Seery, MD, FAAP, FACC
Assistant Professor of Pediatrics
Division of Cardiology
UPMC Children's Hospital of Pittsburgh
Pittsburgh, PA

Kerry Sembera MSN, RN, CCRN-K
Assistant Director,
 Clinical Practice for the Heart Center
Texas Children's Hospital
Houston, TX

S. Kristen Sexson Tejtel, MD, PhD, MPH
Assistant Professor of Pediatrics
 and Pediatric Cardiology
Texas Children's Hospital Heart Center
Baylor College of Medicine
Houston, TX

Rev. Thomas P. Sharon, MDiv, BCC
Assistant Director of Family Advocacy
 and Spiritual Care
Texas Children's Hospital
Houston, TX

Lara S. Shekerdemian, MD, MHA
Professor and Chief, Critical Care
Vice Chair for Clinical Affairs,
 Department of Pediatrics
Baylor College of Medicine,
 Texas Children's Hospital
Houston, TX

Ron Shelton, CCP, LP, FPP
AmSect Fellow of Pediatric Perfusion
Assistant Director, Circulatory Services
Texas Children's Hospital
Houston, TX

Virginia Smith BSN, RN, CCRN
Decentralized Education Coordinator
Cardiac Intensive Care Unit
Texas Children's Hospital
Houston, TX

Cynthia Sturrock, BSN, RN, CCRN
CICU Charge Nurse
CICU Nurse Instructor
Texas Children's Hospital
Houston, TX

Jun Teruya, MD, DSc, FCAP
Professor of Departments of Pathology
 & Immunology, Pediatrics, and Medicine
Baylor College of Medicine
Chief of Division of Transfusion Medicine
 & Coagulation
Department of Pathology
Texas Children's Hospital
Houston, TX

James A. Thomas, MD
Professor, Pediatric Critical Care Medicine
Section Chief, Ethics, Baylor College of Medicine
ECMO Medical Director, Texas Children's Hospital
Houston, TX

Premal M. Trivedi, MD
Assistant Professor of Anesthesiology
Baylor College of Medicine
Division of Pediatric
  Cardiovascular Anesthesiology
Texas Children's Hospital
Houston, TX

Rocky Tsang, MD, FAAP
Assistant Professor of Pediatrics
Baylor College of Medicine
Texas Children's Hospital
Houston, TX

Sebastian C. Tume, MD
Assistant Professor
Department of Pediatrics,
  Section of Critical Care Medicine
Baylor College of Medicine
Houston, TX

Hari P. Tunuguntla, MD, MPH
Assistant Professor, Pediatrics
Division of Pediatric Cardiology,
  Heart Failure & Transplant
Texas Children's Hospital / Baylor College of Medicine
Houston, TX

Santiago O. Valdes, MD
Pediatric Cardiology – Arrhythmia and Pacing
Associate Professor, Pediatrics
Baylor College of Medicine / Texas Children's Hospital
Houston, TX

David F. Vener, MD
Professor of Pediatrics and Anesthesiology
Baylor College of Medicine
Arthur Keats Division of
  Pediatric Cardiovascular Anesthesiology
Texas Children's Hospital
Houston, TX

G. Wesley Vick, III, MD, PhD
Associate Professor
Section of Pediatric Cardiology
Departments of Pediatrics,
  Internal Medicine, and Radiology
Baylor College of Medicine
Texas Children's Hospital
Houston, TX

Saeed M. Yacouby, CRNA, DNP
Department of Anesthesiology
University of Texas – Memorial Hermann Hospital
Houston, TX

Betul Yilmaz Furtun, MD
Assistant Professor
Texas Children's Hospital
Baylor College of Medicine
Houston, TX

David E. Wesson, MD
Professor of Surgery
Baylor College of Medicine
Houston, TX

Jennifer Yborra, RN, AC-PNP
Pediatric Cardiovascular Anesthesia
Texas Children's Hospital
Houston, TX

Justin Zachariah, MD, MPH, FAHA, FAAP
Assistant Professor in Pediatric Cardiology
  Texas Children's Hospital
Baylor College of Medicine
Houston, TX

Foreword

It is with the utmost pride that we write this foreword to the first Texas Children's Handbook of Congenital Heart Disease. It represents the synthesis of more than 60 years of learning within our Heart Center and the work of thousands. The Handbook is written with the full recognition that there are many ways to care for children with heart disease. We hope that a full description of our "way" will provide a useful resource for new clinicians seeking to establish their "way" and for seasoned clinicians interested in reviewing their "way" from another perspective.

We trust that The Handbook adequately reflects our view of the importance of a multidisciplinary approach to the care of the child with heart disease and their family. If we have learned one thing on our continuing journey to excellence, it's that true excellence does not reflect just exceptional performance from an individual surgeon, cardiologist, anesthesiologist, or intensivist, rather it reflects the amalgamation of a vast experience composed of minute-to-minute often seemingly minor management decisions made across the multidisciplinary team. Our "way" reflects meticulous attention to the endless details involved in minute-to-minute patient care and, importantly, a commitment to constantly improve team performance through maintenance of situational awareness, optimal decision-making processes, and multiple types of performance review.

Much of what is written here does not come from an "evidence base" in the strict, traditional sense, but rather from the middle-of-the-night conversations over a sick patient, an astute observation about chest-tube care from the nurse on the intensive care unit, or a student's quality improvement project. To this end, we work under the principle that our Heart Center displays many of the properties of a complex adaptive system, in which everyday interactions between members of the multidisciplinary team and with our patients, result in the emergence of patterns which, when recognized, can be used across the system in order to improve performance.

Central to our ability to recognize these patterns and optimize our learning from them is a robust system of multidisciplinary overcommunication across our Heart Center. All patients for whom a procedure might be considered are presented at twice-weekly multidisciplinary meetings, aimed at explicit decision-making and timeliness of care. All patients are presented again a few days before their surgery in order to provide a final check and to provide situational awareness about their specific needs across the multidisciplinary team. Again, with the aim of providing situational awareness, the multidisciplinary team is informed of every patient who has been admitted to our Heart Center at our daily, early morning meeting. We form a contract with our families that an overall plan of care will be developed for their child by the multidisciplinary team within 24 hours of admission and have a formal "huddle" requirement for urgent decisions. As well as standard "M&M" meetings, we hold weekly, multidisciplinary "performance rounds" to review our delivery of care for every patient's journey and to identify learning opportunities from middle-of-the-night observations. These learnings are consolidated and transformed into improved protocols and processes by "Tiger Teams" assigned to capitalize on each of these learning opportunities. Data related to almost every aspect of our inpatient and outpatient care is shared across the multidisciplinary team and with our external stakeholders.

If we are to optimize the value of these efforts, we need to leverage the intellectual insights of every member of the care team. Because modern leadership strategies have shifted from steep hierarchies to more flexible and resilient decision-making structures based upon communication and collaboration, we have developed focus groups to improve trust and psychological safety across the team. These aspects of team functioning are discussed on a regular basis at "town-hall" meetings and center-wide retreats.

We are proud to thank every member of The Heart Center, who have work over many years to develop our Program. We are extremely grateful to the editors and authors from right across our multidisciplinary team who have worked tirelessly to develop this Handbook and capture the essence of our approach. We thank hospital leadership and the leadership within our College who have provided support for our Heart Center to a degree that none of us could have imagined or expected. Most of all, we thank the thousands of families who have entrusted us to care for their precious children.

We hope that at least some of this handbook will be useful to you as your center continues to develop "your way".

Dan Penny
Chief of Cardiology

Chris Caldarone
Chief of Congenital Heart Surgery

Preface

The Texas Children's Handbook of Congenital Heart Disease is designed as a practical handbook to help clinicians care for children with congenital heart disease on a day-to-day basis. The Handbook is the result of a multiyear effort by a large number of physicians, nurses, and allied staff across a wide variety of disciplines within the Texas Children's Heart Center. It builds on the legacy, mission, and moral imperative of the Heart Center to not only provide unparalleled care to children and adults with congenital heart disease but also to train the next generation of clinicians to care for these patients.

Texas Children's Hospital (TCH) opened its doors in 1954 (Figure 1) as part of St Luke's Episcopal Hospital in Houston with the idea that "any child in the State of Texas in need of medical care and attention – regardless of race, color, creed, or capacity to pay – shall find in Texas Children's Hospital a refuge from the ravages of disease and illness, and the hope for health and happiness" (Leopold Meyer, 1951). The pediatric cardiac program was started that year by Dan McNamara and Denton Cooley (Figure 2). Dr. Cooley had trained under Alfred Blalock at Johns Hopkins, where he was part of the first Blalock-Taussig shunt operation, and joined the faculty of Baylor College of Medicine under Michael E. DeBakey in 1951. He would later become one of the most important pioneers in the history of cardiac surgery. Dr. McNamara had also trained at Johns Hopkins, under the direction of Helen Taussig, and was one of her star mentees. He became the first Chief of Pediatric Cardiology at TCH and would play a leading role in the development of the entire field of pediatric cardiology.

In 1955, Drs. Cooley and McNamara visited Walton Lillehei (at the University of Minnesota) and John Kirklin (at the Mayo Clinic) who had just performed the first intracardiac operations

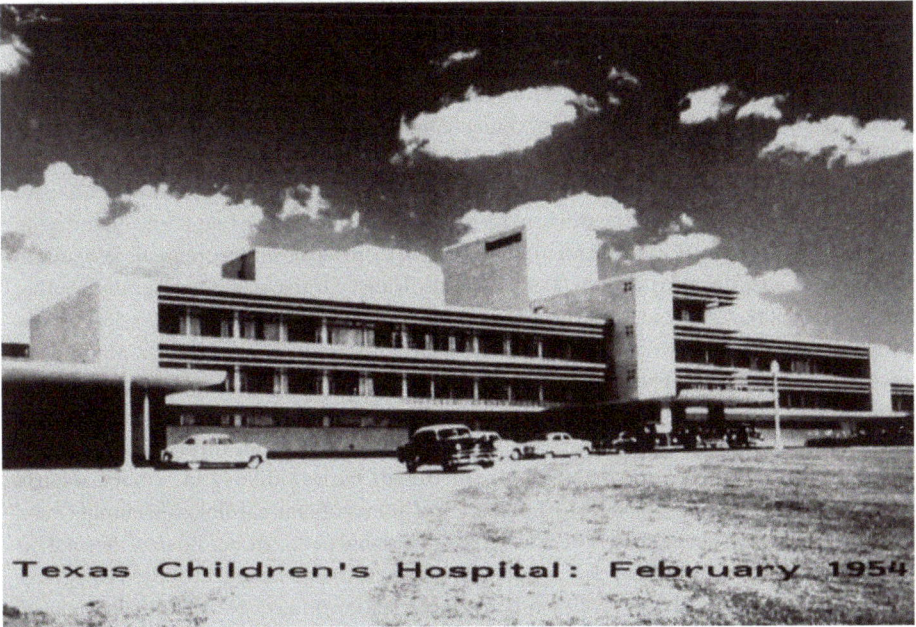

Figure 1. Texas Children's Hospital in 1954.

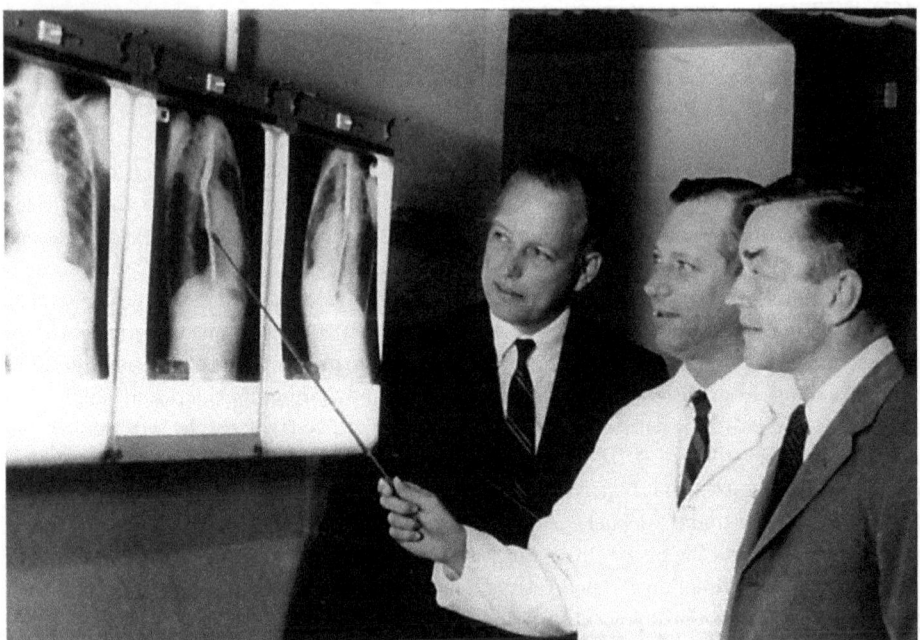

Figure 2. From left to right, Denton Cooley, Edward Singleton (first Chief of Radiology), and Dan McNamara.

using cross-circulation and the first iteration of the cardiopulmonary bypass machine, respectively. Upon returning to Houston, Dr. Cooley assembled a home-grown oxygenator system from parts bought at a restaurant-supply store and started doing open heart surgery. Dr. McNamara, aware of the high mortality of babies with congenital heart disease, encouraged Dr. Cooley to operate on younger and younger babies, challenging the prevailing belief that surgery should be deferred on these patients until later in life. By 1959, they had amassed an impressive series of 120 newborns and infants operated on before one year of life, something previously unheard of. However, as the field of adult cardiac surgery exploded, Dr. Cooley's team, who operated on both adults (at St Luke's Hospital) and children (at TCH), started devoting gradually less time to performing congenital heart surgery. Meanwhile, dedicated cardiac surgical programs at other children's hospitals continued to move the field forward and get better and better surgical results.

During this time, pediatric cardiology at TCH continued to flourish under Dr. McNamara, becoming one of the most prolific academic and training pediatric cardiology programs in the United States. During his tenure, Dr. McNamara trained innumerable pediatric cardiologists that would go on to lead multiple divisions, departments, and hospitals throughout the world. It was also during this time that Dr. McNamara recruited Charles Mullins and Arthur Garson Jr. Dr. Mullins would become a pioneer in the creation of interventional cardiology techniques and eventually be known as the "father of modern interventional pediatric cardiology". Beyond his multiple contributions to patient care, Dr. Mullins is known for developing the series of diagrams that are ubiquitously used to describe cardiac catheterization procedures. Dr. Garson would go on to become one of the fathers of pediatric electrophysiology, and with Dr. McNamara, one of the few pediatric cardiologists to occupy the presidency of the American College of Cardiology. Dr. Garson succeeded Dr. McNamara as Chief of Pediatric Cardiology in 1988 and was followed by J. Timothy Bricker in 1992.

By the mid 1990s, despite the success of TCH in the field of pediatric cardiology, cardiac surgery at TCH (which had separated from St Luke's Hospital in 1987) was provided by surgeons from Dr. Cooley's group who split their time between the care of children and adults. As such, surgical results were suboptimal when compared to other programs that had advanced significantly in the management of newborns and children with congenital heart disease by having dedicated units and personnel. In 1995, Charles Fraser Jr. was recruited by Dr. Bricker and Ralph Feigin (Physician-in-Chief at that time) to create a dedicated and focused congenital heart surgical team. Dr. Fraser had trained under Roger Mee in Melbourne, Australia, where Dr. Mee had achieved unparalleled surgical results by creating a dedicated cardiac surgical unit with meticulous attention to detail through every level of the process of care. Over the ensuing years, Dr. Fraser developed a fully integrated congenital cardiac program with a focus on detailed preoperative, intraoperative, and postoperative management of patients, refinement of processes, careful tracking of outcomes and a managment philosophy that largely persists to this day. Perfusion techniques were borrowed from Dr. Mee's unit in Melbourne and further adapted by Dr. Fraser and a team of dedicated pediatric cardiac perfusionists. Results after congenital heart surgery improved dramatically. Over the ensuing 20 years, Dr. Fraser would train and mentor many congenital heart surgeons from around the globe, many of which now lead congenital cardiac programs in the United States and elsewhere. In 1998, Dean Andropoulos was recruited to build what is now one of the most preeminent pediatric cardiac anesthesiology divisions in the world.

In 2001, a new geographically integrated Heart Center was created occupying contiguous floors within the West Tower of the hospital. This center colocated all patient units, operating rooms, cardiac catheterization labs, clinics, and administrative offices for pediatric cardiology, congenital heart surgery, cardiac anesthesiology, and perfusion. In 2010, Daniel J. Penny was recruited as Chief of Pediatric Cardiology and Lara S. Shekerdemian, a pediatric cardiac intensivist, as Chief of Critical Care for the hospital. Dr. Penny had trained in London and Melbourne, and had most recently been the Chief of Pediatric Cardiology at the Royal Children's Hospital in Melbourne. Dr. Penny would play a significant role in further integration of the different programs for the Heart Center and the participation of TCH on the broader field of pediatric cardiac research as part of the Pediatric Heart Network of the National Institutes of Health. Dr. Shekerdemian had trained in London and Toronto, and was the Director of Intensive Care at the Royal Children's Hospital in Melbourne prior to joining TCH. Under her leadership, not only the cardiac intensive care unit but all critical care services throughout TCH flourished. She led a significant increase in scholarly activity within the Division of Critical Care Medicine, and the creation of subspecialized intensive care units throughout the hospital.

Over the years, TCH has played a significant role in the development of the field of pediatric heart failure and ventricular assist devices (VAD) in children. During this era, under the leadership of Jeffrey Towbin, several of the mechanistic origins of pediatric heart failuire were discovered at TCH. In 2004, TCH had implanted the first dedicated pediatric VAD, the DeBakey child. However, the device presented with critical technological limitations. In 2011, Dr. Fraser led the first-ever prospective multicenter pediatric VAD trial (Berlin EXCOR) that led to FDA approval later that year. In 2015, TCH opened the first-ever dedicated pediatric Heart Failure Unit, an intensive care unit dedicated to children and young adults with structural heart disease and heart failure. TCH also became the first program to use the HeartMate II device for Fontan patients, use the HeartWare VAD as destination therapy in children, and the first to implant the new pediatric Jarvik VAD in the United States. TCH currently implants 20-25 total VADs per year (temporary and durable) and performs 20-30 heart transplants per year, making it one of the largest transplant programs in the country. Other signature clinical programs that have flourished over the history of the Heart Center include Electrophysiology, Interventional Cardiology, Echocardiography, Fetal Cardiology, Adult Congenital, and the Coronary Anomalies Program.

In 2017, TCH was first recognized by U.S. News and World Report as the #1 pediatric cardiology and heart surgery center in the United States. Due to the sustained growth of the cardiac program, the Heart Center moved in 2018 to the brand-new Legacy Tower, encompassing 8 contiguous floors with more than 50 pediatric cardiac intensive care unit beds, 4 operating rooms, and 4 cardiac catheterization labs. That same year, Christopher A. Caldarone was recruited from the Hospital for Sick Children in Toronto to succeed Dr. Fraser as the new of Chief of Congenital Heart Surgery and help lead with Dr. Penny the next chapter for the TCH Heart Center.

Above all, the Heart Center at TCH is recognized for outstanding clinical outcomes. We believe these outcomes are the result of a multidisciplinary team effort that places the patient's needs at the center of care, surrounds the patients with the necessary expertise at all points of their journey, and follows a consistent philosophy with utmost attention to detail. It is our intent with the Handbook to share this philosophy while enumerating the protocols and nuances of care used on a daily basis.

We are infinitely grateful to all the authors and staff that made the creation and publication of this handbook possible. The Handbook is a tribute to the visionary pioneers that laid the foundation and philosophy of the program, to the leaders that have nurtured the environment and allowed the program to prosper, to all clinicians that day in and day out provide unparalleled care to our patients, and especially to our patients that have allowed us to walk with them as they travel their journey.

Carlos M. Mery
Patricia Bastero
Stuart R. Hall
Antonio G. Cabrera

Table of Contents

I. FUNDAMENTALS — 1

1. Segmental Anatomy of the Heart — 2
2. Fetal and Transitional Circulation — 7
3. Diagnostic Imaging — 11
4. Diagnostic Cardiac Catheterization — 15
5. Intraoperative Transesophageal Echocardiography — 20
6. Cardiopulmonary Bypass and Myocardial Protection — 26

II. DISEASES — 33

7. Patent Ductus Arteriosus — 34
8. Atrial Septal Defect — 42
9. Partial Anomalous Pulmonary Venous Return — 48
10. Pulmonary Vein Anomalies — 56
11. Ventricular Septal Defect — 71
12. Atrioventricular Septal Defect — 80
13. Tetralogy of Fallot — 88
14. Transposition of the Great Arteries — 95
15. Congenitally Corrected Transposition of the Great Arteries — 105
16. Double-Outlet Right Ventricle — 115
17. Pulmonary Atresia, Ventricular Septal Defect, Major Aortopulmonary Collaterals — 124
18. Right-Ventricular Outflow Tract Obstruction — 133
19. Absent Pulmonary Valve Syndrome — 144
20. Tricuspid Atresia — 150
21. Ebstein Anomaly — 155
22. Congenital Aortic Stenosis — 163
23. Subaortic Stenosis — 171
24. Supravalvar Aortic Stenosis — 176
25. Aortic Coarctation and Interrupted Aortic Arch — 181
26. Multilevel Left-Heart Hypoplasia — 197

27. Hypoplastic Left Heart Syndrome	201
28. Truncus Arteriosus and Aortopulmonary Window	209
29. Vascular Rings	217
30. Anomalous Left Coronary Artery from the Pulmonary Artery	224
31. Congenital Coronary Anomalies	233
32. Myocarditis and Cardiomyopathy	244
33. Infective Endocarditis	249
34. Arrhythmias	258
35. Inherited Arrhythmia Syndromes	263
36. Kawasaki Disease	267
37. Pericarditis	277

III. SPECIAL CONSIDERATIONS — 281

38. Aortopulmonary Shunts and Ductal Stents	282
39. Single-Ventricle Palliation	289
40. Pulmonary Valve Replacement	302
41. Pacemakers and Defibrillators	308
42. Ventricular Assist Devices	313
43. Extracorporeal Membrane Oxygenation	322
44. Heart Transplantation	333
45. Heterotaxy Syndrome	341
46. Connective-Tissue Disorders	344
47. The Adult Fontan	352
48. Simulation in the Heart Center	359
49. Cardiac Developmental Outcomes	361
50. Genetic Testing	363
51. Transition Medicine in Pediatric Cardiology	372

IV. PERIOPERATIVE CARE — 375

52. Preoperative Evaluation	376
53. Anesthesia for Congenital Heart Disease	382

54. Admission to the Intensive Care Unit	385
55. Sedation and Analgesia in the Cardiac Intensive Care Unit	388
56. Mechanical Ventilation	403
57. Fluids and Electrolytes	408
58. Nutrition	414
59. Anticoagulation	421
60. Intraoperative Hemostasis	428
61. Discharge Education after Congenital Heart Surgery	430
62. Child Life	432
63. The Emotional and Spiritual Components of Congenital Heart Disease	434

V. LINES, TUBES, AND MONITORS — 439

64. Endotracheal Intubation	440
65. Central Venous Catheters	442
66. Left-Atrial Lines	447
67. Chest Tubes	450
68. Peritoneal Dialysis	457
69. Near-Infrared Spectroscopy	461
70. Feeding Tubes	462

VI. POSTOPERATIVE SCENARIOS — 465

71. Low Cardiac Output Syndrome	466
72. Cardiopulmonary Arrest	469
73. Supraventricular Tachycardia	474
74. Junctional Ectopic Tachycardia	477
75. Complete Atrioventricular Block	480
76. Postoperative Bleeding	482
77. Chylothorax	483
78. Pneumothorax	486
79. Pulmonary Hypertension	489
80. Pleural Effusion	492

| 81. Pericardial Effusion | 494 |

VII. APPENDICES 497
A. Drugs 498

Index **511**

Abbreviations **519**

I. Fundamentals

1 Segmental Anatomy of the Heart

William Buck Kyle, Iki Adachi, Debra L. Kearney

Every part of a patient's cardiac care, from native physiology to imaging, sedation strategies, surgical repair, and beyond, is dependent on a fundamental understanding of cardiac anatomy. A systematic approach to evaluating structurally malformed hearts is key to identifying and appropriately diagnosing CHD. While several strategies exist for approaching the examination of the heart, in this review we utilize the sequential segmental approach described by Professor Anderson, often referred to as the "Andersonian approach" (Figure 1-1).

In the Andersonian approach, the heart is divided into 3 components (the atria, the ventricles, and the great arteries) with all four cardiac valves included with the ventricular component. The anatomy is evaluated in terms of their spatial arrangement, morphology, and manner in which components are joined together. Anatomic features systematically assessed include those listed below, in the order described. Fundamental Andersonian terms are *italicized*.

Cardiac Segments

Atrial Arrangement
Atrial arrangement sets the stage for the sequential segmental anatomy, and atrial morphology is the key to the atrial arrangement. Components of each atrium include a venous portion which receives the venoatrial connections, an appendage, and a vestibule leading to the AV connection. The morphologic RA appendage typically has a triangular shape with its broad base originating from the muscle bundle (terminal crest) at the junction with the venous portion of the atrium. The LA appendage is typically narrow and finger-like, with no muscular crest at its base. In contrast to the RA, most of the LA free wall above the AV valve is smooth and devoid of pectinate muscles. As hemodynamics may alter the shape of the appendage, the extent of the pectinate muscles serves as the defining feature for atrial morphology. When the morphologic RA is on the right, the heart exhibits *usual atrial arrangement*. A left-sided, morphologic RA reflects *mirror-image atrial arrangement*. If both atrial appendages are of the same morphologic type, *isomerism of the atrial appendages* (either right or left) exists.

Venoatrial Connections
The pattern of pulmonary venous and systemic venous connection to the atria must be described. The coronary sinus connects with the morphologic RA.

Atrioventricular Connections
There are three major patterns in which the atria may connect (open into) the ventricles. The most common pattern has two atria, each connected to its own ventricle (biatrial-biventricular AV connection). When the morphologic RA connects with the morphologic RV, the AV connections are *concordant*. If the morphologic RA connects with the morphologic LV, the AV connections are *discordant*. In the setting of isomerism, the AV connection is termed *mixed*. The second and rarest pattern has one atrium connected with two ventricles (uniatrial-biventricular AV connection). In these rare hearts, one AV

1. SEGMENTAL ANATOMY OF THE HEART

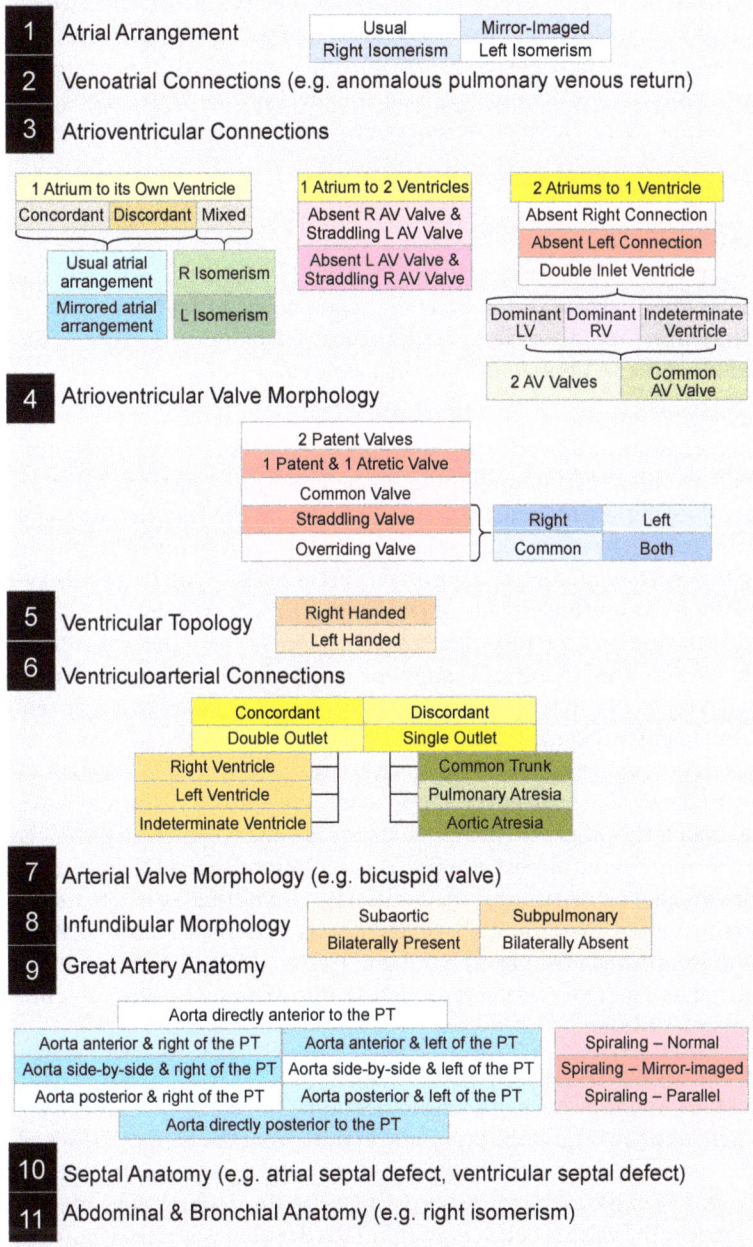

Figure 1-1. Diagrammatic representation of sequential segmental anatomy. Modified with permission from: Ezon D, Goldberg J, Kyle W. Atlas of Congenital Heart Disease Nomenclature: An Illustrated Guide to the Van Praagh and Anderson Approaches to Describing Congenital Cardiac Pathology. Baylor College of Medicine / Texas Children's Hospital; 2015.

valve is *absent* and the other is *overriding and straddling*, with chordal attachments into both ventricles. Note that a straddling valve is assigned to the ventricle which receives greater than 50% of the valve. The third pattern of AV connection occurs when two atria connect to one ventricle (*univentricular AV connection*). This category includes hearts with one absent AV connection (e.g. *absent right atrioventricular connection*) or *double inlet via* either a *common AV valve* or *two AV valves*.

Atrioventricular Valve Morphology

The tricuspid valve (TV) is typically a three-leaflet (anterior-superior, inferior, and septal) valve, defined by chordal attachments of the septal leaflet to the ventricular septum ("septophilic"). The mitral valve (MV) has two leaflets (aortic and mural) with no chordal ventricular septal attachments ("septophobic"). Commissural anatomy with supporting chordae tendinae and papillary muscles should be described. The annulus (hinge point) of the leaflets should also be assessed.

Ventricular Topology

Ventricular topology reflects to the spatial arrangement of the ventricular mass as a consequence of direction of looping of the embryonic heart tube. With normal (rightward) looping, the RV is on the right side and has *right-handed ventricular topology* where only the right hand can be positioned with the palm on the RV septal surface, the thumb in the ventricular inlet, and the fingers in the outlet. With *left-handed ventricular topology*, the RV is on the left side of the heart and will only accept a left hand in a similar orientation. In each instance, the LV will only accept the opposite hand. Even when the RV assumes an anterior-superior position, this assessment remains true. Before topology can be determined, morphology must be assessed. Each ventricle has an inlet, an apical trabecular, and an outlet component. When biatrial-biventricular AV connections are present, the TV is always associated with the morphologic RV, and the MV with the LV. The trabecular component is the most constant and will define the ventricle, even if the other two components are absent. A morphologic RV has coarse apical trabeculations as opposed to fine trabeculations in the LV. One prominent RV trabeculation, the septal band, bifurcates into two limbs that extend to the pulmonary and tricuspid valves, merging with the musculature of the outflow tract. Additional trabeculations between the septal band and free wall (septoparietal trabeculations) may contribute to outflow tract obstruction. In rare instances, ventricular morphology remains indeterminate.

Ventriculoarterial (VA) Connections

There are four major patterns of VA connections. In *concordant VA connection*, the aorta arises from the LV and the pulmonary trunk from the RV. In *VA discordance,* the opposite situation occurs. If both great vessels arise from a single ventricle, *double outlet* (RV or LV) exists. When greater than 50% of the arterial valve diameter arises from a ventricle, the valve is considered committed to that ventricle. If only one arterial valve exists, there is a *single outlet* with either atresia of a semilunar valve or a common arterial trunk. Despite valvar atresia, the VA relationship will still be concordant, discordant, or double outlet.

Arterial Valve Morphology
The number and morphology of the aortic and pulmonary valve cusps should be assessed. The coronary anatomy should be examined, to include the sinus of origin, ostial position and configuration, and branching pattern. The coronary ostia normally arise from the sinuses adjacent to the pulmonary valve (facing sinuses), regardless of the relationship of the great arteries. In an aortic valve with three sinuses, when viewed from the perspective of a person standing in the nonadjacent aortic sinus and facing the pulmonary valve, the aortic coronary sinus to the right-hand side is designated sinus 1 and to the left-hand side, sinus 2. The ostia are positioned in the midpoint of the sinus, slightly inferior to the sinotubular junction.

Infundibular Morphology
The infundibulum is the muscular body that is part of the ventricular outflow, inserted between an arterial and AV valve, typically present in a normal RV. The typical absence of an LV infundibulum permits MV to aortic valve fibrous continuity. The infundibulum may be *bilaterally present* or *bilaterally absent*. If unilaterally present, it should be described as either *subpulmonary* or *subaortic*. Infundibular muscle can cause subarterial outflow obstruction.

Great Artery Anatomy
The great artery arrangement is specified by their orientation relative to one another at the valvar level. The aorta is normally *posterior and rightward* of the pulmonary trunk. The aorta can also be side-by-side and rightward of the pulmonary trunk, anterior and rightward, and so on in a circle around the pulmonary trunk. This relationship is independent of the VA connection. The aortic arch anatomy description should include its size, direction, areas of obstruction, and branches. The branches of the pulmonary trunk and the arterial duct should also be assessed.

Septal Anatomy
The presence of shunting at the atrial and/or ventricular level should be specified to include the size, position, and boundaries of the septal defect. Malalignment of septal structures should also be noted, including the rare atrial to ventricular septal alignment in superior-inferior ventricles. Malalignment between the apical trabecular ventricular septum relative to the outlet septum must be described, to include any resultant RV or LV outflow tract obstruction. Abnormal great artery septation, such as common arterial trunk or aortopulmonary window, should be assessed.

Abdominal and Bronchial Anatomy
Normal abdominal anatomy should be described as usual abdominal arrangement. Variations include mirror-imaged abdominal arrangement, either absence of (asplenia) or multiple (polysplenia) spleens with midline liver. Usual bronchial arrangement, mirror-imaged, or bilateral left or right bronchial anatomy reflecting pulmonary isomerism (sometimes visible on CXR), often correlates with atrial appendage and splenic morphology.

PART I. FUNDAMENTALS

Illustrative Examples

Normal Heart

Usual atrial arrangement with normal superior and inferior caval veins connected to the RA and four pulmonary veins connected to the LA; biatrial-biventricular, concordant AV connections via two patent, structurally normal AV valves; right-handed ventricular topology with concordant VA connections via two patent, structurally normal arterial valves with no outflow tract obstruction; normal coronary ostia and coronary branches; aorta rightwards and posterior of the pulmonary artery; left aortic arch with normal branches and no obstruction; no patency of the arterial duct; no septal defects; usual abdominal and bronchial anatomy.

Hypoplastic Left Heart Syndrome with Aortic and Mitral Atresia

Usual atrial arrangement with absent left atrioventricular connection, concordant ventriculoarterial connections, with aortic atresia, and the aorta posterior and rightward to the PA, with a hypoplastic LV. (Other normal structures described as above.)

Right Isomerism with Complex CHD

Isomerism of the RA appendage; bilateral superior caval veins connected to ipsilateral atria with no bridging innominate vein, absent coronary sinus, total anomalous pulmonary venous connection to right superior caval vein; mixed AV connections via common AV valve and no attachment of the superior bridging leaflet to the ventricular septum; right-handed ventricular topology with double outlet RV via two patent, structurally normal arterial valves and no outflow tract obstruction; normal coronary arteries; aorta rightwards and posterior of the pulmonary artery with normal pulmonary artery spiraling; left aortic arch with normal branches and no obstruction; no patency of the arterial duct; absent spleen with midline liver; right bronchial isomerism.

Suggested Reading

Ezon D, Goldberg J, Kyle W. Atlas of Congenital Heart Disease Nomenclature: An Illustrated Guide to the Van Praagh and Anderson Approaches to Describing Congenital Cardiac Pathology. Baylor College of Medicine / Texas Children's Hospital; 2015.

2 Fetal and Transitional Circulation

Shaine A. Morris, Nancy A. Ayres

Fetal Circulation

Understanding fetal circulation is critical to understanding how children are born alive with severe CHD, and how uniquely altered hemodynamics in the fetus with CHD may compromise cerebral development.

The fetal cardiovascular circulation depends on the presence of 3 structures that typically resolve after birth: the ductus venosus, the foramen ovale, and the ductus arteriosus. Oxygenated, high nutrient blood from the maternal arterial circulation enters the fetus from the placenta via the umbilical vein. The umbilical vein then drains to the IVC via a restrictive connection, the ductus venosus. This highly oxygenated blood is then directed by the Eustachian valve at the right atrial-inferior vena caval junction across the foramen ovale, into the LA. This blood then courses across the mitral valve, aortic valve, and into the upper extremity, cerebral, and then lower body circulation via the aorta. This shunting of oxygenated blood across the foramen ovale to the left side of the heart allows the richest, most highly oxygenated blood to be delivered to the fetal brain.

After oxygenated blood is delivered to the fetal systemic circulation, deoxygenated blood returns via the IVC and SVC to the RA. This blood courses across the tricuspid valve, into the RV, and across the pulmonary valve. After this, a small proportion of blood (<10%) is directed to the fetal lung bed via the branch PAs. The rest of the deoxygenated blood courses across a large ductus arteriosus into the descending aorta. As blood courses inferiorly, it leaves the fetus by entering the umbilical arteries, which arise from the bilateral internal iliac arteries. They course around the fetal bladder and then enter the umbilical cord to run adjacent to the umbilical vein. This deoxygenated blood then returns to the maternal circulation.

In addition to the unique shunting locations in fetal life, fetal circulation differs from postnatal circulation in that PVR and fetal hemoglobin are very high. The increased affinity of fetal hemoglobin for oxygen allows the fetus to extract oxygen from the maternal blood.

Transitional Circulation

At birth, multiple hemodynamic factors change at once. The umbilical cord is cut, removing the maternal oxygen source. The child starts to breathe, and the transition from inhaling amniotic fluid to air acutely drops the PVR and triggers the process of closure of the ductus arteriosus (which may take several days). The flow to the PAs significantly increases. Due to the cessation of placenta-derived flow across the foramen ovale and with the increased pulmonary venous return from the child's lungs, the foramen ovale is typically partially or completely shut over the next few days. PVR continues to fall over the next few days to weeks, ultimately resulting in a mature cardiovascular circulation.

CHD in the Fetus

Given the presence of the ductus arteriosus and minimal blood flow to the lungs, fetuses with severe ductal-dependent heart disease or with obstructed pulmonary venous return are typically very stable in utero. They most often grow normally or with fetal weights slightly below normal, without cardiovascular compromise. Alternatively, fetuses with cardiovascular lesions that result in increased atrial pressure, like Ebstein anomaly or tricuspid valve dysplasia with severe TR, or mitral valve dysplasia with MR, often result in fetal demise.

The heart is completely formed by 8 weeks of gestation. Many lesions can be detected as early as 11-13 weeks of gestation by transvaginal ultrasound. However, given the suboptimal spatial resolution, many lesions can be missed this early. The first study is therefore performed usually at 18-24 weeks of gestation. If termination is a consideration for the family, the fetus may be evaluated as early as at 16 weeks of gestation.

Almost all major CHD lesions can be detected by fetal echocardiography in experienced hands. Failure to detect lesions is typically due to 1 of 3 reasons (Table 2-1): 1) the lesion develops late in gestation, 2) the lesion is too small to be reliably detected given limited resolution of fetal echocardiography, or 3) the lesion is not manifest until transition to postnatal circulation occurs.

For most families with a fetal diagnosis of CHD, the Cardiology team follows the fetus throughout gestation with visits every 4 to 6 weeks after diagnosis. Table 2-2 illustrates what the fetal team is monitoring during gestation in order to best plan the delivery. Some lesions detected in fetal life may be amenable to fetal cardiac intervention. Table 2-3 shows the fetal cardiac interventions offered at TCH.

Table 2-1. CHD lesions that may be missed at the 18-24 week fetal echocardiography by reason.

Lesion may develop late in gestation
Aortic stenosis
Pulmonary stenosis
Cardiomyopathy, myocarditis
Cardiac tumors
Lesion may be too small to detect with current instrumentation or with fetal hemodynamics/low flow
Small VSDs
PAPVR
Bicuspid aortic valve
Secundum ASD
Coronary artery anomalies
Lesions that become relevant with postnatal circulation
PDA
PFO
Coarctation of the aorta (may not be present until ductus arteriosus closes)

ASD: atrial septal defect, PAPVR: partial anomalous pulmonary venous return, PDA: patent ductus arteriosus, PFO: patent foramen ovale, VSD: ventricular septal defect.

Table 2-2. Fetal cardiology monitoring.

CHD Lesion	What to monitor for during gestation
TGA	1. Premature closure or restriction of the atrial septum 2. Secondary signs of postnatal atrial septal restriction: hypermobile atrial septum, bidirectional flow in the ductus arteriosus
cc-TGA	1. Conduction abnormalities/heart block 2. Poor growth of the aortic arch
Truncus arteriosus	Worsening truncal stenosis or regurgitation
Tetralogy of Fallot	Progressive pulmonary stenosis, followed by flow reversal in the ductus arteriosus (signifying need for postnatal PGE)
Pulmonary atresia with VSD	Growth of the branch PAs
DORV	Subvalvar, valvar obstruction
Aortic stenosis	1. Retrograde flow in the aortic arch, suggesting insufficient systemic output and postnatal need for PGE 2. Progressive worsening aortic stenosis→ aortic atresia 3. Growth failure of the LV; progression to HLHS 4. Mitral regurgitation in the common setting of mitral valve arcade or other structural mitral valve anomaly
Coarctation of the aorta	1. Retrograde flow in the distal arch 2. Poor growth of left-sided structures
HLHS	Restriction of the atrial septum (although typically if the septum will be restrictive in classic HLHS, it is evident from the first fetal echo)
Pulmonary stenosis	1. Worsening subvalvar or valvar stenosis 2. Retrograde flow in the ductus arteriosis (signifying need for postnatal PGE)
Pulmonary atresia with intact ventricular septum	1. Growth of the RV, PA, pulmonary valve 2. Development of coronary artery sinusoids
VSD	Often not followed unless large or associated with other lesions
AVSD	1. Worsening AV valve regurgitation 2. Poor growth of the aortic arch
Heterotaxy	1. Tachyarrhythmias and bradyarrhythmias 2. Poor ventricular function 3. Progression of specific CHD lesions
Ebstein anomaly, dysplastic tricuspid valve	Poor prognostic factors, including pulmonary regurgitation, absent antegrade pulmonary flow, retrograde ductal flow, low tricuspid regurgitation velocity Hydrops
TAPVR	Obstruction of the ascending/descending vein
Absent pulmonary valve syndrome	Hydrops
Tricuspid atresia	Progressive restriction at the VSD, subvalvar, valvar region
Vascular rings	Often don't follow unless associated with other lesions
Supraventricular tachycardia	1. Hydrops 2. Monitor/treat until returned to sinus rhythm or infrequent arrhythmia

Maternal lupus, SSA antibodies	Conduction abnormalities → complete heart block
Complete heart block	1. Hydrops 2. Extreme bradycardia
Mitral valve dysplasia	1. Restriction of the atrial septum 2. Hydrops 3. Worsening aortic stenosis/arch obstruction

AVSD: atrioventricular septal defect, cc-TGA: congenitally corrected transposition of the great arteries, CHD: congenital heart disease, DORV: double-outlet right ventricle, HLHS: hypoplastic left heart syndrome, LV: left ventricle, PA: pulmonary artery, PGE: prostaglandin E, RV: right ventricle, TAPVR: total anomalous pulmonary venous return, TGA: transposition of the great arteries, VSD: ventricular septal defect.

Table 2-3. Lesions that may be amenable to fetal intervention.

Lesion	Intervention
Critical AS/evolving HLHS	Fetal aortic valvuloplasty
Critical left-heart obstruction or mitral valve dysplasia with intact or severely restrictive atrial septum	Atrial septoplasty or atrial septal stenting, possibly with use of laser
Small left-heart structures with tubular arch hypoplasia/coarctation and apex-forming LV	Chronic maternal hyperoxygenation
Critical pulmonary stenosis	Pulmonary valvuloplasty
Pericardial teratoma	Open resection
Fetal arrhythmia	Transplacental antiarrhythmic therapy
Ebstein anomaly	1. Indomethacin for ductal restriction 2. Chronic maternal hyperoxygenation

AS: aortic stenosis, HLHS: hypoplastic left heart syndrome, LV: left ventricle.

3 Diagnostic Imaging

Prakash M. Masand, Cory V. Noel, Tobias R. Schlingmann

The main imaging modalities used for evaluation of patients with CHD are transthoracic echocardiography (TTE), cardiac MRI (CMR), and cardiac CT. The indications, contraindications, and weaknesses of each of those modalities are listed in Table 3-1.

Transthoracic Echocardiography (TTE)

TTE is the frontline noninvasive imaging modality used across all age groups and cardiac conditions. Particularly in young patients with good acoustic windows, it allows for the complete delineation of cardiac anatomy, extending all the way to abdominal situs, systemic veins, pulmonary veins, and aortic arch. In addition to anatomic information, 2D echocardiography provides helpful functional data, such as chamber size and quantification of left ventricular systolic function (ejection fraction). RV size and systolic function remain a qualitative estimation.

Color-flow Doppler visualizes the direction and velocity of blood flow, which allows for the detection of intracardiac shunts (e.g., ASD, PFO, VSD, PDA), valvar regurgitation, or flow acceleration and turbulence at sites of obstruction. Spectral Doppler interrogation can further determine the peak and mean velocities of blood flow and, thus, quantify the severity of valvar or vascular obstruction. By measuring the peak velocity of pulmonary or tricuspid valve regurgitation jets, spectral Doppler can help estimate PA and RV systolic pressures, respectively. Furthermore, Doppler evaluation of pulmonary vein flow, AV valve inflow, and tissue Doppler velocities can be helpful in detecting different stages of diastolic dysfunction.

Image quality depends on patient cooperation. In small children (<3 years and <13 kg), consider procedural sedation if the expected diagnostic yield outweighs the risks of sedation.

Cardiac Magnetic Resonance (CMR)

CMR has emerged as a complementary, and often times superior, imaging modality for investigating anatomy, function, and tissue characterization in the pediatric population. CMR is the reference standard for ventricular volumetric, functional quantification, and blood flow, all of which are key components for CHD patients. There are a number of CMR techniques useful in examining the anatomy and physiology of the CHD patient. Through various techniques, the intracardiac anatomy with dynamic motion, quantification of blood flow velocity and volume, depiciton of the extracardiac vascular structures, identification of myocardial scarring and viability, myocardial perfusion during pharmacologic stress, and myocardial edema may all be analyzed during a comprehensive exam.

PART I. FUNDAMENTALS

Table 3-1. Indications, contraindications, and weaknesses of the different diagnostic imaging modalities.

Modality	Indications	Contraindications	Weaknesses
TTE	- Postnatal confirmation of a prenatal diagnosis - Comprehensive anatomic and functional evaluation of new patients with a suspected cardiac anomaly (e.g., central cyanosis, non-functional murmurs, abnormal ECGs, exertional chest pain) - Routine longitudinal follow-up of existing cardiac patients	- None. No known side effects. No radiation exposure.	Image quality and diagnostic accuracy depend heavily on the quality of acoustic windows in each patient. These can be quite limited, particularly in large and/or adult patients. In those cases, advanced imaging modalities, such as cardiac CT or MRI, should be employed.
CT	- Coronary artery evaluation across all age groups - Partial and total anomalous pulmonary venous connection, and intrinsic pulmonary vein stenosis - Aortic evaluation in neonates and infants - Pulmonary atresia with multiple aortopulmonary collaterals (for visualization of mediastinal branch pulmonary arteries, and collateral vessels arising from the aorta) - Vascular ring evaluation with airway-specific views - Dynamic airway studies - Assessment of conduits, stents, and assist devices - Branch PA evaluation prior to single ventricle palliation - Ruling out aortic dissection in aortopathy patients - Midaortic syndrome and renal artery stenosis	- Poor renal function - History of serious allergy to iodinated CT contrast	Exposure to ionizing radiation. Physiologic heart rate of infants may limit scan resolution, particulary of coronaries.

12

3. DIAGNOSTIC IMAGING

CMR	- Complement TTE when it does not provide adequate diagnostic information - Alternative to invasive diagnostic catheterization - Evaluation of arterial and venous anomalies - Quantification of shunts and regurgitant lesions - Quantification of myocardial function and myocardial scarring / tissue characterization - Cardiac tumor characterization - Myocardial iron assessment - Exercise CMR - RV assessment (e.g., patients who have previously undergone repair of tetralogy of Fallot) - Aortopathies (e.g., bicuspid aortic valve, connective tissue disorders, coarctation of the aorta) - Assessment of ventricular volume and function in patients with single ventricle - Evaluation of patients with heterotaxy - Assessment of myocardial scar formation, biomarkers of edema and fibrosis, septal thickness, and ventricular mass and function in patients with myocarditis, hypertrophic cardiomyopathy, muscular dystrophy, and dilated cardiomyopathy to assess - Surveillance in adult patients with CHD due to complex anatomy and often poor acoustic windows - Patients with normal cardiac anatomy but detrimental cardiac effects of disease or treatment (e.g., primary pulmonary hypertension, anthracycline-induced cardiac dysfunction, sickle-cell anemia).	- Devices or material that are not compatible with the magnet, most commonly pacemakers and ICD - Within 6 weeks of device placement, even if the device itself is MRI compatible - Claustrophobia - Gadolinium-based contrast cannot be safely given in the context of renal failure	Although devices and stents may be MRI compatible, their presence may cause artifact which can limit the diagnostic quality. Intracardiac assessment in small infants may be difficult due to limitations in spatial resolution.

13

PART I. FUNDAMENTALS

Cardiac Computerized Tomography (CT)

Multidetector CT is now an established modality for noninvasive evaluation of the cardiac anatomy in children and adults. Cardiac CT scanning in pediatric patients has evolved significantly since the advent of new generation CT scanners. This past decade has seen a revolution in the techniques available on CT scanners, to decrease the amount of radiation exposure. More importantly, they provide an ultrafast scan time (as low as 0.27 seconds for anatomic coverage up to 16 cm on a volume CT scanner), and improved spatial resolution, required to assess complex anatomy in pediatric patients. The current CT technology has allowed "freezing" of cardiac motion for optimal visualization of cardiac morphology.

CT allows comprehensive visualization of the cardiac structures and the entire aorta along with its visceral branches with a single contrast injection. The contrast is typically iodinated and injected via a peripheral extremity line, utilizing a pressure injector system. One of the prerequisites to contrast administration is having normal renal function. The contrast bolus can be adequately timed using a bolus tracking technique available on most CT scanners.

Cardiac CT studies are usually ECG gated, where the scanner is able to read the patient's inherent cardiac rhythm from the ECG leads. There are 2 options for ECG gating: prospective and retrospective triggering. With *prospective triggering*, a systolic or diastolic phase within the R-R interval is utilized. The majority of cardiac CT exams are performed using prospective triggering, which allows for a significant reduction in radiation dose (up to a third of the dose compared with the retrospective option). When evaluating coronary arteries, *retrospective gaiting* is favored since no pharmacologic agents are used to lower the higher pediatric heart rate.

Cardiac CT scanning is performed without sedation in the majority of the patients. The indications to perform cardiac CT under sedation include evaluation of coronary arteries in neonates and infants, since the heart rates are relatively high (greater than 140 bpm), and anatomic evaluation in developmentally delayed patients.

3D post processing techniques are commonly utilized to enhance visualization of the anatomy depicted on a contrast-enhanced CT study. Volume rendering, maximum intensity projection, and surface shading are done on a separate postprocessing workstation, generating 3D data that is easily understood by the cardiologists and cardiothoracic surgeons.

4 Diagnostic Cardiac Catheterization

Athar M. Qureshi, Srinath T. Gowda, Aimee Liou, Wayne J. Franklin

Due to the advances in non-invasive imaging, the vast majority of cardiac catheterizations performed in the current era are for the purpose of interventions. However, diagnostic catheterizations still play a vital role in the management of many patients with CHD. Interventional cardiac catheterization procedures are described elsewhere in this text as part of the management of individual lesions, and many other interventional procedures are beyond the scope of this text.

Indications
Some indications for diagnostic cardiac catheterizations are:
- To ensure suitable candidacy for intended surgical procedures, e.g., prior to Glenn or Fontan operations.
- To better define complex anatomy that is not well delineated with noninvasive imaging or to complement noninvasive imaging of complex lesions. Examples include major aortopulmonary collateral arteries, coronary artery anomalies, and coronary artery fistulous connections that may be difficult to define with noninvasive imaging (particularly small vessels in patients with fast heart rates).
- To assist in management decisions of complex or critically ill patients with regards to medical, surgical, or transcatheter treatment, e.g., in postoperative patients.
- To facilitate hemodynamic assessment and endomyocardial biopsy procedures in patients post-heart transplantation and in patients with myocarditis or cardiomyopathies.
- To assess and test the reactivity of the pulmonary vascular bed in patients with pulmonary hypertension and pretransplant evaluation of end-stage CHD.
- To help differentiate between constrictive pericarditis and restrictive cardiomyopathy.
- As part of most interventional cardiac catheterization procedures to facilitate comparison of hemodynamics and anatomy before and after the intervention.

Preprocedural Considerations
Details of the patient's clinical history/examination, anatomy, physiology, prior cardiac catheterizations and/or surgeries must be known prior to diagnostic cardiac catheterizations. Prior vessels accessed and known vessel occlusions should be documented. A "time out" sheet (Figure 4-1) with essential information must be obtained for every patient undergoing a cardiac catheterization, in addition to a detailed informed consent.

Anesthetic Management
Fasting guidelines for elective catheterization procedures are similar to those used for operative procedures: 8 hours for heavy food, 6 hours for light food, formula or milk, 4 hours for breast milk, and 1 hour for clear liquids. Almost all diagnostic cardiac catheterizations at our institution are performed with general anesthesia supervision.

Texas Children's Hospital®

Baylor College of Medicine

TIME OUT

Team Introductions (Name/Service)

Patient and procedure confirmation

- ❑ Identity Name ______________________ MRN ______________
- ❑ Diagnosis ____

____
- ❑ Procedure(s) ____

____
- ❑ Consent obtained Yes No

Patient weight ____________

Grids ❑ Out (<20 kg) ❑ In (>20 kg)

Patient position

❑ Standard: Supine, arms up ❑ Other ______________________________

Vascular access site and side

- ❑ Groin R L ❑ Neck R L
- ❑ Other ____
- ❑ Known vascular occlusions ______________________________________

Planned implants available	N/A	Yes	No	
Special equipment/personnel available	N/A	Yes	No	
Anesthesia plan				
Intubation, positive pressure ventilation	Yes	No		
Room air	Yes	No		
Extubation upon completion	Yes	No		
Allergies (Drug, Contrast, Latex, Food)	NKA	Yes	____________	
Antibiotic prophylaxis to be given	Yes	No		
Heparin to be given	Yes	No		

Blood Available in lab Yes No Special needs Yes No

Anticipated critical events or concerns ______________________________

____

❑ Backup personnel identified and available ❑ Contact information readily available

Planned disposition ❑ Discharge ❑ Observe on ward ❑ Admit to ICU

v1.0 04.2017

Figure 4-1. Time-out form for cardiac catheterization procedures.

4. DIAGNOSTIC CARDIAC CATHETERIZATION

Whenever possible, it is ideal to perform the procedure in as close to a basline physiologic state as possible, with very light sedation and analgesia, or with moderate sedation. This can be performed in older children, adolescents, and adults with the caveat that sedated patients tend to hypoventilate. In smaller children, critically ill patients, or patients with complex anatomy, endotracheal intubation or airway control with a laryngeal mask airway is performed to facilitate a stable respiratory state for the duration of the procedure.

Cardiac Catheterization Procedure

Vascular Access

The vessels most commonly accessed percutaneously for diagnostic cardiac catheterizations are the femoral vein, femoral artery, and internal jugular vein. A thorough understanding of the landmarks used for percutaneous access of these vessels is mandatory. However, one should be familiar with the use of ultrasound in patients with difficult access, a history of vascular occlusions, smaller patients, or when unconventional vascular access is used (e.g., hepatic or splenic veins, carotid artery, or axillary artery access; mainly used for interventions).

Sheath/Catheter Selection

The smallest-size sheaths and catheters needed to achieve the goals of the procedure should be placed. There are numerous catheters available that facilitate diagnostic catheterizations. Catheters can be broadly classified as torque-directed or flow-directed (with a balloon inflated at the tip with CO_2, not air, in order to prevent air embolism if the balloon ruptures). Pressure measurements are generally made with end-hole catheters that transduce the pressure at the location of the tip of the catheter. Catheters with multiple side holes may result in inaccurate pressure measurement, e.g., if all the holes are not proximal or distal to an area of stenosis.

Hemodynamics

Prior to obtaining hemodynamics, a baseline condition should be verified by obtaining an ABG (or VBG if there is no arterial access). If needed, ventilation/sedation should be adjusted prior to recording baseline hemodynamics. Likewise, the anesthetic delivery should be adjusted prior to obtaining baseline hemodynamics to optimize the patient's BP. By convention, baseline hemodynamics are obtained on room air, but this may not be possible, nor necessary, in critically ill patients.

Pressure transducers should be balanced prior to performing hemodynamics. It is also important to perform the hemodynamic measurements as quickly as possible, as fluctuations in the patient's hemodynamic state may occur during the case (due to fluid administration, etc.) that could make the data difficult to interpret. Knowledge of normal hemodynamic tracings and age-related pressures is important. Systolic gradients are used for stenoses of semilunar valves or arterial vessels. Mean gradients are used for stenotic venous lesions or stenoses across AV valves (in addition to "*a*" wave-to-end diastolic pressure measurements).

There are two main methods for calculating cardiac output. One method uses the concept of *thermodilution*. In this method, cold or room temperature saline is injected

PART I. FUNDAMENTALS

in the proximal port (positioned in the RA) of a thermodilution catheter, and the temperature change is measured by the time it reaches the tip of the catheter that is positioned in the PA, to calculate the cardiac output. This method may not be accurate in the presence of significant TR or in the presence of intracardiac shunts.

Most cardiac output measurements are made using the *Fick principle* (Table 4-1). By convention, cardiac index is calculated, which is the cardiac output indexed to BSA. Indexed oxygen consumption (VO_2) is derived from nomograms using age, sex, and heart rate. Oxygen content is equal to 1.36 x Hemoglobin (g/dL) x saturation. The denominator in the equation is multiplied by 10, to convert deciliters to liters. Normally, the cardiac index (Qs, or systemic blood flow) equals the pulmonary blood flow (Qp). When performing the calculations, the saturations should be entered as a fraction of 1, i.e., 98 percent aortic saturation = 0.98. A normal cardiac index is $\geq$2.5 L/min/m². If one calculates the Qp:Qs ratio, all that is needed are the saturations due to cancelling out of the common numerator and denominator factors (Table 4-1).

Mean *distal* PA pressures should be used to calculate PVR (Table 4-1). Normal PVR should be 2 Woods Units/m² or less, while the SVR normally ranges from 15 to 30 Woods Units/m².

Frequently, a patient will be inspiring an oxygen content more than room air. Testing of hemodynamics is often performed under different conditions, e.g., in patients with pulmonary hypertension by administering 100% oxygen and then 100% oxygen in addition to iNO. **It is vital to include dissolved oxygen content into the equations when the patient is inspiring oxygen content more than room air. Failure to do so will result in significant errors in calculations of both flows and resistances.** The dissolved oxygen is taken into account by multiplying 0.003 by the PaO_2 (on room air this is considered negligible). For example, on oxygen (see abbreviations in Table 4-1):

$$Qp = \frac{VO_2 \, (mL/min/m^2)}{\{(1.36 \times Hb(g/dL) \times PV \, SaO_2) + (0.003 \times PV \, PaO_2)\} - \{(1.36 \times Hb \, (g/dL) \times PA \, SaO_2) + (0.003 \times PA \, PaO_2)\} \times 10}$$

$$Qs = \frac{VO_2 \, (mL/min/m^2)}{\{(1.36 \times Hb(g/dL) \times Ao \, SaO_2) + (0.003 \times Ao \, PaO_2)\} - \{(1.36 \times Hb \, (g/dL) \times MV \, SaO_2) + (0.003 \times MV \, PaO_2)\} \times 10}$$

Angiography

Power angiography is performed with an injector using catheters with side holes. Generally, the goal is to deliver 1 mL of contrast per kg in one heart beat (calculated by the heart rate). For larger patients, the maximum amount of contrast that can be delivered and maximum flow rate of the catheter is used to calculate the contrast amount and rate of injection. In the presence of a significant left-to-right shunt, the contrast amount delivered may need to be increased. The pounds-per-square-inch (PSI) pressure may need to be decreased and the rise time (time until maximum PSI is achieved) increased on injection to prevent recoil of the catheter, staining of a chamber/vessel, or ectopy/arrhythmias in the ventricles. Hand injections (in smaller vessels or in smaller children) can also be performed through end hole catheters or side hole catheters.

Whenever possible, the "store fluoro" option should be used if the image does not need to be of very high diagnostic quality (e.g., to test position of a catheter), as this results in

4. DIAGNOSTIC CARDIAC CATHETERIZATION

much less radiation compared to cineangiograms. When performing cineangiography, it is advisable to use both the anteroposterior and lateral cameras in orthogonal or complimentary views. It is extremely vital to pay attention to all aspects of radiation safety, e.g., shielding the patient and personnel in the room (anesthesiologists, interventional cardiologists, assistants, staff) from radiation.

Complications

Adverse events are rare in diagnostic cardiac catheterizations (<1%) and when they occur, are usually minor. In extreme cases, surgical backup or access to special interventional catheterization equipment up may be necessary, e.g., patients with severe pulmonary hypertension and no shunts, or patients with severely depressed ventricular function.

Postprocedure

After the procedure, patients are transferred to the recovery area and then to the regular floor or discharged home. Some patients will recover in the CICU, depending on their clinical status. Patients are to be maintained on bed rest for 6 hours in the case of femoral arterial access or 4 hours for femoral venous access only. For patients who undergo internal jugular venous access alone, 2 hours of bed rest is sufficient in most cases. Patients are restricted from swimming, bathing, vigorous activity, and exercise for 3-5 days after the procedure.

Table 4-1. Flows and resistances.

Qs (mL/min/m^2)	$\dfrac{VO_2 \ (mL/min/m^2)}{1.36 \times Hb(g/dL) \times (Ao \ SaO_2 - MV \ SaO_2) \times 10}$
Qp (mL/min/m^2)	$\dfrac{VO_2 \ (mL/min/m^2)}{1.36 \times Hb(g/dL) \times (PV \ SaO_2 - PA \ SaO_2) \times 10}$
SVR or Rs (WU/m^2)	$\dfrac{MAP - mSVP}{Qs}$
PVR or Rp (WU/m^2)	$\dfrac{mPAP - mLAP}{Qp}$
Qp/Qs	$\dfrac{Ao \ SaO_2 - MV \ SaO_2}{PV \ SaO_2 - PA \ SaO_2}$
Rp/Rs	$\dfrac{PVR}{SVR}$

Ao: aortic; Hb: hemoglobin; MAP: mean arterial pressure; mLAP: mean left atrial pressure; mPAP: mean pulmonary arterial pressure; mSVP: mean systemic venous pressure; MV: mixed venous; PA: pulmonary artery; PV: pulmonary vein; PVR: pulmonary vascular resistance; Qp: pulmonary blood flow; Qs: systemic blood flow; Rp: indexed pulmonary vascular resistance; Rs: indexed systemic vascular resistance; SaO$_2$: oxygen saturation; SVR: systemic vascular resistance; VO$_2$: oxygen consumption; WU: Woods units.

5 Intraoperative Transesophageal Echocardiography

Betul Yilmaz Furtun, G. Wesley Vick III, Wanda C. Miller-Hance

In transesophageal echocardiography (TEE), the ultrasound transducer, positioned at the end of a flexible probe, is passed into the esophagus so that the heart can be imaged from its posterior aspect along with adjacent vascular structures. Because the probe is out of the operative field, TEE can be readily employed before and after heart surgery. Indeed, the most common indication for TEE in the pediatric and adult CHD populations is for assessment during cardiac surgery.

General Aspects of TEE Imaging

A comprehensive TEE examination includes a systematic evaluation of valves, cardiac chambers, and vascular structures across several windows, using a combination of 2D imaging, spectral Doppler assessment, and color-flow interrogation. Contrast echocardiography, performed by injecting agitated saline into a central or peripheral vein, can be useful for identifying small intracardiac shunts, associated variants/anomalies, and residual septal defects that may impact perioperative management.

TEE imaging devices have evolved significantly over time (Figure 5-1). Improvements in ultrasound probe technology and image processing have recently made 3D TEE feasible in adults, adolescents, and older children. This modality is being increasingly utililized, particularly to assess valve pathologies and complex cardiovascular disease. The algorithm used at TCH for intraoperative imaging in regards to approach and TEE probe selection is outlined in Figure 5-2.

While manipulating the TEE probe (Figure 5-3), the echocardiographic evaluation is performed by navigating various transducer positions in the esophagus and stomach (Figure 5-4). This allows for multiple cross-sections to be obtained (Figure 5-5). A

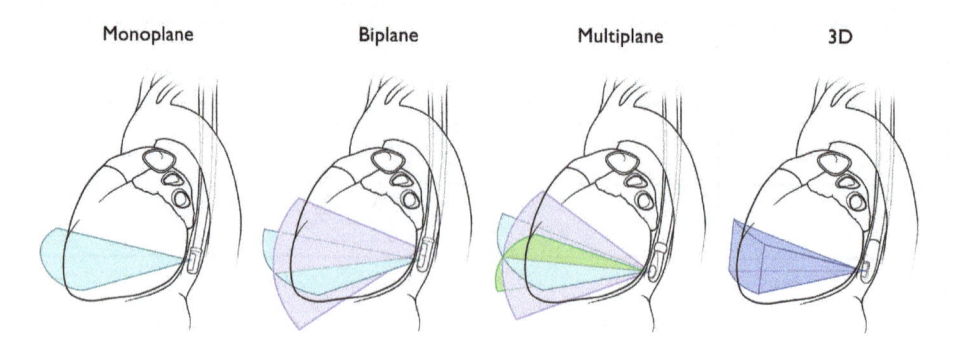

Figure 5-1. Evolution of TEE probe technology. *Monoplane* probes produce a single, transverse scan plane whereas *biplane* probes consist of two sets of transducers, mounted perpendicular to each other allowing for orthogonal (transverse and longitudinal) plane scanning. *Multiplane* probes produce a circular continuum of 2D images. Matrix array transducers allow for 3D real-time imaging and anatomic display from any perspective.

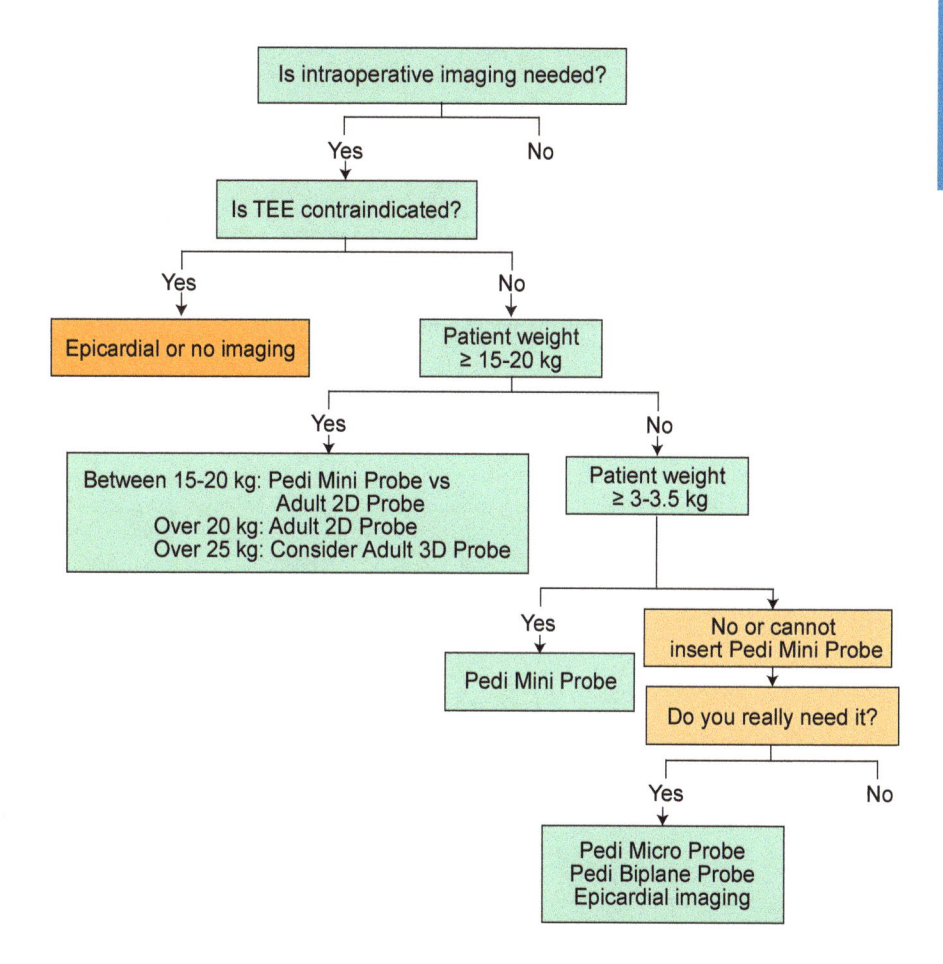

5. INTRAOPERATIVE TRANSESOPHAGEAL ECHOCARDIOGRAPHY

Figure 5-2. Algorithm for intraoperative imaging and TEE probe selection. Outline of TCH's intraoperative echocardiographic imaging approach. TEE probe selection is primarily based on patient weight and probe size. Between a weight of 15 and 20 kg, probe selection is influenced by the information to be obtained during the examination. Pedi micro: pediatric micromultiplane TEE probe, Pedi mini: pediatric minimultiplane TEE probe.

significant portion of the exam takes place at the midesophageal level, however images obtained from other windows complement the examination and in many cases are essential for a detailed structural and/or hemodynamic assessment. The approach to the comprehensive TEE examination in children and all patients with CHD is well outlined in recently published guidelines (Puchalski et al. 2019) and other educational resources (Wong and Miller-Hance 2014, Vegas and Miller-Hance 2015). Although in most cases the goal is a complete examination, the TEE study may be limited by unique patient conditions or specific circumstances in the intraoperative setting. When the

21

PART I. FUNDAMENTALS

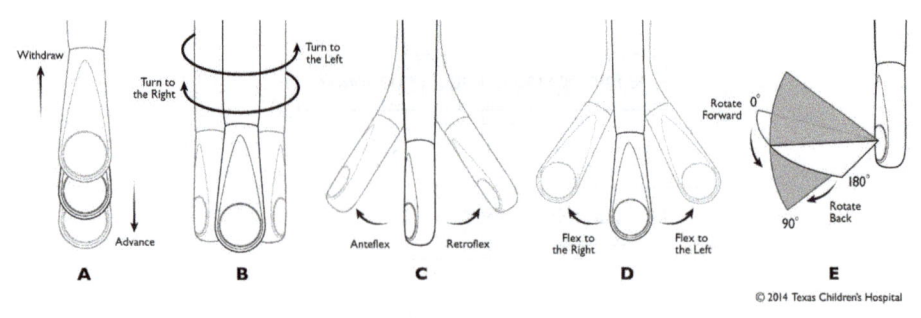

Figure 5-3. TEE probe manipulation. Terminology used to refer to manipulation of the TEE probe.

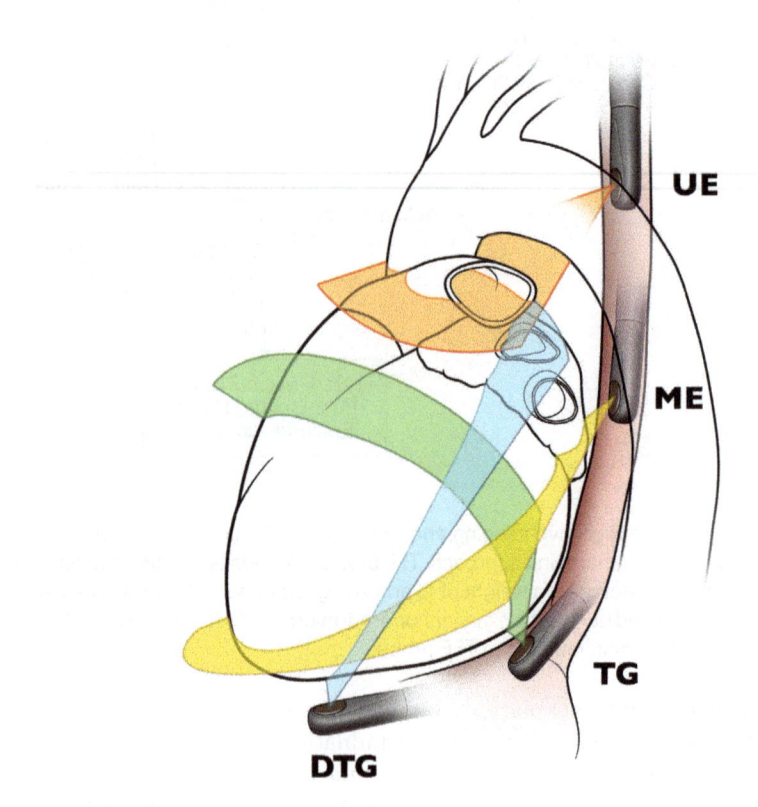

Figure 5-4. TEE imaging windows. Standard positions of the TEE imaging transducer and representative imaging planes. DTG: deep transgastric, ME: mid esophagus, TG: transgastric, UE: upper esophagus.

5. INTRAOPERATIVE TRANSESOPHAGEAL ECHOCARDIOGRAPHY

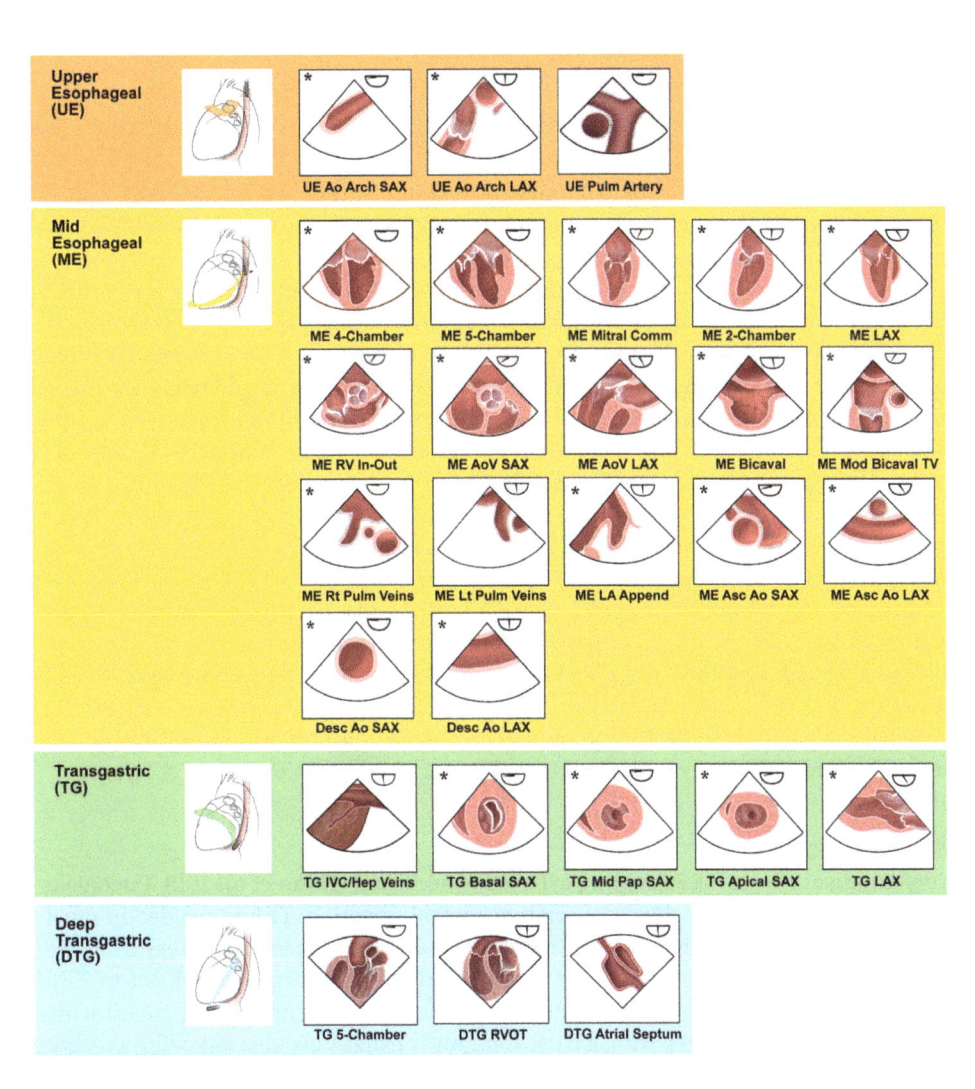

Figure 5-5. TEE views. Suggested TEE imaging views for the comprehensive evaluation in children with or without CHD and in adults with CHD. The windows and representative imaging planes are shown on the left panel and corresponding views in that window on the right panel. Ao: aortic, AoV: aortic valve, Asc: ascending, Comm: commissural, Desc: descending, Hep: hepatic, In-out: inflow-outflow, LAX: long-axis, Lt: left, Pap: papillary, Pulm: pulmonary, Rt: right, SAX: short-axis, TV: tricuspid valve. Panels marked by an asterisk are reproduced with permission from Hahn RT, Abraham T, Adams MS, et al. Guidelines for performing a comprehensive transesophageal echocardiographic examination: recommendations from the American Society of Echocardiography and the Society of Cardiovascular Anesthesiologists. J Am Soc Echocardiogr 2013;26:921-964.

interrogation needs to be limited, all attempts should be made to perform a focused/targeted study to capture all the relevant information expeditiously.

Benefits/Indications of the Technology

The benefits of intraoperative TEE have been well documented as a contributor to the overall excellence in clinical outcomes for CHS over the last several decades. It is considered indicated in most patients undergoing heart surgery, including neonates, infants, children, adolescents, and adults with CHD. In the pediatric age group, TEE also contributes to surgical interventions in acquired pathologies such as endocarditis, abscess, tumors/masses, and those involving mechanical circulatory support. The main goals of intraoperative imaging are to evaluate cardiac anatomy and hemodynamics prior to the procedure and even more importantly, to assess the surgical results. The study allows the perioperative team to review the cardiac findings prior to commencement of the operation and after separation from CPB. Intraoperative TEE also assists cardiac deairing, guides the selection of anesthetic agents and vasoactive drugs, helps in the assessment of preload and ventricular function, and facilitates management plans in the critical care setting.

In addition to perioperative indications, TEE can be used to obtain diagnostic information and to guide nonsurgical interventions. Although used less commonly, TEE can also benefit high-risk cardiac patients undergoing noncardiac operative procedures, to assure that ventricular function remains stable and to optimize hemodynamics. Such patients include those with known cardiac dysfunction, cardiomyopathy, single ventricle, coronary artery pathology, or pulmonary hypertension.

Contraindications

Contraindications to TEE imaging are well established (Hahn et al. 2013, Puchalski et al. 2019). Although considered a relative contraindication, TEE is avoided in most patients with vascular rings. The presence of an aberrant subclavian artery from the descending aorta does not represent a contraindication but may be subject to TEE probe compression, thus impacting the selection of invasive arterial BP monitoring sites. Transgastric and deep transgastric imaging is usually avoided following a recent gastrostomy tube placement and/or Nissen fundoplication.

Safety, Complications, and Populations at Risk

TEE is relatively safe in the pediatric age group and can be performed even in small neonates, however, in all cases the benefit-risk should be assessed as it represents a semi-invasive procedure. Although hemodynamic and respiratory complications rarely occur, the potential for these should be recognized particularly in neonates and small infants.

The TEE transducer should be thoroughly inspected prior to insertion to ensure that all insulating layers are intact. Considerations in patients with Down syndrome, such as potential cervical spine anomalies, large tongue, intrinsic airway narrowing, and risk of bradycardia associated with oropharyngeal instrumentation, require extra diligence during probe insertion. In view of the concern for hemodynamic instability in the neonate with total anomalous pulmonary venous return related to probe compression of the posterior venous confluence, we prefer epicardial imaging in this setting. Endocarditis prophylaxis is not recommended by the AHA for TEE imaging. However, patients routinely receive antibiotics for perioperative surgical prophylaxis, which frequently include the same agents given for bacterial endocarditis prophylaxis.

Limitations

Despite its benefits, TEE should always be considered a complementary imaging modality. Therefore, all diagnostic studies should be reviewed prior to surgery, especially the preoperative TTE. Limitations of TEE include imaging structures such as the transverse aortic arch and isthmus, left and distal PAs, pulmonary and systemic veins, and aortopulmonary collateral vessels. Epicardial imaging may supplement TEE and overcome some of these limitations, particularly during the evaluation of anterior and vascular structures (Stern el al. 2019). Technical limitations of TEE may predispose to suboptimal angles of Doppler interrogation and result in underestimation of severity of disease. Hence, in some cases, additional data such as direct pressure or saturation measurements are obtained in the OR to aid in return to CPB decisions. Additional intraoperative concerns include environmental challenges due to suboptimal ambient lighting and limited study time. A critical aspect of TEE imaging is being able to interpret the findings rapidly and to effectively communicate these to the teams, requiring a high level of expertise.

Suggested Readings

Hahn RT, Abraham T, Adams MS, et al. Guidelines for performing a comprehensive transesophageal echocardiographic examination: recommendations from the American Society of Echocardiography and the Society of Cardiovascular Anesthesiologists. J Am Soc Echocardiogr 2013;26:921-964.

Puchalski MD, Lui GK, Miller-Hance WC, et al. Guidelines for performing a comprehensive transesophageal echocardiographic examination in children and all patients with congenital heart disease: Recommendations from the American Society of Echocardiography. J Am Soc Echocardiogr 2019;32:173-215.

Stern KWD, Emani SM, Peek GJ, et al. Epicardial echocardiography in pediatric and congenital heart surgery. World J Pediatr Congenit Heart Surg 2019;10:343-50.

Vegas A, Miller-Hance WC. Transesophageal Echocardiography in Congenital Heart Disease. In: Andropoulos DB, Stayer SA, Mossad EB, Miller-Hance WC (eds). Anesthesia for Congenital Heart Disease. Wiley-Blackwell; 2015. Pp 250-293.

Wong PC, Miller-Hance WC. Transesophageal Echocardiography for Congenital Heart Disease. Springer; 2014.

6 Cardiopulmonary Bypass and Myocardial Protection

Mary Claire McGarry, Ron Shelton

The perfusion team's primary duty is to support the patient's hemodynamics and vital organs while they undergo CHS. Throughout cardiopulmonary bypass (CPB), good communication between the perfusionist, anesthesiologist, and surgeon is imperative. A cohesive team using meticulous skills and methods ensures excellent outcomes.

Every patient's perfusion is individualized and customized to each patient's unique needs. Infants are not treated as small adults, but rather require specialized techniques and equipment. This customized approach allows for a predictable level of care for each and every patient, every day. The main perfusion strategies at TCH are shown in Table 6-1. CPB is conducted using high flow and low patient pressures. Custom MAPs for individual patients based on age are shown in Table 6-2. Flows are calculated at 150 mL/kg for patients up to 10 kg. Flows for patients >10 kg are based on BSA using the appropriate cardiac index according to age (Table 6-3). BSA is calculated as follows:

$$BSA = \sqrt{\frac{height(cm) \times weight(kg)}{3600}}$$

The use of alpha-1-antagonist vasodilators during CPB can help maintain flows at 100% throughout the duration of CPB. In order to manage these high flows, adequate CPB circuits (Table 6-4), adequate venous drainage, and safe arterial line pressures are imperative. Table 6-5 and Table 6-6 show the appropriate aortic and venous cannulae selection charts, respectively, to allow required flows. For patients with bilateral SVCs, tricaval cannulation is performed unless a large bridging innominate vein is present. Alternatively, the left SVC can be cannulated retrograde through the coronary sinus after cardioplegic arrest. For those situations, the sizes of of the left and right SVC cannulae tend to be smaller than the recommended one for the SVC in bicaval cannulation.

Individualized CPB Prime Preparation

The prime on the pump is created in a way that is as physiologically close as possible to the patient's own pH, electrolyte level, and other chemistry values. Sodium, potassium, calcium, pH, bicarbonate, base excess/deficit, and chloride are kept within normal ranges of each individual patient's levels. There are several basic prime "recipes" that have been developed and that can be used in an emergency to provide good prime values (Table 6-7).

The prime blood gas and electrolytes should be as similar to the patient's ABG as possible. The target hemodilution range should be between 28 and 32% if whole blood or PRBCs are added to the prime.

Anticoagulation Management

ACT is used to measure anticoagulation levels during cardiac surgery. The baseline ACT is measured at the beginning of the case. Heparin is administered by the anesthesiologist

6. CARDIOPULMONARY BYPASS AND MYOCARDIAL PROTECTION

Table 6-1. Principles of perfusion at TCH

High-flow, low-pressure strategy
Individualized circuits, primes, and flow
Meet the metabolic demands of the patient
pH-stat acid-base strategy (keep physiologic)
Effective cardiac preservation
Conventional ultrafiltration

Table 6-2. Custom MAP for individual patients based on age.

Age	Mean pressure on CPB
Neonate	35-38 mmHg
Toddler	38-45 mmHg
Child	40-50 mmHg
Adult	50-60 mmHg

Table 6-3. Patient flows on CPB based on weight.

Weight	Flows on CPB (mL/min)
<10 kg	Weight (kg) x 150 mL/min/kg
≥10 kg	0-2 years: 3.0-3.2 mL/min/m² x BSA (m²) 2-4 years: 2.8 mL/min/m² x BSA (m²) 4-6 years: 2.6 mL/min/m² x BSA (m²) 6-10 years: 2.5 mL/min/m² x BSA (m²) >10 years: 2.4 mL/min/m² x BSA (m²)

Table 6-4. Cardiopulmonary bypass circuits.

Weight	Circuit size Arterial:Venous	Oxygenator	Prime volume
0-7 kg	3/16" : 1/4"	Capiox RX05	350 mL
7-24 kg	1/4" : 3/8"	Capiox RX15	650 mL
24-35 kg	3/8" : 3/8"	Capiox RX15	800 mL
35-45 kg	3/8" : 3/8"	Capiox RX25	950 mL
>45 kg	3/8" : 1/2"	Capiox RX25	1250 mL

to achieve an ACT of at least 350 seconds prior to initiation of CPB (goal ACT >480 seconds). ACT levels are measured throughout the bypass case to ensure constant levels of anticoagulation. Following protamine administration after the completed procedure, the ACT should return to baseline levels. The use of coagulation labs and thromboelastography can also be used to manage anticoagulation and postoperative bleeding (see Chapter 60).

PART I. FUNDAMENTALS

Table 6-5. Aortic cannula sizes based on required flow.

Flow (mL/min)	Aortic cannula size
0-350	6 Fr
350-650	8 Fr
650-1000	10 Fr
1000-1800	12 Fr
1800-2400	14 Fr
2400-4000	16 Fr
4000-5000	18 Fr
5000-6500	20 Fr
>6500	22 Fr

Table 6-6. Venous cannula sizes based on required flow.

Single right atrial cannula		Bicaval cannulation	
Flow (mL/min)	Cannula size	Flow (mL/min)	Cannula size SVC/IVC
0-300	16 Fr	0-300	8/10 Fr
300-500	18 Fr	300-650	10/12 Fr
500-1000	20 Fr	650-1000	12/14 Fr
1000-1500	24 Fr	1000-1250	12/16 Fr
1500-3000	28 Fr	1250-1800	14/16 Fr
3000-4000	32 Fr	1800-2000	14/18 Fr
>4000	36 Fr	2000-2400	16/18 Fr
		2400-3000	18/20 Fr
		3000-4000	20/24 Fr
		4000-4500	24/24 Fr
		4500-5000	24/28 Fr
		>5000	28/28 Fr

Meeting the Metabolic Demands of the Patient

The goal of the perfusion techniques during CPB is to meet the metabolic demands of the patient. Patients that are chronically cyanotic have a much higher baseline metabolic rate and parameters will need to be adjusted appropriately.

The metabolic needs of every patient are monitored during CPB using lactate levels, cerebral oximetry, and mixed venous saturations. If any of these parameters suggest that the metabolic needs of the patient are not being met, several interventions are possible:
- Increase MAP
- Increase blood flow
- Increase hematocrit through transfusion or hemoconcentration (hematocrit on CPB

Table 6-7. Physiologic Prime "Recipes"

Age group (volume)	Dosage	Ingredient
Infant (350 mL)	25 mL 125 mL 200 mL 1500 U 8 mEq 350 mg	0.45% NaCl FFP Fresh PRBCs Heparin NaHCO3 CaCl
Toddler (650 mL)	40 mL 80 mL 200 mL 330 mL 3000 U 17 mEq 650 mg	Plasmalyte A 0.45% NaCl FFP Fresh PRBCs Heparin NaHCO$_3$ CaCl
Adolescent (1025 mL)	600 mL 200 mL 200 mL 25 mL 4000 U 30 mEq 300 mg	Plasmalyte A 0.45% NaCl 25% albumin 5% dextrose Heparin NaHCO$_3$ CaCl
Adult (1230 mL)	800 mL 200 mL 200 mL 30 mL 5000 U 40 mEq 450 mg	Plasmalyte A 0.45% NaCl 25% albumin 5% dextrose Heparin NaHCO$_3$ CaCl

is typically maintained between 30% and 34%, even when profound hypothermia is used)
- Increase or optimize arterial pCO_2, which is a cerebral vasodilator
- Use hypothermia to lower the metabolic needs
- Administer more sedation

Some degree of hypothermia is generally used while on CPB to decrease the metabolic demands of the body. For procedures using CPB but without cardiac arrest, temperature is usually allowed to drift down to 34 °C. The goal temperature on CPB for procedures using cardiac arrest will depend on the complexity of the procedure and the potential need to decrease flows on CPB. Cooling the patient to 18 °C is common practice if circulatory arrest or antegrade cerebral perfusion are utilized. During cooling and warming patients on CPB, a maximum gradient of 6 to 8 °C is used for neonates/infants and of 8 to 12 °C for adolescents/adults.

pH-Stat Acid-Base Strategy of ABG Management

A pH-stat method of managing patient ABG levels is used at TCH. This strategy measures the actual CO_2 and oxygen levels at the current patient temperature. The temperature-corrected arterial CO_2 levels of the patient are kept between 45 and 50 mmHg. Arterial PaO_2 levels are kept between 150 to 250 mmHg. In the premature neonate patient, it is recommended that arterial PaO_2 levels are maintained below 200 mmHg. This strategy optimizes cerebral perfusion and typically results in quality perfusion and low lactate levels.

Myocardial Protection

Appropriate myocardial protection is extremely important during CHS. At TCH, myocardial preservation is achieved by using a cold high-potassium cardioplegia solution to achieve cardiac arrest. Cardioplegia is delivered at a temperature between 6 and 12 °C. Particular attention is placed on the pressure at which the cardioplegia is delivered. In general, it is delivered at a pressure close to the end-diastolic pressure of each individual patient prior to bypass (usually 30-60 mmHg), which corresponds to the normal filling pressure of the coronary arteries for that patient in particular.

The contents of the crystalloid cardioplegia solution that had traditionally been used (Mee cardioplegia) can be found on Table 6-8 and varied between patients <10 kg and >10 kg. The initial dose was administered for a period of 4 minutes and subsequent doses were administered every 20 minutes for a duration of 2 minutes, during cross-clamp.

In April 2019, the myocardial protection protocol was converted to use del Nido solution, which is a standard "off-the-shelf" mixture (Table 6-9). The dosage of del Nido cardioplegia is calculated at 20 mL/kg up to a maximum of 1 L full dose. The administered solution is 1 part of oxygenated patient blood to 4 parts of del Nido solution (4:1). Subsequent half doses are 10 mL/kg and quarter doses are 5 mL/kg. These subsequent doses are given routinely from 40 to 60 minutes after the arresting dose. A conversation with the surgeon during timeout will clarify dose timing. Since the use of del Nido cardioplegia is known to lower ionized calcium levels slightly, the calcium is corrected 10 minutes after removal of the cross-clamp. The corrected calcium level goal is 1.2-1.4 mg/dL. The use of prophylactic lidocaine is not necessary as in with the Mee cardioplegia, since the del Nido solution contains lidocaine.

Neuroprotection

Cerebral oximetry through NIRS is monitored routinely on every case. In general, deep hypothermic circulatory arrest (DHCA) is avoided except for very few procedures. For procedures that require aortic arch reconstruction (e.g., aortic arch advancement, Norwood procedure), antegrade cerebral perfusion (ACP) is used through a graft sutured to the innominate or subclavian artery (the carotid artery if there is an aberrant subclavian artery). ACP allows for continuous perfusion of the brain during the portion of the procedure that requires aortic arch intervention. At TCH, ACP is performed at deep hypothermia (18 °C) and flows are adjusted using a combination of transcranial Doppler (targeting a similar mean flow than that observed while on 100% CPB flow), radial arterial BP, and NIRS. Flows during ACP tend to be between 30% and 40% of calculated 100% CPB flows.

6. CARDIOPULMONARY BYPASS AND MYOCARDIAL PROTECTION

Conventional Continuous Ultrafiltration (CUF) During CPB
CUF is used extensively at TCH while on CPB. CUF is used whenever the patient has extra volume on CPB, blood products are added to the circuit, or potassium levels are high. A series of customized pH-balanced crystalloid solutions are used during the CUF process to normalize the pH as well as electrolytes. In addition, CUF allows removal of inflammatory cytokines, increases the colloid osmotic pressure, increases the hematocrit levels, and prevents body edema during and after CPB.

Preparing the Patient for Weaning Off CPB
The following steps are taken to optimize the patient for successful wean from CPB:
- Slow and even rewarming to a nasal temperature of 36.3 °C and a rectal temperature of 34 °C
- Achieving optimum hematocrit as discussed with the surgeon and anesthesiologist
- All electrolytes are within normal levels
- Optimization of all drips and adequate ventilation by the anesthesiologist
- TEE is present for postoperative assessment

With the surgeon's guidance, the perfusionist fills the heart with the precise amount of volume by occluding the venous line. Simultaneously, the flow of the pump is decreased incrementally until the patient's cardiopulmonary system is functioning independently.

Table 6-8. Mee cardioplegia ingredients by weight.

Weight	Quantity	Ingredient
<10 kg	385 mL 26 mL 100 mL	Cardioplegia Base Solution[a] Cardioplegia Buffer Solution[b] 25% Albumin
>10 kg	385 mL 100 mL 12.5 mL 5 mL	Cardioplegia Base Solution[a] 0.9% NaCl 20% Osmotrol (or 10 ml of 25% mannitol) 8.4% NaHCO$_3$

[a] Cardioplegia Base Solution (385 mL): 0.52 mL NaCl 10%, 5.63 mL dextrose 50%, 10 mL mannitol 250 mg/mL, 7.5 mL KCl 2mEq/mL, 5.82 mL NaCl 4 mEq/mL, 355.53 mL sterile water for injection.
[b] Cardioplegia Buffer Solution: 9.37 g/L Na$_2$CO$_3$, 27 g/L NaHCO$_3$.

Table 6-9. Ingredients of Del Nido cardioplegia.

Ingredient	Quantity
Plasmalyte A	1000 mL
Mannitol 20%	16.3 mL
Potassium chloride 2 mEq/mL	3 mL
Sodium bicarbonate 8.4%	13 mL
Magnesium sulfate 4.06 mEq/mL	4 mL
Lidocaine 2%	6.5 mL

31

II. Diseases

7 Patent Ductus Arteriosus

Christopher J. Rhee, Henri Justino, Saeed M. Yacouby, Carlos M. Mery

Patent ductus arteriosus (PDA) is a postnatal communication between the main PA and the descending thoracic aorta due to the persistence of the fetal ductus arteriosus. In term infants, the ductus arteriosus normally closes at around 72 hours of age; however, in preterm infants, ductal closure is often delayed. In infants between 24 to 28 weeks' gestational age, 80-90% of PDAs remain open at 4 days of age.

Pathophysiology and Clinical Presentation

A PDA results in shunting of blood between the PA and aorta. The degree and direction of shunting depends of the size of the PDA (diameter and length), the pressure difference between the aorta and PA, and the difference between SVR and PVR. Normally after birth, closure is aided due to increased PaO_2 from lung expansion as well as other vasoconstrictive mediators like PGF2-alpha, acetylcholine, and bradykinin. In contrast to term infants, premature infants may have delayed PDA closure. Prenatally, the PDA is normally large and unrestrictive, and the PVR is elevated resulting in shunting of blood from the PA to the aorta. After birth, PVR falls due to factors including lung expansion and pulmonary vasodilation due to increased PaO_2. As PVR falls, the shunt through the PDA changes direction from right-to-left to left-to-right.

Premature infants have incomplete muscularization of the pulmonary arterioles, leading to a very rapid drop in PVR after birth. As such, in premature infants, a large PDA with a large left-to-right shunt can present with pulmonary vascular congestion as early as the first week of life. In addition, diastolic BP may be low due to "runoff" through the PDA, potentially leading to impaired myocardial and coronary perfusion and a "steal phenomenon" from peripheral organs like the kidney and intestine. The presence of retrograde flow in the abdominal aorta is associated with an increased risk for necrotizing enterocolitis (NEC) and feeding difficulties in this population. Unlike premature infants, term newborns experience a delay in the drop in PVR in the presence of a large PDA, such that a substantial left-to-right shunt is only expected to develop in the first 6-12 weeks of life.

Clinical signs and symptoms are dependent on the magnitude of the left-to-right shunt. A PDA with large left-to-right shunt may result in respiratory symptoms due to pulmonary edema, failure to thrive, with moderate-to-severe enlargement of the left-heart chambers (LA and LV) due to increased pulmonary venous return. Physical findings can range from a loud continuous murmur at the left infraclavicular area to a very soft murmur (a *very* large PDA will result in equal aortic and PA pressures with low-velocity flow across the PDA, which may result in a very soft murmur). The precordium is active and a gallop may be audible. The widened pulse pressure results in bounding pulses, with peripheral pulses being especially easy to palpate (e.g., palmar or digital pulses). A PDA with moderate left-to-right shunt may have less prominent pulmonary symptoms, and usually without failure to thrive; all the typical physical findings would be less prominent, but a continuous murmur and moderate left-heart enlargement are the rule. A PDA with small-to-moderate left-to-right shunt may be

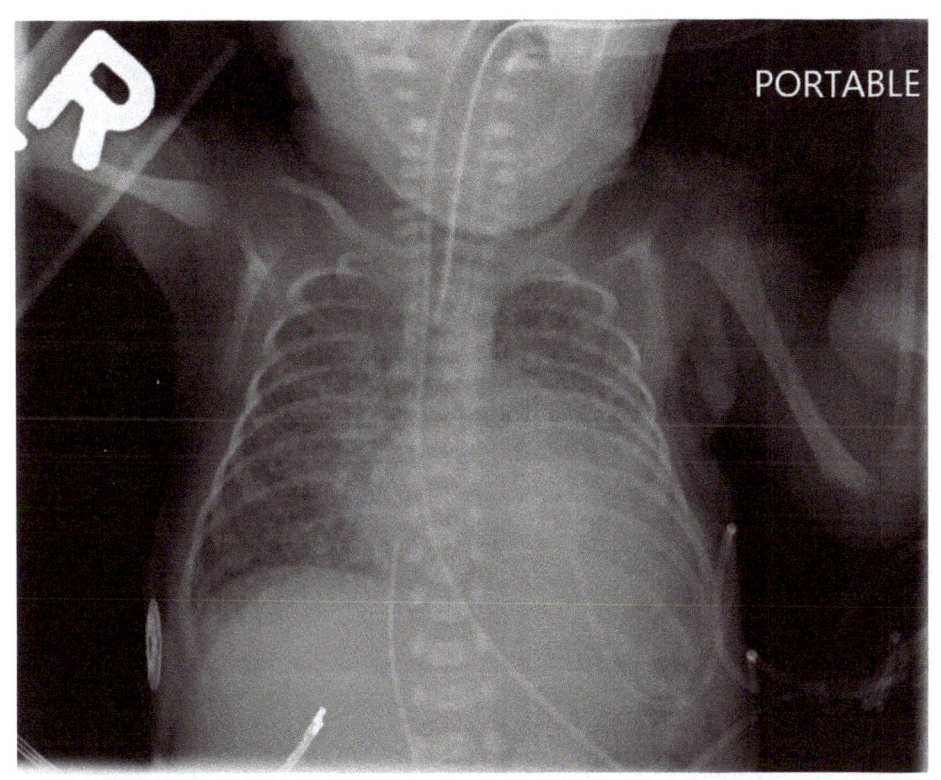

Figure 7-1. CXR of a patient with a large PDA demonstrating pulmonary edema.

asymptomatic, exhibit a continuous machinery murmur with normal precordial activity and normal pulses, and the left heart chambers may be mildly enlarged or normal. Finally, a tiny PDA with insignificant left-to-right shunt may present with either a soft continuous murmur, a soft long systolic-only murmur, or no murmur at all; the latter scenario of a tiny PDA without a murmur is referred to as a "silent PDA". In all cases of a tiny PDA with insignificant left-to-right shunt, patients are asymptomatic and the left heart structures must be of normal size; in fact, left heart enlargement in the setting of a tiny PDA should prompt the search for other causes of left heart enlargement.

PDA in the setting of other cardiac anomalies (e.g., coarctation, ductal-dependent lesions for systemic or pulmonary perfusion) will be considered elsewhere in this text.

Diagnosis
- **CXR (Figure 7-1).** May be normal with a small PDA. However, if moderate-to-large PDA, CXR will show cardiomegaly, increased pulmonary vascular markings, LA enlargement, and in severe cases, frank pulmonary edema.
- **ECG.** Most often normal. It may show LVH and combined ventricular hypertrophy in moderate-to-large PDA.
- **Echocardiogram (Figure 7-2).** The mainstay of diagnosis. In addition to assessing

PART II. DISEASES

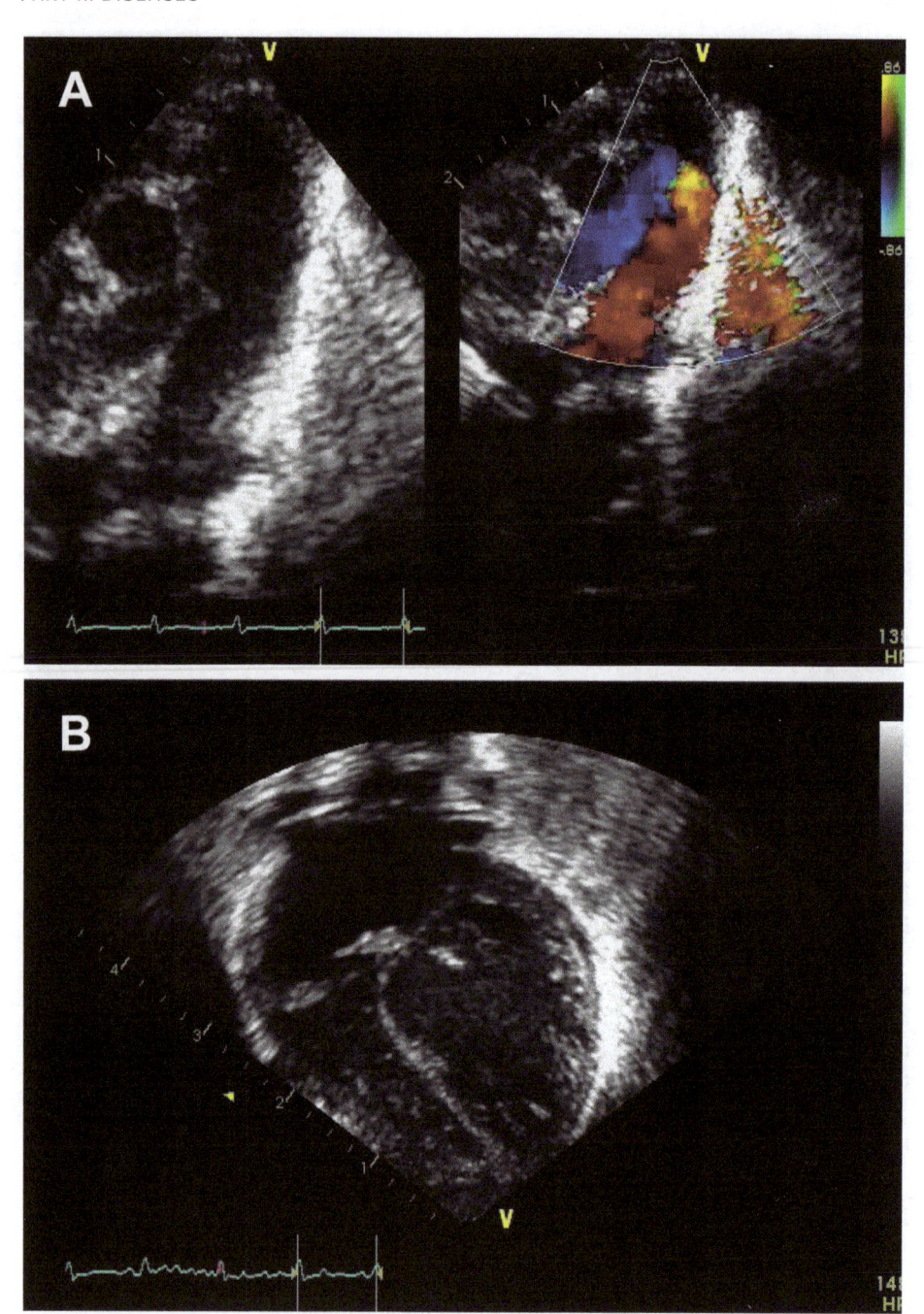

Figure 7-2. Echocardiographic images of a patient with a large PDA. Panel A shows a short-axis view demonstrating a large PDA with left-to-right shunting. Panel B shows left heart enlargement.

the presence and size of the PDA, it is important to ascertain shunt direction, morphology of the duct, arch sidedness, any concerns for aortic coarctation (which could be unmasked after PDA ligation), and origin of the coronary arteries (pulmonary origin of a coronary artery can lead to myocardial ischemia upon PDA ligation if unrecognized). Left heart enlargement is present if there is significant left-to-right shunting.

Medical Management

Medical, transcatheter, or surgical treatment is usually reserved for symptomatic PDAs in premature neonates; in this population treatment reduces the short-term need for mechanical ventilation but no long-term benefits have been established.

In term infants and older children, PDA closure is recommended in symptomatic patients or in asymptomatic patients with left heart enlargement. PDA closure is not required in those with tiny PDAs without left heart enlargement.

Conservative Management in the Premature Infant
- Modest fluid restriction to 120-130 mL/kg/day
- Lasix 0.5-1 mg/kg IV or 1-2 mg/kg PO every 8 to 12 hours
- Avoidance of further decrease in PVR
- Shunt limiting strategies: increased PEEP or permissive hypercapnia
- Use of vasoactive medications

Treatment with Ibuprofen or Indomethacin in the Premature Infant

If conservative management fails, treatment with cyclooxygenase inhibitors is the treatment of choice for pharmacologic closure of a symptomatic PDA. If the PDA closes or is significantly reduced in size >48 hours after the first course, no further doses are required. However, if the PDA fails to close, administration of a second course of treatment may be attempted. Efforts should be made to obtain an interval echocardiogram prior to initiating a second course of treatment.

Ibuprofen treatment:
- First dose: 10 mg/kg
- Second dose: 5 mg/kg (24 hours after first dose)
- Third dose: 5 mg/kg (24 hours after first dose)

If ibuprofen is not available, indomethacin may be used to treat a symptomatic PDA. Recommended dosage depends on the age of the infant at the time of treatment (Table 7-1). All dosages should be based on birth weight if the infant remains below birth weight early in life, or on current weight.

Contraindications to ibuprofen/indomethacin treatment include oliguria (urine output <0.6 mL/kg/hr), renal dysfunction (serum creatinine >1.6 mg/dL), NEC, coagulopathy, thrombocytopenia (platelet count <60,000 /uL), active bleeding, infection, or clinical conditions requiring ductal-dependent blood flow.

If the PDA remains symptomatic after the second course or if unable to provide a second course due to the contraindications noted above, surgical or transcatheter treatment may be considered.

PART II. DISEASES

Table 7-1. Dosing for indomethacin treatment of a PDA.

Age at first dose	First dose	Second dose	Third dose
< 48 Hours	0.2 mg/kg	0.1 mg/kg	0.1 mg/kg
2-7 Days	0.2 mg/kg	0.2 mg/kg	0.2 mg/kg
7 Days or older	0.2 mg/kg	0.25 mg/kg	0.25 mg/kg

Indications for Intervention in the Premature Infant

Surgical PDA ligation or transcatheter device closure may be required for those infants that fail medical management, have clinical instability, fail to wean off mechanical ventilation, or fail to have optimal growth in the setting of a PDA.

Anesthetic Considerations

For infants and children undergoing percutaneous ductal occlusion in the cardiac cath lab, general anesthesia is commonly achieved by a balanced technique utilizing low-dose narcotic, benzodiazepine, and anesthetic gas. This technique requires the establishment of an artificial airway, usually with an endotracheal tube. It is common practice for infants and children undergoing ductal occlusion in the cardiac cath lab to be extubated at the end of the procedure; the anesthetic is geared toward that end.

For those infants and children requiring surgical closure, age and weight determine where such closure takes place. Infants <1.5 kg are typically operated at the bedside in the NICU. For these patients, a standardized checklist is completed by the NICU prior to surgical closure (Table 7-2). Patients are commonly intubated prior to anesthesia team arrival and already have IV access in place. Prior to positioning, the patient is anesthetized and paralyzed to prevent extubation. Anesthesia is administered totally by IV means, as no anesthetic gases are available at the bedside. Prior to giving any narcotic, glycopyrrolate 10-20 mcg/kg IV is administered to prevent bradycardia. Fentanyl is most commonly used and the total dose for a case is often 10-20 mcg/kg. Muscle relaxation is achieved with rocuronium or vecuronium. Fresh or low-potassium blood should always be available at the bedside during surgery. Caution should be taken in these patients, as rapid administration of blood can cause hyperkalemia, hypocalcemia, and myocardial dysfunction due to citrate toxicity.

For patients undergoing surgical closure in the operating room, it is common to insert an arterial line for monitoring BP and evaluating blood gases, and a balanced anesthetic technique (combined IV and inhalational anesthesia) is used. It is uncommon to extubate patients immediately after surgery due to the higher doses of narcotics needed for a thoracotomy.

The ventilatory strategy should be to maintain normocarbia to slight hypercarbia, and minimize supplemental oxygen unless it is required for normal oxygen saturation. This strategy will help maintain PVR, reducing left-to-right shunting and diastolic runoff, which can lead to myocardial ischemia. Efforts to reduce diastolic runoff should include a conservative ventilation strategy, minimize anesthetic concentration, and maintain

SVR. The administration of phenylephrine 0.5-1 mcg/kg IV commonly restores SVR, raises the diastolic BP, and corrects coronary insufficiency if it occurs.

Catheter-Based Intervention

Transcatheter device closure of a PDA is an accepted method of closure in term infants and older children. Recently, availability of novel devices that can be delivered though smaller catheters has rendered percutaneous PDA device closure possible even in extremely low-birthweight infants weighing <1 kg. Device closure in infants <2.5 kg should be performed entirely through a venous (femoral or jugular) approach, with avoidance of placement of a femoral arterial catheter to avoid arterial injury. Upon reaching the ductus from a transvenous approach through the right heart, angiography is performed within the PDA to measure its length and diameter. A variety of devices with different shapes and sizes are available to treat a PDA, and most are delivered with catheters or sheaths <5 Fr in small children. Imaging the aorta during device placement to prevent aortic protrusion can be performed with angiography or echocardiography. It is also possible to perform PDA device closure in small infants entirely using echocardiography at the bedside in the NICU. For larger children >5 kg, arterial injury is much less likely, hence devices can be delivered to the PDA using a transvenous or transarterial (usually femoral) approach. PDA device closure in older children is an outpatient procedure.

Complications

Complications of device closure of PDA in small children less than 2 to 3 kg include device protrusion into the aorta or into the main PA near the left PA ostium. Aortic protrusion is more serious, as it can result in device-induced coarctation. Careful echo imaging of the region of the aortic isthmus should exclude patients with preexisting hypoplasia of the aortic isthmus or a true mild coarctation prior to the procedure, and intraprocedural echo can be used to aid with device placement to avoid this complication. In older children, significant aortic or PA device protrusion is less likely. Device embolization in larger children is typically managed by transcatheter device retrieval followed by placement of a more appropriately sized device. However, in very small children (less than 1.5 to 2 kg) device retrieval can be difficult and consideration should be given to surgical retrieval followed by surgical PDA ligation at the same time.

Surgical Intervention

Surgical ligation or division remains a common method used for PDA closure in premature infants. The standard approach involves a left posterolateral serratus-sparing thoracotomy via the fourth intercostal space using a short incision. The superior and inferior aspects of the ductus are dissected with care not to injure the PDA, which is very friable, especially in premature infants. All structures including the vagus nerve, left recurrent laryngeal nerve, and aortic arch should be readily identified. For small babies, a medium or medium-large titanium clip is used to occlude the PDA. The clip should be tested outside of the body prior to use since it is not possible to reposition or remove the clip once deployed. It is important to ascertain that the clip is all the way

PART II. DISEASES

> **Surgical PDA closures at TCH (1996-2016)**
> Median number of procedures per year: 11 (2-31)
> Median age at surgery: 35 days (1 day - 13 years)
> Median weight at surgery: 2.5 kg (0.5-28 kg)

around the ductus but not including the recurrent laryngeal nerve (that crosses behind the PDA) or the left mainstem bronchus (that also lies behind). A chest tube is placed at the discretion of the surgeon, based upon the friability of the lungs and potential for air leak.

In older patients, the PDA may be circumferentially dissected and either controlled with a silk ligature or divided between polypropelene ligatures. A chest tube is routinely placed in these patients.

It is possible to develop an aortic coarctation after PDA ligation. Patients that have a relatively small isthmus or concerns for developing an aortic coarctation should be carefully evaluated for the need to perform an aortic coarctation repair at the time of surgery. As such, these patients should undergo surgery in the OR rather than the NICU.

Complications

Some of the most critical technical complications that ought to be prevented are:
- Left vocal cord dysfunction from injury of the recurrent laryngeal nerve

Table 7-2. NICU checklist for patients undergoing PDA ligation in the NICU.

NICU Checklist for Bedside PDA Ligations
Day before surgery
- Preoperative orders placed in EPIC by CV Anesthesia NP
- Hematocrit (Hct) checked with goal Hct >30 %. If Hct <30%, transfuse and recheck. NICU team to order blood transfusion and to recheck Hct level.
- Type and screen sent, blood ordered for: 2 quarter units <7 day old blood to be delivered in bag on day of surgery
- NPO orders written
- CV surgeon consultation and consents signed (CHS team to arrange)
12 hours before/day of surgery
- Neobar removed by NICU respiratory therapy
- Dedicated IV placed by NICU team or dedicated IV Port available by the morning of surgery
- 2 suction setups available and working (one for surgeon, one for Anesthesia)
- Blood warmer at bedside
- Baby placed on K-pad (warming pad)
- 2 pulse oximeters – one on right hand, second on either leg
- 2 BP sources – one BP cuff on right arm, second cuff on either leg (leg cuff not needed if patient has UAC or lower extremity arterial line)
- Internal temperature cable to bedside
- Blood ordered from blood bank and brought to bedside in cooler 15 minutes prior to posted start time
- Family at bedside 30 minutes prior to posted start time (for Anesthesia consent)
- Area cleared of non-essential equipment, visitors and non-essential personnel. Toys/extra blankets off bed and "Surgery in Progress: DO NOT enter" sign posted
For any questions, please page the CHS Clinician on call.

- Chylothorax from disruption of lymphatic vessels and lymph nodes
- Aortic coarctation
- Ligation of incorrect structures

Postoperative Management of the Premature Infant

Nearly 50% of preterm infants may develop postligation cardiac syndrome (PLCS) after surgical PDA ligation. This syndrome is characterized by systemic hypotension and oxygenation failure often requiring vasoactive medications and prolonged mechanical ventilation. Low cardiac output is due to an acute increase in SVR and decreased preload. Symptoms usually begin 8 to 12 hours following intervention and tend to resolve 24 hours afterward.

Milrinone has been used to lower the afterload, with some benefit in infants with PLCS. Some other infants may require the use of other inotropes such as dopamine to improve their BP.

8 Atrial Septal Defect

Josh Kailin, Aimee Liou, Iki Adachi

Atrial septal defect (ASD) is a common congenital heart defect, comprising up to 10% of all congenital heart disease. ASDs frequently accompany other CHDs. This chapter focuses on isolated ASDs. Types of defects in the atrial septum include (Figure 8-1):

- **Patent foramen ovale**: persistent flap opening between the septum primum and the limbus of the fossa ovalis.
- **Secundum ASD**: deficiency, absence, or perforation of the septum primum, leaving shunting at the level of the ostium secundum.
- **Primum ASD**: an endocardial cushion defect resulting in deficiency of the AV septum.
- **Sinus venosus ASD**: an interatrial shunt resulting from abnormal incorporation of primitive venous structures into the atrium. This does not represent a deficiency of the atrial septum itself and is usually associated with partial anomalous pulmonary venous return.
- **Coronary sinus ASD**: a rare deficiency of the "roof" of the coronary sinus as it travels behind the LA that allows for interatrial shunting.

Pathophysiology and Clinical Presentation

ASDs allow for shunting between the left and right atria (Figure 8-2). The degree and directionality of shunting is typically determined by relative RV and LV compliance and defect size. Since the RV is typically more compliant than the LV, atrial-level shunting in the absence of other disease is typically left-to-right. Hemodynamically significant left-to-right shunts cause RA and RV dilation.

Patients with ASDs are typically asymptomatic. Large ASDs may occasionally present in the first few years of life with recurrent respiratory infections, generalized fatigue, failure to thrive and tachypnea; or in the 4th to 5th decade of life, when symptoms of right-heart failure develop secondary to chronic right-heart volume overload. Patients may develop atrial arrhythmias or pulmonary vascular disease in late adulthood.

Physical exam reveals a murmur of ejection quality in the pulmonary valve position, a result of extra flow across the pulmonary valve from the left-to-right shunt. The second heart sound may be widely split (fixed split S_2). The apical impulse may be diffuse and laterally displaced. Adult patients with a longstanding ASD may have findings of right-heart failure including hepatomegaly and edema.

Diagnosis

- **CXR.** Cardiomegaly is the result of RA and RV enlargement. The pulmonary vascular markings can be prominent secondary to the left-to-right shunt.
- **ECG.** RA enlargement, RV hypertrophy, and frequently an RSR' pattern in lead V1.
- **Echocardiogram (Figure 8-3).** Confirms diagnosis, size, and type of ASD.

8. ATRIAL SEPTAL DEFECT

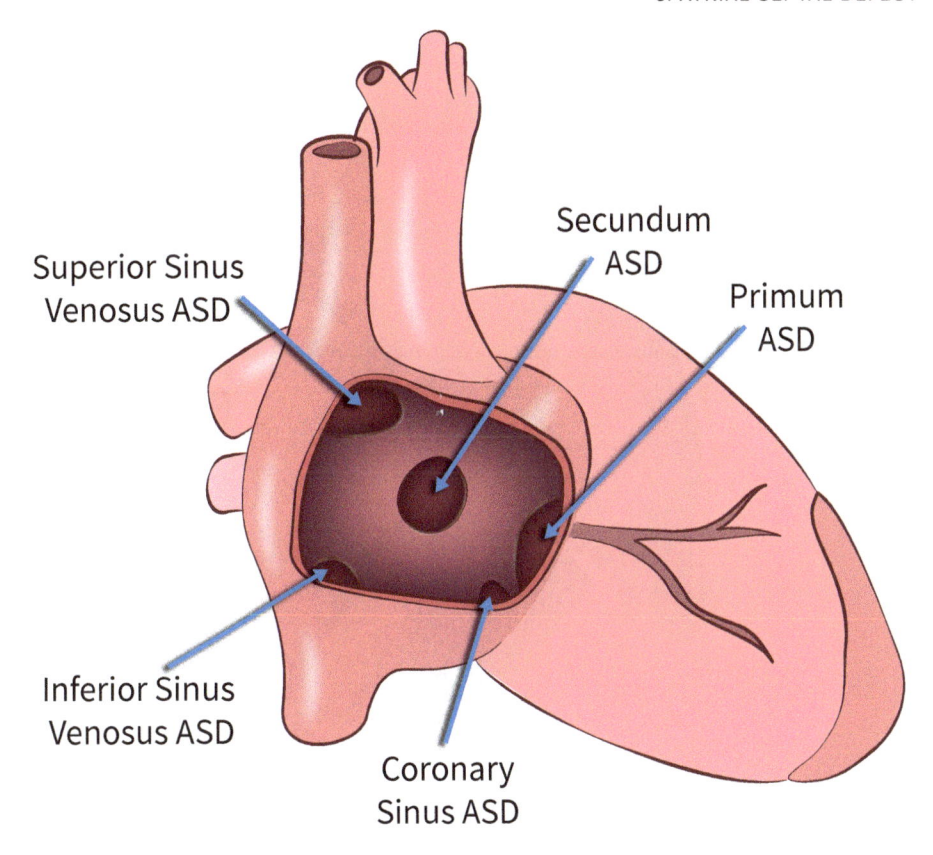

Figure 8-1. Types of ASD. Image courtesy of Dr. Josh Kailin, www.pedecho.org.

Indications/Timing for Intervention
Because of asymptomatic presentation and a high rate of spontaneous closure of smaller defects in young children, referral is typically delayed until patients are 4 to 5 years of age. Additional factors may prompt earlier referral. Indications for referral include:
- Moderate-to-large ASD with right-heart enlargement and diastolic flattening on echocardiogram
- Qp:Qs ≥1.5:1
- Special circumstances when ASD is associated to other problems such as pulmonary hypertension, mitral stenosis, etc.
- Comorbidities such as chronic lung disease and prematurity
- Frequent respiratory infections
- Sequelae of transient right-to-left shunting including cyanosis, embolism, recurrent transient ischemic attacks (TIA)
- Symptoms including fatigue and exercise intolerance (rare)

PART II. DISEASES

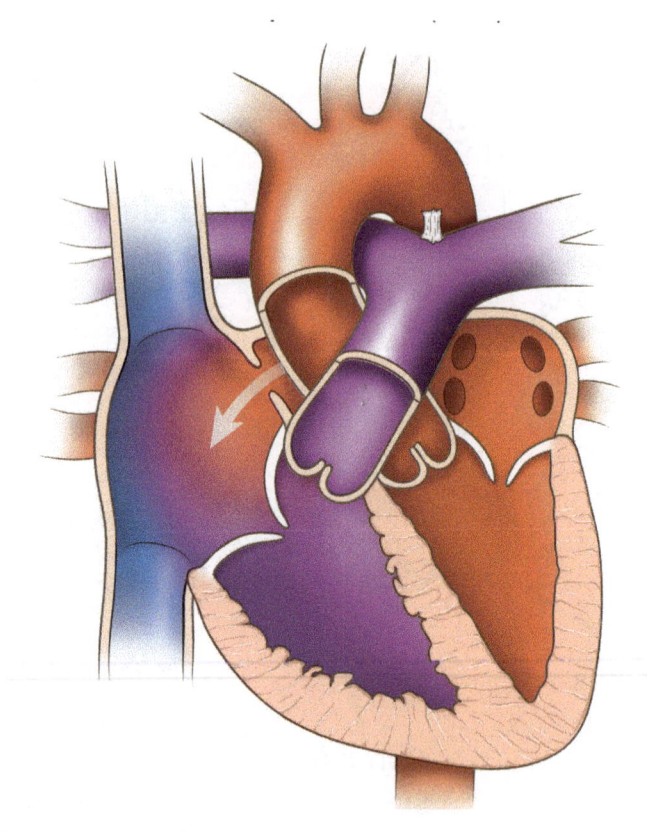

Figure 8-2. Pathophysiology of ASD.

Catheter-Based Intervention
Currently, catheter-based device occlusion is reserved for select patients with secundum ASDs. The transcatheter approach can be used in infants when clinically indicated. In asymptomatic patients without pressing clinical symptoms, allowing the patient to reach a weight of 20 kg can confer additional ease to the procedure.

TEE is performed to fully assess the features of the defect and the feasibility of transcatheter closure; features evaluated include defect size, shape, septal rims, and location of defect. Patients with defects determined by TEE to be unsuitable for catheter-based closure are referred for surgical closure.

The procedure includes a right-heart catheterization with determination of the degree of left-to-right shunting (Qp:Qs). The defect is then balloon-sized using the "stop flow" technique (Carlson et al. 2005).

A device is placed within the defect using TEE, fluoroscopy, and angiography (Figure 8-4). These imaging techniques allow for guidance and assessment for device malposition, residual shunt, or impingement on neighboring cardiac structures. Following device closure, patients are treated with aspirin for 6 months, after which the device is

8. ATRIAL SEPTAL DEFECT

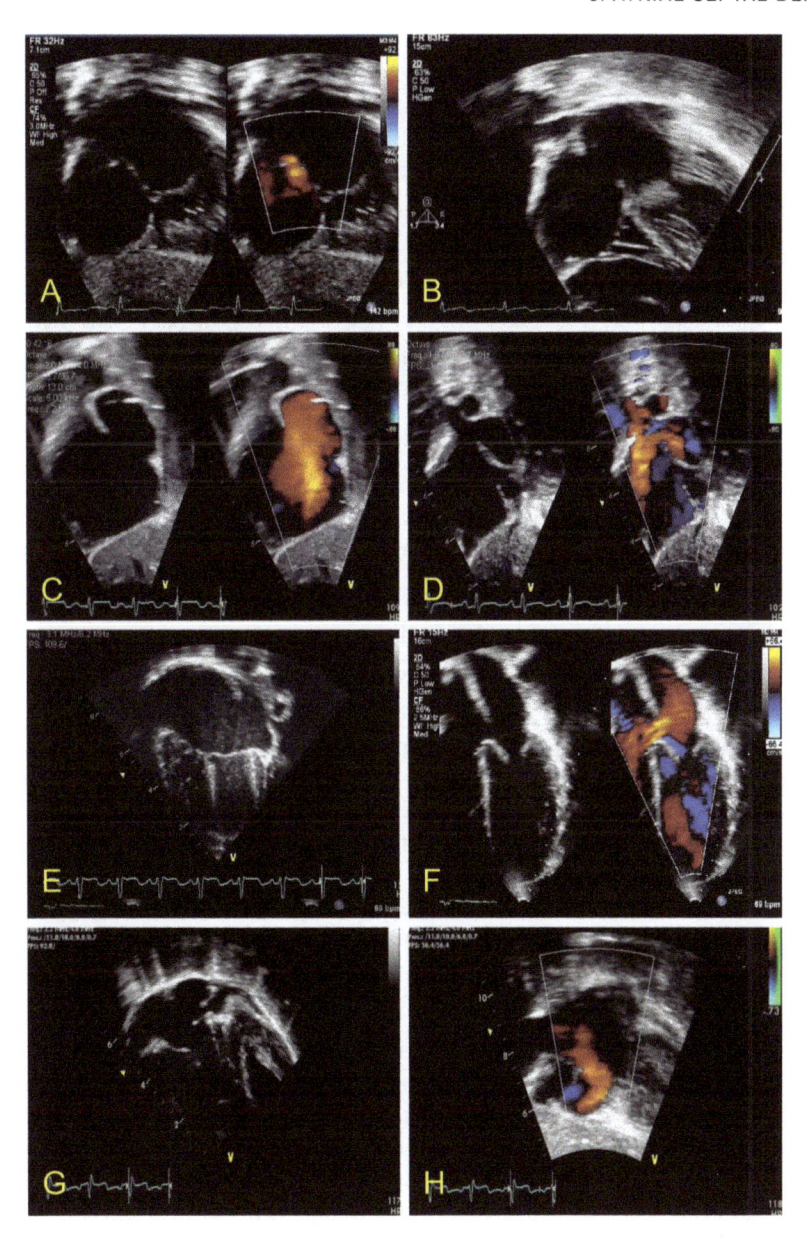

Figure 8-3. Echocardiographic images of ASDs. A) Color-compare image of a PFO with left-to-right shunting, B) 2D image of a large secundum ASD, C) Color-compare image of a large secundum ASD with left-to-right shunting, D) Color-compare image of a superior sinus venosus ASD with left-to-right shunting, E) 4-chamber view demonstrating a large primum ASD, F) 4-chamber view with color-compare showing left-to-right shunting across a primum ASD, G) 4-chamber view demonstrating a coronary sinus ASD due to an unroofed coronary sinus, H) color Doppler image of a coronary sinus ASD showing left-to-right shunting. Images courtesy of Dr. Josh Kailin, www.pedecho.org.

PART II. DISEASES

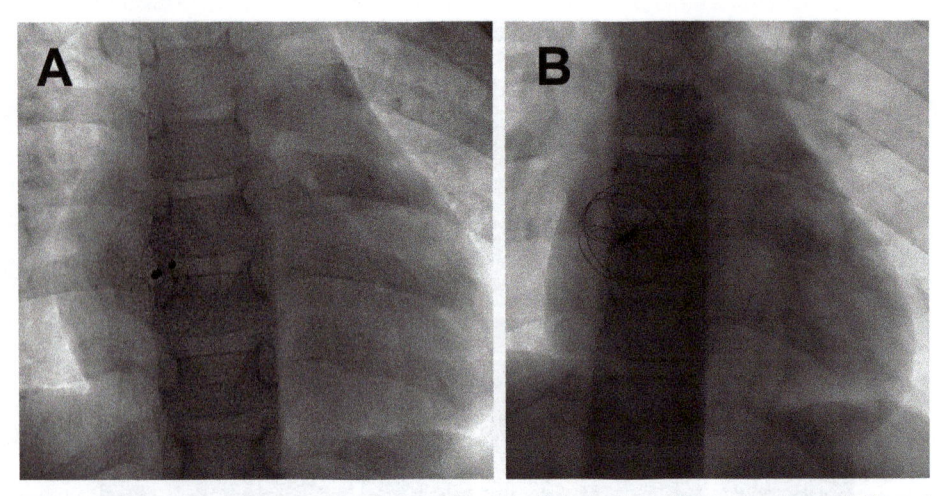

Figure 8-4. Angiographic images of two different ASD devices: A) the Amplatzer™ Septal Occluder (St. Jude Medical Inc., St Paul, MN) and B) the Gore® Cardioform ASD Occluder (W.L. Gore & Associates, Flagstaff, AZ).

likely to have endothelialized; an echocardiogram 6 months after the procedure helps to rule out residual shunt.

Postcatheterization Complications
- **Device embolization.** Can occur secondary to device undersizing or inadequate tissue rims. The device may be retrieved via transcatheter approach or retrieved surgically, with concomitant surgical ASD repair.
- **Device erosion.** May occur secondary to device oversizing or device proximity to the atrial roof or the aorta.
- **Atrial arrhythmias.** Isolated ectopic beats or nonsustained atrial tachycardia can occur but are uncommon.

Surgical Repair
The standard approach for surgical ASD repair is via median sternotomy, although a minimally invasive approach (partial low sternotomy) can be performed in selected secundum ASD cases. CPB is established with bicaval cannulation. The heart is arrested by cross-clamping the ascending aorta while protecting the myocardium with cold cardioplegia administered into the aortic root. The ASD is exposed by opening the RA. Typically, the ASD is closed with a fresh autologous pericardial patch, unless the defect is small, in which case primary closure may be an option.

Surgical Complications
A relatively common complication seen after ASD repair is the development of a pericardial effusion, also known as postcardiotomy syndrome. Patients are often asymptomatic and may present with an increased cardiac silhouette on CXR. Echocardiography is

used to confirm the diagnosis. Depending on the size of effusion and presence or absence of tamponade physiology, treatment includes fluid evacuation (surgical vs. catheter-based) or medical management (diuretics and nonsteroidal anti-inflammatory drugs).

ASD procedures at TCH (2013-2017)
Median number of procedures per year: 37 (33-42)
Perioperative mortality: 0

Long-Term Follow-Up

Patients with unrepaired ASDs require follow-up with a cardiologist. Patients with small ASDs without significant right-heart dilation may follow up every 2 to 3 years. Patients with moderate-to-large ASDs with right-heart dilation should follow up at least annually and sometimes more frequently if <2 years of age to assess for symptoms. Following surgical repair or device closure, patients typically follow up annually with ECG and echocardiogram.

Suggested Reading

Carlson KM, Justino H, O'Brien RE, et al. Transcatheter atrial septal defect closure: modified balloon sizing technique to avoid overstretching the defect and oversizing the Amplatzer septal occluder. Catheter Cardiovasc Interv 2005;66:390-6.

9 Partial Anomalous Pulmonary Venous Return

Alan F. Riley, Iki Adachi

Partial anomalous pulmonary venous return (PAPVR) is a heterogenous group of lesions where at least one, but not all, of the pulmonary veins drain into the right heart or systemic veins. Similar to total anomalous pulmonary venous return (TAPVR), PAPVR can be associated with a wide variety of intracardiac lesions, particularly when associated with heterotaxy syndrome or anomalies of atrial and abdominal arrangement. Individualized multimodality imaging and surgical strategies are often required as a result of the broad anatomical variants of PAPVR.

The most common PAPVR variant is drainage of the right upper pulmonary vein into either the RA, the right atrial-SVC junction, or into the SVC. Other variants include drainage of some of the left pulmonary veins into the innominate vein or all right pulmonary veins into the right atrial-IVC junction via a descending vertical vein ("scimitar" syndrome).

The majority of patients with PAPVR will have an associated ASD, usually of the sinus venosus type. These ASDs are close to the right/posterior wall of the septum with no posterior rim. PAPVR of the right upper pulmonary veins to the SVC tends to be associated with a superior sinus venosus ASD while PAPVR of the right veins into the IVC tends to present with an inferiorly located sinus venosus ASD.

Pathophysiology and Clinical Presentation

The pathophysiology of PAPVR is related to the left-to-right shunt and/or, very rarely, obstruction to pulmonary venous drainage from the lungs. Mechanisms of pulmonary venous obstruction, if present, are similar to TAPVR and due to: 1) stenosis at the connection of the anomalous veins to the RA or systemic vein, 2) mechanical compression from the PAs, bronchi, or diaphragm, and/or 3) intrinsic long segment vessel hypoplasia. Similar to other supraventricular left-to-right shunts, PAPVR results in cardiomegaly with right-heart dilation. The degree of right-heart dilation is proportional to the number of pulmonary venous segments involved and can be additive to any other associated shunts (e.g., ASD). Chronic RA and RV dilation over years or decades can increase the risk for arrhythmias and RV systolic and diastolic dysfunction.

Children with isolated, unobstructed PAPVR are usually asymptomatic. These patients tend to be evaluated due to idiopathic right-heart dilation. Some patients may present with recurrent respiratory infections. On physical exam, patients will have a systolic ejection murmur on the left superior sternal border (related to increased pulmonary valve flow) and a widely split S_2.

Diagnosis

- **ECG.** Patients may have an incomplete right bundle branch block, possible RVH, and possible RA enlargement.
- **CXR.** Will show cardiomegaly and increased pulmonary vascular markings.

9. PARTIAL ANOMALOUS PULMONARY VENOUS RETURN

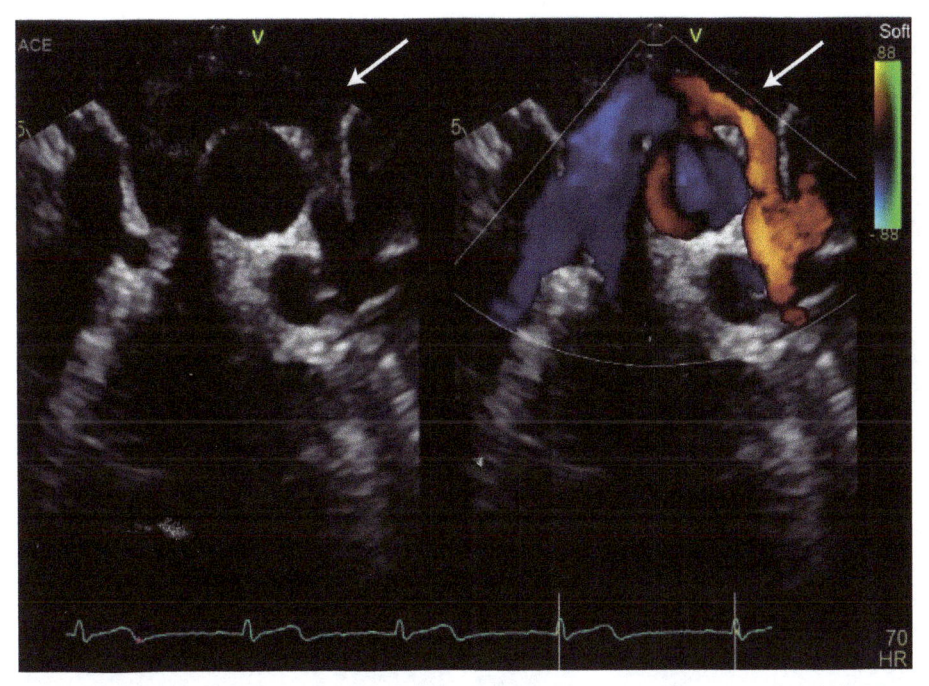

Figure 9-1. Echocardiographic suprasternal color-compare image of an anomalous left upper pulmonary vein draining into the left brachiocephalic vein (arrow). Image courtesy of Dr. Josh Kailin, www.pedecho.org.

- **Echocardiogram.** There is usually right atrial and ventricular dilatation. The defect may not be obvious on the standard parasternal views. Subcostal coronal views can demonstrate the entrypoint of the right upper pulmonary vein. If the defect is higher in the SVC, a high parasternal long axis may demonstrate the defect. Mild-to-moderate TR may be present. Pulmonary valve flow acceleration secondary to left-to-right shunting can mimic mild pulmonary valve stenosis (velocity no more than 2.5-3 m/s) but the valve should have normal appearance. Like in other atrial loading defects, there will be interventricular septal flattening during diastole. If there is additional septal flattening in systole, pulmonary hypertension should be suspected. Echocardiography can also show an anomalous left upper pulmonary vein draining into the left innominate vein (Figure 9-1).
- **CTA and MRI.** Cross-sectional imaging may be helpful to delineate the anatomy of the anomalous veins for surgical planning (Figure 9-2). It is particularly useful for surgical planning in patients with scimitar syndrome to define the location of the vein with respect to the right and left atria.
- **Cardiac catheterization.** Not needed in the vast majority of patients with PAPVR. Cardiac catheterization is indicated in patients with scimitar syndrome in order to embolize aortopulmonary collaterals (that are almost always present in these patients) prior to surgical intervention (see below).

PART II. DISEASES

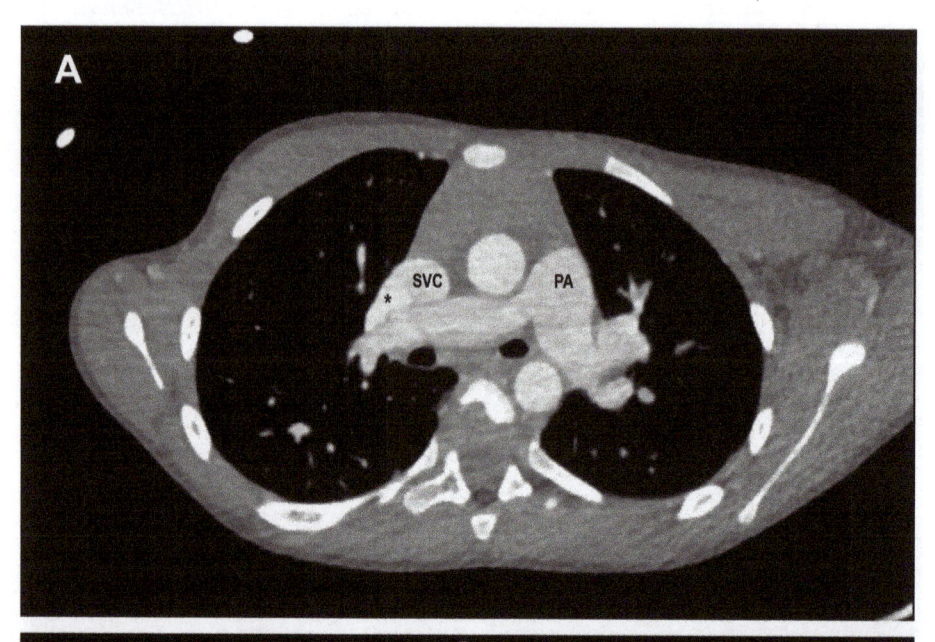

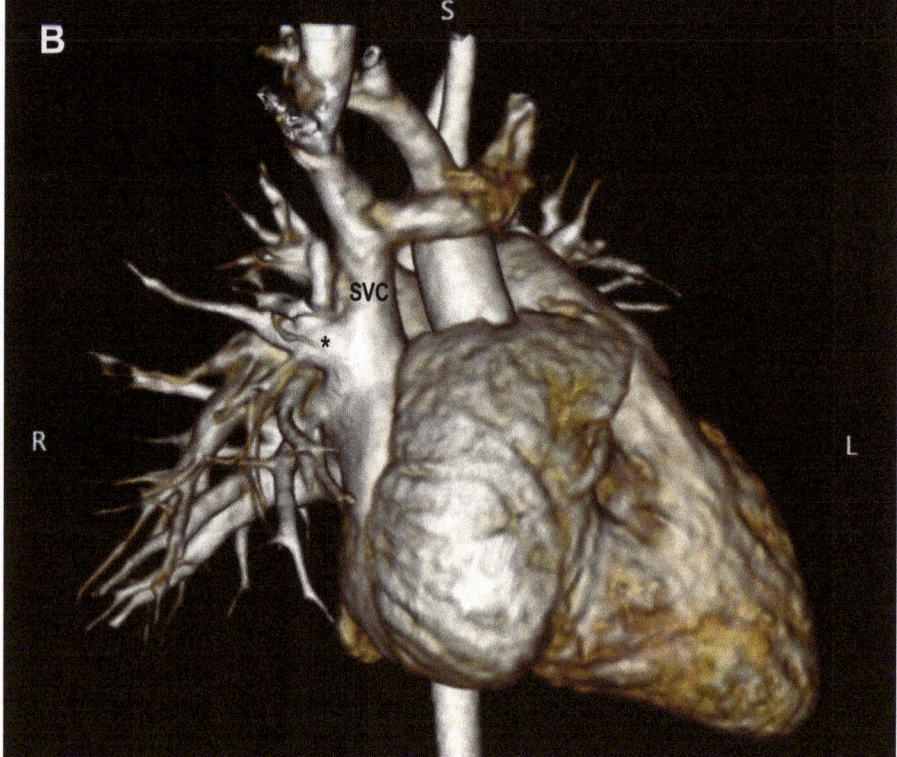

Figure 9-2. Axial (A) and 3D-reconstruction CTA images of a patient with PAPVR of the right upper pulmonary vein (*) to the SVC.

9. PARTIAL ANOMALOUS PULMONARY VENOUS RETURN

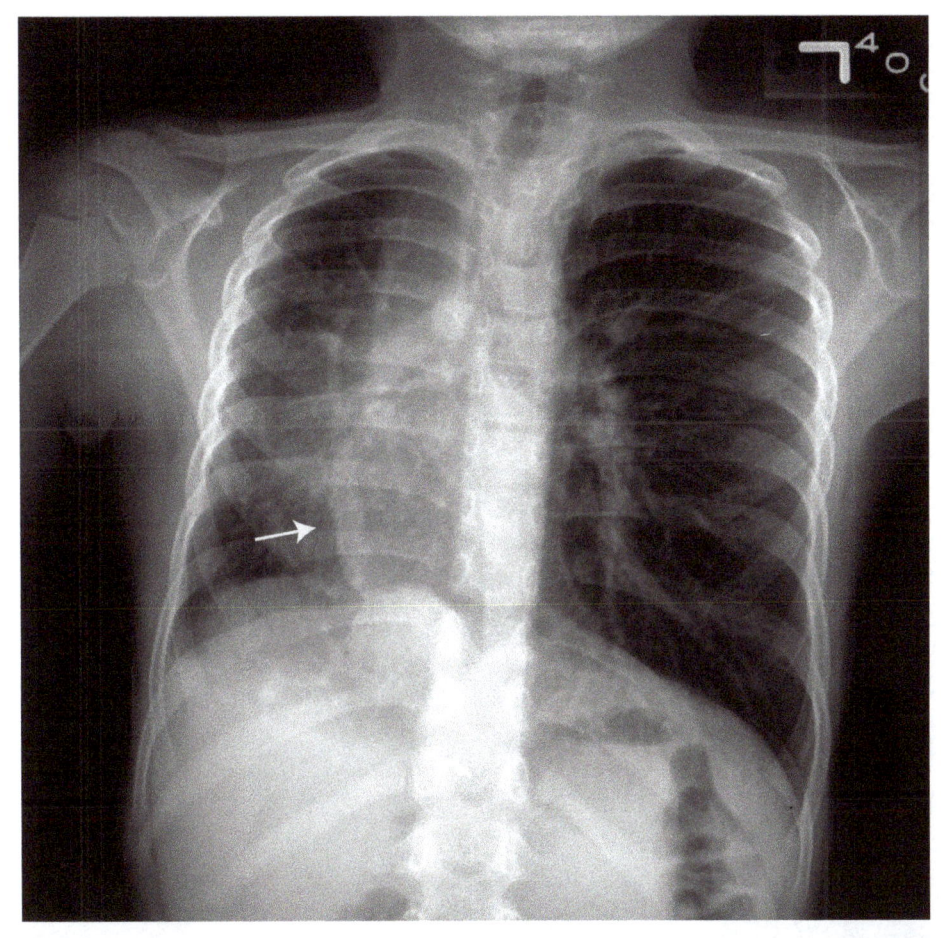

Figure 9-3. CXR of a patient with scimitar syndrome showing right lung hypoplasia and the shadow of the anomalous right upper pulmonary vein descending towards the IVC (arrow).

Indications / Timing of Intervention

Indications for surgical intervention are dependent on the degree of pulmonary overcirculation. Isolated single anomalous pulmonary veins may not result in enough right-heart dilation to warrant intervention. In borderline cases, MRI estimates of Qp:Qs can be helpful in determining indications for intervention. Patients with low-volume pulmonary overcirculation (Qp:Qs <1.5:1) likely do not require surgical correction and long-term cardiology follow-up is needed to evaluate for sequelae of pulmonary overcirculation. On the contrary, little is known regarding the long-term effect of right-heart volume overload. In such borderline cases, it is important to have a balanced view of the natural history of the condition against the surgical risks.

Elective surgical intervention for isolated PAPVR is optimally performed later in life (school age). In patients that require neonatal surgery for other intracardiac lesions,

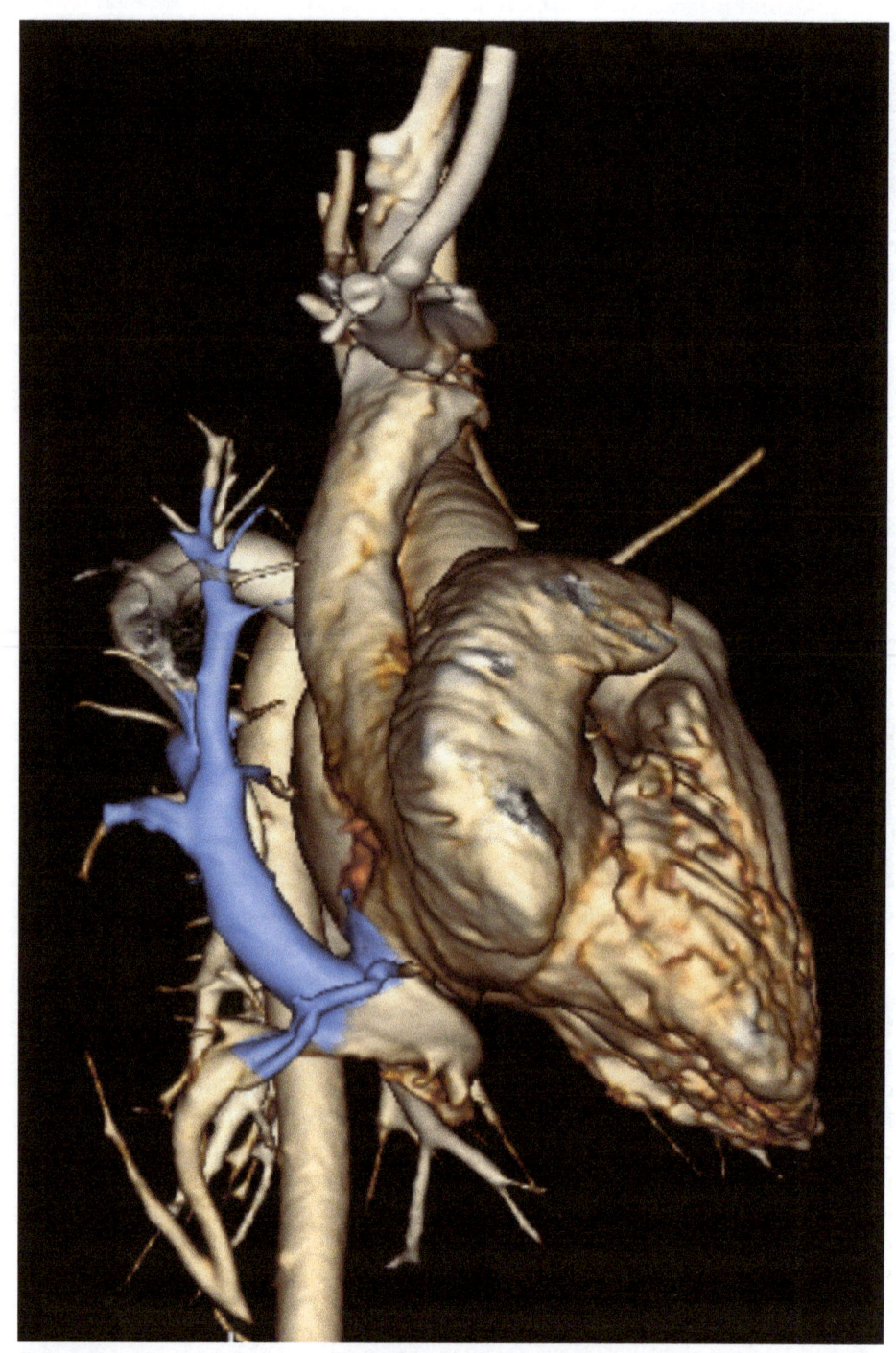

Figure 9-4. 3D-reconstruction CTA image of a patient with scimitar syndrome showing the anomalous right pulmonary vein (blue) descending and inserting into the IVC.

9. PARTIAL ANOMALOUS PULMONARY VENOUS RETURN

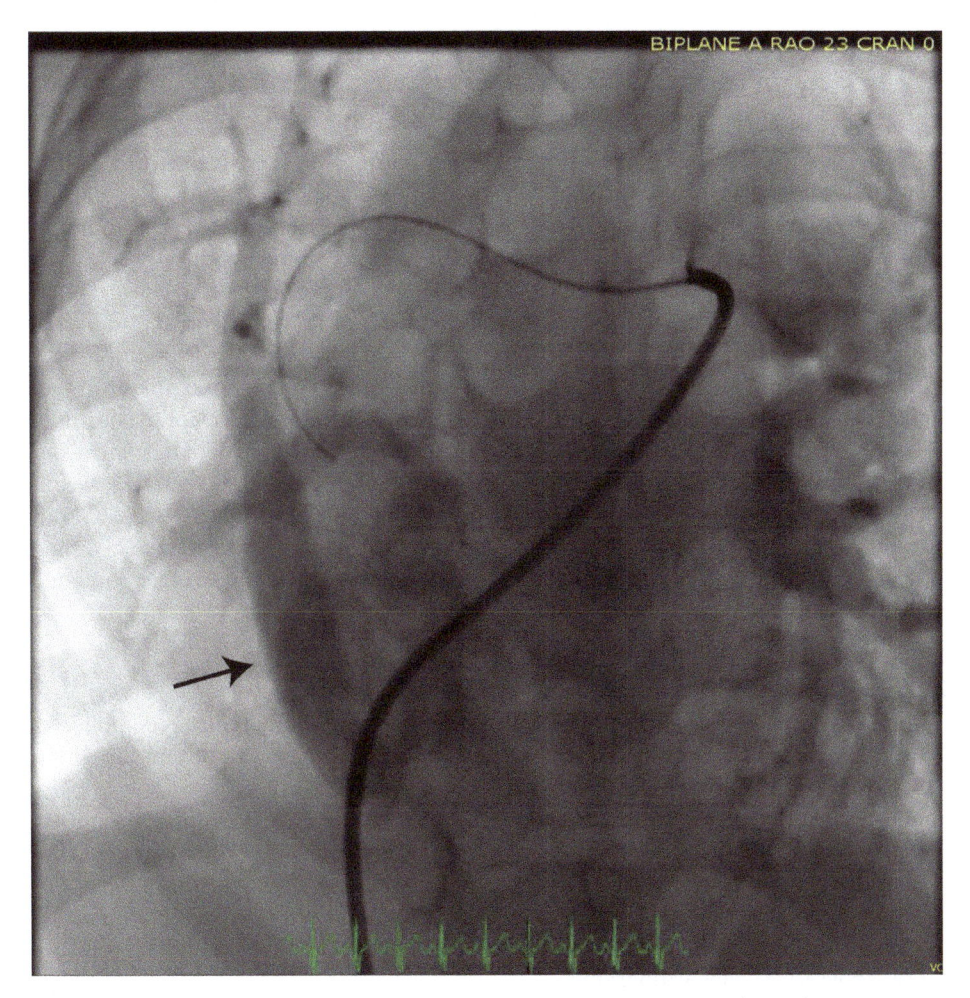

Figure 9-5. Cardiac catheterization showing a prominent scimitar vein (arrow).

PAPVR of a single isolated pulmonary vein may be left alone in order to optimize surgical results of manipulation, redirection, and/or reimplantation of the anomalous vein.

Surgical Repair
The specifics of the surgical repair depend on the particular type of PAPVR. Most procedures are performed via median sternotomy and under cardiopulmonary bypass with cardioplegic arrest.

Anomalous Left Pulmonary Vein Into The Innominate Vein
The anomalous vein may be left in situ, ligated at its entrypoint into the innominate vein, and a longitudinal anastomosis performed between the anterior surface of the pulmonary vein and the left atrial appendage, which is laid on top of the vertical vein.

Alternatively, the anomalous vein may be detached and anastomosed directly to the LA appendage with care not to torque these structures.

Anomalous Right Upper Pulmonary Vein

For patients with anomalous right pulmonary veins into the RA, an intracardiac baffle is created with autologous pericardium to redirect the flow through the sinus venosus ASD (if present) or through a created defect (if no ASD present) toward the LA. If the anomalous veins drain into the SVC and creating a baffle would potentially obstruct the SVC, there are 2 different surgical options: a Warden procedure and a two-patch repair. For the Warden procedure, the SVC is divided just above the entrypoint of the pulmonary veins and sutured close (with or without a patch). The SVC orifice is baffled through the atrial septum towards the LA and the distal SVC is reimplanted into the right atrial appendage to provide drainage of the SVC. If there is significant tension due to a short SVC, a posterior anastomosis may be created and an anterior patch placed on the anastomosis to relieve tension. In the two-patch repair, a baffle is created between the pulmonary veins and the LA, and a second patch is placed to enlarge the SVC and prevent obstruction. This repair may be associated with a higher incidence of sinus node injury (or injury to the blood supply of the sinus node), especially in older patients.

Complications

Potential complications of surgical repair of PAPVR include:

- **Arrhythmias and sinus node dysfunction.** Sinus node dysfunction may complicate PAPVR repair. Long-term freedom from dysfunction appears to be similar when comparing both surgical techniques.
- **Postoperative stenosis.** Patients undergoing repair of PAPVR of the right upper pulmonary veins can develop postoperative stenosis in the baffle between the anomalous pulmonary veins and the LA. Additionally, the connection between the SVC and the RA in a Warden procedure is also vulnerable to developing postoperative stenosis. Both potential complications should be evaluated with routine postoperative echocardiograms.
- **Reintervention.** Smaller size and younger age are the dominant predictors of reintervention after repair of PAPVR for both, the two-patch technique and the Warden procedure.

Scimitar Syndrome

Scimitar syndrome is rare variant of PAPVR with a wide variety of presenting scenarios. It is characterized by right pulmonary veins draining anomalously into the IVC and associated variable degrees of right-lung hypoplasia. Additional findings can include pulmonary hypertension and/or pulmonary sequestration with an aortopulmonary collateral from the descending aorta. An inferior sinus venosus or secundum ASD is often present. Some patients present early in life or infancy with pulmonary hypertension and symptoms out of proportion to the PAPVR. Some patients are incidentally diagnosed in adolescence or adulthood, often when a CXR identifies the characteristic scimitar vein, which appears like the 8th century Turkish sword of the same name (Figure 9-3).

9. PARTIAL ANOMALOUS PULMONARY VENOUS RETURN

The pathophysiology of scimitar syndrome is secondary to a combination of the left-to-right shunting (PAPVR, ASD, aortopulmonary collateral) and pulmonary vascular disease, which is likely secondary to a combination of the pulmonary overcirculation, pulmonary hypoplasia, and pulmonary venous obstruction.

Diagnosis and procedural planning depend on a multimodality imaging strategy. TTE usually makes the diagnosis of scimitar syndrome and estimates right heart pressures. Cardiac MRI or CTA is needed to characterize the PAPVR, particularly the insertion into the IVC and the relationship with the RA or LA (Figure 9-4). Cardiac catheterization can measure PA pressures directly and confirm the anatomy of the PAPVR (Figure 9-5). However, cardiac catheterization is best used for coiling of the aortopulmonary collaterals that are commonly present from the descending aorta to the right lung.

Supracardiac PAPVR repairs (1996-2019)
(Binsalamah et al. 2020)
Number of patients: 158
- Warden procedure: 122 (78%)
- Single-patch repair: 26 (22%)

Median age at operation: 6.3 years
Median length of stay: 4 days
Perioperative mortality: 1 (0.6%)
Long-term outcomes (median follow-up 3.8 yrs):
- Cath-based interventions: 10 (6%)
- Reoperation (patch dehiscence): 1 (0.6%)

Scimitar syndrome diagnoses (1995-2019)
(Bonilla-Ramirez C, Salciccioli KB, et al. 2020)
Number of patients: 61
Median age at diagnosis: 1.3 years
Surgical repair: 23 (38%) patients:
- Intracardiac baffle: 13
- Reimplantation: 9
- Other: 1

Postoperative 5-year freedom from stenosis: 70%
Postoperative 5-year survival: 95%

Indications for surgical intervention can be controversial, particularly in asymptomatic older patients with no significant pulmonary overcirculation (Qp:Qs <1.5:1). Younger presentation is typically associated with more severe disease and neonatal presentation tends to be associated with poor outcome, with or without surgical intervention. Timing of intervention can also be controversial, weighing the consequences of ongoing pulmonary hypertension and left-to-right shunting versus the benefits of somatic growth and improved surgical outcomes.

Surgical intervention is individualized for each particular patient. Options include creation of a long baffle between the entrypoint of the scimitar vein into the LA (through an existing or created ASD), reimplantation of the scimitar vein higher into the RA followed by creation of a shorter baffle, creation of a side-to-side anastomosis between the vein and the RA with creation of a baffle, or reimplantation of the anomalous vein directly into the LA. Baffle stenosis is a long-term consideration after these surgical repairs, especially if a long baffle is created.

Suggested Readings

Binsalamah ZM, Ibarra C, Edmunds EE, et al. Younger age at operation is associated with reinterventions following the Warden procedure. Presented at AATS 2019. Submitted for publication, 2020.

Bonilla-Ramirez C, Salciccioli KB, Adachi I, et al. Smaller right pulmonary artery is associated with longer survival time without scimitar vein repair. Presented at CHSS 2019. Submitted for publication, 2020.

Pulmonary Vein Anomalies

Heather A. Dickerson, Erin A. Gottlieb, Athar M. Qureshi, Christopher A. Caldarone, Antonio G. Cabrera, Carlos M. Mery

This chapter encompasses 2 different lesions of the pulmonary veins: total anomalous pulmonary venous return (TAPVR) and isolated pulmonary vein stenosis. Partial anomalous pulmonary venous return (PAPVR) is covered in Chapter 9.

TAPVR

TAPVR is a lesion characterized by the anomalous drainage of all pulmonary veins into the RA or a systemic venous structure, instead of into the LA. Embryologically, TAPVR is due to a failure of fusion of the pulmonary venous lung buds with the posterior outpouching of the LA. As a consequence, there is no connection between the pulmonary veins and the LA, but the veins usually maintain a connection to the systemic veins through an ascending or descending "vertical vein".

Anatomical Considerations

In most cases of TAPVR, pulmonary veins drain into a pulmonary venous confluence that then drains into either the RA or a vertical vein. TAPVR is classified into 4 categories depending on the site of drainage:

- **Supracardiac (45%).** There is usually a horizontal pulmonary venous confluence behind the LA that drains into a vertical vein that ascends and connects to either the SVC or more commonly, the innominate vein. The vertical vein may travel anterior to the left PA or between the left PA and the left bronchus, where it may become compressed by these structures. Compression at this level may lead to obstructed physiology and pulmonary hypertension, which in turns dilates the PA and causes of further obstruction (hemodynamic "vise").
- **Cardiac (25%).** The anomalous veins drain directly into the RA or via a dilated coronary sinus. In general, cardiac TAPVR is unobstructed and often presents later in infancy.
- **Infracardiac (25%).** The veins usually drain into a vertical pulmonary venous confluence that drains into a vertical vein that travels down through the diaphragm and drains into the IVC or into the portal venous system or hepatic veins. The vast majority of these patients have obstruction of the pulmonary venous return due to the high resistance of the hepatic sinusoids, compression at the level of the diaphragm, and/or stenosis at the entrypoint into the IVC and as such, require emergent intervention.
- **Mixed (5%).** Different pulmonary veins have different types of drainage.

Pathophysiology and Clinical Presentation

The clinical presentation of patients with TAPVR depends whether there is significant obstruction of the pulmonary veins or not. Since pulmonary veins normally drain into the LA through a large and unobstructed confluence, having all pulmonary veins drain into a smaller vertical vein is not optimal. As such, it is safe to assume that every patient

10. PULMONARY VEIN ANOMALIES

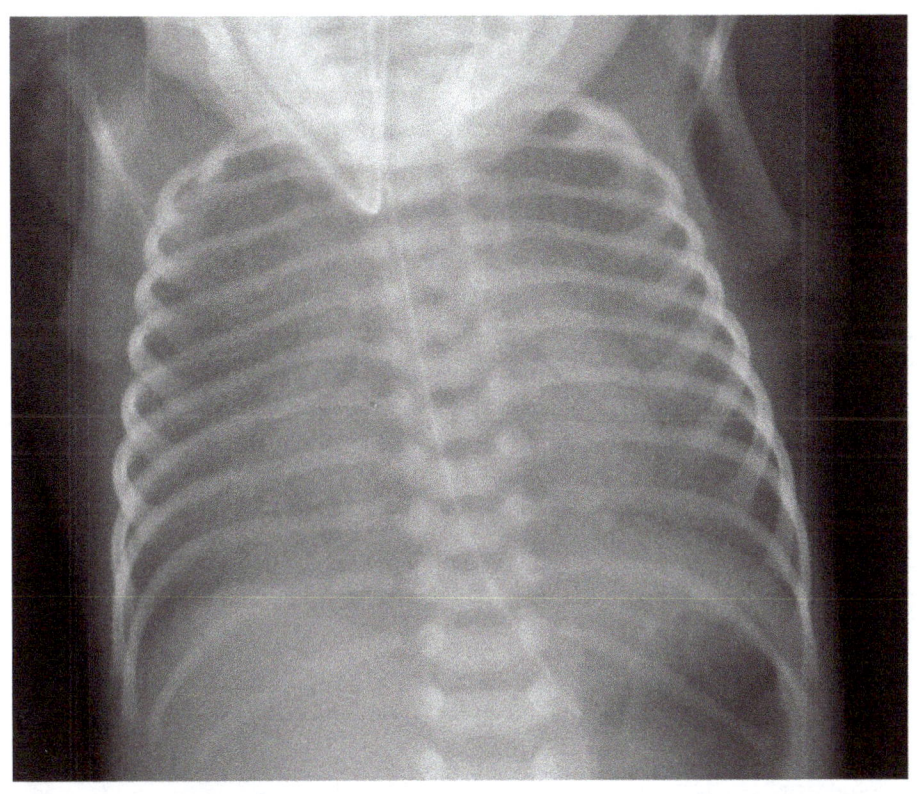

Figure 10-1. CXR of a patient with obstructed TAPVR showing severe pulmonary edema.

with TAPVR has some degree of obstruction, even if the obstruction is not clinically significant.

Fetal diagnosis of TAPVR is often difficult as the blood is shunted away from the lungs and oxygenated through the placenta. There is therefore little flow through the pulmonary veins and thus they are difficult to delineate. At times, anomalous pulmonary veins will be diagnosed in utero when there are other cardiac defects such as in patients with heterotaxy syndrome. Due to the difficulty of prenatal diagnosis, patients with TAPVR often present postnatally.

Patients with significant obstruction will present immediately after birth with significant pulmonary edema, severe and progressive cyanosis, pulmonary hypertension, metabolic acidosis, and frequently cardiogenic shock. Often, these neonates are treated as having persistent pulmonary hypertension of the newborn (PPHN) and are found to have TAPVR when an echocardiogram is performed as part of their workup. If the pulmonary veins are not obstructed, these children present in the first few months of life with signs of heart failure due to pulmonary overcirculation (increased left-to-right shunt) and cyanosis due to intracardiac mixing.

PART II. DISEASES

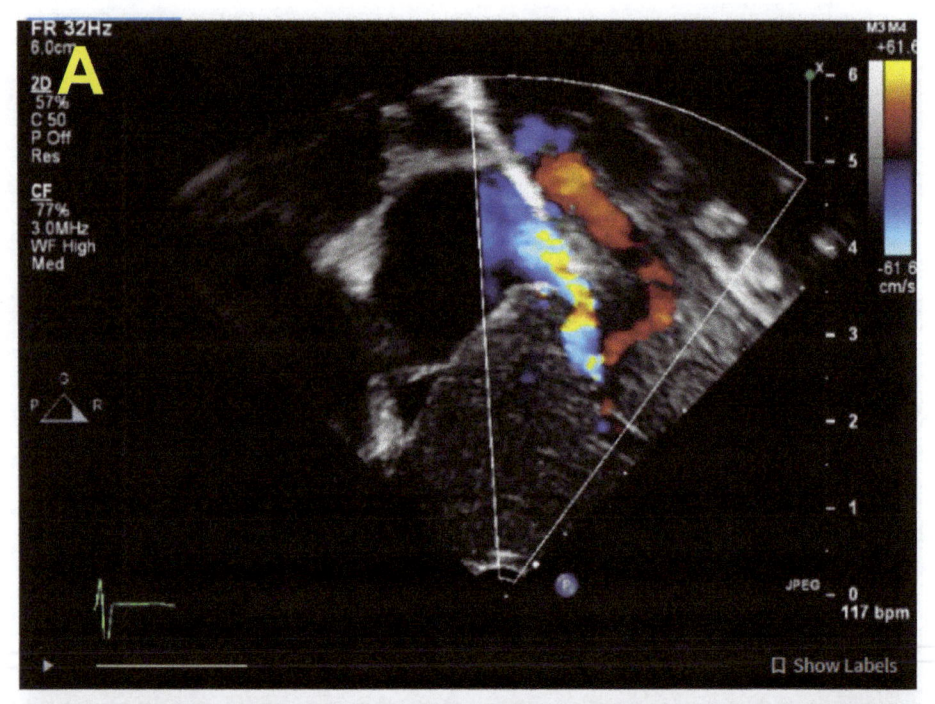

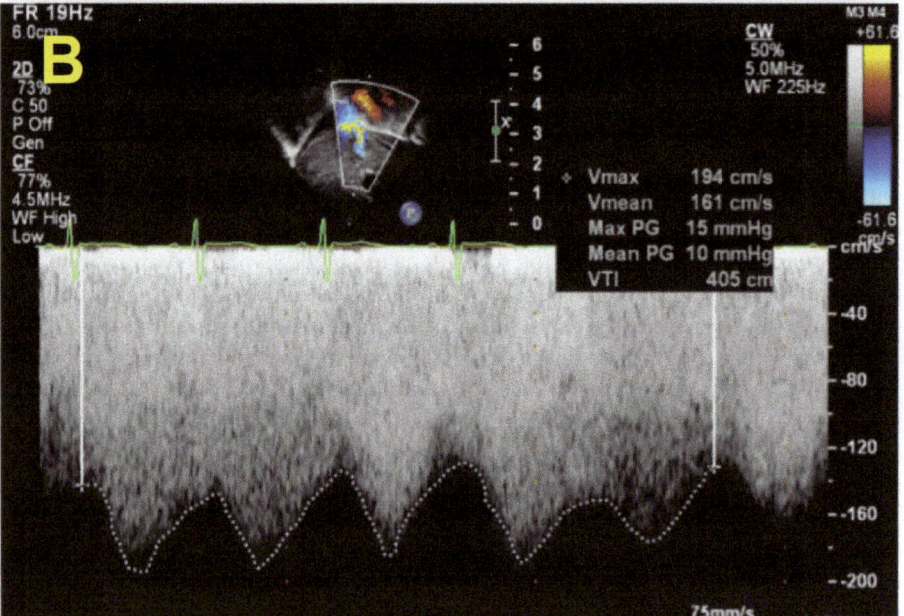

Figure 10-2. Echocardiogram of a patient with infracardiac TAPVR. The descending vein is shown coursing through the diaphragm and turning into the hepatic venous system and then into the right atrium (A). Spectral Doppler pattern of stenotic connection from descending vertical vein to hepatic venous system (B). Images courtesy of Dr. Josh Kailin, www.pedecho.org.

10. PULMONARY VEIN ANOMALIES

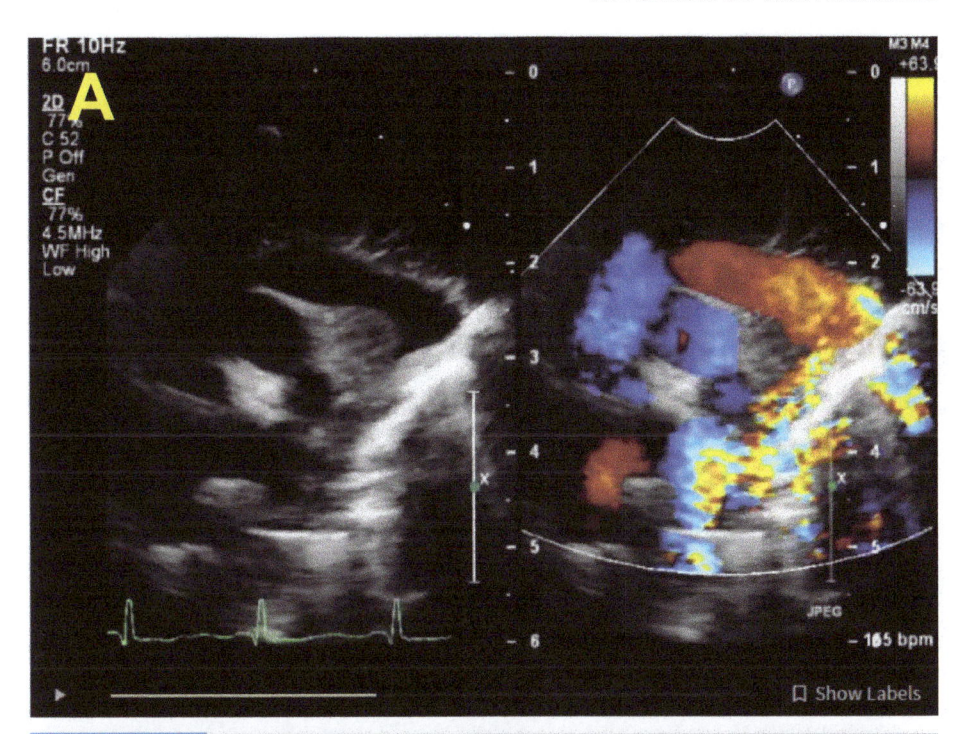

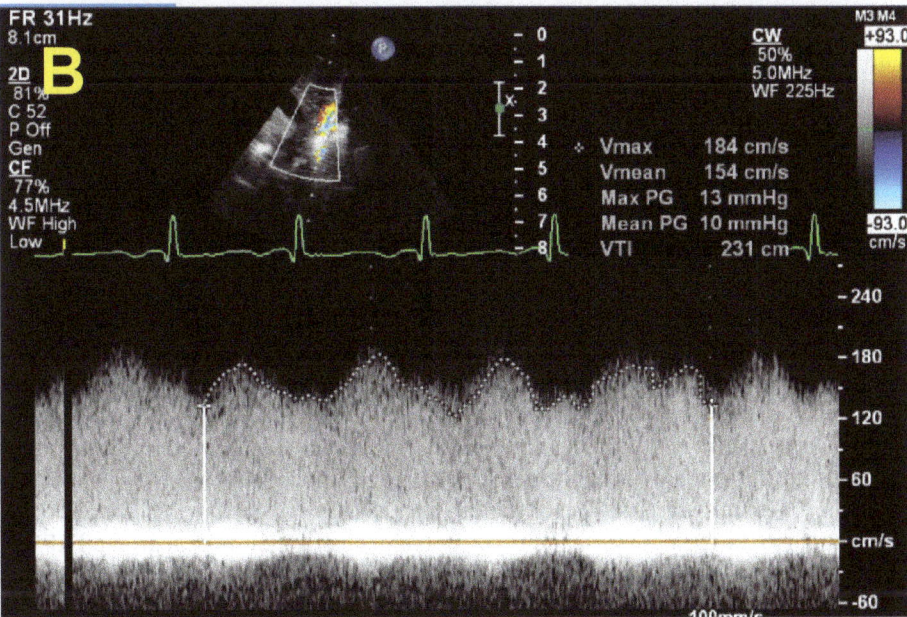

Figure 10-3. Echocardiogram of a patient with supracardiac TAPVR. The ascending vein is noted entering into the left innominate vein, which in turn drains into the SVC (A). There is obstruction between the left PA and left bronchus, as noted in the Doppler pattern (B). Images courtesy of Dr. Josh Kailin, www.pedecho.org.

59

PART II. DISEASES

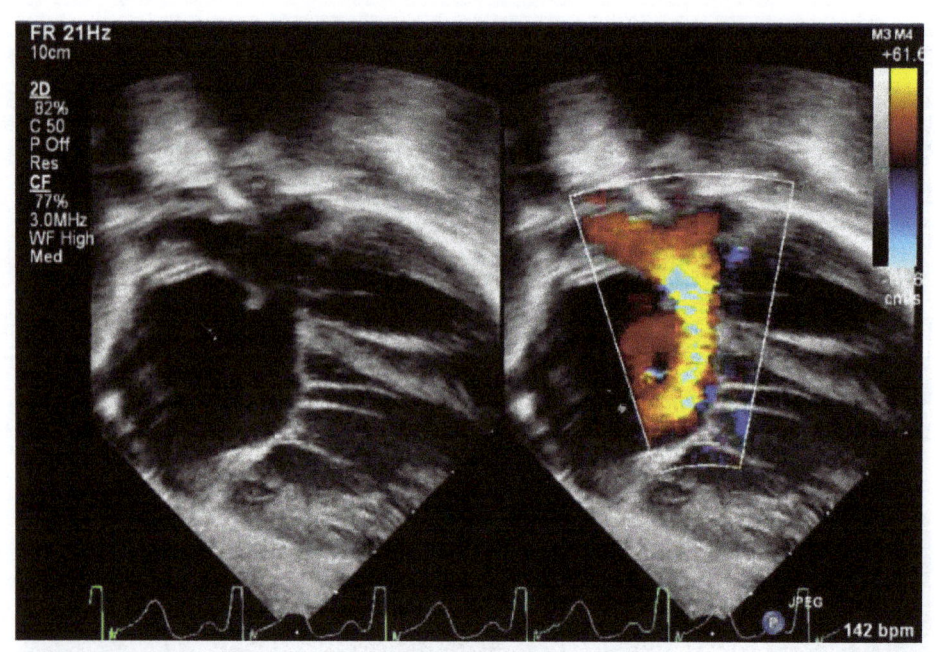

Figure 10-4. The classic "whale's tail" seen in anomalous pulmonary veins draining into the coronary sinus with flow into the RA.

Diagnosis
- **CXR.** Patients with significant obstruction will show severe pulmonary edema (Figure 10-1) whereas patients with no obstruction will demonstrate evidence of pulmonary overcirculation (cardiomegaly and increased pulmonary vascular markings). Older patients with supracardiac TAPVR to the innominate vein may show what has been described as the "snowman sign" with the upper silhouette formed by the vertical vein on the left and the dilated SVC on the right.
- **Echocardiography.** Diagnosis usually relies on the initial echocardiogram. A sign that there is TAPVR is purely right-to-left shunting across the atrial level communication (PFO or ASD). There needs to be delineation of whether the TAPVR is supracardiac, infracardiac, cardiac (to the coronary sinus or to the right atrium directly), or mixed. Each pulmonary vein should be imaged, the insertion into the confluence or ascending/descending vein described, and the course of the ascending or descending vein should be traced to localize areas of obstruction. By definition, patients with infracardiac TAPVR (Figure 10-2) are obstructed due to the long course to return to the RA and multiple sites of potential obstruction. Supracardiac TAPVR (Figure 10-3) can be obstructed, most frequently where the ascending vein courses between the bronchus and left PA. The image on echocardiography of cardiac TAPVR to the coronary sinus (Figure 10-4) is termed a "whale's tail" due to the similarity of appearance. In supra- and infracardiac TAPVR, the ascending or descending vein is noted by echocardiography as a venous structure coursing away from the heart. In

10. PULMONARY VEIN ANOMALIES

supracardiac TAPVR often the ascending vein is noted coursing into the innominate vein (flow toward the transducer in suprasternal notch views) and in infracardiac TAPVR a vein is noted descending through the diaphragm rather than the expected venous course toward the heart (the sine qua non is "red" venous flow through the diaphragm when imaging in subcostal windows). Echocardiography should also focus on delineating other intracardiac lesions as TAPVR is frequently associated with heterotaxy syndrome and single-ventricle cardiac disease. In isolated TAPVR, RV pressure can be evaluated and the size of the LV, LVOT, and aortic arch should be assessed as there can be associated hypoplasia of left-heart structures due to limitations of in utero flow through the left side of the heart.
- **CTA.** If the pulmonary veins cannot be adequately delineated by echocardiography, they can be imaged using cardiac CTA, provided that the patient is stable. Surgical intervention should not be delayed in a patient in extremis in order to obtain a CTA unless there is a high suspicion of complete pulmonary venous atresia (uncommon). Timing of contrast administration must account for the fact that flow through the pulmonary veins may be significantly delayed if severely obstructed.

Preoperative Management

Preoperative management of obstructed TAPVR involves hemodynamic stabilization and expedited progression to the OR for repair. Patients are often acidotic and can have hemodynamic compromise due to severe cyanosis. Prolonging preoperative medical management can lead to worsening of end-organ dysfunction. Significant ventilation and treatment of pulmonary hypertension can even worsen the clinical picture by worsening pulmonary edema. Inotropic support is indicated to maintain end-organ perfusion. Preoperative management of unobstructed TAPVR involves diuresis due to the increasing left-to-right shunt as neonatal PVR decreases.

Indications / Timing of Intervention

The diagnosis of TAPVR is an indication for surgical intervention. Patients with obstructed TAPVR require emergent intervention. Patients with a diagnosis of unobstructed TAPVR undergo semielective repair prior to initial discharge of the hospital (if diagnosed in utero or in the neonatal period) or shortly after diagnosis, if diagnosed as an outpatient.

Anesthetic Considerations

The anesthetic management of TAPVR is very dependent on patient anatomy and on the degree to which the anomalous pulmonary veins are obstructed.

Preoperative

Obstructed TAPVR is a true neonatal emergency. The preoperative evaluation should focus on the patient's anatomy, intravenous and intraarterial access, and the degree of pulmonary venous obstruction and resulting pulmonary edema. Medications should be reviewed, as many of these patients may require infusions of epinephrine, dopamine, vasopressin, and PGE. The echocardiogram should be reviewed for associated anomalies, as the anatomy will dictate whether the patient may need a systemic-to-pulmonary artery shunt, a PA band, arch advancement, or other procedure in addition to the repair of the TAPVR. The CXR should be reviewed with special attention to the appearance of the lungs and the position of the umbilical arterial and venous lines. A recent arterial blood gas should be reviewed and the degree of hypoxemia and/or acidosis should be noted, as well as the lactate. Ventilator settings may also yield important information regarding the condition of the lungs.

Intraoperative
A TEE is usually avoided during TAPVR repair because it can cause obstruction of the pulmonary venous confluence and make the operation more challenging. In the pre-CPB period in patients with obstructed TAPVR, oxygenation can become increasingly difficult and inhaled nitric oxide may be necessary to bring the PO_2 to minimally acceptable values. Post-CPB, pulmonary hypertension and poor pulmonary mechanics may be encountered. iNO, milrinone, and epinephrine may be required to augment RV function and decrease PA pressures.

Surgical Repair
The goal of surgical repair of TAPVR is to create a large anastomosis between the left atrial structures and the pulmonary venous confluence. The procedure is performed through a median sternotomy. Aaorto-bicaval cannulation is preferred.

Circulatory arrest is uncommonly required, but cooling after initiation of CPB can be helpful if a short period of circulatory arrest is anticipated. While cooling, the pulmonary venous confluence is dissected from behind the pericardium and the pulmonary veins are identified. It is useful to place fine marking stitches on both the pulmonary venous confluence and the posterior aspect of the atrium while slightly filling the heart in order to define the optimal position of the anastomosis.

Once the goal temperature is reached, the heart is arrested. A right atriotomy is performed to visualize the atrial anatomy. The heart is usually retracted rightward in order to allow for visualization. Using intermittent DHCA, the vertical vein is ligated, an incision is performed on the anterior aspect of the pulmonary venous confluence, and a corresponding incision is created on the posterior aspect of the LA, sometimes extending into the LA appendage. An anastomosis is carefully created between the LA and the pulmonary venous confluence with running fine Prolene suture. Partial or full CPB flows may be intermittently used during this portion of the procedure. After the anastomosis is created, full CPB is reinitiated and the patient is rewarmed. The ASD is closed either primarily or with a small pericardial patch. An LA line may be placed through the LA appendage (if not used for the anastomosis) or through the RA and the sutureline of the ASD closure. The cross-clamp is removed and the right atriotomy closed.

It is important to note that the left heart in patients with TAPVR tends to be relatively small and noncompliant. As such, administration of even small amounts of fluid can significantly increase LAP and push the left heart beyond its Starling curve. An LA line allows judicious management of intracardiac volume. As such, CPB is carefully weaned making sure that LAP is kept low, even if that means tolerating a relatively lower BP. It is common for the left heart to slowly improve its output as one usually sees significant improvements in BP at the same intracardiac volume over the first 30-60 minutes off CPB.

Postoperative Management

Much of the postoperative management of patients with obstructed TAPVR is dealing with the residual end-organ dysfunction caused by preoperative instability. Patients with obstructed TAPVR have elevated PVR and very reactive pulmonary vascular beds. In addition, they often require significant preoperative ventilation and may have suffered barotrauma, making ventilation more difficult. Some of these patients may require treatment of pulmonary hypertension with oxygenation, iNO, and sildenafil. Patients initially remain sedated and at times require neuromuscular blockade in the initial postoperative period until the reactive component of their elevated PVR improves.

> **TAPVR repairs at TCH (1995-2019) (Spigel et al. 2020)**
> Number of patients: 336
> Patients with heterotaxy: 118 (35%)
> - Single ventricle patients: 106/118 (90%)
> - Obstructed TAPVR: 48/118 (41%)
> - TAPVR repair: 94/118 (80%)
> Patients without heterotaxy: 218 (65%)
> - Single ventricle: 14/218 (6%)
> - Obstructed TAPVR: 87/218 (40%)
> - TAPVR repair: 213/218 (98%)
> Median follow-up time: 6.6 years
> Mean number of pulmonary vein interventions:
> - Heterotaxy, obstructed TAVPR: 2.5
> - Heterotaxy, unobstructed TAPVR: 1.3
> - No heterotaxy, obstructed TAVPR: 1.3
> - No heterotaxy, unobstructed TAPVR: 1.3
> 30-day survival: 97% (95-99%)
> 5-year survival: 86% (83-91%)

Patients with TAPVR have relatively small left hearts due to limitations of fetal blood flow. Patients are managed with relative hypotension initially to not add undue strain to the LV. As mentioned above, patients are intolerant to volume administration, which can significantly increase LAP due to a noncompliant LV. This can reflect back onto the pulmonary venous pressure and lead to pulmonary hypertensive crises. Patients are monitored with an LA line to guide intravascular volume and hemodynamic/inotropic management. Patients are also managed with peritoneal dialysis for volume and cytokine removal. Monitoring for neurologic sequelae of preoperative instability is also important in the postoperative management.

Complications and Long-Term Follow-Up

The development of postoperative complications in these patients is directly related to their preoperative status. Patients with obstructed TAPVR are at a higher risk of end-organ dysfunction as a consequence of their preoperative course. As mentioned above, pulmonary hypertension episodes are not unusual in patients with preoperative obstructed TAPVR. However, pulmonary vascular reactivity tends to improve over the first few days after repair.

One of the most significant and vexing long-term complications after TAPVR repair is the development of pulmonary venous stenosis. This complication occurs in approximately 10% of patients after TAPVR repair (Morales et al. 2006) and usually presents within the first 6 months after repair. Patients with heterotaxy syndrome who present with obstructed TAPVR are at a higher risk of developing postrepair pulmonary vein stenosis (Spigel et al. 2020). Even though the stenosis can occur at the site of the anastomosis, some patients present with more diffuse fibrotic involvement of the upstream pulmonary veins. Initial intervention for postrepair pulmonary venous stenosis is usually surgical and entails a "sutureless" repair in which the affected pulmonary veins are opened into the pericardial well and the atrium is sutured to the pericardium around the pulmonary veins. Recurrence of pulmonary venous stenosis is a challenging problem and pulmonary venous stenting in the cardiac catheterization lab may be required.

Isolated Pulmonary-Vein Stenosis

Patients with pulmonary vein stenosis comprise one of the most critically ill and challenging groups of patients we treat. Pulmonary vein stenosis may be broadly divided into 2 categories: primary (congenital) or secondary (e.g., post-TAPVR repair) pulmonary vein stenosis. Primary (congenital) pulmonary vein stenosis carries a worse outcome. In either category, survival for patients with progressive pulmonary vein stenosis is approximately 50% at 1 year.

Pathophysiology and Clinical Presentation

The origin of primary stenosis of the pulmonary veins relates to incomplete incorporation of the common pulmonary vein into the posterior wall of the LA. Pulmonary vein stenosis may be localized or diffuse. Diffuse stenosis of individual pulmonary veins has been seen in children with pulmonary atresia or hypoplastic left heart syndrome and TAPVR in the presence of heterotaxy.

Patients usually present with tachypnea or recurrent pneumonia. If present, right-heart failure in infants will manifest as vomiting and abdominal distention from pulmonary hypertension and hepatomegaly. Hemoptysis is less frequently observed in infants but it tends to be present in older children with individual pulmonary vein stenosis. Due to the combination of pulmonary venous desaturation and right-heart failure, patients can be cyanotic or desaturated.

On examination, there is an RV impulse with narrowing of S2, making it at times single with an accentuated P2. There might be a murmur of TR manifested as a holosystolic murmur that is high frequency (similar to MR) and localized in the midsternal border.

Diagnosis

- **ECG.** It is common to see RV hypertrophy with RA enlargement.
- **CXR (Figure 10-5).** May show significantly increased pulmonary vascular markings or pulmonary edema, with or without cardiomegaly. Pulmonary vascular markings may be asymmetric if there is regional/segmental obstruction.
- **Echocardiogram (Figure 10-6).** The echocardiogram should focus on detailing the individual distal portions of the pulmonary veins using high parasternal views or subcostal windows. Abnormal pulmonary venous Doppler will manifest as continuous, high-velocity turbulent flow with loss of phasic variation. The RV should be examined as it may be dilated and dysfunctional as a consequence of pulmonary hypertension. Indirect measures of pulmonary hypertension (e.g., septal configuration, TR jet) are important.
- **CTA (Figure 10-7).** CTA plays a significant role in diagnosis and management

10. PULMONARY VEIN ANOMALIES

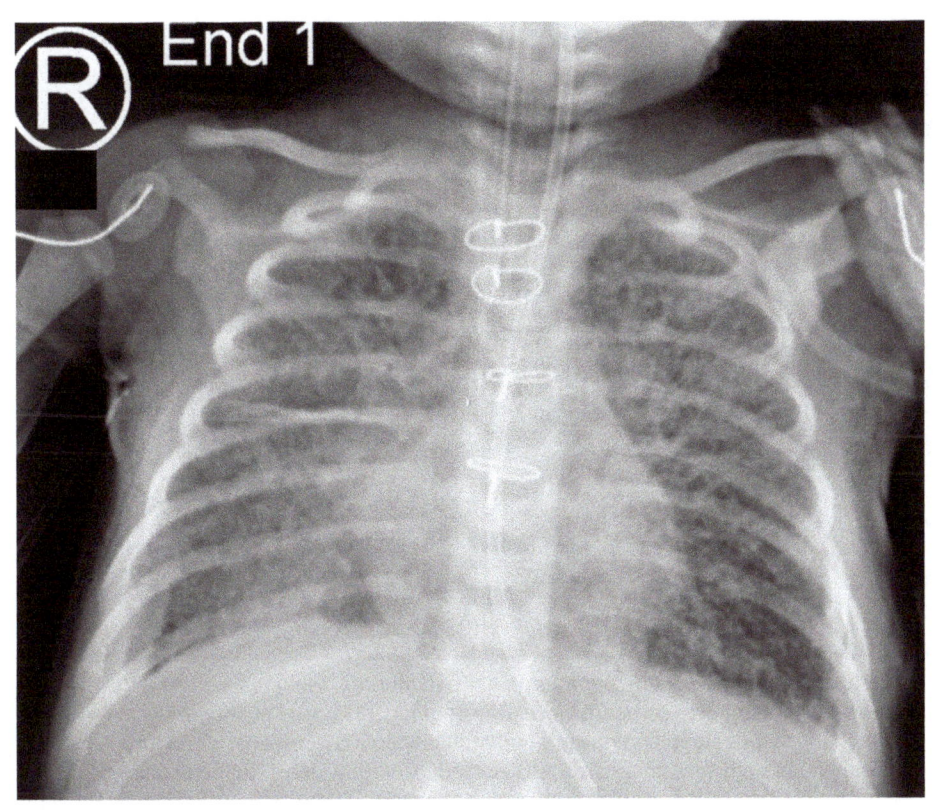

Figure 10-5. CXR of an infant with pulmonary vein stenosis (diffuse) after surgical correction for TAPVR. There is bilateral pulmonary edema with fluid in the fissure and bilateral pleural effusions (more right than left). Of note, there is no obvious cardiomegaly.

of patients with pulmonary vein stenosis. It is useful in assessing the degree and length of stenoses, the differential involvement of each pulmonary vein, and the morphology of the upstream segments. CTA not only helps to provide a roadmap for intervention but is also helpful for patient follow-up.
- **Cardiac catheterization.** Diagnostic and therapeutic cardiac catheterization play a critical role in the management of these patients (see below).

Management
The management of patients with pulmonary vein stenosis requires coordination of care within the context of a multidisciplinary team. At TCH, a dedicated Pulmonary Vein Stenosis team consists of cardiothoracic surgeons, interventional cardiologists, noninvasive cardiologists, pulmonary hypertension specialists, intensive care specialists, anesthesiologists, nurses, and other specialists. Cases are reviewed and therapeutic plans, which integrate catheter-based and surgical interventions, are orchestrated with the expectation that patients will receive multiple interventions, aggressive surveillance, and medical management of pulmonary hypertension and remodeling of pulmonary arteriopathy.

PART II. DISEASES

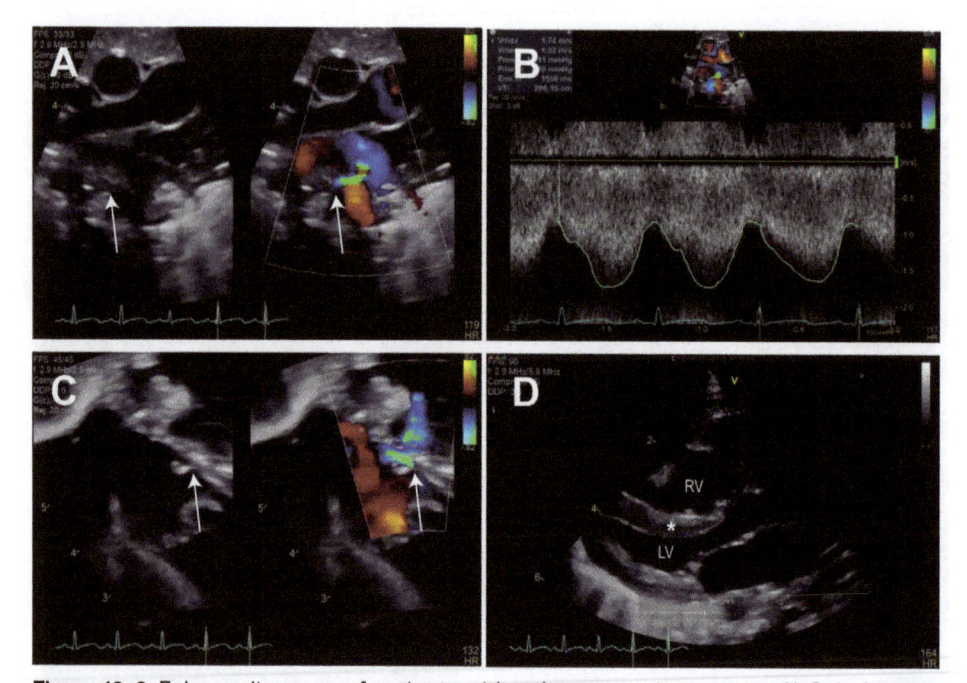

Figure 10-6. Echocardiograms of patients with pulmonary vein stenosis. A) Side-by-side supra-sternal notch color-compare views of a stenotic left upper pulmonary vein (arrows). B) Pulmonary venous Doppler of the left upper pulmonary vein demonstrating turbulent flow with a continuous and abnormal increased velocity. C) Side-by-side 4-chamber color-compare views of a stenotic left lower pulmonary vein (arrows). D) Dilated and dysfunctional RV with a shifted interventricular septum (*) due to pulmonary hypertension from pulmonary vein stenosis. Images courtesy of Dr. Josh Kailin, www.pedecho.org.

Medical Management

Although the management of pulmonary vein stenosis is either catheter-based or surgical, diuretics can be used to mitigate the effects of pulmonary congestion on respiratory mechanics. However, preload changes should be carefully managed since RV dilation and restricted pulmonary blood flow will also impact LV preload and potentially reduce systemic output.

When right-heart failure is present, inotropic support with catecholamines may be required. Several pharmacological strategies have been used to reduce proliferation of the intimal layers of the pulmonary veins. The addition of sirolimus or everolimus to the treatment regimen of these challenging patients is still under investigation.

Catheter-Based Intervention

Indications for intervention include severe anatomic pulmonary vein stenosis (especially multivessel involvement) with significant hemodynamic compromise due to pulmonary hypertension, cyanosis in the presence of a shunt, right-heart failure, respiratory symptoms (e.g., tachypnea with need for respiratory support), recurrent pneumonias, hemoptysis, and failure to thrive. For high-risk patients, planning consists of appropriate

10. PULMONARY VEIN ANOMALIES

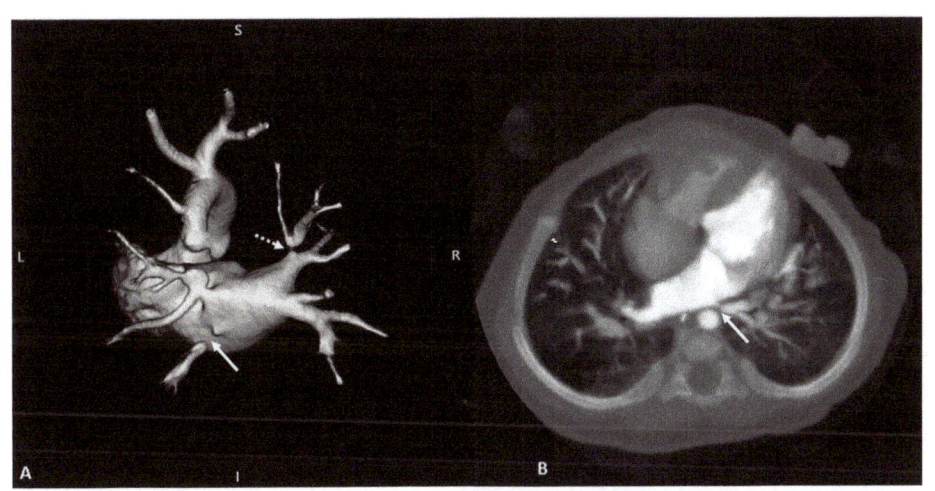

Figure 10-7. CT scan in a 4-month-old, ex-premature infant with a chromosomal abnormality, postsurgical VSD closure and newly discovered severe pulmonary vein stenosis with pulmonary hypertension. A) 3D imaging shows severe left lower lobe pulmonary vein stenosis (solid arrow) and severe right upper pulmonary vein stenosis (dotted arrow). The left upper pulmonary vein and its subsegments can also be seen to be stenotic. B) Axial imaging demonstrates severe left lower pulmonary vein stenosis (arrow).

surgical backup and the potential use of ECMO or other forms of mechanical support if a patient's condition deteriorates in the cardiac catheterization laboratory. In some instances, the procedure may have to be performed with the patient already on ECMO support.

Cardiac catheterization is performed with general anesthesia and biplane fluoroscopy. Arterial access is obtained for pressure monitoring. Femoral venous access is the preferred route for intervention.

In critically ill children considered to be at high risk for an impending cardiac arrest, the first portion of the procedure should be the creation of an ASD to improve hemodynamics. The ASD is created with a transseptal needle in standard fashion or by using radiofrequency energy/electrocautery. Transseptal puncture should be carried out using biplane fluoroscopy. However, echocardiography (transthoracic or transesophageal) may be necessary for difficult transseptal punctures, such as those in patients with prior surgical patches or challenging anatomy because of leftward bowing of the atrial septum from severe pulmonary hypertension.

For standard-risk patients, complete right-sided hemodynamics are performed (and left-sided, if indicated) and all PA wedge positions are entered. After hemodynamics are measured, PA wedge angiography is performed to delineate the pulmonary veins on levophase (both upstream and ostial pulmonary veins) and provide anatomic diagnostic information and a roadmap for the intended interventions on stenotic/occluded pulmonary veins. In addition to delineating stenotic pulmonary veins, PA wedge angiography may identify a small channel of a pulmonary vein that was felt to be occluded by noninvasive imaging. If indeed the pulmonary vein is occluded, PA

PART II. DISEASES

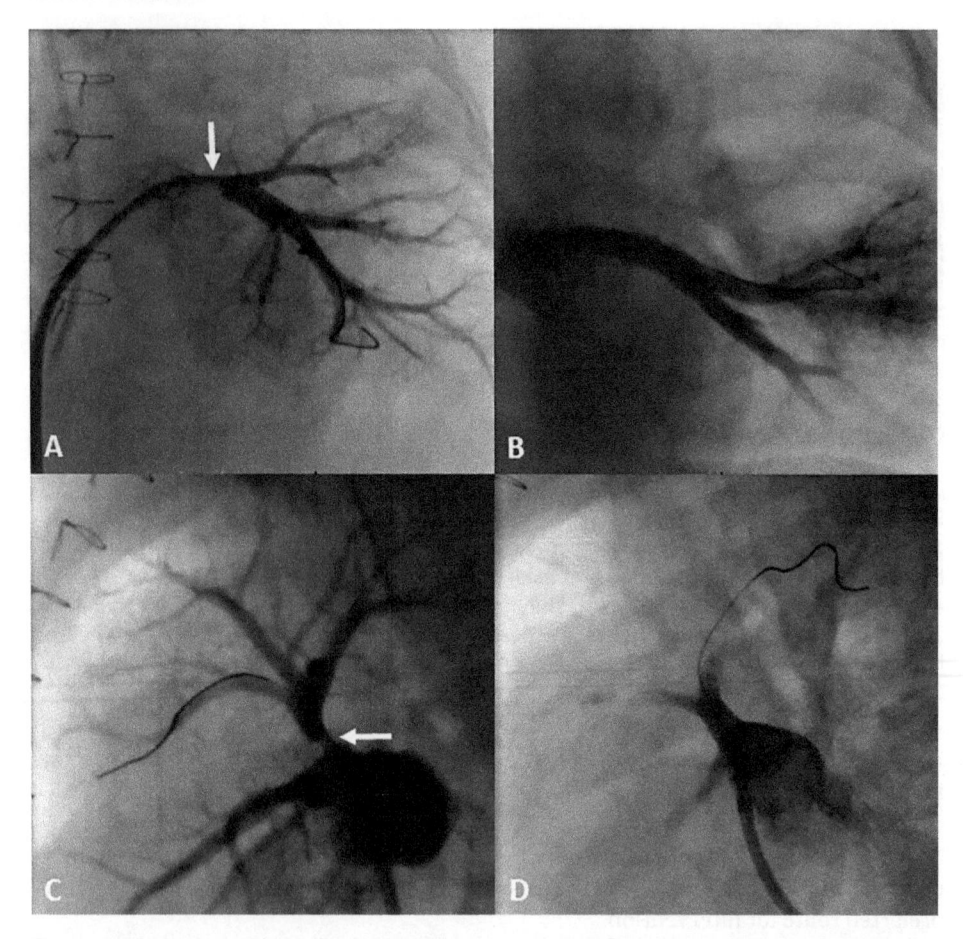

Figure 10-8. Angiography in the same patient described in Figure 10-7 shows severe stenosis of the left lower pulmonary vein at 4 months of age in a left anterior oblique/cranial projection (arrow) (A). A follow-up catheterization at 11 months of age shows an unobstructed left lower pulmonary vein after stenting with a drug-eluting stent and dilation to 5 mm (B). The right upper pulmonary vein is also severely stenotic at 4 months of age (C) on the lateral projection (arrow). An unobstructed right upper pulmonary vein is seen at 7 months of age after implantation of a 4 mm drug-eluting stent (D).

wedge angiography still provides an anatomic target for recanalization, if feasible. In some instances, a more focused diagnostic cardiac catheterization may be performed based on findings from a CTA (Figure 10-7).

After transseptal puncture, the patient is heparinized to maintain an ACT ≥250 seconds for the duration of the procedure. Once the pulmonary veins are entered, balloon angioplasty is performed (standard or high-pressure angioplasty). A cutting balloon may be used, if needed, to treat resistant lesions. In general, an appropriately sized stent is implanted. It is preferable to insert a large diameter stent (bare metal stent), if possible. If the vessel is small, which is frequently the case in pediatric pulmonary vein stenosis, a coronary stent is implanted (usually 4-5 mm, but smaller in some instances). These stents can be redilated later and intentionally fractured to accommodate implantation of a larger-diameter stent. "Kissing" stents or intentional vessel jailing with dilation/ stenting through stent side cells may be needed to treat pulmonary veins in close proximity. While some centers perform balloon angioplasty (standard, high-pressure, and cutting-balloon angioplasty) for pulmonary vein stenosis, we prefer to implant stents whenever possible. This may be associated with a higher likelihood of maintaining vessel patency and achieving the largest lumen diameter possible in follow-up. We prefer to implant drug-eluting stents (Figure 10-8) in small-diameter pulmonary veins. Over a 24-year period at TCH, drug-eluting stents (implanted in 105 lesions) have been found to result in a significantly less rate of lumen loss than bare metal stents (implanted in 58 lesions) (Khan et al. 2019).

An ASD is usually created with a large balloon to facilitate subsequent interventions and decrease procedure times (in addition to providing a pop-off mechanism). Meticulous attention to central venous access is important. Due to repeated procedures, transhepatic venous access and recanalization of femoral/internal jugular veins may be needed for future interventions.

Operators should have the ability to treat infrequent, but significant complications (e.g., cardiac perforation, pulmonary vein tears, thrombotic events, stent dislodgement) with appropriate surgical backup.

Surgical Intervention

Surgical therapy for established pulmonary vein stenosis should be performed within the context of a multidisciplinary program to manage a highly lethal condition, which frequently recurs despite adequate decompression in the OR. The concept of a "one-and-done" operation that cures the problem should not be expected. With aggressive surveillance and a low threshold for repetitive reintervention, the state of the art suggests that the prognosis can be improved.

The anatomic profile of disease in an individual patient has a strong influence on the likelihood of a durable surgical result. The group with the most favorable prognosis includes patients with stenosis at the site of anatomic repair after correction of TAPVR, where the stenosis is largely related to stricture at the site of the anastomosis between the atrium and the pulmonary veins. This complication occurs in approximately 10-15% of TAPVR repairs. The most likely etiology is a failure to create a sufficiently large anastomosis at the TAPVR repair or a pursestring effect due to inappropriate tension during construction of the anastomosis. Both problems may be avoided using a sutureless repair technique when repairing TAPVR. This type of pulmonary vein stenosis is termed post-repair pulmonary vein stenosis (PR-PVS).

When evaluating a patient with PR-PVS, a key feature to evaluate is the size of the upstream pulmonary veins. Typically, patients with PR-PVS with early detection will have dilated upstream pulmonary veins and are amenable to surgical decompression with a sutureless approach. When the upstream pulmonary veins are small, however, the likelihood of recurrent stenosis within the smaller pulmonary veins is high and aggressive surveillance is indicated. The sutureless approach can be used to reestablish continuity with atretic pulmonary veins, but the size of the upstream pulmonary veins is also an important predictor of postoperative restenosis.

Another important subset of patients are patients with primary (congenital) pulmonary vein stenosis. In these patients, the size of the upstream pulmonary veins is also an important predictor of need for future reintervention and ultimate survival.

Patients who are brought to the OR after stent-based therapy can undergo resection of the stents as part of a sutureless repair or intraoperative stent dilation in those with either small upstream pulmonary veins or stents that extend significantly into the upstream segments.

Long-Term Follow-Up

Patients are followed after catheterization or surgical therapy by the Pulmonary Vein Stenosis team. Surgical patients undergo a surveillance CT scan within a month of repair. Catheterization-based interventions are typically followed with a repeat catheterization after 3 months. In both tracks, there is a low threshold for subsequent reinterventions.

Pulmonary vasodilators and pulmonary vascular remodeling therapy may be considered for patients in the interim period between surgical or catheterization-based decompression and the expected recurrence of pulmonary vein stenosis.

For patients with relentless progression and/or poor upstream pulmonary vein development, adjunctive medical therapy with rapamycin (found to be effective in a very small clinical experience) or losartan (efficacy demonstrated in an animal model) may be considered. Efficacy of these and other medications in large clinical cohorts of patients with pulmonary vein stenosis is lacking.

Suggested Readings

Khan A, Qureshi AM, Justino H. Comparison of drug eluting stents versus bare metal stents for pulmonary vein stenosis in childhood. Catheter Cardiovasc Interv 2019;94:233-242.

Morales DLS, Braud BE, Booth JH, et al. Heterotaxy patients with total anomalous pulmonary venous return: improving surgical results. Ann Thorac Surg 2006;82:1621-1628.

Spigel ZA, Edmunds EE, Binsalamah ZM, et al. Heterotaxy syndrome and obstructed pulmonary veins. Accepted for presentation at AATS 2020. Manuscript in preparation.

11 Ventricular Septal Defect

Antonio G. Cabrera, Patricia Bastero, Athar M. Qureshi, Carlos M. Mery

A ventricular septal defect (VSD) is a communication between both ventricles. There are different types of VSDs based on anatomy (Figure 11-1):

- **Perimembranous.** Underneath the tricuspid valve and with continuity between the tricuspid and aortic valves. The septal leaflet of the tricuspid valve forms one of the rims of the defect.
- **Muscular.** Completely surrounded by muscular tissue. It can be subclassified into outlet, inlet, mid-muscular, and apical, depending on the area of the muscular septum where it is mainly located.
- **Inlet.** Analogous to the VSD seen in patients with AV septal defects. Both the right and left AV valves are in continuity and form the posterior border of the defect. It may be associated with a mitral cleft.
- **Doubly committed juxta-arterial (DCJA).** Also called supracristal or subpulmonary VSD. The defect is bordered by both arterial valves (aortic and pulmonary), which are in continuity. There is a lack of infundibular septum and the pulmonary valve lies at the same level as the aortic valve. The defect can have perimembranous extension, in which case there is continuity between the aortic and tricuspid valves.

Pathophysiology and Clinical Presentation

The magnitude and direction of shunting depends on the size of the defect and the relationship between the resistance of the systemic and pulmonary circulations. Classically, since SVR is higher than PVR, shunting occurs from left to right (Figure 11-2). In situations in which the defect is very small (pressure-restrictive), shunting will be relatively small and the RV and PA pressures will remain normal (i.e., much lower than the LV and aortic pressures). In a large VSD, there is significant left-to-right shunting and the LV and RV pressures are equalized (non-restrictive VSD).

In newborns, given the transitional circulation after birth, there is a gradual decrease in PVR that translates into progressive left-to-right shunting. Once the PVR has found its lowest point during the first 6 weeks of life, symptoms of CHF become evident. In newborns and infants, these symptoms include tachypnea and diaphoresis with feeds, failure to thrive, and tachycardia.

If the defect is large and left untreated, the patient will eventually develop pulmonary vascular changes that will translate into a high PVR with eventual reversal of shunting and development of cyanosis. The development of irreversible pulmonary vascular disease (Eisenmenger syndrome) is variable but may happen early, especially in patients with genetic syndromes such as trisomy 21.

The physical exam findings relate to the amount of shunting, the size of the defect, the relative pulmonary and systemic vascular resistances, and the presence of secondary abnormalities such as MR (from significant left-heart dilation) or AI (from prolapse of the aortic valve into the defect). The diagnosis of a VSD is usually made prenatally during echocardiographic screening or after birth when a murmur is detected. Children

PART II. DISEASES

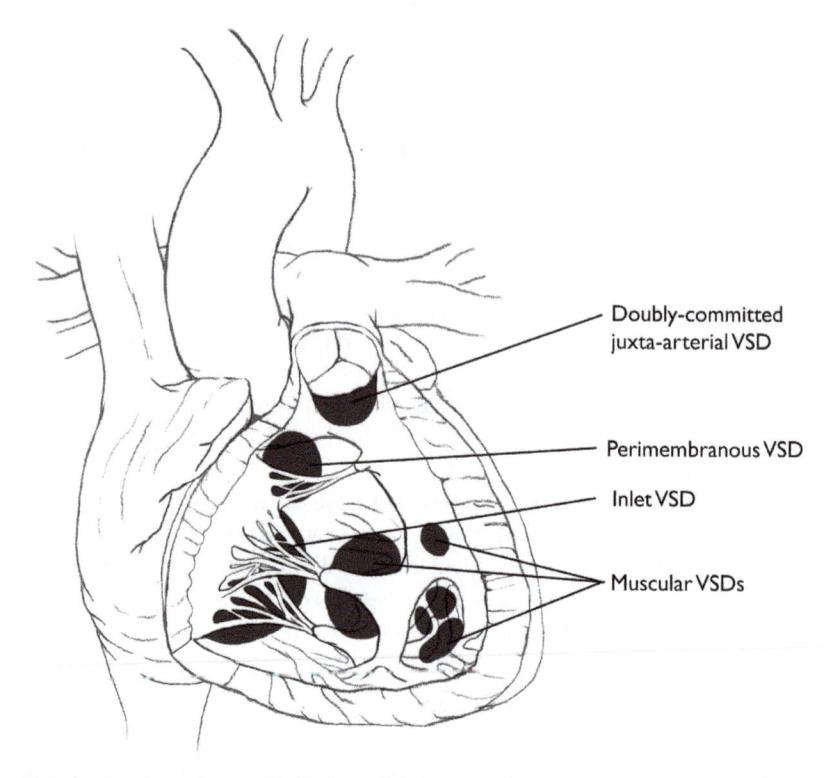

Figure 11-1. Anatomic variants of VSD based on location.

with significant volume overload will present with respiratory distress, tachypnea, and in many cases with emesis (usually from hepatomegaly-associated compression of the stomach).

Usually, there is a hyperdynamic LV impulse and a harsh holosystolic high-frequency murmur at the left lower sternal border. The murmur is well heard in the back. When PA pressures are normal, the second heart sound (S_2) will be split with a normal pulmonary component (P_2). When PA pressures are elevated, the S_2 will be narrowly split or single, with a loud P_2. The frequency of the murmur depends on the pressure drop between the LV and RV. A low-frequency diastolic rumble (absence of silence during diastole) heard at the left lower sternal border usually means that there is at least 2:1 shunting from left to right. At times, an S_3 gallop may be heard at the apex. A high-frequency end-diastolic murmur will be a sign that there is concomitant AI.

Diagnosis
- **ECG (Figure 11-3).** There can be LV and sometimes RV hypertrophy and occasional atrial enlargement.
- **CXR (Figure 11-4).** Helpful in the initial evaluation and follow-up of children with VSDs, particularly while titrating diuretics or when trying to establish the nature of

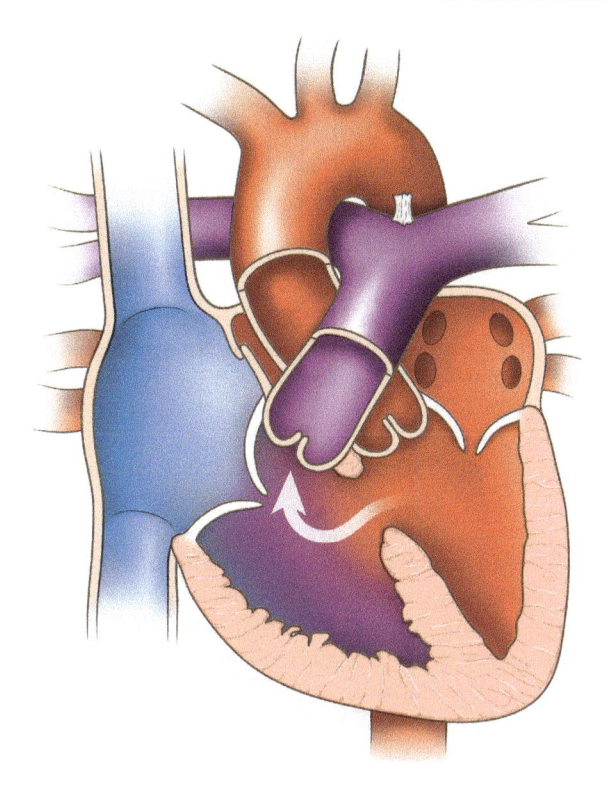

Figure 11-2. Pathophysiology of VSDs with left-to-right shunting.

their respiratory distress. It tends to show cardiomegaly and increased pulmonary vascular markings due to left-to-right shunting.
- **Echocardiogram (Figure 11-5).** Mainstay of diagnosis. It is important to obtain complete sweeps to demonstrate the location and size of the defect, measure chamber dilatation (atrial and/or ventricular), profile MR, and interrogate the aortic valve for potential prolapse. It is also important to obtain additional imaging to demonstrate the Doppler velocity of the defect to indirectly estimate the size of the defect and the PVR. In older children, with long standing defects, the presence of a double-chamber RV should be investigated.
- **Cardiac catheterization.** Rarely needed. However, in patients who present late, it may be indicated to assess PVR for suitability of VSD closure and/or the need for pulmonary vasodilator therapy.

Medical Management
Loop diuretics are effective at mitigating congestion symptoms and allowing for better feeding in patients with VSDs. Furosemide 1-2 mg/kg/dose scheduled up to every 6 hours tends to be enough to manage moderate-to-large defects. Chlorothiazide 5-10 mg/kg/dose given twice a day can be a helpful adjuvant in cases of significant volume loading or when there is some degree of diuretic resistance. Spironolactone in doses of 0.5-1 mg/

PART II. DISEASES

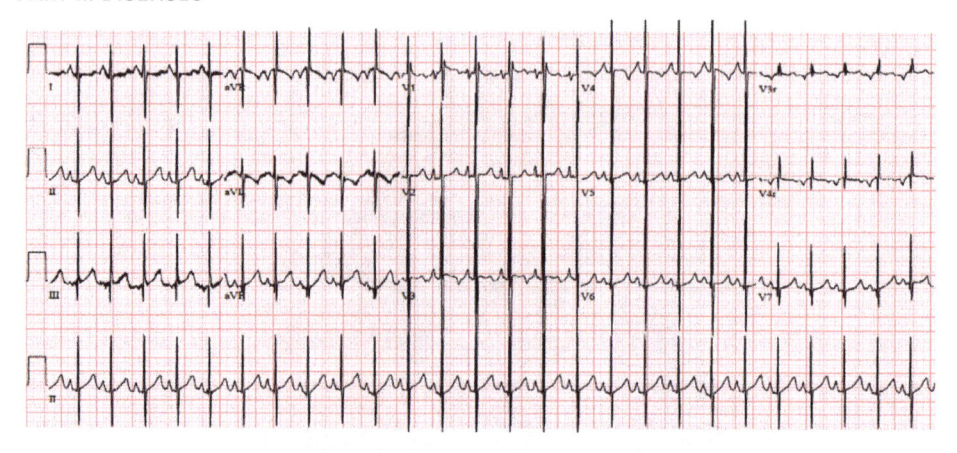

Figure 11-3. ECG on a patient with VSD demonstrating right atrial enlargement and biventricular hypertrophy.

kg/dose given twice a day can help with potassium sparing and mitigate loop diuretic resistance. Afterload reduction with angiotensin-converting enzyme (ACE) inhibitors can also be helpful by decreasing SVR and potentially reducing left-to-right shunting.

Large perimembranous VSDs can be initially managed with diuretics and ACE inhibitors. If there is no aortic valve prolapse on echocardiography and the child is gaining weight, medical management can be continued. If the S_2 becomes single and there is rapid improvement of CHF signs with weight gain and no change on the size of the defect on echocardiography, one should suspect increased PVR. In these cases, early surgical intervention should be undertaken, or if later in life, a cardiac catheterization should be considered to evaluate pulmonary vascular reactivity.

Muscular VSDs tend to close spontaneously by 2 years of age. As such, conservative management is usually indicated, unless the defects are large and the patient fails medical management. Patients with multiple apical muscular VSDs ("Swiss-cheese" septum) can have significant shunting and placement of a PA band may be necessary to control CHF symptoms. It is thought that Swiss-cheese VSDs may be a part of the LV non-compaction spectrum and if LV function decreases, cardiomyopathy should be suspected.

Indications / Timing for Intervention

The vast majority of VSDs (80%) will close spontaneously. However, some defects should be repaired in order to prevent long-term complications such as AI, endocarditis, and development of pulmonary vascular disease. In asymptomatic patients requiring intervention, repair is usually delayed until later in infancy.

Indications for intervention include:
- **Failure of medical management.** Patients with large VSDs and symptoms resistant to medical management are usually repaired in infancy.
- **Left-heart dilation.** VSDs that have a large left-to-right shunt as manifested by

11. VENTRICULAR SEPTAL DEFECT

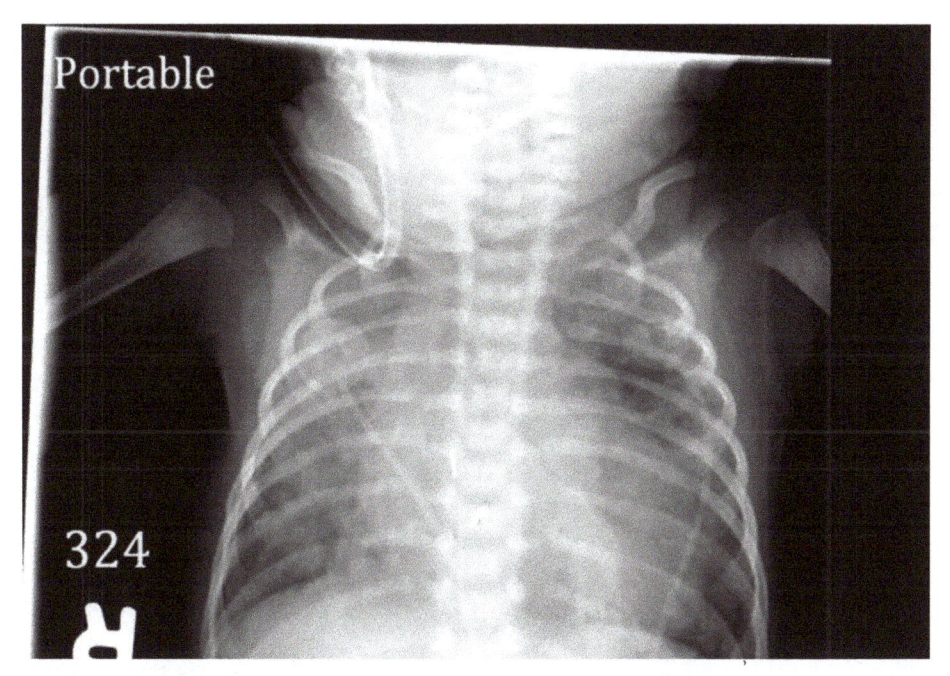

Figure 11-4. CXR on an 8-week-old patient with a large and symptomatic VSD, in addition to prematurity-associated lung disease. The CXR shows cardiomegaly with increased pulmonary vascular markings.

left-heart dilation may benefit from intervention if they have not closed spontaneously after infancy.
- **DCJA defects.** DCJA defects are associated with aortic valve prolapse and virtually all patients will develop AI before childhood or adolescence. In addition, these defects tend to not close spontaneously.
- **Aortic valve prolapse.** With or without AI.

The likelihood of spontaneous closure decreases with age and is <10% in VSDs that are patent beyond 2-3 years of age. True inlet VSDs rarely close spontaneously; strong consideration should be made for early intervention.

Catheter-Based Intervention
Device closure can be performed in patients with muscular VSDs, either as primary therapy (Figure 11-6) or as an adjunct to surgical closure, as some muscular VSDs may be not be able to be closed surgically due to the difficulty in distinguishing them from trabeculations on the RV side. The procedure frequently involves the creation of an arteriovenous loop to facilitate delivery of the VSD device from the venous side. Retrograde deployment of VSD devices can also be performed in some instances without the creation of an arteriovenous loop. Transesophageal and transthoracic echocardiography provide vital imaging guidance during the procedure.

In some very small patients, or when a concomitant operation is being performed

PART II. DISEASES

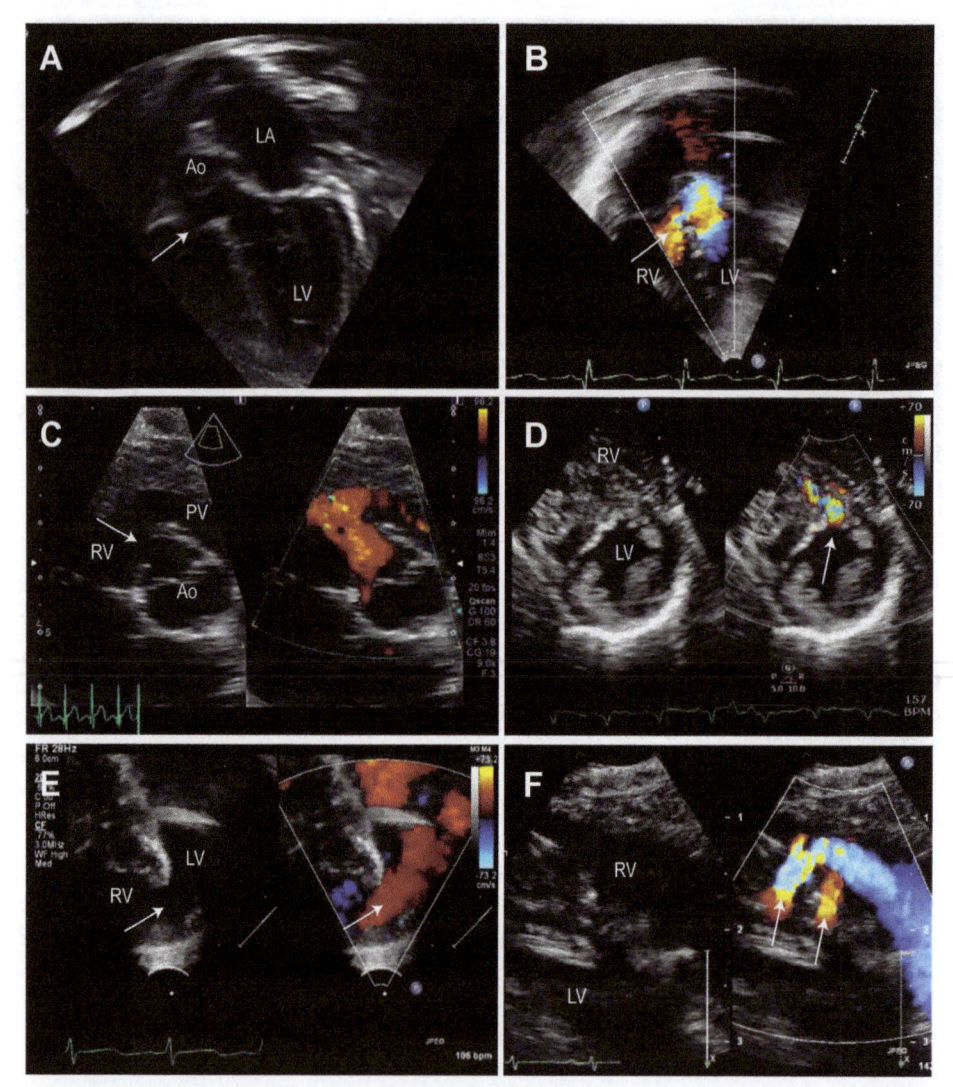

Figure 11-5. Echocardiography for diagnosis of VSD. A) 5-chamber view of a perimembranous VSD (arrow). B) 5-chamber view with color Doppler of a perimembranous VSD (arrow). C) Parasternal short-axis color-compare view of a large perimembranous VSD (arrow). D) Short-axis color-compare view of a mid-muscular VSD (arrow). E) 4-chamber color-compare view of a large apical muscular VSD (arrow). F) Parasternal long-axis color-compare view of several mid-muscular VSDs (arrows). Ao: aorta, PV: pulmonary valve. Images courtesy of Dr. Josh Kailin, www.pedecho.org.

(e.g., PA band takedown), a hybrid approach can be used (direct "perventricular" VSD closure) in the OR or cardiac catheterization laboratory with a surgeon and an interventional cardiologist.

Patients with perimembranous VSDs are currently not suitable candidates for

11. VENTRICULAR SEPTAL DEFECT

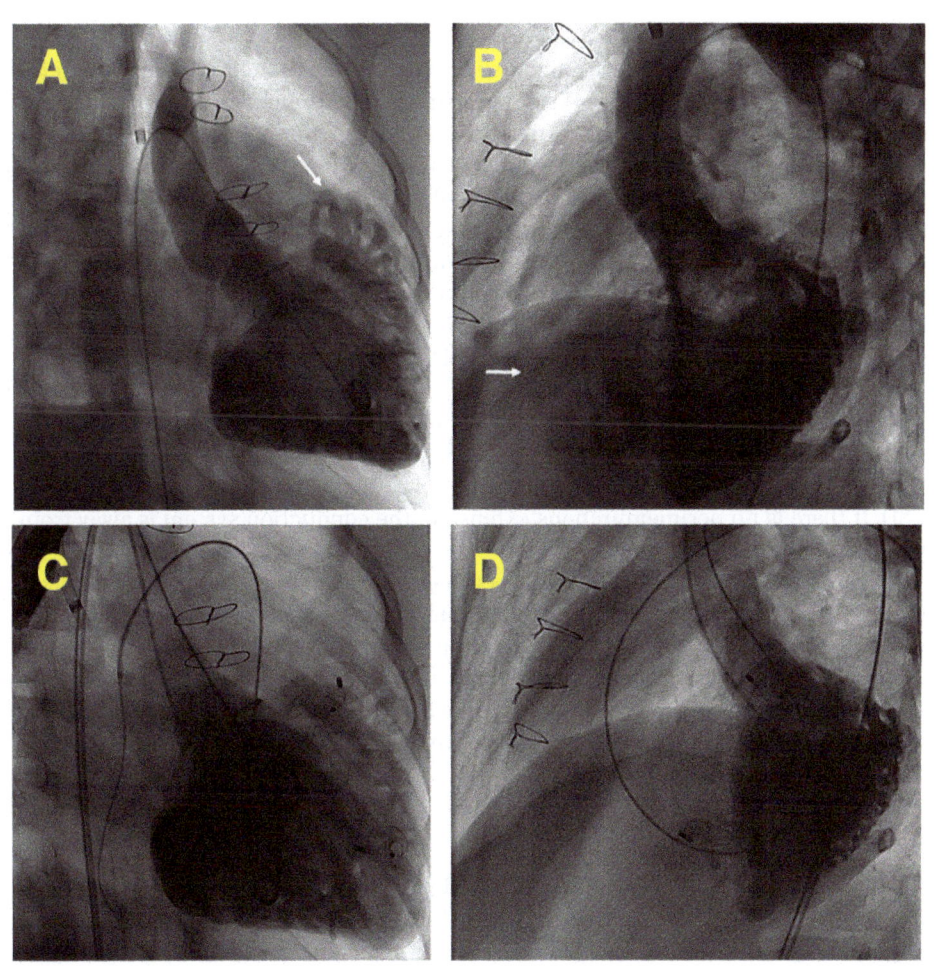

Figure 11-6. LV angiogram in a 6-year-old girl with multiple muscular VSDs. Left-to-right shunting via multiple defects in the anterior muscular septum (arrow) can be seen on a right anterior oblique/caudal projection (A). Significant shunt via apical/mid muscular VSDs to the body of the right ventricle (outlined by arrow) is also seen on the left anterior oblique/cranial projection (B). After placement of percutaneous devices in the anterior and apical muscular septum, a significant reduction in left to right shunt is seen in the corresponding post procedure angiograms (C and D).

catheter-based closure of their defects in general, due to the proximity of the defect to the AV node (with risk of heart block after device closure), and the tricuspid and aortic valves. Exceptions are patients with perimembranous defects and aneurysmal tricuspid valve tissue, which may allow a device to be placed within the defect(s), away from the AV node and surrounding valves.

Surgical Repair

Surgical repair of VSDs is performed using standard aorto-bicaval cannulation for CPB and mild-to-moderate hypothermia. Most perimembranous, inlet, and muscular defects are approached through a right atriotomy. If there is significant aneurysmal tricuspid valve tissue covering a perimembranous or inlet VSD, the tricuspid valve may be partially detached to allow full visualization of the defect. VSDs are usually repaired using glutaraldehyde-treated autologous pericardium and either interrupted pledgeted sutures or a combination of running and interrupted pledgeted sutures. In the case of perimembranous or inlet VSDs, the bundle of His travels on the posteroinferior margin of the defect, mainly towards the LV side. Care is taken to place sutures superficially and away from the rim of the VSD. Small defects may be closed primarily with interrupted double-plegeted sutures.

DCJA defects are approached through a transverse pulmonary arteriotomy. Interrupted sutures with pericardial pledgets are placed through the pulmonary valve annulus and into the rim of the defect. A pericardial patch is then used to close the VSD. If there is no perimembranous extension, the conduction system is away from the VSD on these patients.

Apical defects and those muscular defects below the moderator band can be difficult to visualize through an atriotomy and alternative approaches should be considered (cath intervention vs. ventriculotomy). In some patients with multiple VSDs (i.e., Swiss-cheese septum), early closure is challenging and placement of a PA band may allow symptom control and growth. These patients can be brought back to the OR later in life for PA band takedown and VSD repair; some patients may require cath closure of the VSD at the same time.

Postoperative Management

Older patients are usually extubated in the OR. Neonates and small infants tend to be left intubated and are then extubated within the first few hours of arrival to the CICU. These patients have usually a very uncomplicated postoperative course where the most common event to manage is hypertension secondary to a hyperdynamic LV.

In patients with significant CHF symptoms preoperatively, optimization of preload, contractility, and afterload is key. These patients are commonly managed with a milrinone infusion to optimize cardiac output, and a tight fluid control, including diuretic treatment on postoperative day 1 to prevent and improve pulmonary congestion. Extubation within 24 hours of surgery is expected.

It is not unusual for the TEE to show mild-to-moderately depressed LV function after repair of a large VSD, usually due to volume unloading of the heart. This decreased function tends to have no clinical significance and is usually improved a few days after repair.

Patients tend to stay in the CICU 1-2 days. Patients that had significant overcirculation preoperatively tend to show dramatic improvements in oral intake, tachypnea, and weight gain immediately after surgery.

Complications

Potential complications after surgical closure of VSDs include:

- **Heart block.** Variable or complete heart block may complicate surgical VSD repair due to direct injury to the AV node or the bundle of His. If the patient remains in complete heart block 7-10 days after surgery, consideration should be made to placing a permament pacemaker.
- **Arrhythmias.** Arrhythmias, such as JET, may develop in small children, likely from traction of the conduction system during repair.

> **TCH experience with VSD repairs** (Scully et al. 2010)
> Median number of repairs per year: 29 (22 – 43)
> Median age at surgery: 10 months (20 days – 18 years)
> Median ICU length of stay: 2 days (1 – 14 days)
> Median hospital length of stay: 5 days (2 days – 6 months)
> Perioperative mortality: 0.5%
> Bleeding requiring reoperation: 1%
> Perioperative complete AV block: 0

Suggested Reading

Scully BB, Morales DL, Zafar F, et al. Current expectations for surgical repair of isolated ventricular septal defects. Ann Thorac Surg 2010;89:544-9.

12 Atrioventricular Septal Defect

Antonio G. Cabrera, Jordana Goldman, Premal M. Trivedi, Carlos M. Mery

Atrioventricular septal defects (AVSD) are a spectrum of anatomic defects that originate due to the lack of complete septation of the atria, the ventricles, and incomplete separation of the AV valves. The endocardial cushions are the embryologic precursor that promotes the closure of the septae and separation of two distinct AV valvar structures. The result is a series of defects that span from primum ASDs to complete AVSDs in which the crux of the heart is underdeveloped or absent with resultant large atrial and ventricular septal communications and significant left-to-right shunting. There is clockwise and downward insertion of the AV valves with resultant increase in the number of leaflets (five or more), leaving a defective area of apposition or "cleft" that its commonly the source of valvar regurgitation before, and sometimes after surgery.

Classification

There are several different classifications of AVSDs. AVSDs can be classified into *complete* (primum ASD, common AV valve, large unrestrictive inlet VSD), *transitional* (primum ASD, common or separate AV valves, restrictive inlet VSD), and *partial* (primum ASD, separate AV valves with a "mitral cleft", and no inlet VSD) defects. In addition, they can be classified as *balanced* if both ventricles are similar in size and the AV valve is balanced between both of them, or *unbalanced* if one of the ventricles is larger than the other or the AV valve preferentially opens to one ventricle or the other.

Instead of separating AVSDs into complete, transitional, and partial, Anderson defines an AVSD as a defect that allows for shunting between atria and ventricles. He does not differentiate between complete and partial AVSDs because they both include a common AV junction. He divides AVSDs based on a single AV valve orifice or two AV valves orifices (separated or not by a tongue of tissue connecting the bridging leaflets). AV valves are not considered tricuspid or mitral but should be described as right and left AV valves.

The Rastelli classification, which is used for complete AVSDs, divides these defects depending on the characteristics of the superior bridging leaflet of the AV valve. There are 3 types:

- **Type A (most common):** The superior bridging leaflet is divided into a left and a right components, and there are chordal attachments between these components and the crest of the ventricular septum.
- **Type B (rare):** The superior bridging leaflet has anomalous chordal attachments that straddle the ventricular septum. This is associated with unbalanced defects.
- **Type C:** The superior bridging leaflet is complete and free-floating with no chordal attachments to the crest of the interventricular septum.

Pathophysiology and Clinical Presentation

Pathophysiology will depend on the size of the atrial and ventricular septal communications, balance or hypoplasia of the ventricles, and the degree of AV valve regurgitation. There is almost always atrial-level shunting due to the presence of a primum ASD. When the ASD is large or the septum is essentially absent, there will be significant mixing at the atrial level and the patients may present with some degree of cyanosis. If the VSD is large and unrestrictive, shunting will be governed by the difference between the relative resistances of the systemic and pulmonary vascular beds.

The diagnosis tends to be made either prenatally or after a murmur evaluation. In children with Down syndrome, a screening echocardiogram should be performed during the neonatal period because of the high association (40-60%) with CHD, of which approximately half will have an AVSD.

As PVR decreases after birth, signs and symptoms from volume overload will be apparent. Tachypnea, subcostal retractions and difficulty feeding will worsen until producing failure to thrive and in some cases, predisposing children to recurrent respiratory infections.

In children with a partial AVSD, the clinical findings will be similar to an ASD. On physical exam, there will be a widely split S_2 without variation during inspiration. This finding is more common in older children. Patients with a complete AVSD will present with failure to thrive and CHF symptoms. There will be tachypnea and tachycardia with hepatomegaly. There is usually a narrowly split S_2 with accentuation of P_2 from increased pulmonary pressures. The murmur arising from the large VSD tends to be holosystolic and low/mid frequency. The holosystolic murmur from left AV valve regurgitation is usually high frequency and peaks late. Cyanosis occurs when there is abnormal systemic venous return or when the PVR is significantly elevated. However, some degree of cyanosis is not unusual in patients with complete AVSD.

Diagnosis

- **ECG (Figure 12-1.** Classically shows left-axis deviation with RVH.
- **CXR (Figure 12-2).** Shows cardiomegaly with increased pulmonary vascular markings and air trapping due to bronchial wall edema from elevated LAP. The left mainstem bronchus may appear elevated due to LA dilation.
- **Echocardiogram (Figure 12-3).** Cornerstone of diagnosis. Attention should be paid to the morphology and size of the ASD and VSD, the elongated and unwedged position of the aorta (most evident on the anterior sweep of the 4-chamber and the subcostal coronal views), the presence of LVOT obstruction, the morphology of the AV valves (including whether they are separated or not), and the degree of AV valve regurgitation. An en-face view of the AV valve is useful to assess the morphology of the valve and whether there is deficiency of any of the leaflets. Associated lesions such as the presence of a persistent left SVC or coarctation of the aorta should also be thoroughly investigated. Some conotruncal abnormalities such as tetralogy of Fallot and double-outlet RV may coexist with AVSD.
- **Cardiac catheterization.** Usually not necessary for the diagnosis. It may be useful in late-presenting patients with concerns for suspected high PVR.

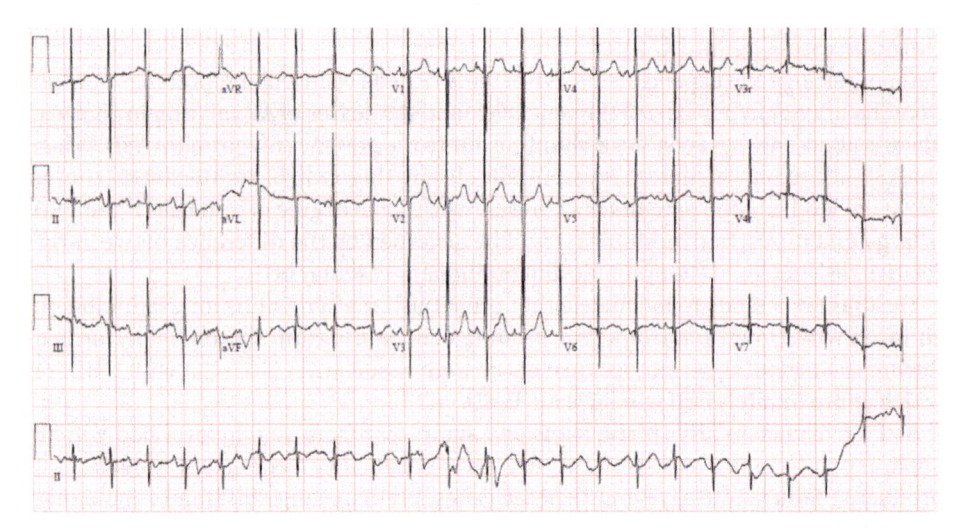

Figure 12-1. ECG in a 3-month-old patient with AVSD demonstrating left-axis deviation and RVH.

Indications / Timing for Intervention

The presence of an AVSD is an indication for surgical intervention. Repair tends to be easier outside of the newborn period, especially due to the thin and friable nature of the AV valves in neonates. As such, if possible, patients with complete AVSD are repaired electively at 4-6 months of age (Figure 12-4). Early intervention (in infancy or neonatal period) may be necessary in patients with CHF symptoms that are resistant to medical management and those with significant AV valve regurgitation. Older patients with concerns for high PVR should undergo cardiac catheterization prior to repair.

Patients with partial or transitional AVSDs are usually asymptomatic and repair is undertaken electively at 3-4 years of age, unless they have significant AV valve regurgitation or symptoms from a significant shunt.

Anesthetic Considerations

Anesthetic goals common to the spectrum of AVSDs include minimizing left-to-right shunting and left AV valve regurgitation in the pre-CPB period, and preventing post-repair hypertension to reduce stress on the newly repaired left AV valve.

Partial and Transitional AVSDs

In the absence of significant left AV valve regurgitation, anesthetic management is similar to that of a large secundum ASD. Extubation in the OR is reasonable. Patients with moderate-to-severe left AV valve regurgitation may have CHF symptoms and present earlier in life. For these patients, phentolamine may be needed on CPB if the child is an infant, inotropic support (milrinone and/or low-dose epinephrine) may be required postoperatively, and afterload reduction with nicardipine or nitroprusside may be required at the end of the procedure.

12. ATRIOVENTRICULAR SEPTAL DEFECT

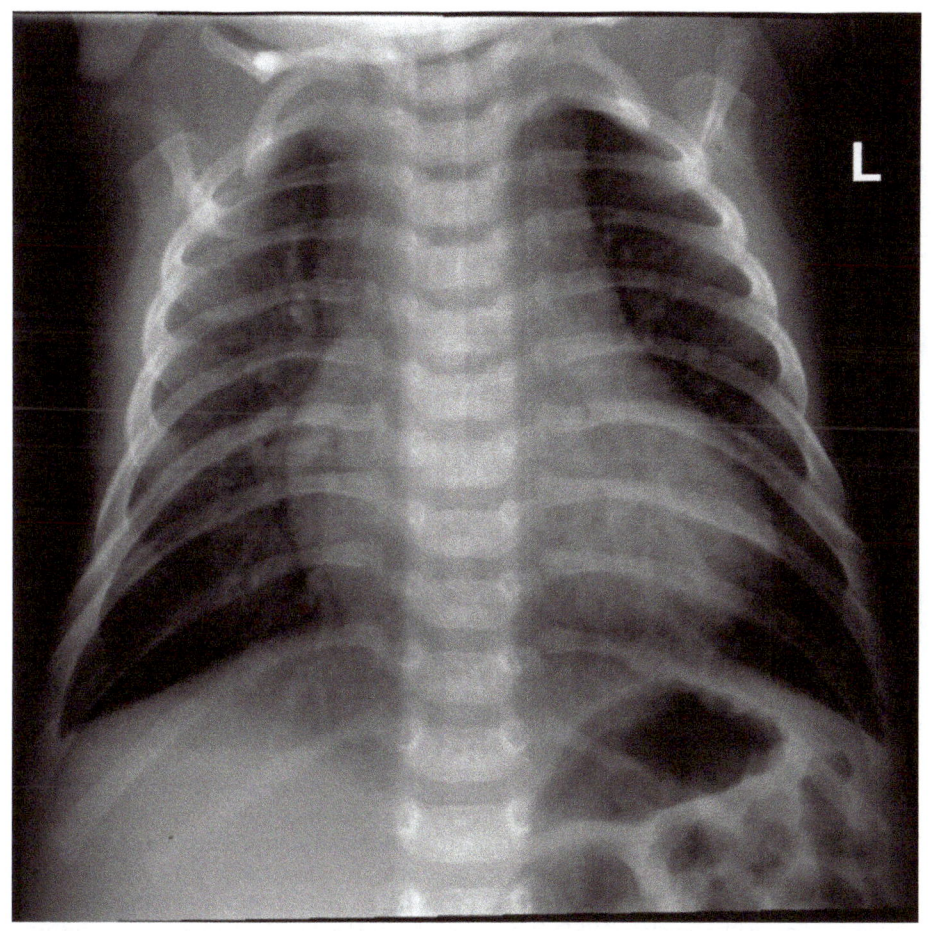

Figure 12-2. CXR in a 3-month-old patient with a complete AVSD and large atrial and ventricular components. The CXR shows cardiomegaly and increased pulmonary congestion consistent with overcirculation.

Complete AVSDs

Patients with significant overcirculation are often on multiple diuretics and occasionally on HFNC or CPAP to decrease work of breathing. One can anticipate that these patients may be "dry" prior to induction, have poor lung compliance with lung hyperinflation, and may desaturate more rapidly once apneic.

Patients with trisomy 21 pose additional concerns: 1) a propensity for bradycardia with anesthesia, particularly with volatile agents; 2) potential for upper airway obstruction and abnormal lungs; 3) potential difficulty with vascular access; and 4) hypothyroidism (thyroid labs should be sent preoperatively and liothyronine, or T3, should be available if there are concerns for hypothyroidism). Cervical spine injury during infancy is uncommon.

PART II. DISEASES

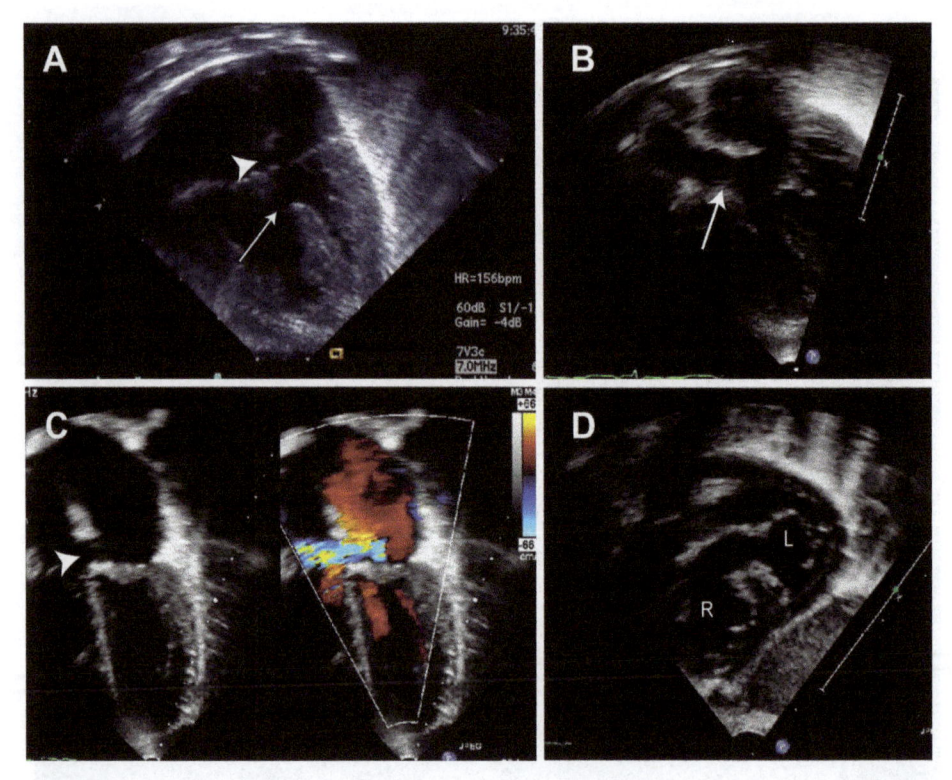

Figure 12-3. Echocardiograms on patients with AVSD. A) 4-chamber view of a complete AVSD showing a large inlet VSD (arrow), a large primum ASD (arrowhead), and a common AV valve. B) 5-chamber view showing an elongated LVOT (arrow) consistent with a "gooseneck" deformity seen in patients with AVSD. C) Color-compare view of a patient with a partial AVSD, showing left-to-right shunting across the primum ASD (arrowhead). D) En-face view of a common AV valve in a patient with complete AVSD. Images courtesy of Dr. Josh Kailin, www.pedecho.org.

The periods of induction and intubation represent a high-risk time during which overcirculation may worsen (due to the use of a higher FiO_2), or right-to-left shunting may occur (if PVR were to increase due to hypoxia or the stimulus of intubation). Based on the patient's preoperative state, volume resuscitation and inotropy and/or pressor support may be needed to support hemodynamics pre-CPB.

Phentolamine (max total dose of 200 mcg/kg administered incrementally to effect) is often needed to achieve full CPB flow (150 mL/kg/min). We target a MAP in infancy of ~40 mmHg and use bilateral cerebral NIRS to guide flows, CO_2 levels, and hemoglobin. ROTEM® can be used to guide the need for additional blood products (pump is primed with 1 unit of PRBC and 1 unit FFP for infants, with goal hematocrit prior to ending CPB of at least 40%).

Patients are usually weaned off CPB on low-dose epinephrine (0.02-0.05 mcg/kg/min) and low-dose milrinone (0.375 mcg/kg/min). Milrinone is not bolused. iNO is not routinely used unless there was preoperative or immediate post-CPB concern for

12. ATRIOVENTRICULAR SEPTAL DEFECT

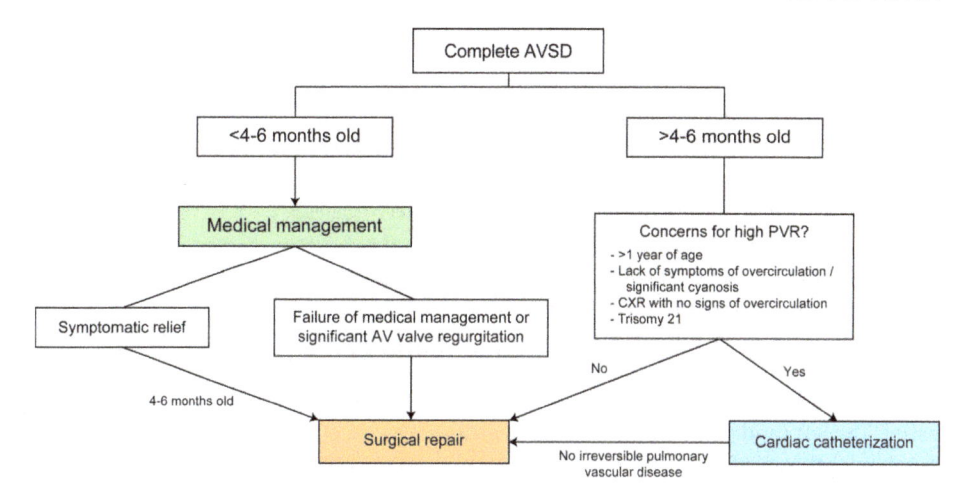

Figure 12-4. Algorithm for management of patients with AVSD.

elevated PVR. Platelets and/or cryoprecipitate (or RiaSTAP®) are used to achieve hemostasis. Care is taken not to volume overload the left heart during this process (an LA line is often present as a guide), and if needed, blood can be removed from the patient to allow administration of these products. Invariably, afterload reduction is needed to treat hypertension (nicardipine or nitroprusside). For sedation, dexmedetomidine is often started once normal sinus rhythm is present, and continued to the CICU. Total fentanyl administered for the case generally ranges between 100 and 200 mcg/kg, with most of it given during the onset of CPB and upon rewarming.

Surgical Repair

AVSD repair is performed using standard aorto-bicaval cannulation and mild-to-moderate hypothermia. The repair is performed through a right atriotomy. Repair of a partial AVSD consists on closure of the left zone of apposition (mitral cleft) and repair of the primum ASD using fresh autologous pericardium. It is important to carefully probe the ventricular septum underneath the AV valves to ascertain that no VSD is present. Repair of transitional AVSDs is similar but involves identification of the VSD or VSDs, and repair. Depending on the number and morphology of the defect(s), repair may be achieved by primary closure with interrupted pledgeted sutures, a small pericardial patch, or by placing a series of interrupted pledgeted sutures on the crest of the septum and bringing those sutures through the AV valve and the base of the ASD patch (Australian technique).

Repair of a complete AVSD is achieved using a two-patch technique. Once the atriotomy is performed, the AV valve is "floated" by instilling saline into the ventricles, and the ideal coaptation point between superior and inferior bridging leaflets, and left and right sides, is defined. A glutaraldehyde-fixed pericardial patch is sutured to the crest of the ventricular septum using either interrupted pledgeted sutures or a running

PART II. DISEASES

suture. It is important to trim this patch appropriately; leaving it too short or too high may lead to AV valve regurgitation or LVOT obstruction. A series of horizontal-mattress sutures are placed through the superior portion of the VSD patch, the AV valves, and the base of the pericardial ASD patch. The ASD patch is lowered and all sutures tied down. Both AV valves are tested. The left (and sometimes also the right) zone of apposition ("cleft") is reapproximated with interrupted sutures. If the left component is small (as occurs when the left mural leaflet is deficient or the valve is unbalanced), the zone of apposition may not be able to be completely closed. In general, the valves should accept a Hegar dilator corresponding to at least 70-80%

Complete AVSD repair at TCH (1995-2016) (Mery et al. 2018)
Number of isolated complete AVSD repairs: 350
Median number of repairs per year: 17 (9 – 28)
Patients requiring PA band prior to full repair: 17 (5%)
Median age at surgery: 5 months
Median ICU length of stay: 5 days
Median hospital length of stay: 10 days
Perioperative mortality: 2% (6/350)
Perioperative need for permanent pacemaker: 0.3% (1/350)
Survival at 10 years: 93%
Reoperation at 10 years: 9%
Median time to reoperation: 3 years

Partial / transitional AVSD repair at TCH (1995-2017)
(Mery et al. 2019)
Number of partial/transitional repairs: 265
Median number of repairs per year: 13 (5 – 17)
Median age at surgery: 2 years
Median ICU length of stay: 2 days
Median hospital length of stay: 5 days
Perioperative mortality: 0.7% (2/265)

of the predicted size for the child. Depending on the appearance of the valves upon testing, more complex repairs (such as annuloplasty sutures or closure of additional fenestrations) may be required. The ASD patch is then sutured in place.

Due to the deficient inlet segment, the AV node and bundle of His are displaced inferiorly. The AV node lies between the coronary sinus and the atrioventricular valve prior to giving rise to the bundle of His, which travels on the left side of the ventricular septum. It is therefore important to suture the VSD patch superficially to the right side of the ventricular crest. There are 2 ways to avoid injury to the AV node during repair of the primum ASD component: 1) bringing the ASD sutureline around the coronary sinus thus leaving the sinus draining into the left atrium, or 2) taking very superficial bites on the edge of the left AV valve at the level of the coronary sinus, thus leaving the sinus draining normally into the RA.

Postoperative TEE is necessary to assess for residual shunting and AV valve stenosis or regurgitation. An LA line and a peritoneal dialysis catheter are routinely placed on these patients. The LA pressure and tracing may be helpful to assess the significance of left AV valve stenosis or regurgitation.

Postoperative Management

All patients undergoing CPB are at risk for LCOS, bleeding, and arrhythmias. AVSD repairs have their own subset of potential challenges, some of them related to specific aspects of the anatomy. Important anatomical aspects to consider are whether the AVSD was balanced or unbalanced, and in the latter case, whether it was RV- or LV-dominant. Patients with an RV-dominant AVSD that undergo a biventricular repair may be particularly sensitive to fluid resuscitation due to the small size of the LV and the restrictive physiology from ventricular hypertrophy.

AVSDs are pressure- and volume-loading lesions (left-to-right shunting), and as such, postoperative care should focus on managing pulmonary and systemic vascular resistances, and intravascular volume. Patients are usually kept sedated their first night after surgery, avoiding acidosis, optimizing oxygenation, and managing potential low-cardiac output with vasoactive drugs instead of volume resuscitation. Our vasoactive drug of choice for LCOS management is milrinone (inodilator and lusotropic agent), if the patient's BP allows. It is important to understand the postoperative status of the AV valves. In general, we aim for lower SVR while maintaining adequate perfusion pressures (monitored by lactate, urine output, NIRS, etc.) in order to prevent undue stress on the repaired left AV valve.

Postoperative AVSD patients will have CVP and LAP monitoring. The goals are to keep both pressures in the single digits. The TEE report regarding the postoperative gradient across the AV valves is useful to guide intracardiac pressures and heart rate goals.

The extubation time frame varies among patients, but it is important to avoid acute elevations on SVR during this time to preserve the integrity of the AV valve repair. Whenever possible, patients will be extubated under some degree of conscious sedation (usually dexmedetomidine drip) for this reason.

Patients with trisomy 21 may have a somewhat elevated PVR after surgery. In addition, these patients have special airway considerations and their natural hypotonic state may affect the extubation strategy (it may be useful to extubate to noninvasive ventilatory support). If there is a need for reintubation, hyperextension should be avoided due to the possibility of atlanto-occipital instability.

Complications

Potential postoperative complications include:
- **AV block.** Due to the location of the conduction system, it can be injured during repair. If there is persistent complete heart block 7-10 days after surgery, consideration should be made to place a permanent pacemaker.
- **AV valve regurgitation or stenosis.** Patients may develop progressive AV valve stenosis or regurgitation after surgery. The AV valves in newborns are very thin and friable, putting them at risk for dehiscence of the closure of the left zone of apposition ("cleft"). An echocardiogram should be performed in patients that are not progressing appropriately after surgery to rule out AV valve complications.

Suggested Readings

Mery CM, Zea-Vera R, Chacon-Portillo MA, et al. Contemporary outcomes after repair of isolated and complex atrioventricular septal defect. Ann Thorac Surg 2018;106:1429-1437.

Mery CM, Zea-Vera R, Chacon-Portillo MA, et al. Contemporary results after repair of partial and transitional atrioventricular septal defects. J Thorac Cardiovasc Surg 2019;157:1117-1127.

13 Tetralogy of Fallot

Antonio G. Cabrera, Patricia Bastero, Stuart R. Hall, Carlos M. Mery

Tetralogy of Fallot (TOF) is the most common cyanotic congenital anomaly. It is characterized by anterosuperior deviation of the infundibular septum, leading to 4 components: a large anterior malalignment conoventricular VSD, RVOT obstruction (valvar and subvalvar), aortic override, and RVH (Figure 13-1).

Coronary anomalies are present in up to 10-15% of patients with TOF, most commonly an LAD that arises from the right coronary and crosses the RVOT inferiorly. Approximately 25% of the patients have a right-sided aortic arch. TOF is associated with genetic syndromes in 20% of the patients, most notably DiGeorge syndrome (22q11 deletion), trisomy 21, and VACTERL association (vertebral anomalies, imperforate anus, cardiac anomalies, tracheoesophageal fistula, renal anomalies, and limb abnormalities).

Pathophysiology and Clinical Presentation

Progressive subpulmonary obstruction causes shunting of deoxygenated blood across the VSD into the LV (right-to-left shunting) leading to a decrease in systemic oxygen saturation. The degree of shunting is related to the degree of RVOT obstruction and the relative SVR. As such, children may present with cyanosis at birth (rare) or may develop progressive cyanosis as the subpulmonary stenosis progresses.

On physical exam, in addition to varying degrees of cyanosis, patients present with a high-pitched systolic ejection murmur at the left sternal border. Clubbing can be seen in advanced cases, usually after 2-3 years of age.

Children with TOF may present with a hypercyanotic spell ("tet spell"), an acute and sustained episode of profound cyanosis, hyperpnea, agitation, and acidosis. It is the result of complete or near complete obstruction of pulmonary blood flow with worsening right-to-left shunting. This profound cyanosis can lead to acidosis due to poor oxygen delivery. Acidosis may then reduce SVR, thus worsening right-to-left shunting and causing further acidosis. Clinically, patients present with muffling or shortening of the systolic ejection murmur. Treatment of hypercyanotic spells involves:

- Have a family member hold the patient in a quiet room to calm the patient
- Oxygen administration
- Use alpha-agonists (phenylephrine) to increase SVR
- Treat acidosis with sodium bicarbonate replacement
- Decrease agitation/sedation with morphine and/or ketamine

Diagnosis

- **CXR (Figure 13-2).** RVH will produce a "boot-shape" appearance with oligemic lung fields from decreased pulmonary blood flow.
- **ECG.** RA enlargement, RVH, or dominant right-sided forces.
- **Echocardiogram (Figure 13-3).** Important features to assess include details on the VSD (perimembranous vs. doubly-committed juxta-arterial defect), degree of

13. TETRALOGY OF FALLOT

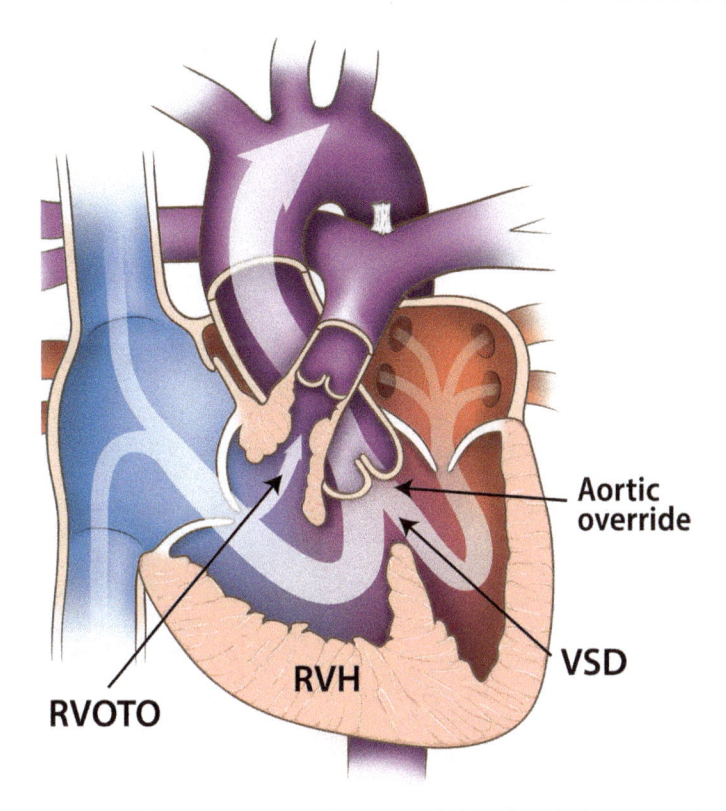

Figure 13-1. Elements of TOF. Anteroseptal deviation of the infundibular septum leading to: 1) a large anterior malalignment conoventricular VSD, 2) valvar and subvalvar RVOT obstruction (RVOTO), 3) aortic override, and 4) right ventricular hypertrophy (RVH).

valvar/subvalvar pulmonary stenosis, aortic arch anatomy, coronary anatomy, and associated anomalies.
- **Cardiac catheterization.** Not necessary for diagnosis. Can be helpful in small children in which stenting of the arterial duct can provide a stable source of pulmonary blood flow as an alternative to a modified Blalock-Taussig-Thomas shunt (mBTTS).

Indications / Timing for Intervention
TOF is repaired using an infundibular-sparing transatrial/transpulmonary repair. This repair is best performed after 4-6 months of age due to the technical difficulty in smaller children and the possibility of JET from surgical retraction in neonates.

Indications for early intervention (mBTTS vs. full repair) include progressive cyanosis (oxygen saturation <85%) or the occurrence of a cyanotic spell (Figure 13-4). Otherwise, patients are repaired electively after 4-6 months of age.

PART II. DISEASES

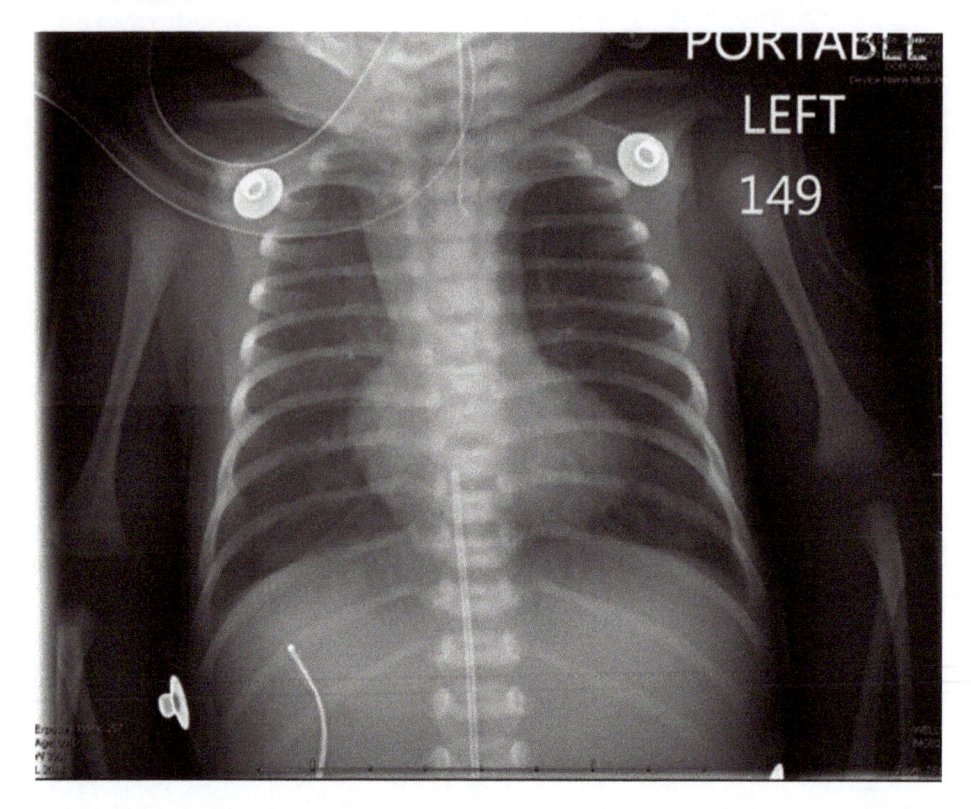

Figure 13-2. Classic CXR on TOF showing a "boot-shaped" heart with oligemic lung fields.

Anesthetic Considerations
The main goals of the pre-CPB period are to maintain adequate preload and SVR to prevent hypercyanotic spells. Should a hypercyanotic spell occur: increase the FiO_2, give phenylephrine 5-10 mcg/kg, increase preload, and deepen the anesthetic. Abdominal compression or surgical compression of the aorta can also augment SVR and force more blood into the pulmonary circulation. Esmolol, starting at 50-200 mcg/kg/min, can also help relieve infundibular spasm and is easily titrated. If all measures fail, rapid cannulation and initiation of CPB may be needed.

Post-CPB, inotropic agents are rarely necessary. Given the possible presence of some dynamic narrowing after repair (see below), esmolol is routinely used to slow down the heart rate and allow adequate time for RV filling. Milrinone can be considered for its lusitropic effects but its concomitant decrease in SVR may make the child more hypotensive than desired.

Surgical Repair
The main goal of the TOF infundibular-sparing repair is to relieve RVOT obstruction while preserving as much contractile infundibular muscle as possible. A ventriculotomy

13. TETRALOGY OF FALLOT

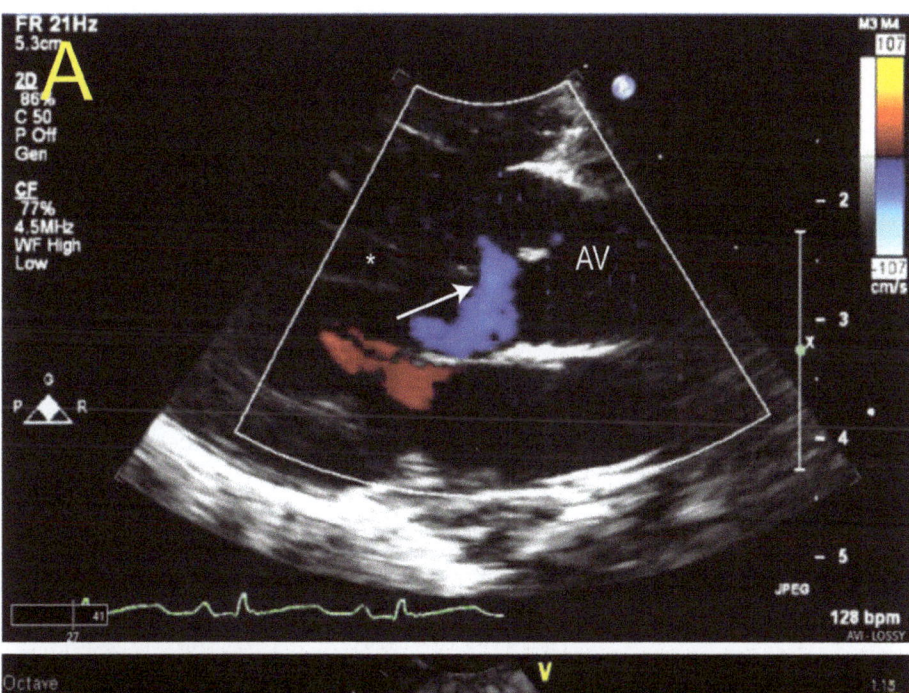

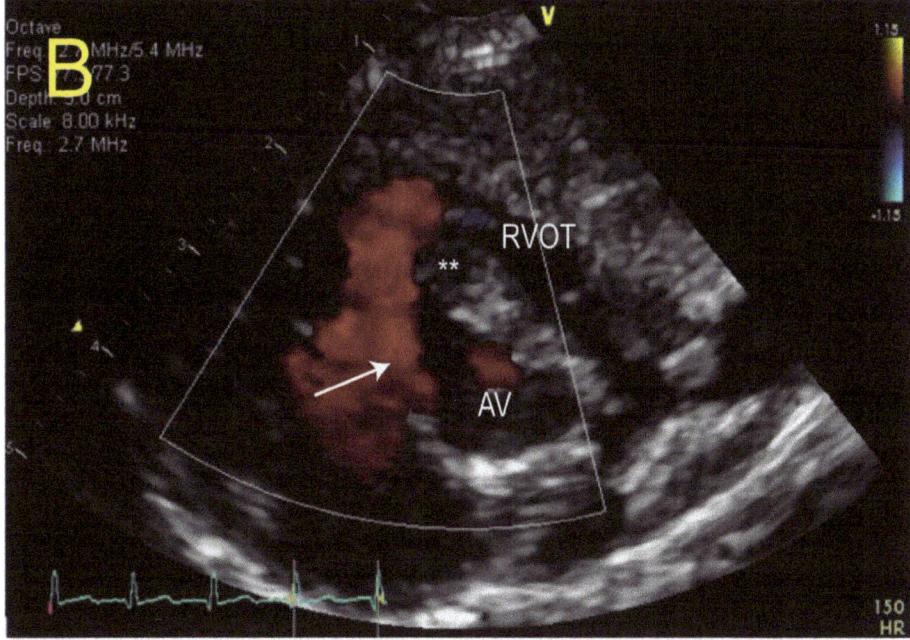

Figure 13-3. Echocardiography in TOF. The parasternal long-axis view (A) shows a conoventricular septal defect (arrow) with override of the aortic valve (AV) on the interventricular septum (*). The short-axis parasternal view (B) shows an anteriorly deviated infundibular septum (**) causing significant narrowing of the RVOT. Flow is seen from the VSD (arrow) toward the RVOT.

PART II. DISEASES

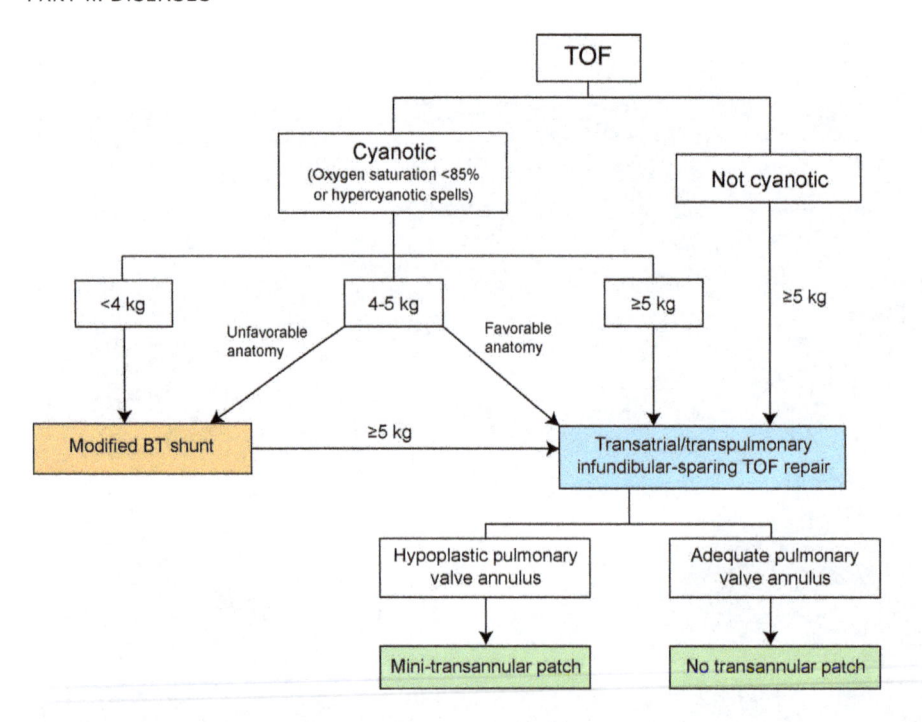

Figure 13-4. Decision process for surgical intervention on TOF.

is avoided to prevent substituting functional muscle for a noncontractile patch. The preservation of the infundibulum may lead in the long term to improved function and better tolerance against PI.

The procedure is performed using standard aorto-bicaval cannulation and moderate hypothermia (28 °C). Working through the tricuspid valve, the hypertrophied septoparietal trabeculations are excised from the free wall of the infundibulum. The infundibular septum is left alone to serve as the anchor for the VSD baffle. The anterior and septal leaflets of the tricuspid valve may be taken down for visualization. Significant traction is avoided to prevent postoperative JET.

The VSD is repaired by creating a baffle between the LV and the anteriorly displaced aortic valve using an autologous pericardial patch tanned on glutaraldehyde. The conduction system (bundle of His) travels on the posteroinferior edge of the VSD and can be injured during repair.

A longitudinal incision is performed on the main pulmonary artery and the pulmonary valve is inspected. If after performing a pulmonary valvotomy the valve accepts a Hegar dilator corresponding to the normal size of the pulmonary valve based on BSA, the valve is preserved (25%). Otherwise, the longitudinal incision is extended proximally across the pulmonary annulus for a few millimeters, creating a transannular incision (75%). The incision is extended minimally until the corresponding Hegar dilator is allowed to pass, therefore leaving the infundibulum intact. An autologous pericardial patch is used to reconstruct the main PA.

> **TCH experience on TOF (2007-2014)**
> TOF repairs performed at TCH: 22-35 per year
> Median age at surgery: 9 months
> Patients that require mBTTS prior to full repair: 17%
> Median ICU length of stay: 3 days
> Median hospital length of stay: 7 days
> Perioperative mortality: 0.9%

An LA line is placed in all patients to help with postoperative management (Chapter 66). Since these patients have diastolic RV dysfunction due to RV hypertrophy, CVP is not an accurate reflection of volume status. Temporary atrial pacing wires are placed in all patients (for postoperative management of JET or other arrhythmias). Ventricular wires are placed selectively based on AV conduction.

Mild dynamic RVOT obstruction at the subvalvar area (<2.5 m/s) is tolerated and expected to improve within a few weeks as the RV remodels. If the obstruction is more significant on postoperative TEE, RV pressure may be directly measured. If the RV pressure is greater than 2/3 systemic, the patch is further extended proximally.

Postoperative Management

The postoperative management is mainly directed to address diastolic dysfunction, for which volume resuscitation and heart rate control are key.

General Management
- **Fluids.** 25% maintenance with D5%/0.45% NS is standard. However, these patients will require volume resuscitation due to diastolic dysfunction.
- **Analgesia and sedation.** Analgesics and sedatives are adjusted for patient's comfort. A fentanyl infusion is used for intubated patients and morphine PCA and/or intermittent morphine is used for short-term mechanical ventilation needs or extubated patients. Scheduled acetaminophen q6h (enteral, rectal, or IV) is used as an adjuvant. *Sedation* is achieved with a combination of dexmedetomidine (both intubated and extubated patients) and/or intermittent benzodiazepines. Midazolam as a drip (only for intubated patients) or intermittently is commonly used; lorazepam is used for longer-term benzodiazepine needs.
- **Vasoactive drugs.** Most patients will arrive from the OR on an esmolol infusion 25-400 mcg/kg/min and a low-dose milrinone infusion 0.25 mcg/kg/min.
- **Mechanical ventilation.** Usually ventilated on SIMV-VC with pressure support and Vt 8-10 ml/kg, aiming for a pH of 7.35-7.45 and SaO_2 >93%. Postoperative TOF patients are expected to be extubated within 12-24 hours after surgery (usually within 6 hours), unless a significant respiratory comorbidity or postoperative complication prevents extubation.

What to Expect in the First 24 Hours Postoperatively
- **Vasoactive drugs.** Patient on no vasoactive drugs or a low-dose of milrinone and/or low-dose esmolol, ready to be started on propranolol if esmolol infusion cannot be stopped. Patients who were on propranolol preoperatively are usually placed on

the same dose of propranolol in the CICU once the esmolol drip has been stopped and slowly weaned off in the next few weeks.
- **Ventilation.** Extubated on regular nasal cannula with low O_2 requirements.
- **Fluids.** Positive fluid balance ~300-350 ml.
- **Nutrition.** Clear fluids are started PO 4 hours after extubation if the patient is stable. Progress to regular diet ad lib.

Complications
The most common postoperative complication after TOF repair is LCOS, usually related to diastolic dysfunction.
- **LCOS.** It will present with tachycardia, normal or low BP, high CVP with normal LAP (low LAP if low intravascular volume), lactic and/or metabolic acidosis, oliguria, low cerebral NIRS, and increased core-toe temperature gradient. Management consists in optimizing RV preload (volume administration, usually no more than 40 mL/kg), improving ventricular filling time (rate control with esmolol), and optimizing lusitropy (milrinone) to optimize RV output, as well as optimizing RV afterload (milrinone and early extubation).
- **Arrhythmias.** Arrhythmias compromising cardiac output are not common among our patients; they include JET (2%) and complete heart block (0.3%). For the management of these arrhythmias, see Chapters 74 and 75. Right-bundle-branch block is a common finding after TOF repair and has no hemodynamic impact.

Suggested Readings
McKenzie ED, Maskatia SA, Mery CM. Surgical management of tetralogy of Fallot: in defense of the infundibulum. Semin Thorac Surg 2013;25:206-212.

Morales DL, Zafar F, Heinle JS, et al. Right ventricular infundibulum sparing (RVIS) tetralogy of Fallot repair: a review of over 300 patients. Ann Surg 2009;250:611-617.

Niu MC, Morris SA, Morales DL, et al. Low incidence of arrhythmias in the right ventricular infundibulum sparing approach to tetralogy of Fallot repair. Pediatr Cardiol 2014;35:261-269.

14 Transposition of the Great Arteries

Antonio G. Cabrera, Paul A. Checchia, Dean B. Andropoulos, Charles D. Fraser Jr.

Transposition of the great arteries (TGA, simple transposition of the great arteries, or D-transposition of the great arteries) is a common cause of prostaglandin-dependent cyanosis and the most common cause of cyanosis in the newborn. It occurs when there is ventriculoarterial discordance and there is recirculation of pulmonary and systemic blood flows. The most common anatomical presentations are with an intact ventricular septum (IVS), a VSD, and VSD with LVOT obstruction (LVOTO) (Figure 14-1). In the absence of intracardiac mixing (PDA, ASD, or VSD), it is rapidly fatal. In the current era, expectations for effective treatment (neonatal surgical repair) should be very high.

Pathophysiology and Clinical Presentation

During fetal life, oxygenated blood from the placenta will cross the PFO and through the main PA and PDA, perfuse the distal aorta. The highly deoxygenated blood from the SVC that enters the RV through the tricuspid valve will perfuse (through the aortic valve) the aortic arch and neck vessels.

After birth, circulation will be in parallel (Figure 14-2). While patent, the arterial duct promotes the pressure differential to enhance atrial mixing by increasing LAP. When there is a marked difference (>5%) in upper/lower extremity saturations and postductal saturations are higher than preductal, the clinician should suspect aortic arch obstruction. When the atrial communication is small or restrictive, infants will be profoundly desaturated (oxygen saturation in the 60s). Given that atrial mixing takes place due to the pressure differential between both ventricles in diastole, it is possible that even in the presence of a large unrestrictive ASD, mixing could be insufficient. A large unrestrictive VSD may be an effective place for mixing when is part of the presenting anatomy, but smaller defects may also be insufficient.

On physical exam, the child will become tachycardic and tachypneic. Grunting can be present when there is acidosis and/or pulmonary edema. The precordium is hyperactive with an RV impulse. The second heart sound will be single from elevated PA pressures.

Diagnosis

- **CXR.** Usually without cardiomegaly immediately after birth. The upper mediastinum may be narrow due to the anteroposterior relationship of the great vessels ("egg-on-a-string" sign).
- **ECG.** Usually normal.
- **Echocardiogram (Figure 14-3).** Echocardiogram is the cornerstone of diagnosis. On the parasternal long-axis view, the great arteries will appear in parallel with the great artery arising from the LV (PA) taking a posterior turn (pathognomonic). One should then detour from the standard echocardiogram protocol to switch to coronal subcostal imaging and demonstrate the atrial septal communication. Thereafter, the focus should be on the arterial duct and its patency. This information

PART II. DISEASES

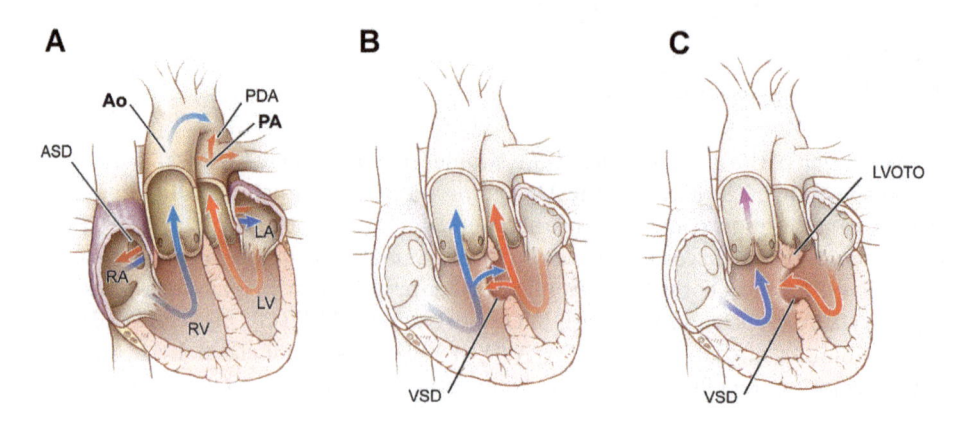

Figure 14-1. Anatomical variants of TGA. A: TGA with IVS. B: TGA with VSD. C: TGA with VSD and LVOTO. Ao: Aorta.

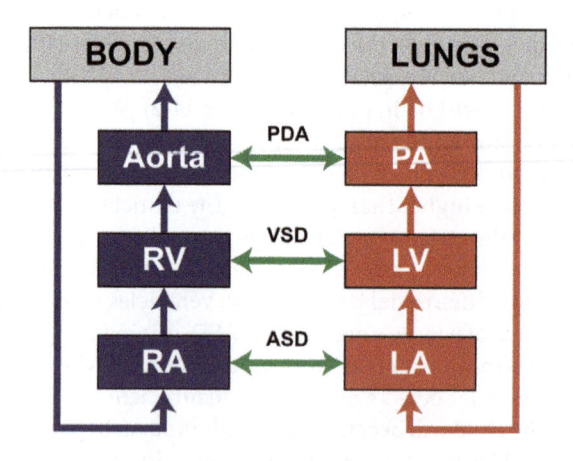

Figure 14-2. Physiology in TGA. The systemic and pulmonary circulations run in parallel, relying on the presence of patent communications (PDA, ASD, or VSD).

is the most relevant when trying to establish the initial diagnosis and to mobilize the interventional cardiology staff for a potential bedside balloon atrial septostomy (BAS). As usual, the echocardiogram laboratory protocol should be completed before making final determinations about interventions. The coronary arteries should be resolved by echocardiogram. The most common coronary artery patters are the following: right and left coronaries (including LAD and circumflex) from usual sinuses (Yacoub A), left circumflex origin from the right coronary artery (Yacoub D), and single origin of the right or left systems (Yacoub B) (Figure 14-4).
- **Cardiac CT.** Usually not necessary. Postoperatively, if there is a concern about the patency of the coronary arteries, the child should undergo cardiac catheterization or return to the OR without delay.

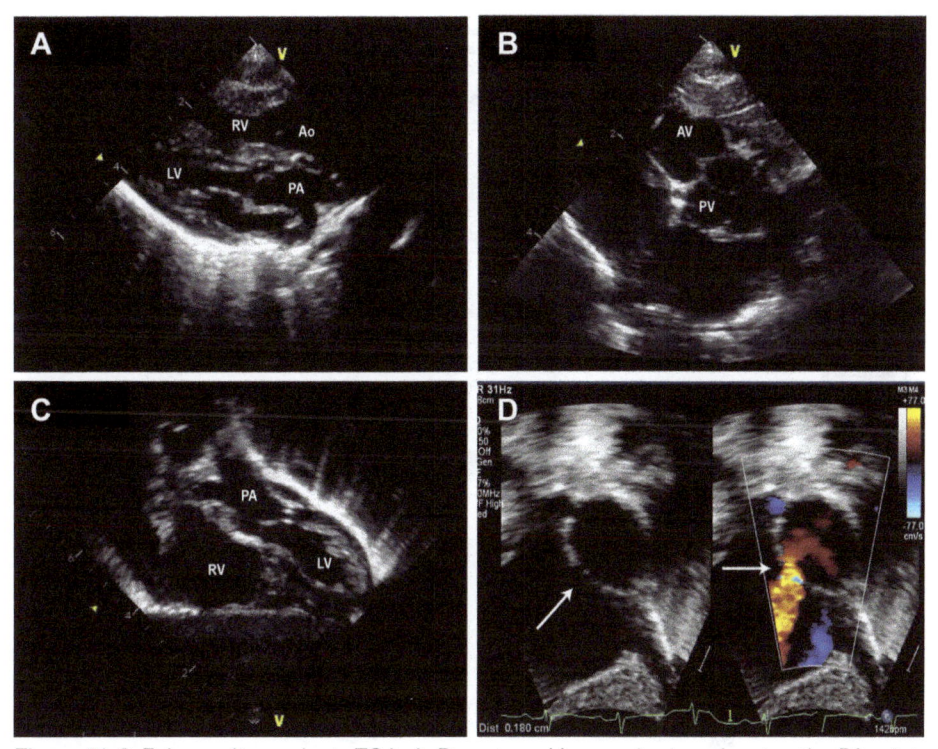

Figure 14-3. Echocardiography in TGA. A: Parasternal long-axis view showing the PA originating from the LV and the aorta (Ao) from the RV. B: Parasternal short-axis view showing the aortic valve (AV) located anterior and rightward to the pulmonary valve (PV). C: Subcostal view again showing the PA originating from the LV. D: Subcostal color-compare image depicting a restrictive atrial septum (arrow). Images courtesy of Dr. Josh Kailin, www.pedecho.org.

- **Cardiac catheterization.** Although the hemodynamic definition of TGA is when the saturation in the PA is higher than the aorta, cardiac catheterization is seldom necessary for diagnosis. After birth, most children will undergo BAS to improve mixing at the atrial level (unless the defect is large and unrestrictive). If there are concerns/questions about coronary artery anatomy, an extreme caudal down-to-barrel angiogram may be performed, although in the current era, precise delineation of the coronary anatomy is not necessary prior to surgery.

Indications / Timing for Intervention

A BAS should be performed in most patients to allow adequate mixing and stabilization of the infant, unless the defect is large and unrestrictive. It is generally performed at the bedside or cardiac catheterization laboratory with either a Rashkind or a Braun catheter. There should be a visible tear on the septum primum allowing for bilateral motion of the remaining flap by echocardiogram and an improvement in oxygen saturations.

The arterial switch operation (ASO) is usually performed after the PVR has decreased

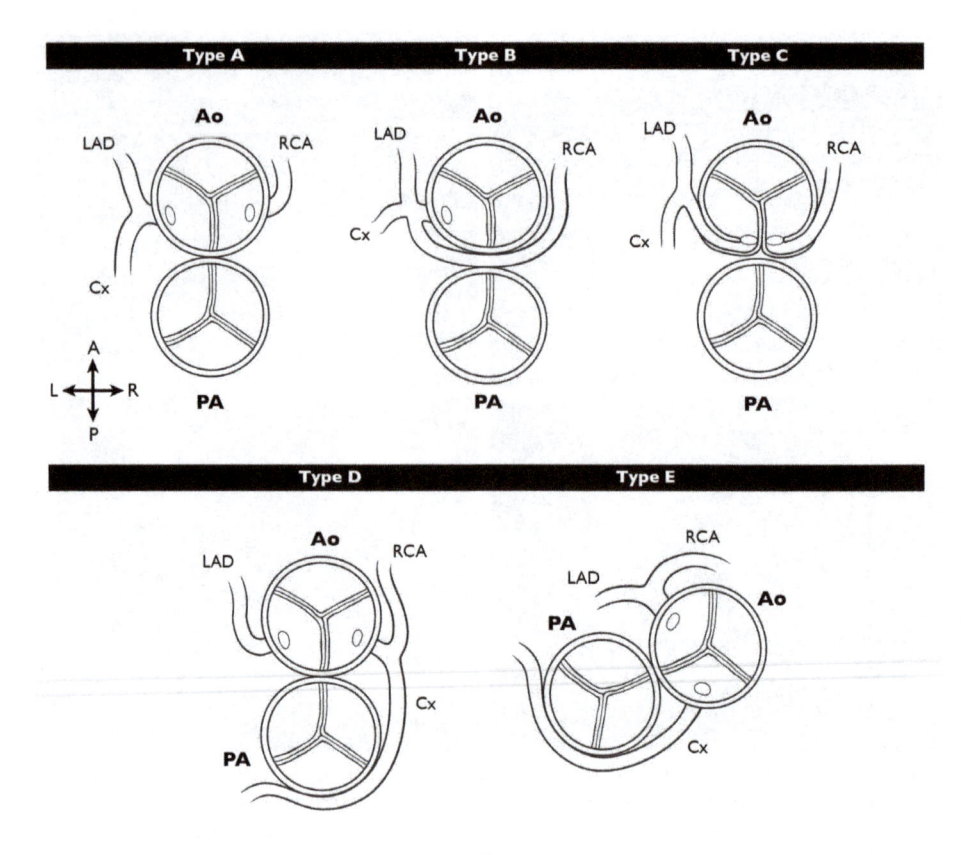

Figure 14-4. Common coronary patterns in TGA (Yacoub and Radley-Smith classification).

(>48 hrs), although a rare patient may present with intractable cyanosis requiring a more urgent ASO. Children with a restrictive ASD/PFO have a slower transition of the PVR and may present with persistent cyanosis even after the BAS. Timing of the ASO is usually on the first week of life. In patients with adequate saturations and non restrictive VSDs, the morphologic LV will not decondition and the ASO may be deferred to a semielective status but within the same hospital admission.

Anesthetic Considerations
Typical anesthetic agents for ASO include fentanyl at 25-100 mcg/kg total dose, isoflurane at any required dose, low-dose midazolam at 0.2-1 mg/kg total dose, and dexmedetomidine, either started before incision with a loading dose, or after aortic cross-clamping, at reduced doses of 0.2-0.5 mcg/kg/hour because of reduced clearance in the neonate.

The anesthetic approach will depend on whether there is adequate mixing (i.e., BAS performed with large ASD, PDA with prostaglandin still infusing, or VSD). If there is significant oxygen desaturation (i.e., SaO_2 <80%) at baseline, there is a significant risk of further desaturation, lower cardiac output, and decreased mixing with the induction

14. TRANSPOSITION OF THE GREAT ARTERIES

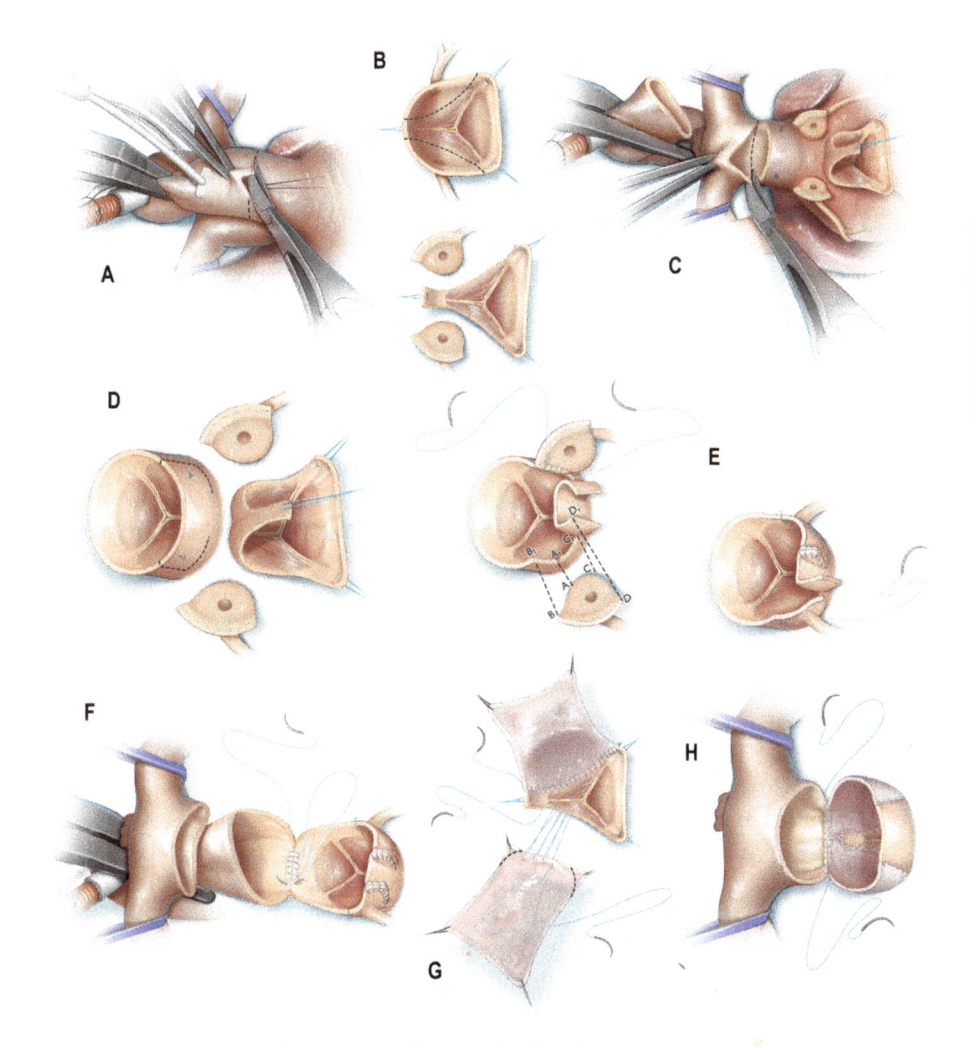

Figure 14-5. Arterial switch operation. See text for details.

of anesthesia. If this is the case, increasing cardiac output with inotropic support (epinephrine 0.02-0.03 mcg/kg/min), increasing FiO_2 to 1.0, and increasing hemoglobin to 13 g/dL or higher with PRBC transfusion is usually effective. Patients with multiple sources of mixing and SaO_2 >90% will often require low FiO_2 of 0.21-0.3 before CPB, and other measures to increase PVR, such as mild hypercarbia and positive end-expiratory pressure of 5-8 cm H_2O. Establishing a baseline cerebral rSO_2 with baseline conditions is important, and treating rSO_2 <50% absolute values, or >20% relative decrease from baseline is an effective approach.

During CPB for the arterial switch operation, the anesthesiologist works closely with the perfusionist and surgeon to optimize conditions of oxygen delivery to the brain and other vital organs. Flow rates of 150 mL/kg/min are normally used, with CPB MAPs usually around 40 mmHg for neonates. Phentolamine at 0.05-0.15 mg/kg in divided doses is often used to maintain high flows with low perfusion pressures. rSO_2 is monitored bilaterally and pH-stat CPB management used, with hematocrit goals at about 30%, to maintain rSO_2 well above baseline during CPB. Weaning from CPB is accomplished gradually using an LA catheter for guidance; LAP is kept at 0-5 mmHg during the weaning process, with a usual goal of 4-8 mmHg immediately after CPB. LV distention (LAP >10 mmHg), particularly in the patient with preoperative IVS, is to be assiduously avoided, because excessive preload will not be tolerated. If during the weaning process LAP is >10 mmHg, intravascular volume is taken from the patient, either into the CPB circuit, or by removal of blood by the surgeon or anesthesiologist.

After CPB, low-dose epinephrine (0.02-0.05 mcg/kg/min), nitroglycerine at 1 mcg/kg/min, and calcium chloride infusion at 5-10 mg/kg/hr are standard infusions. Vasopressin at 0.02-0.04 units/kg/hour can be utilized to increase perfusion pressure, and sodium nitroprusside at 0.5-2 mcg/kg/min can be utilized to decrease BP. Pressure-controlled ventilation with FiO_2 1.0 is utilized to wean from CPB, and FiO_2 can later be reduced, if appropriate.

TEE is often utilized to assess for any residual defects such as VSD, and for myocardial function and sequential wall motion abnormalities of the LV. However, in smaller neonates, TEE may not always be used and clinical status, ST-segment changes, and appearance of the heart are assessed to judge adequacy of repair. In those cases, an epicardial echocardiogram may be utilized if there are questions about anatomy or myocardial function.

The goals of low LAP, MAP in 40s-50s, normocarbia, and maintaining adequate cardiac output are meticulously pursued. After protamine administration, platelet infusion of 10-15 mL/kg is often sufficient to decrease bleeding. Cryoprecipitate at 5-10 mL/kg is the next choice of coagulation products, followed by FFP 10-20 mL/kg. Coagulation product administration can be guided by ROTEM® during rewarming on CPB. If bleeding continues after ruling out surgical causes and administration of 2 or more doses of platelets, cryoprecipitate, and FFP, activated factor VII in doses of 45-90 mcg/kg can be considered after thorough discussion. Although there is theoretical risk of thrombosis from this agent, in practice this has not been observed. The activated factor VII dose can be repeated in ~90-120 minutes if bleeding is ongoing.

Surgical Repair

Anatomic repair (ASO) (Figure 14-5) is now the standard of care for treatment of the majority of TGA patients with IVS, VSD, and aortic arch obstruction (in addition to patients with Taussig-Bing anomaly, see Chapter 16). In developed countries, it is now very unusual for a baby with TGA to present beyond the newborn period for primary treatment, however in some areas of the world, this is more common. In patients presenting with TGA/IVS beyond 6 weeks of life, the LV may have involuted and thereby will not be capable of managing a systemic workload immediately after the ASO. One option is to place a PA band (PAB) to rapidly retrain the LV (in small infants, this usually can happen in a period of approximately 1 week but will frequently require a systemic-to-PA shunt to provide adequate pulmonary blood flow), followed by an ASO. Retraining the morphologic LV, however, is not only time-consuming, but is a risk-laden proposition. As such, some centers recommend an atrial switch operation (Senning or Mustard) for the late-presenting patient with TGA/IVS. Yet another option is to proceed with an ASO in the first 3 months of life with the understanding that temporary mechanical assistance (VAD) may be needed postoperatively.

For the typical newborn patient with TGA/IVS, the ASO is performed within the first week of life, although we have successfully performed a primary ASO up to 8 weeks of life with good results. The ASO is performed via median sternotomy on CPB support. We have favored separate caval venous cannulation in all except the very smallest of babies (<2 kg) along with a single aortic cannula placed in the distal ascending aorta (in patients with severe aortic arch obstruction, a second arterial cannula in the ductus may be needed for perfusion of the lower body). In TGA/IVS, mild hypothermia (nasopharyngeal temperature of ~32 °C) as an adjunct to myocardial and brain preservation. As noted previously (see Chapter 6), we favor a high-flow, low-pressure perfusion strategy individualized to the patient's needs.

During preliminary dissection, fresh, autologous pericardial patches are harvested and prepared for later use in reconstructing the neo-pulmonary sinuses of Valsalva. The coronary ostial locations are noted and marking sutures are placed on the pulmonary root (neoaortic root) to help with coronary ostial translocation. This coronary movement is the key element of the ASO and maneuvers have been well-described to facilitate accurate translocation of all coronary branching patterns including single coronary ostium and intramural coronaries. The surgeon must be prepared for all contingencies.

After the establishment of safe CPB, the patient is gradually cooled. During this phase, the ductus is ligated and divided and the branch PAs are widely mobilized to facilitate anterior positioning of the PAs after reconstruction (maneuver of LeCompte). Following standard cardioplegic arrest, the ascending aorta is transected just at or above the sinotubular junction (mindful of anomalous aortic origins or intramural coronaries) and the ostia inspected (Figure 14-5, A). The coronary ostia are then mobilized as liberal buttons of aortic wall (Figure 14-5, B) and the proximal coronaries are also mobilized with great care not to skeletonize the actual coronary artery. Next, the main PA is transected (also just at or above the sinotubular junction) (Figure 14-5, C). For the majority of patients, we create appropriate, medially based, trapdoor flap incisions in the neoaortic sinuses to facilitate ostial translocation with minimal axial rotation (the key concern in problematic ostial transfer) (Figure 14-5, D). The coronary buttons are anastomosed using very fine monofilament suture (7-0 or 8-0 polypropylene) (Figure 14-5, E). After the maneuver of LeCompte, aortic continuity is reestablished by a primary anastomosis between the ascending aorta and neoaortic root (Figure 14-5, F). As this is occurring, gradual warming of the patient is commenced and the heart is vigorously deaired. The ASD is then completely closed (typically can be done primarily although in some cases, a patch may be needed). The heart is vented through the anterior ascending aorta and reperfused. A normal sinus rhythm should resume spontaneously and the ECG should rapidly normalize. Persistent ST-segment changes may be related to intracoronary air or the more concerning possibility of coronary ostial malpositioning.

PART II. DISEASES

This latter concern is critical and must be assessed at this point. Once the surgeon is satisfied with the coronary translocation, the neopulmonary sinuses are individually reconstructed (deficiencies that were created by the coronary ostial mobilization) with liberal patches of the previously harvested, fresh autologous pericardium (Figure 14-5, G). Finally, PA continuity is reestablished by a primary anastomosis between the neopulmonary root and PA bifurcation (Figure 14-5, H). In patients with side-to-side great vessel relationship (such as Taussig-Bing anomaly), the neopulmonary-to-main-PA anastomosis may need to be placed out onto the right PA to prevent distortion or compression of the translocated coronary buttons.

> **ASO experience (<18 months old) at TCH (1995-2018)**
> Anatomy:
> - TGA/IVS: 204 (52%)
> - TGA/VSD: 137 (35%)
> - TGA/VSD/LVOTO: 17 (4%)
> - Taussig-Bing anomaly: 36 (9%)
>
> Median age at surgery: 8 days (1 day – 17 months)
> Median ICU length of stay: 6 days (5-8 days)
> Median hospital length of stay: 11 days (9-16 days)
> Perioperative mortality: 1.3%
> 5-year survival: 98.2%, 10-year survival: 97.8%, 15-year survival: 97.8%
> Postoperative mechanical circulatory support / ECMO: 2%

In cases where there is a VSD, it is our practice to proceed with VSD closure prior to the ASO. There are several reasons for this sequence. First, in cases with a degree of malalignment of the great vessels to the ventricular septum (very important in cases of Taussig-Bing anomaly, it is critical for the surgeon to be certain that the VSD closure can be committed to one or the other great vessel. Secondly, it is best not to place traction on the reconstructed great vessels after the ASO. Another concern may be the status of the semilunar valves or LVOT, which may often be assessable through the VSD before committing to the ASO. We favor autologous pericardium for VSD closure(s). It is not uncommon for us to reperfuse the heart (by removing the cross-clamp while making the tricuspid valve incompetent and venting the aortic root) for 10-15 minutes between VSD closure and the ASO in order to limit continuous cross-clamp time.

In cases of aortic arch obstruction, the patient will be cooled to a more profound level (nasopharyngeal temperature ~18-20 °C) and then repair the arch primarily (see Chapter 25). Following arch reconstruction, the patient is partially rewarmed while the VSD is closed and the ASO performed.

In patients with significant LVOTO, the ASO may still be possible if the subaortic area is amenable to resection. In patients with congenitally bicuspid pulmonary (neoaortic) valves, the ASO is still feasible, assuming the valve caliber is adequate.

In patients with Taussig-Bing anomaly, there may be an enormous size discrepancy between the aortic root and the pulmonary root (with the pulmonary root being much larger). In this setting, reconstruction of the ascending aorta may require augmentation for an effective anastomosis. Since these patients also often have actual or impending RVOT obstruction, it is often wise to perform a prophylactic RVOT resection prior to reconstruction of the neopulmonary root.

Prior to weaning from CPB, an LA catheter is placed. Information about the LAP

14. TRANSPOSITION OF THE GREAT ARTERIES

is critical to individualized patient management. Intraoperative assessment of the coronary arteries by transesophageal or epicardial echocardiography is obtained to confirm adequate coronary blood flow. A peritoneal dialysis catheter is routinely placed. Hemostasis must be achieved prior to leaving the OR. It is very unusual to need to leave the sternum open.

Postoperative Management

The chief concerns on the postoperative period include the effectiveness of coronary blood flow and the ability of the LV to accommodate to systemic workload. Children with a restrictive ASD preoperatively will be at higher risk of persistently higher PVR and in rare circumstances may require iNO in the early postoperative period.

General Management
- **Fluids.** 25% maintenance with D5%/0.45%NS is standard. Careful attention should be paid to managing the patient with the minimal necessary preload. Unnecessary preload increases may produce increases in myocardial wall stress and lead to ventricular dysfunction and hypotension. This may occur with very small volumes of excess fluid administration (as small as <5 mL total in a single bolus) and is another reason to emphasize the proper use of LAP in perioperative management.
- **Analgesia and sedation.** Analgesics and sedatives are adjusted for patient's comfort. Fentanyl (1-3 mcg/kg/hr) infusion is commonly used for analgesia. *Sedation* is achieved with a combination of dexmedetomidine (both intubated and extubated patients) and/or benzodiazepines. Midazolam as a drip is preferred, as significant shifts in afterload or BP may produce instability.
- **Vasoactive drugs.** Most patients will arrive from the OR on milrinone (0.25-0.75 mcg/kg/min) and sometimes epinephrine (0.02-0.05 mcg/kg/min). Hypotension should be primary managed with inotropes when LV filling pressure (LAP) is higher than 5-10 mmHg.
- **Mechanical ventilation.** Patients are usually ventilated on SIMV-VC with pressure support, at Vt of 8-10 ml/kg and PEEP of 5-7 mmHg, and aiming for pH 7.35-7.45 and SaO_2 >95%. After the ASO, patients may be extubated in the first postoperative day if hemodynamics are adequate.

What to Expect in the First 24 Hours Postoperatively
- **Vasoactive drugs.** It is reasonable to manage milrinone and low-dose epinephrine (<0.03 mcg/kg/min) through extubation to support the LV, as extubation will lead to high SVR, increase in transmural pressure, and consequently higher afterload.
- **Ventilation.** Transitioning from the OR, the lungs will be significantly improved from the preoperative period secondary to continuous ultrafiltration.
- **Fluids.** Even to slightly negative. The peritoneal dialysis catheter should be used starting on the day of surgery.
- **Nutrition.** If considering extubation within 24 hrs, it is not necessary to write for TPN. If longer periods of mechanical ventilation are anticipated, full TPN should be ordered. Oral feeds should be reinstated once successfully extubated.

Complications

The most common post-operative complications after TGA repair are LCOS and cardiac arrhythmias.

- **Coronary artery issues.** Although all coronary artery patterns are able to be managed with the ASO, several multicenter studies have shown that there is increased mortality in complex patterns, in particular intramural coronaries. A low index of suspicion is necessary as coronary issues may present with increased LAP and LCOS, without clear ECG changes.
- **LCOS** (see Chapter 71). Primarily treated with inotropes. A combination of low-dose epinephrine and standard-dose milrinone. High inotrope doses increase the likelihood of arrhythmias. If prolonged, severe, or associated with significant volume requirements, it should prompt reopening of the sternum, visual and echocardiographic inspection of the coronary arteries and either return to the OR or coronary artery evaluation by cardiac catheterization.
- **Arrhythmias.** Arrhythmias or heart block are unusual. Persistent atrial tachycardia or JET (see Chapter 74) may decrease cardiac output.
- **Bleeding** (see Chapter 76).
- **Prolonged mechanical ventilation.**
- **Chylothorax** (See Chapter 77). Potentially from high RV pressures, pulmonary hypertension, or increased tricuspid valve regurgitation in the presence of branch PA stenosis.
- **Mechanical circulatory support.** Any need for mechanical circulatory support after the ASO should prompt cardiac catheterization and coronary artery evaluation. In patients presenting for a primary ASO after 6 weeks of life in the setting of TGA/IVS, one should be prepared for temporary LV mechanical support in the acute perioperative period.

Long-Term Follow-Up

Despite excellent LV recovery and long-term survival rates after TGA repair, surveillance for ongoing complications including aortic root dilation, coronary insufficiency, and branch PA stenosis are necessary for life. In addition, prolonged deep-hypothermic circulatory arrest time, prematurity, and associated genetic syndromes are risk factors for suboptimal short- and long-term neurodevelopmental outcomes.

Suggested Reading

Dibardino DJ, Allison AE, Vaughn WK, et al. Current expectations for newborns undergoing the arterial switch operation. Ann Surg 2004;239:588-596.

15 Congenitally Corrected Transposition of the Great Arteries

Nancy A. Ayres, Emad B. Mossad, Charles D. Fraser Jr.

Anatomical Considerations

Congenitally corrected transposition of the great arteries (ccTGA) is an uncommon congenital cardiac lesion characterized by atrioventricular and ventriculoarterial discordance ("discordant transposition"). While the most frequent segmental anatomic arrangement in ccTGA is usual atrial arrangement, left-handed ventricular topology, and posterior and leftward position of the aorta with respect to the PA (atrial situs solitus, L-looped ventricles, and L-malposed great vessels {S,L,L} according to the van Praagh classification), the condition may also present with complete mirror-image anatomy: mirror-image atrial arrangement, right-handed ventricular topology, and rightward location of the aorta with respect to the PA (atrial situs inversus, D-looped ventricles, and D-malposed great vessels {I,D,D}) (Figure 15-1).

The hallmark of ccTGA is the association of the *morphologic* RV with the systemic circulation. While the coronary anatomy is "mirror-image" in most patients, the coronary origins and branching may be highly variable. In ccTGA, the morphologic tricuspid valve (TV or systemic atrioventricular valve) is often apically displaced with septal attachments leading to it often being referred to as "Ebsteinoid". In fact, this is an incorrect designation in that the apical displacement is not associated with an atrialized portion of the morphologic RV.

The cardiac conduction system is abnormal in ccTGA. The AV node is displaced in an anterior and superior location in most patients, and the bundle of His is elongated. There may be two AV nodes and the incidence of an accessory atrioventricular pathway (as in Wolff-Parkinson-White syndrome) is significant.

Pathophysiology and Clinical Presentation

Clinical presentation of ccTGA is highly variable and relates to anatomic substrate and ventricular function. This leads to a complex set of diagnostic and management considerations. Historically, many individuals with ccTGA with intact ventricular septum (IVS) lived well into adult life undetected, presenting later in life with left AV valve (tricuspid) regurgitation, depressed systemic RV function, or spontaneous AV block (frequent in this condition). In current practice, many patients are now presenting for management consideration in the absence of overt symptoms. This is often the case in patients picked up on screening fetal echocardiography or some other form of prophylactic postnatal assessment (murmur evaluation, serendipitous CXR revealing abnormal cardiac silhouette, screening ECG).

Symptomatic presentation typically relates to the presence of associated cardiac defects, which occur in more than 85% of patients, or ventricular dysfunction. The most common associated cardiac defects are a perimembranous VSD (70%), pulmonary stenosis (PS) or LVOT obstruction (LVOTO, 56%), or AV conduction abnormalities (5%). The left AV valve (tricuspid) is abnormal in more than half the patients, with apical displacement being common.

PART II. DISEASES

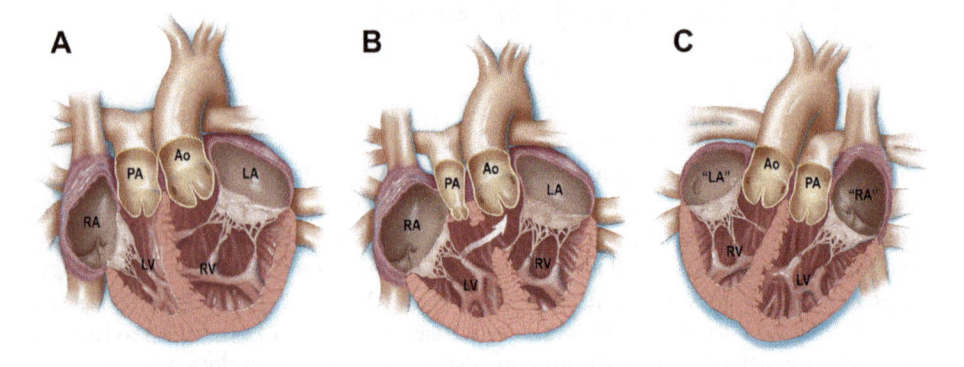

Figure 15-1. Morphological variants in ccTGA. A) Usual arrangement in ccTGA with IVS (levocardia). The morphologic RA is connected to the morphologic LV, which is connected to the PA, and the morphologic LA is connected to the morphologic RV, which is connected to the aorta. B) ccTGA with VSD and LVOTO (PS). The arrow indicates the direction that the baffle would need to take if connecting the LV to the aorta. C) ccTGA with mirror-image anatomy and dextrocardia. The morphologic RA is on the left and the morphologic LA is on the right (atrial situs inversus). Ao: Aorta.

Symptomatic Presentation

Patients with ccTGA and a large VSD may present early in life with signs/symptoms of CHF. The VSD may be nonrestrictive or pressure-restrictive. The latter concern is of importance in determining the conditioning of the morphologic LV (to be discussed below).

A common association of lesions in ccTGA includes VSD with some degree of LVOTO or even true pulmonary atresia. In the absence of other sources of pulmonary blood flow, the degree of LVOTO correlates with systemic arterial desaturation/cyanosis. In patients (newborns) with true pulmonary atresia, pulmonary blood flow is dependent on ductal patency.

Systemic (tricuspid) AV valve regurgitation (TR) may be found in association with the other cardiac lesions or as an "isolated" phenomenon in patients with ccTGA with intact septum. Significant TR leads to symptoms of CHF and is an important clinical marker of concern (see below).

Systemic RV dysfunction may present early or late in life. Progressive reduction in RV ejection fraction (RVEF) in the setting of a small VSD or intact ventricular septum (IVS) leads to RV dilation and secondary tricuspid annular dilation, which will exacerbate TR. Many believe that absent a morphologic problem with the TV, TR becomes an early indicator of RV dysfunction.

Asymptomatic Presentation

Given the widespread use of screening prenatal ultrasound (and subsequent fetal echocardiography when an anatomic issue is identified), there are increasing numbers of children presenting early in life for consideration of intervention for ccTGA. In asymptomatic individuals, this becomes a very complicated management scenario, particularly in the setting of "normal" RV function, IVS or small pressure-restrictive VSD, or trivial TR.

Some individuals present with minimal or no symptoms despite apparently significant hemodynamic lesions. Patients in this category may have significant reduction in RV function with or without significant TR before overt symptoms appear.

Diagnosis

- **CXR.** May show levocardia, mesocardia, or dextrocardia. In the setting of depressed RV function and/or significant TR, there may be cardiomegaly and congested lung fields. Patients with significant LVOTO (PS) may exhibit oligemic lung fields.
- **ECG.** There may be an abnormal P-wave and increased P-R interval. Early repolarization (delta waves) may indicate an accessory AV conduction pathway. Third-degree AV block may occur spontaneously or as a complication of catheter or surgical intervention.
- **Echocardiography.** Mainstay of clinical diagnosis. Important elements of a thorough echocardiographic examination include:
  - Status of the interatrial septum.
  - Systemic and pulmonary venous connections.
  - Status of the interventricular septum. Presence, size, and location of VSDs. Estimated pressure gradient between ventricles.
  - AV valve anatomy and function. In the setting of significant TR, careful delineation of morphologic substrate is critical to decision making (displaced leaflets, annular dilation, dysmorphic leaflets, prolapse, chordal rupture). Morphologic MR is also possible and there are rare cases of a mitral cleft in ccTGA. The status of the mitral valve and need for repair become critical in the consideration of a "double switch" (see below).
  - Ventricular function. Estimated ejection fraction (shortening fraction) of both ventricles. Location/geometry of the interventricular septum provides inferential evidence of RV/LV pressure ratio (see also "double switch"). Status (thickness) of the LV free wall may be useful in situations of LV conditioning ("retraining").
  - Right and left ventricular outflow tract assessment. LVOTO in the setting of a large VSD is frequent. Organic RVOT obstruction (RVOTO) may be associated with aortic arch hypoplasia/coarctation.
  - Semilunar valve morphology and function. Critical in the consideration of anatomic or physiologic repair.
  - Aortic arch anatomy and evaluation for obstruction/coarctation.
- **Cardiac catheterization.** *Diagnostic* catheterization may be an important adjunct to clinical decision making in association with other diagnostic modalities. In the setting of multiple muscular VSDs, cath may be very useful in discerning anatomic detail (and also offers the option of interventional device closure where appropriate). Typically, echo Doppler estimates of pressure gradients are adequate for decision making in most scenarios, but any uncertainty should be careful assessed by hemodynamic cath. Assessing PVR is critically important in settings where there is suspected elevation. This latter scenario is particularly important if a Fontan

PART II. DISEASES

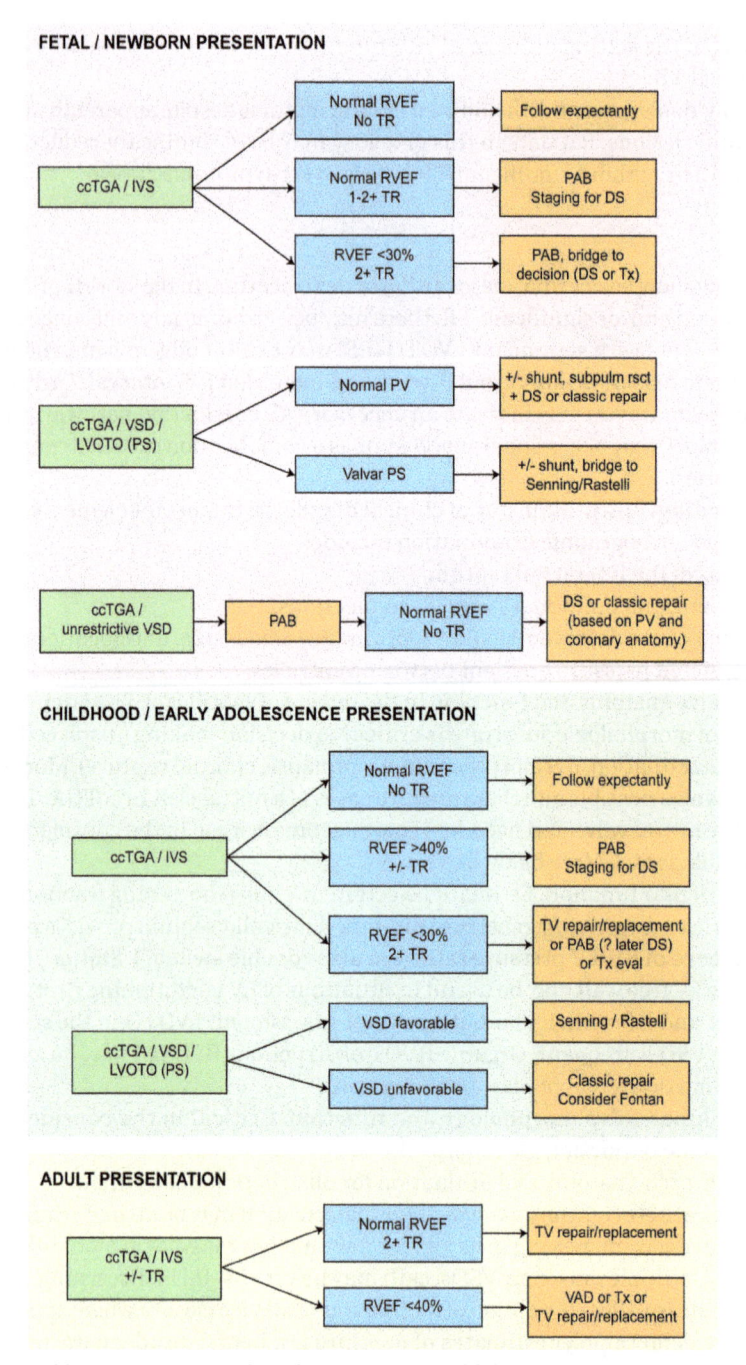

FETAL / NEWBORN PRESENTATION

ccTGA / IVS
- Normal RVEF, No TR → Follow expectantly
- Normal RVEF, 1-2+ TR → PAB Staging for DS
- RVEF <30%, 2+ TR → PAB, bridge to decision (DS or Tx)

ccTGA / VSD / LVOTO (PS)
- Normal PV → +/- shunt, subpulm rsct + DS or classic repair
- Valvar PS → +/- shunt, bridge to Senning/Rastelli

ccTGA / unrestrictive VSD → PAB → Normal RVEF, No TR → DS or classic repair (based on PV and coronary anatomy)

CHILDHOOD / EARLY ADOLESCENCE PRESENTATION

ccTGA / IVS
- Normal RVEF, No TR → Follow expectantly
- RVEF >40%, +/- TR → PAB Staging for DS
- RVEF <30%, 2+ TR → TV repair/replacement or PAB (? later DS) or Tx eval

ccTGA / VSD / LVOTO (PS)
- VSD favorable → Senning / Rastelli
- VSD unfavorable → Classic repair Consider Fontan

ADULT PRESENTATION

ccTGA / IVS +/- TR
- Normal RVEF, 2+ TR → TV repair/replacement
- RVEF <40% → VAD or Tx or TV repair/replacement

Figure 15-2. Management algorithm of patients with ccTGA depending on anatomy and age at presentation. DS: double-switch operation, PV: pulmonary valve, RVEF: RV ejection fraction, Tx: transplant.

palliation is being considered or in cases of late presentation of a patient with a large VSD and unprotected pulmonary vasculature. Diagnostic cardiac catheterization is also a useful adjunct when assessing preparation of a formerly deconditioned morphologic LV in the setting of preparation (PA banding) for a "double switch" or anatomic repair (see below). *Therapeutic* cardiac catheterization may be helpful in settings where there are difficult to reach, apical muscular VSDs that are amenable to catheter-delivered device closure. In the setting of patients who have undergone an atrial switch operation, remedial cardiac catheterization and intervention may be useful and necessary in the settings of baffle limb obstruction or leakage.
- **Cardiac MRI.** The utility of MRI for the majority of patients with ccTGA is debatable; most questions can be answered with echocardiography. An interesting scenario that has gained increasing popularity is the assessment of LV wall thickness over time in patients who are undergoing LV preparation for a double switch. Investigators have also used MR viability studies as an adjunct to this decision tree.

Surgical Considerations

There is ongoing debate among surgeons and centers concerning the optimum surgical strategy for various forms of ccTGA. Categorical options include a "classic" repair in which the morphologic RV is maintained as the sole systemic ventricle, the "double switch" where the morphologic LV is aligned with the systemic circulation, and single-ventricle palliation. To date, there are no definitive data to clarify the issue of which operation offers the patient not only the best short-term outcome, but also the greatest opportunity for a durable long-term solution. However, it is clear that when the RV is aligned with the systemic circulation, the presence of significant TR portends ultimate RV failure and as such, mandates careful attention and justifies surgical intervention. Figure 15-2 provides an overall guide of the management approach at TCH.

Classic Repair

The term "classic" repair has been typically associated with a biventricular reconstruction in which the morphologic RV is relegated to remain the *systemic ventricle*. This arrangement may place the patient at risk of early or late systemic RV failure and/or progressive morphologic TR. As such, assigning the morphologic RV to the systemic circulation has important, often irreversible consequences. There are certain settings in which choosing a classic repair may be the wisest option:
- In certain patients with ccTGA/VSD/LVOTO (PS or pulmonary atresia) with an *inlet VSD* or remote *muscular VSD*, constructing an unobstructed pathway from the morphologic LV to the aorta (Senning-Rastelli) may be problematic. We have believed that in such settings, if the morphologic RV and tricuspid valve have good function (minimal or no TR, and no significant apical displacement), a classic repair may represent a better alternative.
- In cases of ccTGA with IVS, the morphologic LV may not be capable of supporting the systemic circulation if it has not been working at systemic pressure (involuted LV). In this context, if the LV has not responded to reconditioning (PA banding), it is imprudent to proceed with a "double switch".

- Patients with an abnormal pulmonary (neoaortic) valve that would be suboptimal as the systemic semilunar valve.
- An additional and very important consideration is whether or not the family is willing to take on the significant perioperative and ongoing risk of choosing the double switch. It has been well-documented that in large series, the ability to predict the ability of the morphologic LV to durably sustain the systemic circulation after a double switch, particularly if the LV had to undergo a period of reconditioning, is imperfect. The sobering series from Birmingham, England (Winlaw et al. 2005) indicated that after a period of LV retraining and subsequent double switch, the probability of freedom from death or transplant at approximately 10 years of follow-up is in the range of ~75%. Therefore, in counseling families, the team is justified and more specifically responsible for being circumspect about the option of a double switch.

In closing the VSD as part of a classic repair, the surgeon must be knowledgeable about the anterior AV node and His bundle. In the typical outlet/perimembranous-type VSDs, sutures should be carefully placed on the RV side of the septum to avoid surgical AV block. If an LV-to-PA conduit is necessary, care must be exercised to avoid major epicardial coronary arteries and undermining or avulsing important papillary muscle support for the morphologic mitral valve.

The Double Switch

The term "double switch" has been loosely applied to 2 very different physiologic and anatomic situations. The most straightforward situation is in the setting of ccTGA, outlet/perimembranous VSD, PS or pulmonary atresia. In these situations (including patients with situs inversus), a Senning-Rastelli operation can be accomplished to commit the morphologic LV to the systemic circulation. The basic principles include a strategically placed right ventriculotomy, construction of an LV-to-aortic tunnel (we favor autologous pericardium), a Senning atrial switch (Figure 15-3), and placement of a valved conduit from the RV to the PAs. A variation of this proposition that has been promoted by Hanley at Stanford University (Malhotra et al. 2011) is to perform a bidirectional Glenn shunt and a "Hemi-Mustard Rastelli" (Figure 15-4). In either event, results with this operation have proven to be very predictable and durable.

The more challenging situation occurs in the setting of either ccTGA/IVS or ccTGA/VSD in which the goal is aligning the morphologic LV with the systemic circulation. This is achieved by performing an arterial switch operation (ASO), Senning atrial switch, and VSD closure, if applicable. Each scenario is briefly described below.

ccTGA with "Prepared" Morphologic LV

If the morphologic LV has never had the opportunity to involute, it is arguably well prepared to support the systemic circulation. Scenarios include ccTGA with non-restrictive VSD where the morphologic LV has always worked at systemic pressure and the more controversial setting of *newborns* with ccTGA/IVS. In the former situation, the surgeon needs to close the VSD, noting the displaced AV node and His bundle as per above, followed by ASO and Senning operation. The procedure is complex and the heart is arrested for extended periods of time. As such, we have often chosen intermittent

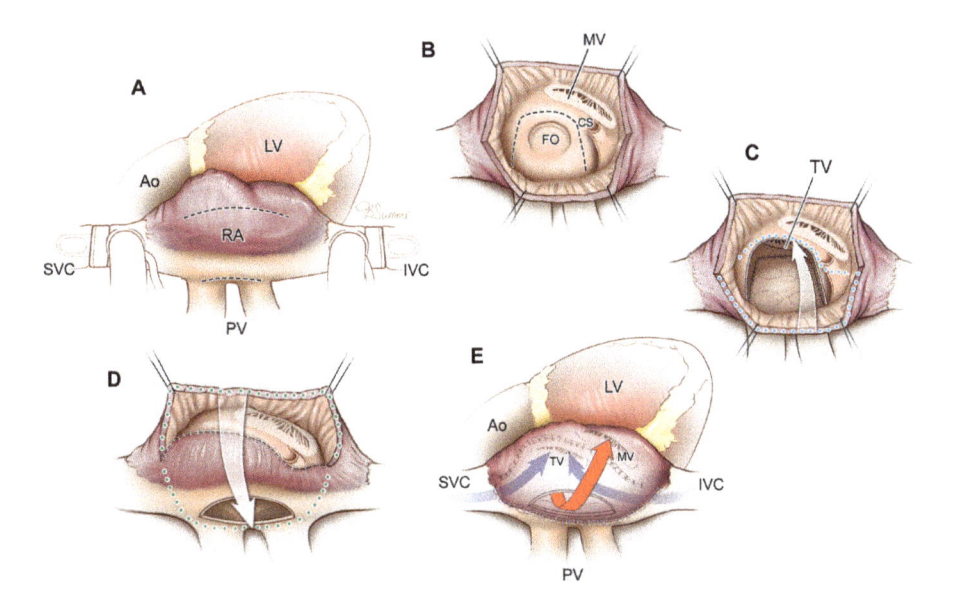

Figure 15-3. Senning atrial switch. Using a series of autogenous flaps, the pulmonary venous flow is directed to the anteriorly located LV, while the SVC and IVC flows are directed into the posteriorly located RV. Incisions are made in the RA and the LA just anterior the pulmonary veins (A), a flap of atrial septum is created (dashed line in B) and sutured posteriorly around the pulmonary veins (C). The posterior free wall flap of the RA is sutured around the atrial septal defect (dotted line in C), therefore redirecting the flow from the SVC and IVC down towards the posteriorly located TV. The anterior free wall flap of the RA is sutured around the incision made anterior to the pulmonary veins (D) to redirect the flow from the pulmonary veins to the anteriorly located mitral valve. Panel E shows the resulting flow redirection. Ao: aorta, CS: coronary sinus, FO: foramen ovale, MV: mitral valve PV: pulmonary veins.

periods of aortic cross-clamp interspersed with periods of myocardial reperfusion to optimally provide predictable myocardial protection.

In the setting of ccTGA/IVS, the morphologic LV (subpulmonary ventricle) will start to involute soon after birth when the PVR and PA pressure naturally drop. This scenario is very analogous to the setting of simple or D-transposition of the great arteries (D-TGA) with IVS. As such, some surgeons have advocated for a very aggressive newborn approach for ccTGA/IVS by performing an ASO and Senning operation to align the LV with the systemic circulation before it has the opportunity to become deconditioned. We believe this aggressive strategy is unfounded. Although there are scattered published reports with favorable outcomes using the neonatal double switch, this approach has not been widely adopted and is currently not recommended for newborns at TCH.

ccTGA with "Unprepared" Morphologic LV

This is arguably the most challenging and controversial situation in the management of patients with ccTGA. Patients with ccTGA/IVS or pressure-restrictive VSD beyond

PART II. DISEASES

the newborn period will have an LV that is incapable of performing adequately at systemic workload if a double switch is performed. For this reason, the idea of "retraining" or reconditioning the morphologic LV by placing a PA band (PAB) has been applied to patients with ccTGA who may benefit from a double switch. As a basic concept, we believe that embarking on the challenging proposition of retraining the LV through PAB (often serial banding) followed by the ultimate double switch must be justified through objective evidence that the morphologic RV is incapable of remaining a durable systemic ventricle. Objective evidence of RV compromise includes RV ejection fraction decline, TR greater than mild (or progressing over time), a grossly displaced TV, or other evidence of impending RV dysfunction.

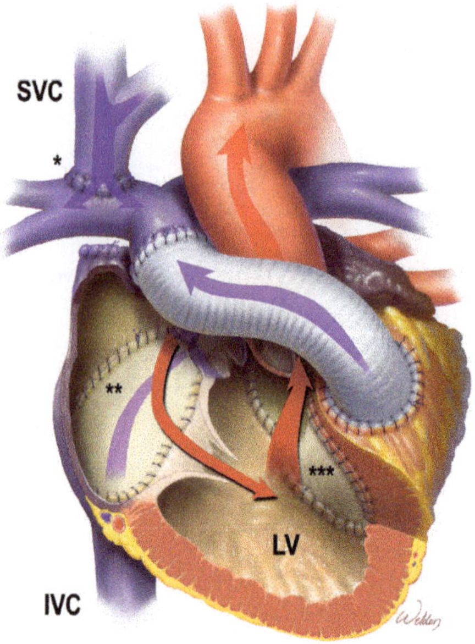

LV retraining is a very controversial subject and there is considerable inter-practitioner/interinstitutional debate about the optimal strategy. The prospect of retraining the LV is rather unpredictable and the long-term results of reconditioned LV performance after the double switch are inconsistent. As such, we have adopted a moderately conservative approach that

Figure 15-4. Hemi-Mustard/Rastelli operation. A bidirectional Glenn is created by connecting the SVC to the right PA (*), a "hemi-Mustard" baffle is created to redirect the flow from the IVC to the LA (**), and a baffle is created to redirect the flow from the right-sided LV to the aorta (***). A conduit is then placed to connect the left-sided RV to the PA. The pulmonary valve, if previously patent, is sewn shut.

includes careful and thorough consultation with the parents during which the various scenarios and potential risks are thoroughly discussed. If the parents agree to the recommendation of PAB retraining of the LV, the patient undergoes diagnostic testing to include TTE, MRI (to assess LV mass, LV wall thickness, and ejection fraction), and cardiac catheterization (to assess LV hemodynamics including peak LV systolic pressure and LV end-diastolic pressure). Of note, a coronary angiography is not required as ASO is able to be performed for all coronary artery branching patterns and ostial relationships.

Following diagnostic testing, the patient is taken to surgery for the initial PAB procedure. Under adequate general anesthesia and mechanical ventilation, and without inotropic support, the pericardium is opened (we usually just open the superior pericardium to facilitate subsequent sternal reentry) and a flexible pressure monitoring catheter is introduced retrograde from the main PA, through the pulmonary valve, and into the LV chamber. In the setting of ccTGA/IVS, it is typical to find a peak LV systolic pressure of

15. CONGENITALLY CORRECTED TRANSPOSITION OF THE GREAT ARTERIES

well less than 1/3 systemic at the outset. A Dacron® tape is passed around the main PA (must be kept above the sinotubular junction to avoid impingement on and distortion of the pulmonary valve). The PAB is sequentially tightened while the surgeon, anesthesiologist, and echocardiographer carefully observe LV function, systemic hemodynamics, and LV systolic pressure. Our experience is that at the primary banding, it is typical that the LV cannot withstand or produce an LV systolic pressure >50-60% systemic in most cases. It is common to see the LV start to fail (dilation, low systemic BP) with bands that are tightened beyond this level. Once the PAB has been adjusted to its final tightness, it is prudent for the team to carefully observe the patient in the OR with the chest open for at least 30 minutes. We have seen situations in which an initial PAB tightness appears to be well tolerated only to find that the LV function starts to decline after some period of time.

> **TCH ccTGA experience (1995-2016)** (De Leon et al. 2017)
> Number of patients: 97
> Median age at presentation: 2 months (0 days – 69 years)
> Median follow-up: 10 years
> 10-year transplant-free survival:
> - Classic (or no) repair (systemic RV) (n=45): 93%
> - Anatomic repair (systemic LV) (n=26): 86%
> - Fontan operation (n=9): 100%
> - Ongoing palliation (PAB, shunt) (n=17): 79%

The next level of controversy relates to the basic questions of how tight a band is tight enough (level of peak LV systolic pressure) and how long to retrain the LV. There is significant variability among institutions concerning answers to both of these questions. Given the uncertainty of the currently available methods to assess adequacy of LV retraining (LV systolic pressure, ejection fraction, LV wall thickness), we have favored a conservative approach. Our goal has been to achieve an LV systolic pressure of at least 80% systemic for a minimum of 6 to 12 months. At this point, if the LV appears to be managing the workload, we will offer the double switch.

The technical issues related to the double switch in ccTGA are somewhat different than the ASO for D-TGA. Typically, the aorta is anterior and leftward in ccTGA and it is not unusual for the great vessels to be almost side-by-side. This may make the coronary translocation more challenging. Furthermore, after a period of banding, the pulmonary sinuses of Valsalva may become very dilated. In this circumstance, it may be prudent to excise as much of the PA sinus as possible while translocating the coronary buttons. The surgeon should mobilize the coronary ostia as very liberal buttons of aortic wall and must be prepared to deal with all variations of coronary ostial origin and branching. Given the relationship of the great vessels, reconstructing continuity between the neopulmonary root and branch PAs may require an anastomosis that is extended out onto the left PA. The details of the atrial switch operation are also beyond the scope of this brief chapter. Given the fact that many surgeons have little experience with the Senning operation, several units have preferred to create a bidirectional Glenn shunt and "hemi-Mustard" connection under the premise that this may be more readily constructed with less potential for baffle limb obstruction.

PART II. DISEASES

The Fontan Operation

Given the various technical and management challenges we have outlined in preceding sections, many surgeons have argued that a Fontan operation may offer a much more straightforward management strategy, particularly for patients with cyanotic variants and in the setting of cardiac malposition (mesocardia or dextrocardia). There is no doubt that the Fontan operation is less technically demanding and in the current era, *acute operative risk is very low*. Whether a Fontan circulation represents a more favorable long-term strategy, however, is debatable. Exposing the liver and abdominal viscera to the obligate increases in systemic venous pressure initiates a relentless cascade of secondary consequences, the timing of which and the degree of derangement, are highly variable among individuals. Nonetheless, given the scope of the complexity of management options in ccTGA, a Fontan operation remains a viable option for selected individuals.

Suggested Readings

DeLeon LE, Mery CM, Verm RA, et al. Mid-term outcomes in patients with congenitally corrected transposition of the great arteries: a single center experience. J Am Coll Surg 2017;224:707-715.

DiBardino DJ, Heinle JS, Fraser CD. The hemi-Mustard, bidirectional Glenn, and Rastelli operations used for correction of congenitally corrected transposition, achieving a "ventricle and a half" repair. Cardiol Young. 2004;14:330-332.

Malhotra SP, Reddy VM, Qiu M, et al. The hemi-Mustard/bidirectional Glenn atrial switch procedure in the double-switch operation for congenitally corrected transposition of the great arteries: rationale and midterm results. J Thorac Cardiovasc Surg 2011;141:162-170.

Rutledge JM, Nihill MR, Fraser CD, et al. Outcomes of 121 patients with congenitally corrected transposition of the great arteries. Pediatr Cardiol 2002;23:137-145.

Winlaw DS, McGuirk SP, Balmer C, et al. Intention-to-treat analysis of pulmonary artery banding in conditions with a morphological right ventricle in the systemic circulation with a view to anatomic biventricular repair. Ciruclation 2005;111:405-411.

16 Double-Outlet Right Ventricle

Wanda C. Miller-Hance, Antonio G. Cabrera, Carlos M. Mery

Double-outlet right ventricle (DORV) is a heterogeneous congenital cardiovascular malformation defined by both great arteries arising mainly (>50%) from the RV. In almost all cases a VSD is present. In general, there is also discontinuity between the AV valves and semilunar valves with presence of a small muscular apron (conus) underneath the semilunar valves. DORV fits within the spectrum of conotruncal anomalies that includes on one end normally related great arteries and tetralogy of Fallot (TOF), and on the other end, transposition of the great arteries (TGA). DORV can also occur within the context of a functional single ventricle and other complex malformations, such as heterotaxy syndromes. The discussion that follows addresses mainly DORV in a biventricular circulation.

Classification

DORV can be anatomically classified based on the relationship of the VSD to the great arteries into (Figure 16-1):
- **Subaortic VSD.** The VSD is mainly related to the aortic valve.
- **Subpulmonary VSD (Taussig-Bing).** The VSD is mainly related to the pulmonary valve. The great vessels are usually malposed with the aortic valve anterior and rightwards to the pulmonary valve or a side-by-side arrangement is present.
- **Doubly committed VSD.** There is a lack of infundibular septum, both aortic and pulmonary valves are at the same level and in continuity, and the VSD is related to both great vessels.
- **Noncommitted VSD.** The VSD is remote to the great arteries.

Pathophysiology and Clinical Presentation

The clinical presentation in DORV is extremely variable, reflecting the underlying pathology. The physiology and clinical features are mainly determined by the anatomic relationship of the VSD to the great arteries and the presence or absence of outflow tract obstruction. These factors account for the classification of the morphologic variants into four physiologic types, each displaying clinical features that resemble those of other malformations as follows:
- **VSD-type:** mimics VSD (Chapter 11)
- **TOF-type:** mimics TOF (Chapter 13)
- **TGA-type:** mimics TGA (Chapter 14)
- **Remote VSD:** mimics VSD or AVSD (Chapters 11 and 12)

The relationship between the physiologic and anatomic classifications is shown in Table 16-1.

Coexistent pathology in DORV can also influence the physiology. Associated defects include pulmonary stenosis (PS) (common finding occurring at the valvar and/or subvalvar levels), secundum ASD, PDA, additional VSDs, AV valve anomalies, subaortic

PART II. DISEASES

DORV with Subaortic VSD

DORV with Subpulmonary VSD

DORV with Noncommitted VSD

DORV with Doubly Committed VSD

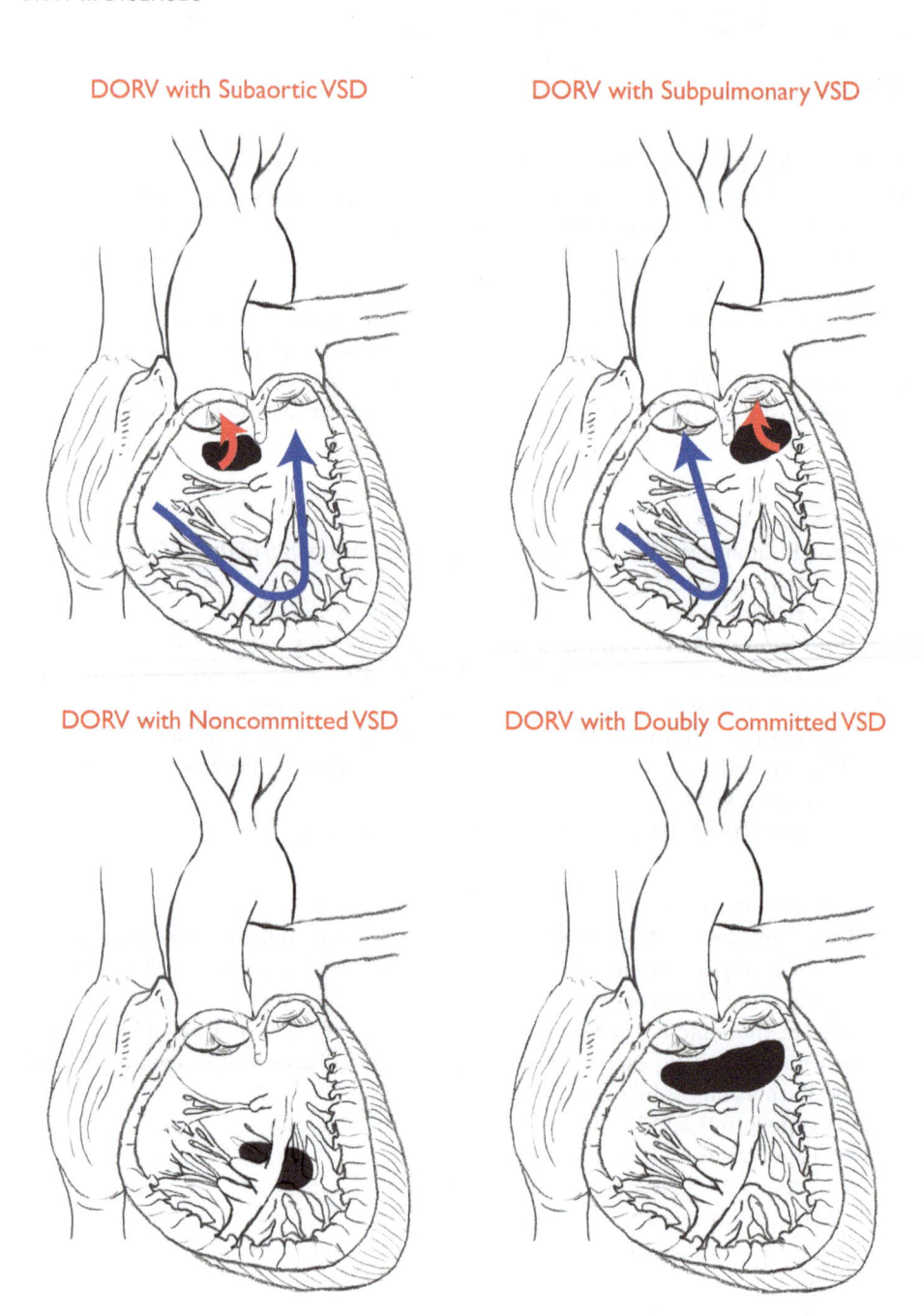

Figure 16-1. Anatomic classification of DORV based on the relationship of the VSD to the great vessels.

16. DOUBLE-OUTLET RIGHT VENTRICLE

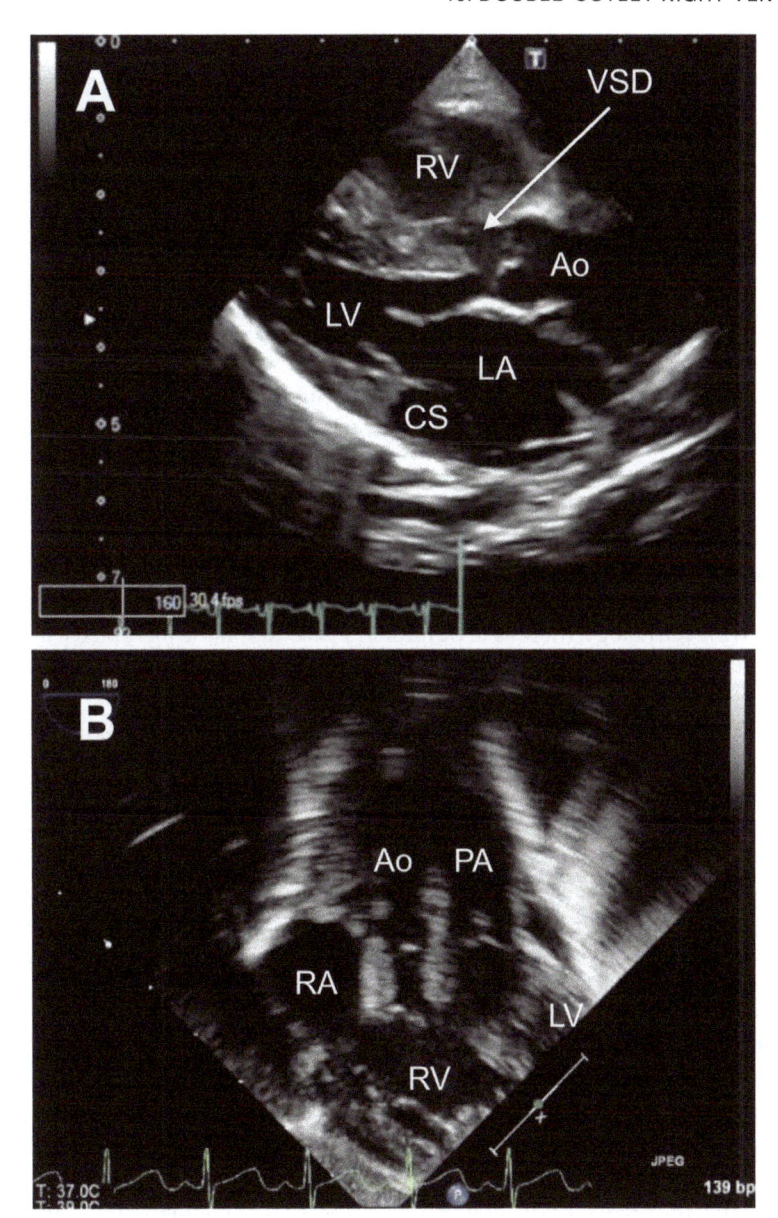

Figure 16-2. Echocardiographic diagnosis of DORV. A) TTE parasternal long-axis image of a patient with DORV and subaortic VSD showing the position of the aortic root over both ventricles, a VSD, and aortomitral discontinuity related to conal tissue. A dilated coronary sinus (CS) is seen related to a left SVC draining into the CS. The patient also had pulmonary stenosis (not shown). B) TEE deep transgastric image in a patient with DORV and subpulmonary VSD (Taussig-Bing) showing the origin of both great arteries from the RV, bilateral conal tissue, and narrowing of the subaortic region. There was associated aortic arch obstruction.

117

Table 16-1. Clinical and anatomic classifications of DORV.

Clinical classification	Anatomic classification	Pulmonary stenosis
VSD-type	Subaortic VSD Doubly committed VSD	-
TOF-type	Subaortic VSD Doubly committed VSD	+
TGA-type	Subpulmonary VSD	+ / -
Remote VSD	Non committed VSD	+ / -

stenosis (e.g., in the Taussig-Bing anomaly), aortic arch obstruction (may be associated with subaortic stenosis in the Taussig-Bing variant), right aortic arch, and coronary artery anomalies.

Diagnosis
- **ECG.** Frequently displays right-axis deviation, RA enlargement, and RVH.
- **CXR.** Findings are variable and not of significant diagnostic value in terms of the underlying pathology. Increased pulmonary vascular markings and cardiomegaly are consistent with an unrestrictive VSD. In contrast, the presence of oligemic lungs is suggestive of pulmonary outflow tract obstruction.
- **Echocardiogram (Figure 16-2).** Fetal echocardiography is diagnostic in most cases. Initial TTE focuses on the size and location of the VSD and its relationship to the arterial outlets, great artery relationships, morphology and patency of the outflow tracts, assessment of the AV valves, and characterization of associated anomalies. Noninvasive imaging guides balloon atrial septostomy (BAS) when indicated. TEE is used in most cases for intraoperative monitoring, to assist in surgical planning, and to evaluate the adequacy of the repair. This technology plays an important role in the exclusion of potential hemodynamically significant residual lesions such as intracardiac shunts, baffle obstruction, and valvar regurgitation. TTE remains the primary imaging modality for long-term surveillance.
- **Cardiac catheterization.** Not necessary in most cases. May be used to facilitate BAS in the Taussig-Bing variant. Angiography can be helpful in patients with complex anatomy. Hemodynamic measurements that include PA pressure and PVR are rarely needed, unless there is a late presentation or clinical concerns following a palliative procedure.
- **CTA/MRI.** May assist in the delineation of associated complex aortic arch anomalies and much less commonly, in the characterization of the anatomy that may impact surgical management (i.e., relationship of semilunar valves to the VSD). Postoperatively, it can be helpful during long-term surveillance.

Medical Management
The preoperative management of the patient with DORV is primarily influenced by the anatomic type and associated physiology.

Subaortic and Doubly Committed VSD
If a subaortic or doubly committed VSD is present and there is no PS, the clinical presentation is typically that of pulmonary overcirculation within the first few weeks of life. After the gradual expected decrease in PVR, PS may become apparent. If PS is of mild severity or nonexistent, tachypnea, intercostal retractions, hepatomegaly, and feeding difficulties are likely to ensue. Diuretic therapy is indicated in these cases (furosemide 1 mg/kg/dose every 6-12 hours). Overcirculation will follow the management of a large VSD (see Chapter 11).

TOF-Type
Children with TOF-type physiology require close monitoring depending on the degree of PS. Progressive cyanosis related to increasing subpulmonary obstruction or hypercyanotic episodes may develop (see Chapter 13). A hypercyanotic spell meets indication for hospital admission with consideration for surgical intervention (complete repair vs. palliation by means of systemic-to-pulmonary artery shunting).

TGA-Type
The neonate with TGA-type anatomy requires evaluation to ensure adequate intercirculatory mixing and aortic arch patency. PGE therapy may be necessary. Given that the VSD and PDA are usually not adequate sites for mixing, a BAS is recommended prior to surgical intervention in most cases unless shunting at the atrial level is unrestrictive.

Remote VSD
These patients usually present with signs and symptoms of pulmonary overcirculation. The VSD tends to be large enough to allow outflow from the LV and mixing of the systemic and pulmonary circulations. Overcirculation is managed medically until PA banding is performed.

Indications / Timing of Intervention
All patients with DORV require cardiac surgery. The majority of these procedures are undertaken during the first year of life. However, the specific type and timing of the surgical intervention depends on the pathophysiologic variant of DORV (see "Surgical Intervention" and Figure 16-3).

Anesthetic Considerations
The anesthetic management during the initial approach to this lesion hinges primarily on the particular physiologic variant and the planned surgical intervention.

Anesthetic goals may include balancing the pulmonary and systemic circulations and maintaining ductal patency by means of a PGE infusion as required to support pulmonary or systemic blood flow. Palliative procedures in the neonate and young infant such as PA banding or aortopulmonary shunting may be favored over initial corrective interventions. These usually require full invasive monitoring and adequate preparation for the respective procedure, however there is rarely a need for CPB. In contrast, corrective interventions imply the use of CPB. These procedures can be complex requiring a long aortic cross-clamp period. Main considerations during the

PART II. DISEASES

post-CPB phase include managing hemodynamics and the coagulation system. Efforts revolve around optimizing: (1) ventricular preload, assisted by TEE and guided by LAP monitoring, (2) myocardial performance and systemic vascular tone, with the use of inotropic/vasoactive agents, (3) pulmonary mechanics, by selecting suitable ventilation strategies, and (4) hemostasis, by the administration of blood products.

Surgical Intervention

VSD-Type

The repair entails creation of an intracardiac baffle between the LV and the aorta. For *subaortic* VSDs, since the defect is in close proximity to the aortic valve, the repair is very similar to closure of a perimembranous/outlet VSD. Ideally, the repair is performed between 6 and 8 months of age although it may take place earlier in life (including the neonatal period) if symptoms are not controlled with medical treatment. Repair of a subaortic VSD is performed through a right atriotomy using glutaraldehyde-fixed autologous pericardium for the baffle. The pericardium is secured to the rim of the defect and the tricuspid valve using either interrupted pledgeted sutures or a combination of running and interrupted pledgeted sutures. Analogous to perimembranous VSDs, the conduction system travels on the posteroinferior rim of the defect and is at risk of injury during the repair.

DORV with *doubly committed* VSDs are analogous to doubly committed juxta-arterial VSDs. Since the defect is underneath the semilunar valves, the repair is usually performed through a transverse pulmonary arteriotomy. A series of interrupted pericardial pledgeted sutures are placed through the pulmonary valve annulus and into the rim of the defect. A glutaraldehyde-fixed autologous pericardial patch is used to close the defect, therefore creating an intracardiac baffle between the LV and the aorta. The conduction system is usually away from the rim of these defects unless they extend into the perimembranous area. Due to the location of the semilunar valves mainly arising from the RV, it is possible for the baffle to impinge into the RV causing RVOT obstruction. The procedure is therefore ideally performed between 8 and 12 months of age. If patients require earlier intervention due to symptoms, placement of a PA band may be useful to delay surgical repair.

TOF-Type

Repair of TOF-type DORV is similar to repair of simple TOF, although it tends to be technically more difficult due to the more anterior location of the aorta. The procedure entails resection of RV muscle bundles and creation of an intracardiac autologous pericardial baffle through a right atriotomy followed by further resection of RV muscle bundles through a longitudinal pulmonary arteriotomy. If the pulmonary valve annulus is significantly hypoplastic, the incision is extended for a few millimeters through the annulus into the RV (transannular incision). The pulmonary arteriotomy is closed with a second autologous pericardial patch (see Chapter 13). The repair is ideally performed after 4-6 months of age. Younger patients with symptoms (significant cyanosis or hypercyanotic spells) may require placement of a modified Blalock-Taussig-Thomas shunt (mBTTS) prior to surgical repair.

16. DOUBLE-OUTLET RIGHT VENTRICLE

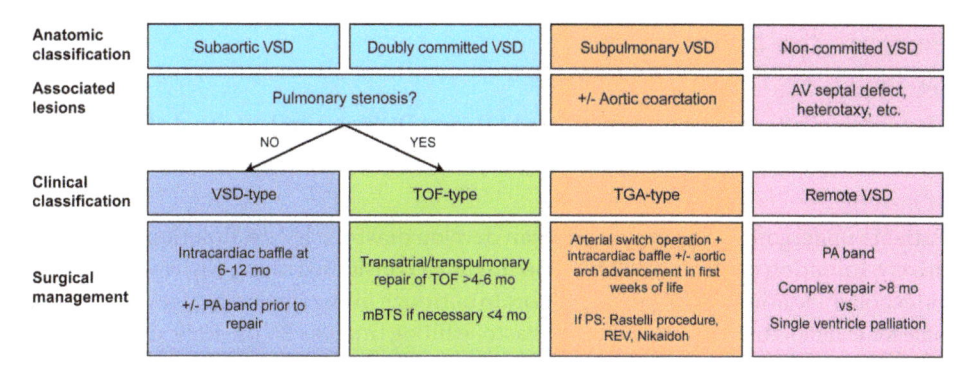

Anatomic classification	Subaortic VSD	Doubly committed VSD	Subpulmonary VSD	Non-committed VSD
Associated lesions	Pulmonary stenosis?		+/- Aortic coarctation	AV septal defect, heterotaxy, etc.
	NO YES			
Clinical classification	VSD-type	TOF-type	TGA-type	Remote VSD
Surgical management	Intracardiac baffle at 6-12 mo +/- PA band prior to repair	Transatrial/transpulmonary repair of TOF >4-6 mo mBTS if necessary <4 mo	Arterial switch operation + intracardiac baffle +/- aortic arch advancement in first weeks of life If PS: Rastelli procedure, REV, Nikaidoh	PA band Complex repair >8 mo vs. Single ventricle palliation

Figure 16-3. Algorithm for surgical intervention in patients with DORV.

TGA-Type

Repair of TGA-type DORV (Taussig-Bing anomaly) entails creation of an autologous pericardial baffle between the LV and the pulmonary valve (the semilunar valve closer to the VSD) and an arterial switch operation (see Chapter 14). Aortic arch hypoplasia or aortic coarctation are not unusual in this setting, requiring arch reconstruction in the form of an aortic arch advancement (see Chapter 25). Surgical intervention is usually undertaken in the first few weeks of life.

Some patients with subpulmonary stenosis may still be candidates for an arterial switch operation and subpulmonary resection. However, an arterial swtich operation may not be possible in some patients with severe PS, as it would translate into LVOT obstruction. The favored approach in these cases consists of a Rastelli procedure that includes creation of an intracardiac baffle between the VSD and the aortic valve with insertion of an RV-PA conduit. The native pulmonary valve is oversewn and the PA stump sutured closed. The conus between the aortic and pulmonary valves, which can be quite prominent, may be excised in order to allow a more direct connection between the VSD and the aorta ("reparation a l'etage ventriculaire" or REV procedure). In certain circumstances, a Nikaidoh procedure may be performed. This operation consists of translocating the aortic root posteriorly (to the previous position of the stenotic pulmonary valve) and reconstructing the RVOT with an RV-PA conduit or a patch. The coronary arteries are usually not translocated and therefore at risk of torsion during this procedure. Repair of TGA-type DORV with PS is usually performed later in life, ideally after infancy.

Remote VSD

Management of patients with a remote or noncommitted VSD is individualized depending on the anatomy. Since the outcomes of creating a very complex intracardiac baffle are suboptimal, a large proportion of these patients may be managed with single ventricle palliation. If so, placement of a PA band (see Chapter 39) is performed within the first few weeks of life to protect the pulmonary vascular bed, followed by subsequent creation of a bidirectional Glenn connection with the goal of eventual total cavopulmonary (Fontan) completion (see Chapter 39).

Postoperative Management

VSD-Type
Management after surgical treatment of VSD-type DORV is similar to that after closure of a large simple VSD (see Chapter 11).

TOF-type
Patients undergoing TOF-type repair can develop diastolic RV dysfunction postoperatively. Initiation of an esmolol infusion might be considered along with avoidance of catecholamine administration in an effort to optimize filling (preload) times. The rationale for esmolol therapy is to enhance diastolic filling times as RV diastolic dysfunction is transient, and to reduce the risk of dynamic RVOT obstruction from tachycardia (see Chapter 13). Diastolic dysfunction may require volume resuscitation. Intravascular volume is better assessed by LAP, as CVP may be elevated due to poor compliance of the RV. These patients are usually 200-300 mL positive after their first postoperative night.

TGA-Type
Following an arterial switch operation, concerning findings include increased LAP, arrhythmias, or ST-segment changes as these suggest myocardial dysfunction and/or coronary insufficiency (see Chapter 14). Perioperative management usually includes infusion of inotropes, agents that influence systemic/pulmonary vascular tone, and calcium. Ventricular dysfunction is in most cases systolic in nature, and therefore, is treated with inotropic support. Volume administration should be minimized. Nitroglycerin is routinely added to potentially limit coronary vascular reactivity given the necessary manipulations of the coronary arteries.

After the Rastelli or REV operation, RV systolic or diastolic dysfunction can be present, which tends to improve after a period of 24-48 hrs. Inotropic support with milrinone and low-dose catecholamine is customary in these patients.

If the operation was a Nikaidoh procedure, one should be vigilant about potential coronary torsion and/or AI. Inotropic support should be maintained until LCOS is resolved (usually the first 24 hours postoperatively). Careful attention to LAP, diastolic BP, and ST segments aid in the recognition of potential complications.

Remote VSD
If the operation was a PA band, the balance to achieve optimal arterial oxygen saturations will depend on minimizing pulmonary venous desaturation and maintaining moderate levels of oxygen provision (<60% FiO_2). Given that the increased afterload is seen by the two ventricles in parallel, it tends to be well tolerated. For details on PA band management and subsequent palliation, refer to Chapter 39.

Complications
- **Pleural effusions.** When there is important RV diastolic dysfunction, increases in CVP could prevent adequate clearance of pleural fluid and drainage of lymph/chyle into the innominate vein from the thoracic duct. Initial diuresis in conjunction with fluid restriction may stave off the accumulation of pleural effusions.
- **JET.** Although the incidence of JET at TCH is very low (atrial tachycardia is the most

16. DOUBLE-OUTLET RIGHT VENTRICLE

common postoperative arrhythmia), it can affect some patients, particularly related to more extensive/complex intracardiac repairs. Addressing all potential triggers or exacerbating factors could "cool off" the automatic focus in JET. If these efforts are not successful (including cooling, lowering doses of catecholamine infusions, sedation, magnesium administration, overdrive pacing), antiarrhtymic treatment with amiodarone, esmolol, sotalol, or procainamide may be necessary (see Chapter 74).

> **TCH experience with biventricular repair of DORV (1995-2016)**
> Number of patients: 151
> - VSD-type: 65
> - TOF-type: 46
> - TGA-type: 40
>
> Perioperative mortality: 1.3%
> 5-year survival: 95%
> 5-year incidence of reintervention: 20-25%

- **Coronary translocation/torsion issues.** These tend to present early with regional segmental wall motion abnormalities on echocardiography, ECG changes (ST- and T-wave abnormalities), and increased LAP, accompanied by hemodynamic alterations and need for high inotropic support. In this setting, volume administration will only increase ventricular wall stress, further accentuating myocardial ischemia. Inotropic / vasoactive drugs are the agents of choice for hemodynamic optimization while diagnostic investigation is undertaken or interventions are considered to address coronary problems.
- **Complete heart block.** This represents an extremely rare complication. If AV dissociation is initially present in the patient receiving dexmedetomidine, the infusion should be discontinued, as it could cause or contribute to the conduction abnormalities. If high-grade block is still present 10 days after surgery (Mobitz II or third-degree AV block), implantation of a permanent pacemaker should be considered (see Chapter 75).
- **LCOS/LV dysfunction.** Usually transient and managed with epinephrine +/- milrinone infusions. Rarely, the epinephrine dose would exceed 0.05 mcg/kg/min. (see Chapter 71).

Long-Term Follow-Up

Close follow-up of patients with DORV undergoing either biventricular repair or single ventricle palliation is mandatory as long-term reintervention is not uncommon. The 5-year incidence of any reintervention (surgical or catheter-based) after biventricular repair is between 20-25%. Reinterventions most commonly include subaortic resection, pulmonary valvotomy/RVOT resection, conduit replacement, and branch PA intervention, depending on the type of DORV repair.

17 Pulmonary Atresia, Ventricular Septal Defect, Major Aortopulmonary Collaterals

Aimee Liou, Carlos M. Mery, Patricia Bastero, Pablo Motta

Pulmonary atresia with ventricular septal defect (PA/VSD) and major aortopulmonary collateral arteries (MAPCAs) is a cyanotic CHD on the spectrum of tetralogy of Fallot (TOF) with ultimate pulmonary obstruction in the form of valve atresia; it is therefore also referred to as tetralogy of Fallot with pulmonary atresia. The PA tree is much more likely to be abnormal in PA/VSD than in TOF.

There is a wide variability in the anatomy of patients with PA/VSD/MAPCAs. On one end of the spectrum, a patient will have well-formed confluent branch PAs supplied by a ductus arteriosus and no MAPCAs, while at the other end of the spectrum, the patient will have no native PAs and all pulmonary supply will be dependent on MAPCAs. The main PA (MPA) segment may be absent, may present as a fibroelastic cord without a lumen, or may have varying degrees of hypoplasia. The native branch PAs may be confluent or discontinuous, and may be normal, hypoplastic, or absent. Ductal origin of one or both branch PAs may be present. Segmental and subsegmental arteries may likewise be present or absent.

MAPCAs arise from the descending thoracic aorta (or the brachiocephalic vessels) as vestiges of the primitive PA supply and, in the absence of native PA branches, comprise the sole source of blood flow to some lung segments. In this disease, some lung segments may have native PA supply, other segments may only have MAPCA supply, and yet others may have dual supply from both MAPCAs and native PA branches. The ductus arteriosus may be present or absent; rarely, bilateral PDAs are present. The RV is typically normal or dilated in size.

As with other conotruncal defects, there is a strong association between PA/VSD and DiGeorge (22q11 deletion) syndrome. A right aortic arch is a common associated anatomic variant.

Pathophysiology and Clinical Presentation

The patient symptomatology and clinical presentation is dictated by the amount of pulmonary blood flow (Qp) through the MAPCAs and the native PAs (via a PDA or communication with MAPCAs). In infants, Qp can be highly dynamic due to changes in PVR, changes in the nature of the MAPCAs, and ductal closure (if applicable).

All neonates with a diagnosis of PA/VSD are admitted to the CICU or NICU and their management will vary based on the source and amount of pulmonary flow. Patients that are dependent on a PDA for adequate pulmonary blood flow are treated with PGE until a procedure is performed to secure a stable source of pulmonary blood flow. Patients that have robust MAPCAs may develop symptoms of pulmonary overcirculation, especially as PVR drops in the first few weeks of life, and will thus require diuretic therapy. If there is no PDA and MAPCAs are inadequate, the patient will be cyanotic and will require an early procedure to improve pulmonary blood flow. Patients that

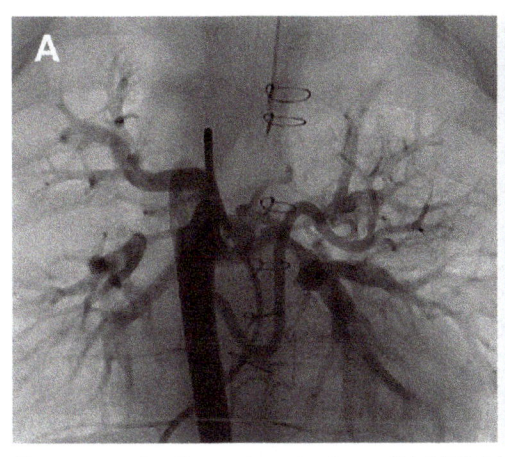

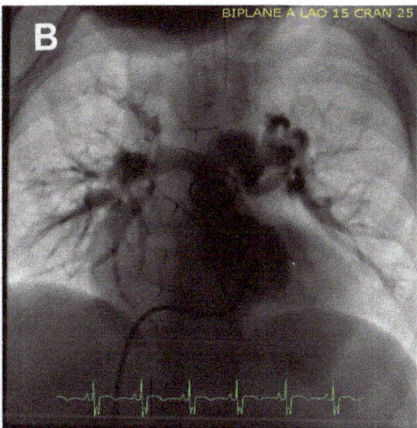

Figure 17-1. Cardiac catheterization on PA/VSD/MAPCAs. A) Catheterization showing multiple MAPCAs arising from the descending aorta. B) Catheterization showing MAPCAs unifocalized into the branch PAs with good overall pulmonary arborization.

develop stenosis of MAPCAs prior to unifocalization will experience a decrease in total Qp resulting in worsening hypoxemia or if they presented with overcirculation, improvement in symptoms.

The physical exam findings will depend on the overall Qp and status of the MAPCAs. A continuous murmur may be heard over lung segments supplied by MAPCAs. Infants with pulmonary overcirculation will develop failure to thrive, a gallop, pulmonary edema, and hepatomegaly. Hypoxemic patients will present with the expected sequelae including cyanosis and clubbing.

Diagnosis
- **CXR.** The cardiac silhouette takes on a boot shape, as seen in TOF. The quality of the pulmonary vascular markings is reflective of PA or MAPCA supply.
- **ECG.** RA enlargement and predominance of right-sided forces is common. Findings of left-heart enlargement (i.e., LA enlargement, biventricular hypertrophy) are seen in patients with large amounts of pulmonary blood flow.
- **Echocardiogram.** The appearance of the cardiac anatomy is similar to that in TOF, with a large VSD typical of conotruncal defects and aortic override. PA anatomy can be delineated to some degree but the images are frequently limited to the proximal native PAs (if present) and proximal MAPCAs. The presence or absence of a PDA should be documented. Aortic arch anatomy and coronary anatomy should also be assessed.
- **Cardiac catheterization (Figure 17-1).** Cardiac catheterization is performed on every patient with PA/VSD and MAPCAs prior to surgical intervention. Angiography is useful to demonstrate the number, size, and distribution of MAPCAs. Selective injection of each individual MAPCA is particularly helpful for mapping the pulmonary segmental supply. In the absence of a ductus arteriosus, pulmonary-vein

PART II. DISEASES

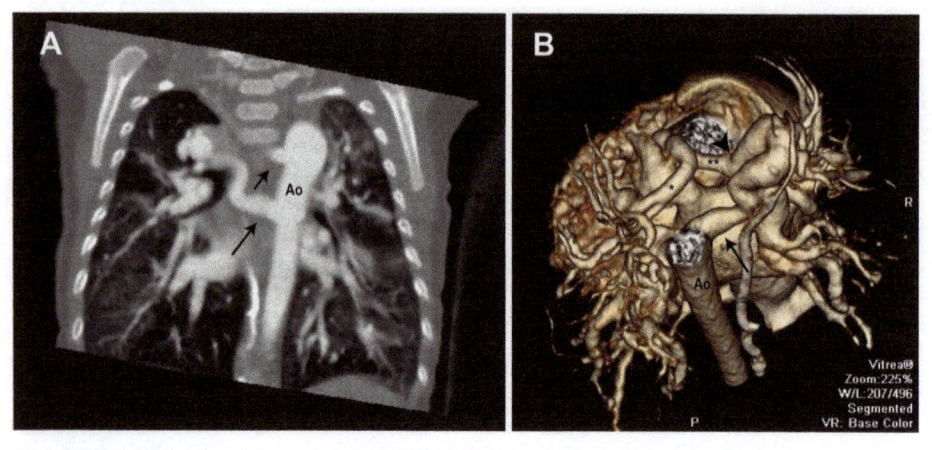

Figure 17-2. CTA of a patient with PA/VSD/MAPCAs. A) Coronal view showing 2 large MAPCAs (arrows) arising from the descending thoracic aorta (Ao). B) 3D reconstruction showing a large MAPCA (arrow) arising from the descending thoracic aorta and bifurcating into several large branches. One of the branches anastomoses to the left PA (arrowhead). * denotes the right PA and ** denotes the left PA.

wedge angiography is very important to define the presence and quality of the native PAs, as many patients will have diminutive but confluent branch PAs that go unrecognized with echocardiogram or CTA. The blood supply of all pulmonary segments must be accounted for. Lung segments with dual supply can be identified and associated MAPCAs intervened on. In some patients, especially those between stages of intervention, cardiac catheterization may also be useful to assess pressures within various MAPCAs. It is sometimes difficult to calculate Qp, the relationship between pulmonary and systemic blood flow (Qp:Qs), and PVR due to the presence of multiple sources of pulmonary blood flow.
- **CTA (Figure 17-2).** Very useful to demonstrate the nature, course, and distribution of MAPCAs and native PAs. CTA is particularly useful as a complement to cardiac catheterization for surgical planning as it shows the course of the MAPCAs and their relationship with surrounding structures (e.g., trachea, bronchi, atria).

Management Strategy

The ultimate goal in the therapeutic pathway for most patients with PA/VSD/MAPCAs is to achieve a biventricular circulation with a single PA tree that arises from the RV and supplies all pulmonary segments. In some patients, a fully unifocalized PA tree supplying all lung segments is not achievable secondary to poor quality of PAs or MAPCAs. An abundance of severely stenotic pulmonary vessels or a limited number of pulmonary segments included in the pulmonary circulation may represent excessive afterload for the RV, precluding VSD closure.

Due to the heterogeneity of this lesion, management is individualized for each particular patient. However, the overall philosophy of management at TCH follows some general guidelines (Figure 17-3):

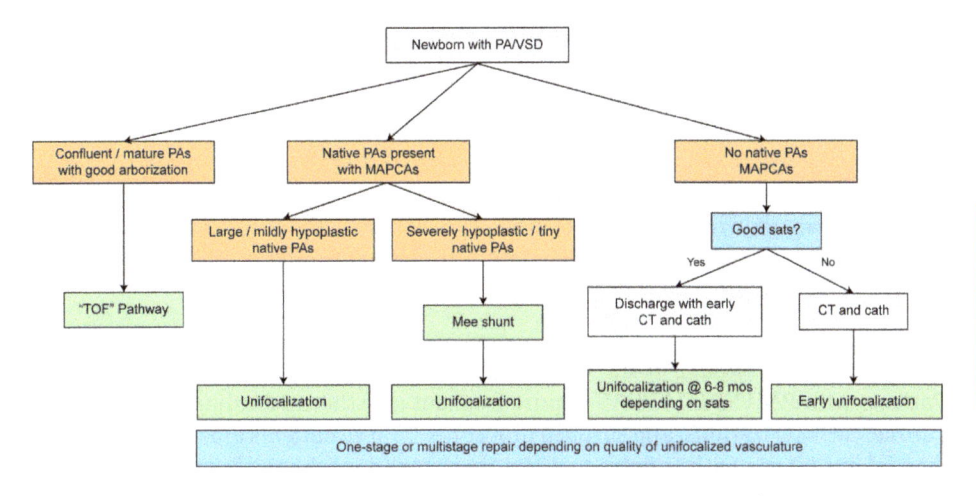

17. PULMONARY ATRESIA, VENTRICULAR SEPTAL DEFECT, MAJOR AORTOPULMONARY COLLATERALS

Figure 17-3. General algorithm for management of patients with PA/VSD/MAPCAs.

- **Patients with well-formed confluent branch PAs supplied by a PDA.** These patients are analogous to patients with tetralogy of Fallot. They will be maintained on PGE and will then undergo a procedure to secure a stable source of pulmonary blood flow. Options include placement of a PDA stent or creation of a modified Blalock-Taussig-Thomas shunt (mBTTS) (see Chapter 38). Later in infancy, patients will undergo biventricular repair with a Rastelli procedure (see below). In some circumstances, the patients may undergo a single-stage repair with a Rastelli procedure at the newborn stage.
- **Patients with hypoplastic branch PAs and MAPCAs.** A large proportion of patients with PA/VSD/MAPCAs will have diminutive branch PAs that may not be seen on CTA due to the lack of contrast flow into them. This is why a good pulmonary-venous angiography in the cardiac catheterization lab is very important. The overall strategy for these patients is to promote the growth of the confluent branch PAs in order to use as a scaffold to unifocalize relevant MAPCAs. These patients generally present with oxygen saturations that can vary from the 70s to the 90s, depending on the quality of the MAPCAs. As such, it is not usually necessary to perform any procedure during the newborn period. Patients are usually discharged home and undergo assessment of PAs and MAPCAs with a combination of cardiac catheterization and CTA. If the branch PAs are diminutive, a central shunt (Mee shunt) is performed (see below), usually at 3-6 months of age. An mBTTS may be used in patients that have slightly larger PAs in order to avoid overcirculation but still promote PA growth. The PA anatomy is reassessed later in in infancy and the patient is then put forward for surgical repair in the form of a Rastelli procedure with or without unifocalization (see below).
- **Patients with no native central PAs and sole MAPCA supply to the lungs.** This is the most challenging group of patients with PA/VSD/MAPCAs. Despite the lack of visualized central PAs, many patients will actually have diminutive central

PAs that were not seen on preoperative imaging but may be usable as part of the surgical strategy. After full assessment of MAPCAs with CTA and angiography, patients are taken to the OR, usually in late infancy. If diminutive central PAs are found on mediastinal exploration, a Mee shunt may be performed. Otherwise, all unifocalizable MAPCAs are brought together to create a central confluence that is then connected to either an mBTTS or a nonvalved conduit arising from the RV. Patients are then reassessed later in life with cardiac catheterization and CTA, and depending on the pulmonary arborization, the decision is made whether to proceed with a Rastelli procedure or not.

Anesthetic Considerations

Patients with PA/VSD/MAPCAS require frequent anesthetics for diagnostic studies, cardiac catheterizations, and surgical procedures. These patients are managed under general anesthesia with endotracheal intubation and mechanical ventilation due to the little pulmonary reserve secondary to the low Qp.

Preoperative Considerations
- **Difficult airway.** Patients with 22q11 deletion syndrome have micrognathia with the potential of a difficult airway. In addition, the trachea is usually short and mainstem bronchial intubation is possible.
- **Cyanosis.** It is important to assess for polycythemia as part of the preoperative evaluation. A hematocrit >65% is linked to impaired microvascular perfusion, hyperviscosity syndrome, and thrombosis.
- **Increased bleeding risk.** Cyanosis is associated with an increased bleeding risk due to thrombocytopenia and factor deficiencies.

General Anesthetic Considerations
The speed of inhalation induction of anesthesia is slower in patients with right-to-left shunting due to the low Qp. On the other hand, IV induction bypasses the first-pass pulmonary uptake, making IV induction faster. Due to the decreased Qp, there are lung areas that are ventilated but not perfused, causing a ventilation/perfusion (V/Q) mismatch. The use of $ETCO_2$ monitoring to assess ventilation may become unreliable due to the mismatch and lead to respiratory acidosis. As such, it is important to monitor arterial blood gases in longer procedures.

Spasm of MAPCAs during surgical manipulation and/or catheter interventions is possible and can lead to profound cyanosis. Stopping the stimulation, deepening anesthesia, treating acidosis, and increasing BP usually relieves the spasm.

Procedure-Specific Anesthetic Considerations
- **Cardiac catheterization.** Interventional rehabilitation of PA branches is associated with 2 dreaded complications for the anesthesiologist: intrapulmonary bleeding and lung reperfusion injury. Intrapulmonary bleeding is easily diagnosed by red blood in the airway and decreased lung compliance. Lung reperfusion injury also manifest with decreased lung compliance and mostly pink, frothy secretions. Most of the time, these complications are self-limited and can be medically managed with

100% FiO$_2$ and an increase in PEEP. Occasionally, one-lung ventilation is needed to protect the healthy lung. The last resort, if unable to ventilate and oxygenate, is the use of rescue ECMO.
- **Unifocalization procedures.** Unifocalization procedures performed through a thoracotomy require lung isolation techniques when feasible (>10 kg). This can lead to alterations in dead space and respiratory acidosis. The use of regional anesthetic techniques (i.e., thoracic epidural or paravertebral blocks) are useful adjuvants to general anesthesia in order to minimize postoperative pain.
- **Complete repair and PA augmentation.** The risk of bleeding is high in these procedures due to repeated surgeries, multiple suture lines, and underlying cyanosis. Antifibrinolytic use and point-of-care coagulation testing are useful to minimize the use of blood products. Postrepair RV dysfunction is common despite the use of inotropic therapy (milrinone and low-dose epinephrine) to wean off CPB. iNO should be available, especially in high-risk patients. In addition to TEE, direct PA pressure measurement is usually performed at the surgical field.

Catheter-Based Intervention

As mentioned above, diagnostic catheterization plays an important role in defining the anatomy of the MAPCAs, the supply of each of the different pulmonary segments, and the anatomy of the PAs (via pulmonary venous wedge angiography).

Catheter-based therapy in PA/VSD/MAPCAs is focused on ensuring adequacy of pulmonary blood flow and PA architecture. Prior to surgical intervention, areas of dual supply that involve small MAPCAs may be identified and can be occluded.

Ductal stenting may be appropriate in patients with a PDA and clinical evidence of inadequate Qp during a trial of ductal closure (see Chapter 38).

MAPCAs may become stenotic before or after unifocalization. Angioplasty or stenting of unifocalized MAPCAs is performed when stenosis is clinically significant, as this can result in cyanosis (if the VSD remains patent) or RV hypertension (if the VSD has been closed). A discussion with the surgical team is paramount to discuss what the best strategy for stenotic MAPCAs may be for a particular patient. Many patients require serial catheterizations to "rehabilitate" stenotic unifocalized MAPCAs. Cutting-balloon angioplasty is sometimes used in stenotic lesions that are particularly resistant to standard balloon angioplasty.

Patients who receive a conduit in the RV-PA position frequently require catheter-based interventions (angioplasty, stenting, or transcatheter valve placement) on the conduit.

In specific clinical scenarios, for patients possessing rare anatomic variants with patent MPA segments and isolated valve atresia, pulmonary valve perforation and valvuloplasty may be useful.

Surgical Intervention

As mentioned above, patients with this disease are managed in a multidisciplinary fashion and the therapeutic approach is individualized based on anatomy and physiology.

PART II. DISEASES

A series of surgical procedures can be performed on these patients, depending on the overall strategy (Figure 17-3).

Aortopulmonary Shunts

Patients that have diminutive native PAs can benefit from growth of those PAs by augmenting flow with the use of an aortopulmonary shunt. The shunt that we commonly use for patients with significantly hypoplastic PAs is the Mee shunt. This shunt involves detaching the main PA from the heart and creating an end-to-side anastomosis between the distal main PA and the ascending aorta. The procedure may be performed through a median sternotomy or a lateral thoracotomy. The pericardium is opened and the optimal location for the shunt on the ascending aorta is marked with a fine suture. The proximal main PA is ligated and the vessel is divided after controlling the branch PAs with fine tourniquets. A side-biting clamp is placed on the previously selected site on the ascending aorta, an incision is performed and enlarged with an aortic punch, and the anastomosis is performed with either a running fine suture or a set of interrupted sutures. The branch PAs are released and the sidebiting clamp is removed from the aorta. It is important to keep an adequate orientation of the branch PAs in order to avoid twisting of the diminutive PAs, in particular the right PA. The location of the shunt is usually located on the posterior aspect of the aorta and slightly to the left.

A Mee shunt is not a good alternative for patients with only mild or moderate hypoplasia of the PAs since they may become quite overcirculated. These patients are better served by an mBTTS (see Chapter 38).

Unifocalization

An important consideration in the workup of patients with MAPCAs is which MAPCAs are relevant and which MAPCAs are not. In general, the purpose is to achieve a pulmonary vascular bed that includes all or as many pulmonary segments as possible. A combination of CTA and cardiac catheterization usually allows to define whether each of the different 19 pulmonary segments is supplied by a native PA, only by a MAPCA, or have "dual supply", meaning supply from both a native PA and a MAPCA. In general, MAPCAs that solely supply pulmonary segments should be unifocalized (unless they are very small and unifocalization is not technically feasible). MAPCAs that provide dual supply to pulmonary segments may be unifocalized (if they are large and accessible) or occluded (either in the cath lab or surgically). As a rule of thumb though, large MAPCAs are usually important sources of pulmonary blood supply and one should think twice before occluding them. It is important for the imaging (cardiac catheterization or CTA) to be recent (<3 months) in order to accurately reflect the status of the MAPCAs.

Unifocalization of MAPCAs can be performed either as part of a complete repair or as a separate procedure via either a median sternotomy or a thoracotomy. Ideally, MAPCAs are unifocalized into a native PA scaffold after allowing the native PAs to grow. However, MAPCAs may need to be unifocalized into a shunt or into a confluence that is supplied by a shunt or a conduit from the RV. The decision regarding the most optimal strategy is made depending on the individual characteristics of the patient and how this operation fits on the overall surgical and interventional roadmap designed for the particular patient. Another consideration is whether temporary occlusion of the involved MAPCAs will be feasible without the need for CPB.

A preoperative CTA is very useful to define the particular location and course of MAPCAs and the relationship between the MAPCA and surrounding structures. If the procedure is performed as part of an intracardiac repair, it is useful to perform as much of the dissection as possible prior to administering heparin and instituting CPB. However, complete dissection of the MAPCAs may be challenging due to the location of the vessels, usually behind the cardiac mass and the airway. Due to the size of the MAPCAs, it is desirable to control them with fine tourniquets immediately after CPB is instituted in order to reduce the usually massive amount of pulmonary venous return. If the MAPCAs have not been completely dissected on institution of CPB, the body is kept at normal temperature to allow the heart to eject the blood that is returning through the pulmonary veins (cooling decreases the effectiveness of the heart's contractility and can lead to cardiac distention). Once all MAPCAs are controlled, the patient is cooled down for the intracardiac portion of the procedure.

> **TCH experience with PA/VSD/MAPCAs (1995-2013)**
>
> Number of patients: 107 (does not include patients without MAPCAs)
> - Single ventricle palliation: 9 (8%)
> - Single-stage repair: 17 (16%)
> - Staged repair: 61 (57%)
> - Awaiting intervention: 20 (19%)

Rastelli Repair

The ultimate goal of the treatment strategy for these patients is a biventricular repair. The Rastelli repair involves the creation of a baffle between the LV and the aorta (therefore closing the VSD) and placement of an RV-PA conduit to allow the RV to eject blood into the lungs. The Rastelli procedure may be performed as part of a large operation involving unifocalization of MAPCAs or as a separate procedure.

The Rastelli procedure is performed through a median sternotomy with regular aortobicaval cannulation, using moderate hypothermia (25-28 °C). After cardioplegic arrest, a right atriotomy is performed and the left heart is vented through the atrial septum. Working through the atriotomy, the VSD is closed by creating an autologous pericardial (or Dacron®) baffle between the LV and the aorta. It is important to create the baffle in a way that allows it to bulge in order to prevent LVOT obstruction. This is achieved by advancing more on the patch and less on the heart tissue. A right ventriculotomy is then performed for placement of the conduit. Performing the VSD closure via the atriotomy allows the conduit to be placed more lateral on the heart and away from the sternum. The ventriculotomy should be created close to the shoulder of the heart (the obtuse margin) and away from the LAD and any large conal branches. It is important to excise RV muscle in order to allow unimpeded flow from the RV into the conduit. Options for conduits include cryopreserved aortic and pulmonary homografts, bovine jugular vein conduits (Contegra®), and composite porcine-valved Dacron® conduits (Hancock® conduits). Our preference for small children has been to implant cryopreserved homografts. In these cases, a small hood is created proximally between the RV and the homograft, using homograft tissue, autologous pericardium, or Gore-Tex® material. The placement of the RV-PA conduit can be performed either after ASD

PART II. DISEASES

closure and removal of the cross-clamp (with the heart beating), or prior to removal of the cross-clamp (with the heart stopped), depending on the expected difficulty and the length of the cross-clamp period. It is not customary for us to leave an ASD in place. An LA line and peritoneal dialysis catheter are routinely placed.

PA pressures are routinely measured after weaning off CPB. Some degree of pulmonary hypertension is not unusual. However, if PA pressures are significantly increased despite the use of iNO and there is no evidence of mechanical obstruction of the conduit or the branch PAs, one has to assume that the pulmonary vascular bed is not adequate enough to support a biventricular circulation at this time. It may be necessary to create a VSD fenestration or remove the VSD patch (and possibly place a PA band) in order to avoid RV failure.

Postoperative Management
The postoperative management depends on the procedure performed.
- **Aortopulmonary shunts.** Based on the size of the shunt, SVR, PVR, and intravascular volume-controlling strategies will be key to optimizing Qp:Qs. Special attention must be placed on appropriate pain control in patients with thoracotomies, as these are more painful than sternotomies and have a higher risk for atelectasis and possible longer ventilatory support requirements. See Chapter 38 for specific postoperative management of patients with aortopulmonary shunts.
- **Unifocalization.** It is important to know the size and anatomy of MAPCAs in order to provide adequate management to optimize Qp. Long, tortuous MAPCAs unifocalized into small PAs will need PVR-optimizing maneuvers such as deep sedation, consideration of neuromuscular blockade, achievement of FRC, oxygen supplementation, and iNO. Volume resuscitation may be useful in some instances. If not all MAPCAs have been unifocalized, the use of vasopressors to increase the driving pressure into the lungs (systolic BP) may be needed.
- **Full repair (Rastelli procedure, PA plasty).** RV systolic and diastolic dysfunction is common in the early postoperative stages. Medical strategies to support systolic function (milrinone and/or epinephrine infusions) and reduce afterload (achieving FRC, oxygen supplementation, and iNO) are needed. These patients also tend to benefit from lower heart rate and increased filling to manage their RV diastolic dysfunction. Manipulation of PVR and SVR for cardiopulmonary interactions and ventricular interdependence will be key the first 24-48 hours postoperatively. Most patients will remain sedated the first night postoperatively. LAP allows adequate fluid management over the first few days. Peritoneal dialysis should be started on the first postoperative night.

18 Right-Ventricular Outflow Tract Obstruction

Antonio G. Cabrera, Athar M. Qureshi, Charles D. Fraser Jr.

Both pulmonary atresia with intact ventricular septum (PA-IVS) and isolated pulmonary stenosis (PS) represent variations within the spectrum of RVOT obstruction. These lesions vary significantly in terms of clinical and morphological characteristics, and thus management strategy. As such, PA-IVS and isolated PS will be discussed in separate sections of this chapter.

PA-IVS

PA-IVS is a lesion characterized by an atretic pulmonary valve, a muscularized and variably hypoplastic RV with no ventricular septal communication, and a variably hypoplastic and tethered tricuspid valve (TV). An ASD is obligatory for survival. This lesion is associated with coronary abnormalities which may make catheter and surgical procedures significantly risky.

PA-IVS is a highly heterogeneous lesion. As such, the decision-making process and management of these patients is quite complex and has been subject of much controversy. Many patients are able to achieve a biventricular circulation (through different stages) while others will benefit from single-ventricle palliation. In certain circumstances, a "1.5-V repair" can be achieved in patients that would otherwise not be candidates for a biventricular circulation.

Pathophysiology and Clinical Presentation

PA-IVS presents with variable degrees of TV and RV hypoplasia. TV annular dimension is moderately associated with the degree of RV hypoplasia. The TV leaflets may vary from normal to severely thickened with the subvalvar apparatus matted with indistinct chordae and fibrotic, and at times infarcted, papillary muscles. In a small number of cases (5-10%) there is significant TV dysplasia with apical displacement of

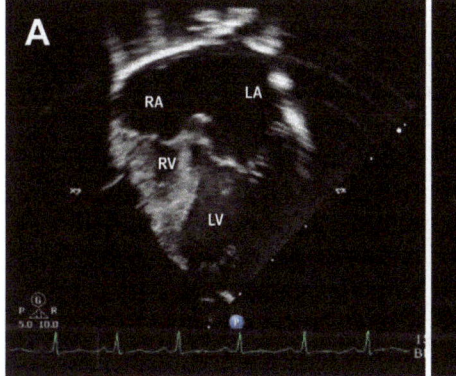

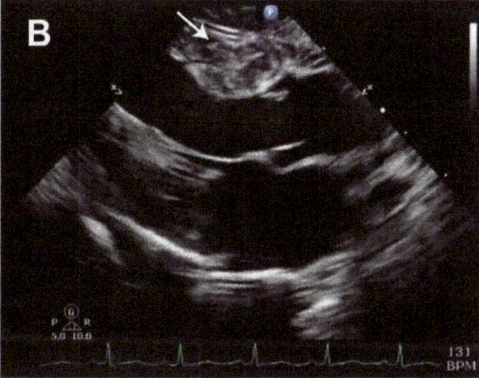

Figure 18-1. Echocardiography in PA-IVS. A) 4-chamber view showing a small, muscularized, and hypertrophied RV with a small TV. B) Parasternal long-axis view showing a normal-sized LV with a small and muscularized RV (arrow). Images courtesy of Dr. Josh Kailin, www.pedecho.org.

PART II. DISEASES

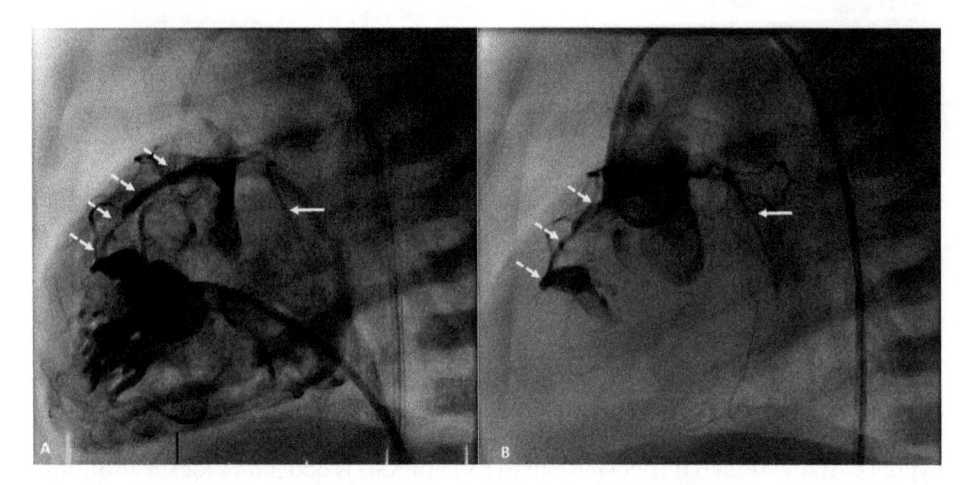

Figure 18-2. A) Right ventricular angiogram in a newborn with PA-IVS. Interruption of the mid left anterior descending coronary artery (dotted arrows) with a fistulous connection to the RV is seen. A small circumflex coronary artery (solid arrow) is also seen. B) Direct angiography in the left main coronary artery confirms interruption of the left anterior descending coronary artery (dotted arrows) and a small circumflex coronary artery (solid arrow).

the valve (Ebstein-like), which can lead to severe TR, massive RA dilation, a dilated RV, and concomitant LV dysfunction. Mortality in these patients may exceed 50-55%; heart transplantation should be considered.

In PA-IVS, since there is some inflow through the TV into the RV but no outflow, the RV becomes significantly pressurized. This phenomenon can lead to abnormal development of the coronary circulation and the presence of coronary sinusoids or fistulas between the RV and the coronary arteries. The flow dynamics of these fistulas can lead to the development of proximal coronary stenoses, making the coronary perfusion dependent on flow from the hypertensive RV through the fistulas and into the coronary arteries (RV-dependent coronary circulation, RVDCC). RVDCC is specifically defined as myocardial perfusion that is at least partially dependent on RV fistulas due to proximal epicardial coronary obstruction of two or more major coronary branches or ostial atresia. Intimal fibromuscular hyperplasia often occurs in the coronary arteries associated with fistulas and may be responsible for myocardial ischemia and infarction. The presence of RVDCC has significant implications not only for the management but the long-term prognosis of this lesion.

The factors that are mainly associated with long-term outcomes in PA-IVS are:
- Presence or absence of RVDCC
- Size and morphology of the RV
- Size and function of the TV

Patients with PA-IVS are dependent on a PDA and an ASD for early survival. If a patient has not been diagnosed prenatally and the duct is allowed to close, the patient will present with severe hypoxemia and acidosis. Once PGE has been started for ductal patency, the patient will have some cyanosis (due to the obligatory right-to-left shunt at

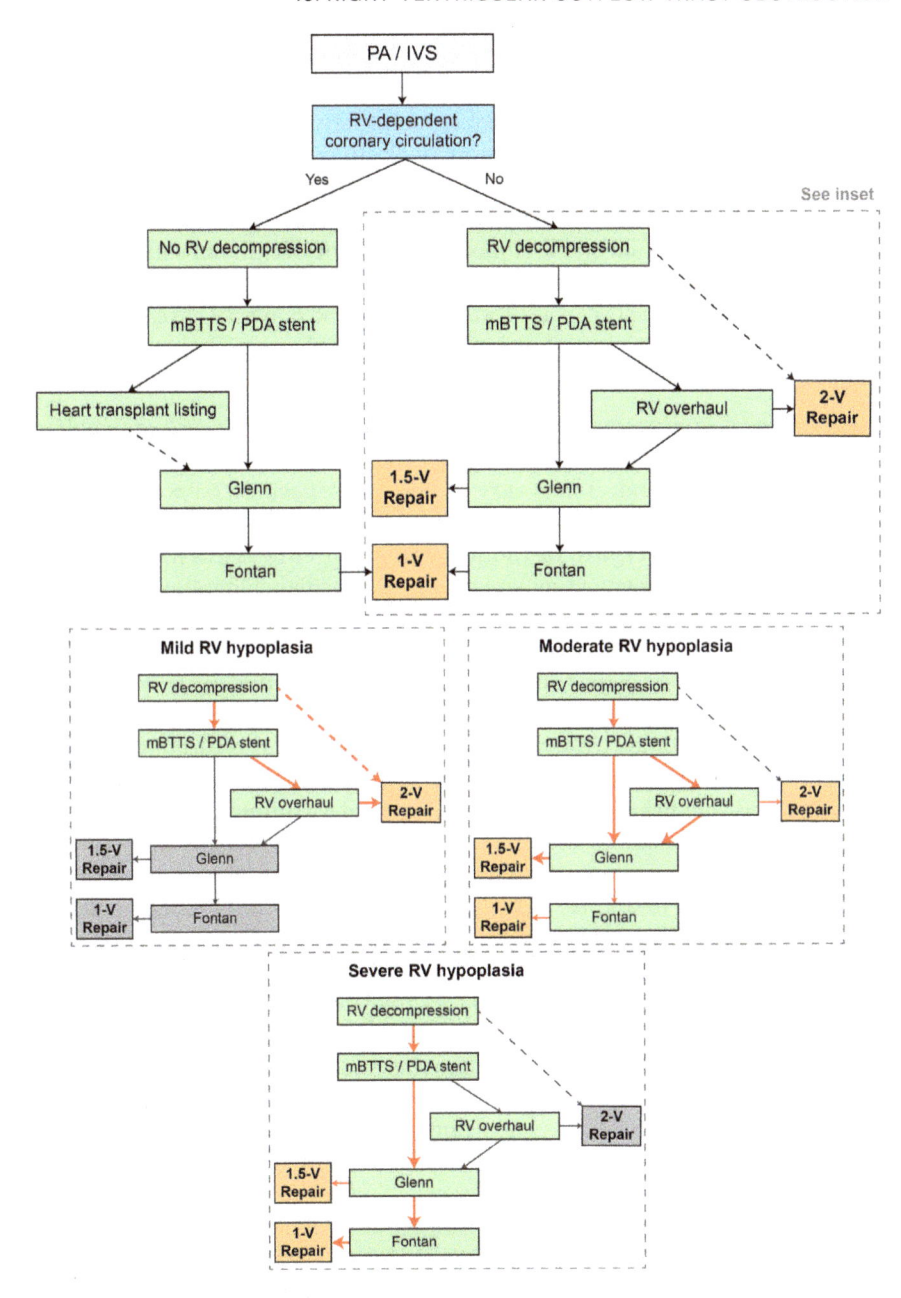

18. RIGHT-VENTRICULAR OUTFLOW TRACT OBSTRUCTION

Figure 18-3. Management algorithm for patients with PA-IVS. Management depends on whether the patient has RVDCC and the degree of RV and TV hypoplasia. The treatment is individualized for each particular patient. Red solid arrows indicate the most common direction for each scenario, followed by less prominent red arrows, and then dashed red arrows. Grey arrows indicate very unlikely directions for that particular scenario.

135

the atrial level). As PVR decreases, patients will become more tachypneic and exhibit signs of overcirculation. On cardiac exam, there is usually a mid-precordial impulse. The second heart sound is single and sometimes there could be an S_3 gallop. When the TV is significantly hypoplastic and stenotic, a diastolic rumble may be heard. There is a harsh high-frequency holosystolic murmur at the right midsternal border when there is significant TV insufficiency. This could be misinterpreted as MV regurgitation or a VSD.

There is a wide spectrum on the clinical presentation of children with RVDCC. Some children may have overt ischemia with shock and poor ventricular function, others may have ventricular tachycardia/fibrillation, but the majority have subtle episodes of angina/inconsolability with transient ST-segment changes.

Diagnosis
- **CXR.** Ranges from normal-sized cardiac silhouette to cardiomegaly with pulmonary edema and hyperinflation.
- **ECG.** RA enlargement. It may vary between nonspecific ST-T wave changes and significant ST-depression/elevation if there is significant coronary ischemia.
- **Echocardiogram (Figure 18-1).** Important features to assess include the type of pulmonary atresia (membranous/plate like or muscular obliteration), the characteristics of the TV (size, mobility, function), and the size and morphology of the RV. The size and character of the tricuspid valve mechanism are important, although in most cases, the actual size of the tricuspid orifice may be very difficult to determine in the setting of the very hypertensive RV. Much has been said of determining whether the RV is "tripartite" (inlet, trabecular, and infundibular portions), but this is probably overstated. The most important determinant in predicting an effective RV in the long term is whether or not there is a well-formed RV infundibulum in the newborn period. It is important to assess the function of both ventricles and the presence of any segmental wall motion abnormalities. Coronary artery anatomy should also be assessed. To-and-fro flow through the coronary arteries demonstrated by color Doppler suggests coronary-RV fistulas although it does not establish whether there is RVDCC or not. A subcostal/coronal view will demonstrate the presence of an atrial communication with obligatory right-to-left shunting. The atrial septum usually appears elongated and aneurysmatic.
- **Cardiac CTA.** Rarely necessary unless there are particular questions that arise from the echocardiogram. CTA does not identify the presence or absence of RVDCC.
- **Cardiac catheterization.** It is important to perform a cardiac catheterization in all patients with PA-IVS shortly after birth in order to define the presence or absence of RVDCC, evaluate the RV chamber size, and potentially establish a source of pulmonary blood flow. Cardiac catheterization is not only diagnostic but plays a significant role in the management strategy of these patients. Cardiac catheterization with an RV injection is critical to determine the presence and character of RV to coronary communications. Many patients will have RV to coronary sinusoids and, as such, when the RV is injected, one may observe extensive filling of the epicardial coronary arteries (Figure 18-2A). It is also critical to perform antegrade coronary angiography (ideally with direct ostial injection) to critically assess the nature of the RV communication, to ascertain whether or not there is ostial atresia, to determine

whether there are interrupted segments of the epicardial coronary arteries (and whether the interruptions/stenosis are located in the proximal or distal coronary arteries), and to answer the critical question of whether or not there are RVDCC (Figure 18-2B). The presence of extensive RV-to-coronary communications alone (in the absence of ostial atresia and/or interrupted segments of the epicardial coronaries) *does not* equate with the diagnosis of RVDCC. Furthermore, it must be noted that if one leaves the RV without decompression over the long term, these sinusoidal communications, which are by definition hypertensive relative to normal coronary artery pressure, will often lead to distortion of otherwise normal coronary arteries and may ultimately lead to an acquired RVDCC.

Indications / Timing for Intervention

All patients should undergo a diagnostic cardiac catheterization after stabilization. In addition, all patients will require a stable source of pulmonary blood flow in the newborn period. This can be accomplished by RVOT perforation in the cath lab, placement of a PDA stent, a modified Blalock-Taussig-Thomas shunt (mBTTS), creation of a transannular RVOT patch, or a combination of these techniques (see below).

Management

The management of patients with PA-IVS is complex due to the heterogeneity of the disease. Figure 18-3 shows the algorithm used for decision-making in this disease.

RVDCC

In babies with true RVDCC, the RV cannot be decompressed as this will lead to critical ischemia. Unfortunately, many of these babies are at risk for progressive stenoses of not only the connections, but the epicardial coronaries themselves. As such, critical ischemia and sudden cardiac death are important ongoing risks. In these babies, the next step in management is to establish a stable source of pulmonary blood flow. This is typically achieved by either placing a PDA stent or creating an mBTTS (see Chapter 38). Placement of a PDA stent often requires discontinuation of the PGE to allow for ductal constriction prior to placement of the stent. Whether one places a PDA stent or surgically creates a shunt, it is very important to avoid "over-shunting" the patients, which may exacerbate the propensity for ischemia. An advantage that ductal stenting may offer is the option of performing a balloon atrial septostomy which may be an important adjunct to management in babies with marginal atrial-level communications. It is critically important to note that in the setting of RVDCC, an attempt to decompress the RV may be a fatal proposition.

In those children with true RVDCC, the next step in the management algorithm is to consider cardiac transplantation. It must be noted (and thereby shared with the patient's parents), that the prospect for neonatal transplantation in terms of suitable donor organ availability is a statistically improbable consideration. This does *not* mean that newborns cannot be successfully transplanted; it does mean that listing does not equate with successful transplantation. As such, we have recommended urgent listing of appropriate candidates at the earliest appropriate time. While candidates are waiting, we have for the most part required the patients to stay in the hospital in an advanced care unit. While unheralded decompensations do occur (acute shunt occlusion, dysrhythmia), in

> **TCH experience with PA-IVS (1995-2017)**
> Number of patients: 89
> Median age at first intervention: 4 days (0-64 days)
> Median weight at first intervention: 3 kg (1-5 kg)
> Median TV Z-score at presentation: -2.5 (-5.3 – -2.2)
> Presence of RV-coronary fistulas: 42 (55%)
> RVDCC diagnosed at presentation: 20 (22%)
> Final strategy for patients (median follow-up 8 years):
> - 1-V Repair: 37%
> - 1.5-V Repair: 17%
> - 2-V Repair: 24%
> - Transplant: 3%
> - Death: 20%
>
> 10-year survival: 82%

most patients there are subtle warning signs that may signal impending decompensation (declining NIRS, declining SaO_2, poor weight gain, new ECG changes, etc.) that are potentially reversible if rapidly addressed. As the children get older, they may become eligible for second- (bidirectional Glenn shunt) or even third- (Fontan) stage palliation. We have had a number of children with RVDCC who have been successfully progressed through all stages of palliation. As an important intraoperative management point, children with RVDCC typically cannot tolerate complete RA (and thereby RV) decompression on CPB. As such, perfusion techniques designed to maintain RV filling (partial CPB or SVC-to-RA shunt with an oxygenator) are important along with very careful intraoperative assessment for ischemia, primarily as demonstrated by important ECG changes. It is also important to recognize that even after palliation with Glenn and Fontan circulations, these patients are at risk for coronary events and even sudden death, due to progressive distortion (or progression of stenoses/occlusions) of the coronary arteries. As such, routine surveillance and testing as an outpatient over time with a particular emphasis on the coronary arteries is mandatory.

RV Decompression

In patients without evidence of RVDCC, we have moved forward with efforts to open the pulmonary valve to promote prograde RV ejection, even in the setting of RV sinusoids. The first step is typically to perform a radiofrequency perforation (or perforation using chronic total occlusion guidewires) of the atretic pulmonary valve in the cardiac catheterization lab followed by serial balloon dilation. In some cases, this may be all that is needed and the patients may eventually be weaned from PGE with adequate prograde pulmonary blood flow provided by the RV. In patients in whom the RV cannot generate adequate blood flow, either a PDA stent or mBTTS is constructed. It has generally been our approach to allow the PDA to constrict and accept slightly low saturations in some patients in whom RV remodeling (with resultant improvement in saturations) can take months. If it is evident that a patient will require another source of pulmonary blood flow, this is usually performed 1-2 weeks later after a trial off PGE. However, in some cases, it is obvious at the initial cardiac catheterization that another source of pulmonary blood flow will be needed. In those instances, a PDA stent may be placed at the time of the initial procedure, or an mBTTS created soon afterward in the OR. If percutaneous pulmonary valvotomy is not successful, our management algorithm is to then perform an open pulmonary valvotomy with at most a minimal transannular incision. While we may then perform an RVOT resection, we do not favor a transmural infundibulotomy (RVOT incision) as some centers do. At the primary operation, we will usually perform an atrial septectomy and inspect the tricuspid valve, but do not attempt tricuspid valvuloplasty in most cases at this time.

RV "Overhaul"
In the presence of a well-formed infundibulum, even very diminutive RVs are amenable to promotion and may grow significantly. In shunted patients, the RV and PA morphology is carefully followed by echocardiography and catheterization or CTA. If the RV is muscle bound and not progressing in size, an intermediate operation is often necessary; typically around 3-6 months of life. This operation was initially described as an RV "overhaul" and consists of tricuspid valvuloplasty, RV endocardial and trabecular resection, and RVOT resection. This operation is done on CPB and the systemic-to-PA shunt is temporarily occluded. The patient is then left with a partially shunt-dependent circulation and RV progress is carefully monitored.

1.5-Ventricle Repair
In some patients, the RV never progresses to the degree that it is capable of handling the entire cardiac output. Our experience suggests that often, the rate-limiting feature is the TV dimension. It is unwise to attempt to "force" more flow through the TV than it can accommodate. If the true tricuspid orifice (not the annular dimension, but the actual effective orifice) is 50% or less than what it should be for the patient's BSA, one should strongly consider a 1.5-ventricle repair. This operation includes RV endocardial/trabecular resection, partial or complete ASD closure, takedown of the systemic-to-PA shunt, and creation of a bidirectional Glenn anastomosis. This can be a very effective circulation, which provides reasonable pulmonary blood flow (SaO_2 usually in the mid-to-high 90s even if there is a small ASD left), and low hepatic venous pressures. Of note, we have not typically placed a pulmonary valve in most cases.

Biventricular Repair
The decision to proceed with a septated circulation may be challenging in cases of a truncated RV or marginal TV. If the right-sided structures are believed to be adequate, the ASD is completely closed and CPB weaned while measuring RA pressures. If the measured CVP is <10-12 mmHg with good cardiac output, the chest is closed. If it is greater than this, CPB is reinstituted and a small (4-5 mm) fenestration is created in the atrial septum. Later in life, test occlusion and even permanent closure of the ASD can be performed in the cardiac catheterization laboratory.

Fontan Circulation
Other than patients with RVDCC, there are some patients with a previously decompressed RV in whom a Fontan operation may ultimately be necessary. This occurs in cases of a very small TV, an RV that fails to progress, and inadequate pulmonary blood flow to maintain adequate oxygen saturations. In such cases, the additional flow provided by a total cavopulmonary connection Fontan is warranted. In the setting of PI, it may be

necessary to place a patch over the TV (carefully avoiding the AV node) to prevent a circular shunt after the Fontan connection.

Isolated Pulmonary Valvar and Supravalvar Stenosis

Isolated PS is the most common valvar abnormality that requires intervention in the neonatal period. Valvar PS has been associated with Allagille and DiGeorge syndromes, while supravalvular PS has been associated with Williams and Noonan syndromes.

Pathophysiology and Clinical Presentation

Overall, there are 3 distinct types of valvar PS: critical neonatal PS, typical PS, and dysplastic PS. *Critical PS* presents in the newborn period as cyanosis, and is defined as PS that is ductal-dependent for pulmonary blood flow. Cyanosis is the result of right-to-left shunting at the atrial level. These patients will present with decreased pulmonary blood flow and may have variable degrees of diastolic dysfunction from severe RV hypertrophy. Patients who have *typical PS* have leaflets that are fused and the main PA demonstrates poststenotic dilation. Patients with *dysplastic pulmonary valves* have thicker leaflets than those with typical PS, and little or no leaflet fusion. The main PA segment is small and frequently, the branch PAs are also small. This form of PS is seen in patients with Noonan syndrome, Williams syndrome, and other genetic conditions.

On clinical exam, there will be a prominent RV impulse with or without a thrill, a systolic ejection click, and a harsh systolic ejection murmur. The murmur frequency will vary depending on the degree of valvar stenosis and the PVR. At birth, the murmur will likely be low frequency, and as PVR decreases, the frequency of the murmur will increase. In cases of supravalvular PS, the exam will be similar, with the exception of the systolic ejection click, which will be absent. Depending on the degree of obstruction, there can be hepatomegaly secondary to a combination of high RV afterload and diastolic dysfunction.

Diagnosis

- **ECG.** Significant RVH and possible RA enlargement.
- **CXR.** Nonspecific. In severe cases, it will show decreased pulmonary blood flow (oligemic lungs).
- **Echocardiogram (Figure 18-4).** There is typically fusion of the valvar commissures that prevents complete opening or "doming" during systole, leaving a small orifice for ventricular stroke volume ejection. There are variable degrees of RV hypertrophy and/or hypoplasia. It is important to perform a careful assessment of the size and z-score of the branch PAs, the presence or absence of collaterals, and the presence of a PDA.

Indications / Timing for Intervention

Patients with severe PS (and some with moderate PS) require intervention to relieve the obstruction. Indications for intervention include patients with critical PS and patients with a peak gradient >40 mmHg by TTE or a peak-to-peak systolic gradient >40 mmHg in the cardiac catheterization laboratory. Lesser gradients may be an indication to intervene in the presence of RV dysfunction or poor cardiac output.

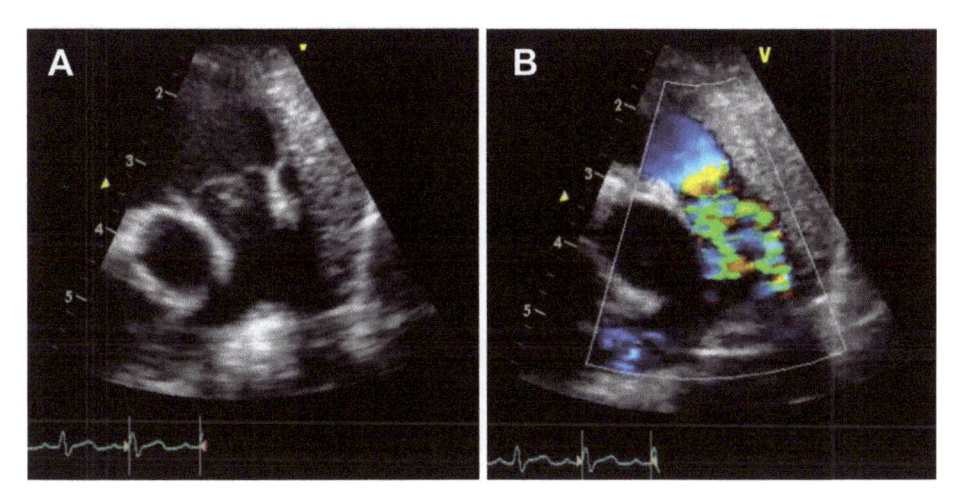

Figure 18-4. Parasternal short-axis 2D (A) and color-Doppler (B) echocardiographic views showing a doming pulmonary valve with PS.

Catheter-Based Intervention

Percutaneous balloon valvuloplasty is the treatment of choice for isolated valvar PS. Neonates with critical PS may require intervention to be able to stop PGE administration and improve oxygen saturations. In our experience, roughly 20-30% of patients with critical PS will need reintervention after balloon valvuloplasty (either an alternate source of pulmonary blood supply, or repeat balloon pulmonary valvuloplasty or RVOT surgery) in the first 4 months of life. A small minority of patients will not exhibit adequate RV growth and may require a Glenn or an RV overhaul operation later on.

The fused valves in patients with typical PS are very amenable to balloon valvuloplasty with nearly all procedures being successful, as the areas of fusion can be easily torn with a balloon. These patients typically present a large main PA due to poststenotic dilation (Figure 18-5A).

For patients with dysplastic pulmonary valves (Figure 18-5B), the success rate for balloon valvuloplasty is less (approximately 50%). These patients may require more than one catheter procedure, larger balloons, and inflations at higher pressure to relieve the obstruction. Those who do not respond with these catheter-based interventions require surgical relief of the obstruction.

Catheterization Procedure

During the cardiac catheterization procedure, careful pullback measurements are made to discern the exact level of obstruction and to ensure there are no other obstructions present in the branch PAs or RVOT. Angiography with delineation of the anatomy and pulmonary valve annulus is made. Generally, a balloon is initially chosen that is 1.2-1.3 times the pulmonary valve annulus. With a properly selected balloon (exception being dysplastic pulmonary valves), a waist is seen at the narrow segment within the leaflets, that yields with inflation. After inflation, pressure measurements are made to determine whether further intervention is warranted. The goal of the procedure is

PART II. DISEASES

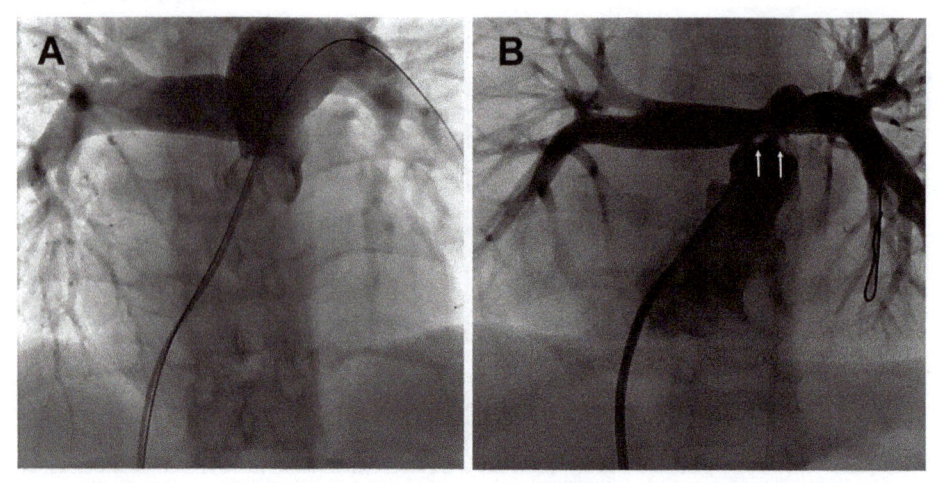

Figure 18-5. A) Main PA angiogram in a 15-year-old with typical valvar PS. Note the dilated main PA segment. B) Main PA angiogram in an infant with a dysplastic pulmonary valve. The small main PA can be seen, as can the very thick dysplastic pulmonary valve leaflets (arrows).

not to completely abolish the gradient, as more than desired PI (requiring treatment later in life) may develop. Mild-to-moderate PS is tolerated well for many years, if not for one's entire life.

Postcatheterization Management
PGE may be maintained in the immediate post-balloon-valvuloplasty period. Cyanosis and desaturations may still be present secondary to significant RV diastolic dysfunction and right-to-left shunting through the PFO. Diastolic dysfunction, especially when there is RV hypoplasia, tends to improve after several days and more than one attempt at weaning PGE.

Postcatheterization Follow-Up
Repeat balloon valvuloplasty may be needed in some patients, particularly younger patients or patients with dysplastic pulmonary valves. PI is common in follow-up and a small subset of patients may require pulmonary valve replacement later in life. For patients with critical PS, PGE can be stopped after the procedure, and patients should be monitored for the need for another source of pulmonary blood flow or reintervention on the RVOT. In these patients, remodeling of the RV may take months, and some degree of cyanosis is expected during this timeframe.

Surgical Intervention
Surgical intervention is reserved for patients who fail percutaneous balloon valvuloplasty or those in which the annulus of the pulmonary valve is significantly hypoplastic. Patients with isolated valvar PS and a reasonable annulus may benefit from surgical valvotomy (carefully incising into each of the commissures to enlarge the effective orifice of the valve) and/or debridement of thickened and dysplastic pulmonary valve leaflets. Patients with a significantly hypoplastic pulmonary annulus may require a

transannular pulmonary patch to enlarge the RVOT. In cases of supravalvar PS, patients may undergo patch enlargement of the supravalvar area with either a single patch or a pantaloon patch (analogous to supravalvar aortic stenosis repair, see Chapter 24). Patients with critical PS may require placement of an aortopulmonary shunt to supplement pulmonary blood flow (see Chapter 38).

In patients with long-standing PS, secondary muscular infundibular obstruction develops over time and may result in residual obstruction after open valvotomy. Our practice has been to carry out a careful infundibular resection through the pulmonary valve if there appears to be the potential for residual muscular obstruction.

19 Absent Pulmonary Valve Syndrome

Judith A. Becker, Ashraf Resheidat, Carlos M. Mery

Absent pulmonary valve syndrome (APVS) is a rare congenital heart disease that is characterized by a large conoventricular VSD, aortic override, and either absence or severe underdevelopment of the pulmonary valve leaflets, usually with a small pulmonary valve annulus. Even though APVS is sometimes described as a variant of tetralogy of Fallot, the anatomy and pathophysiology of these diseases are quite different. Due to the absence of a competent pulmonary valve and the presence of a stenotic pulmonary valve annulus, there is typically both significant obstruction and severe insufficiency of the pulmonary valve. Classically, these patients do not have a ductus arteriosus. The infundibulum is long and muscularized, and contrary to tetralogy of Fallot, these patients tend not to have significant infundibular muscular obstruction. In utero, patients with APVS have to-and-fro flow between the RV and the PAs, which in turn results in significant aneurysmal dilation of the main and branch PAs. Because of PA enlargement, patients can have significant extrinsic compression of the trachea and bronchi. Chronic compression can lead to significant tracheobronchomalacia, which may persist for a long time after repair, and may impact patient survival. APVS can be associated with genetic syndromes including DiGeorge syndrome and other extracardiac abnormalities such as single umbilical artery, abnormal brain development, omphalocele, skeletal anomalies, and polydactyly.

Pathophysiology and Clinical Presentation

Clinical presentation is variable. The most important determinant of presentation is the degree of PA dilation and compression of the tracheobronchial tree. Nowadays, a large proportion of children with APVS are diagnosed in utero, allowing for delivery in a tertiary care center where teams can develop an appropriate management strategy. Patients with severe main and branch PA dilation and airway compression will present with respiratory distress, hypercarbia, and respiratory acidosis in the newborn period requiring mechanical ventilation. Some patients require high ventilatory pressures to overcome the airway compression or may even require prone positioning to help alleviate the gravitational effect of the large PAs compressing the airway. Pulmonary hyperinflation can be significant and can cause mediastinal shift or contribute to further compression of mediastinal structures. Patients will have variable degrees of cyanosis from right-to-left shunting across the VSD in the setting of high PVR and PI. With adequate ventilation, as PVR decreases, some of these children (in particular those with larger pulmonary annuli) will develop a net left-to-right shunt. Patients with less significant PA dilation may present with milder respiratory symptoms.

On exam, patients tend to have a hyperdynamic precordium with a single S_1 and S_2. There is a systolic and diastolic (to-and-fro, rather than continuous) murmur heard best at the mid-to-upper left sternal border, with wide radiation.

19. ABSENT PULMONARY VALVE SYNDROME

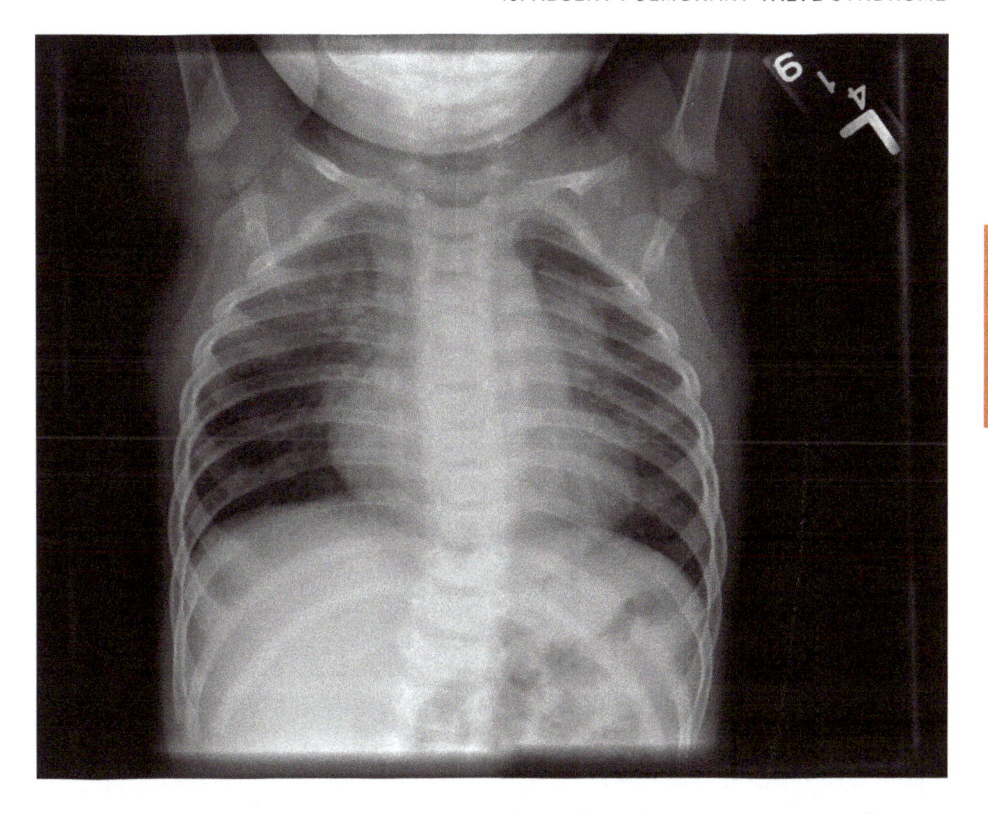

Figure 19-1. CXR showing hyperinflated lungs, a boot-shaped heart, and prominent PAs.

Diagnosis
- **Fetal echocardiogram.** The presence of dilated branch PAs should raise the suspicion of APVS. In addition, the RV is usually dilated, there is some narrowing at the level of the pulmonary annulus, and to-and-fro flow can be documented across the RVOT by color and spectral Doppler. A ductus arteriosus is usually absent; the presence of a duct worsens the prognosis.
- **CXR (Figure 19-1).** Demonstrates hyperinflation with diffuse or localized air trapping. The prominent aneurysmal branch PAs can be visualized at the hilum. The cardiac silhouette has a boot-shape appearance due to RV hypertrophy.
- **ECG.** May demonstrate LVH as well as RVH, in contrast to the child with tetralogy of Fallot that does not typically present LVH.
- **Echocardiogram (Figure 19-2).** Demonstrates a large conoventricular VSD, a narrow infundibulum and pulmonary valve with to-and-fro flow through a rudimentary pulmonary valve or thickened annulus. The dilation of the MPA and branch PAs can be observed on echocardiography. Windows may be limited due to pulmonary hyperinflation. As PVR drops, the antegrade velocity across the RVOT increases.
- **CTA (Figure 19-3).** Cross-sectional imaging with CTA (or less likely MRI) is useful

PART II. DISEASES

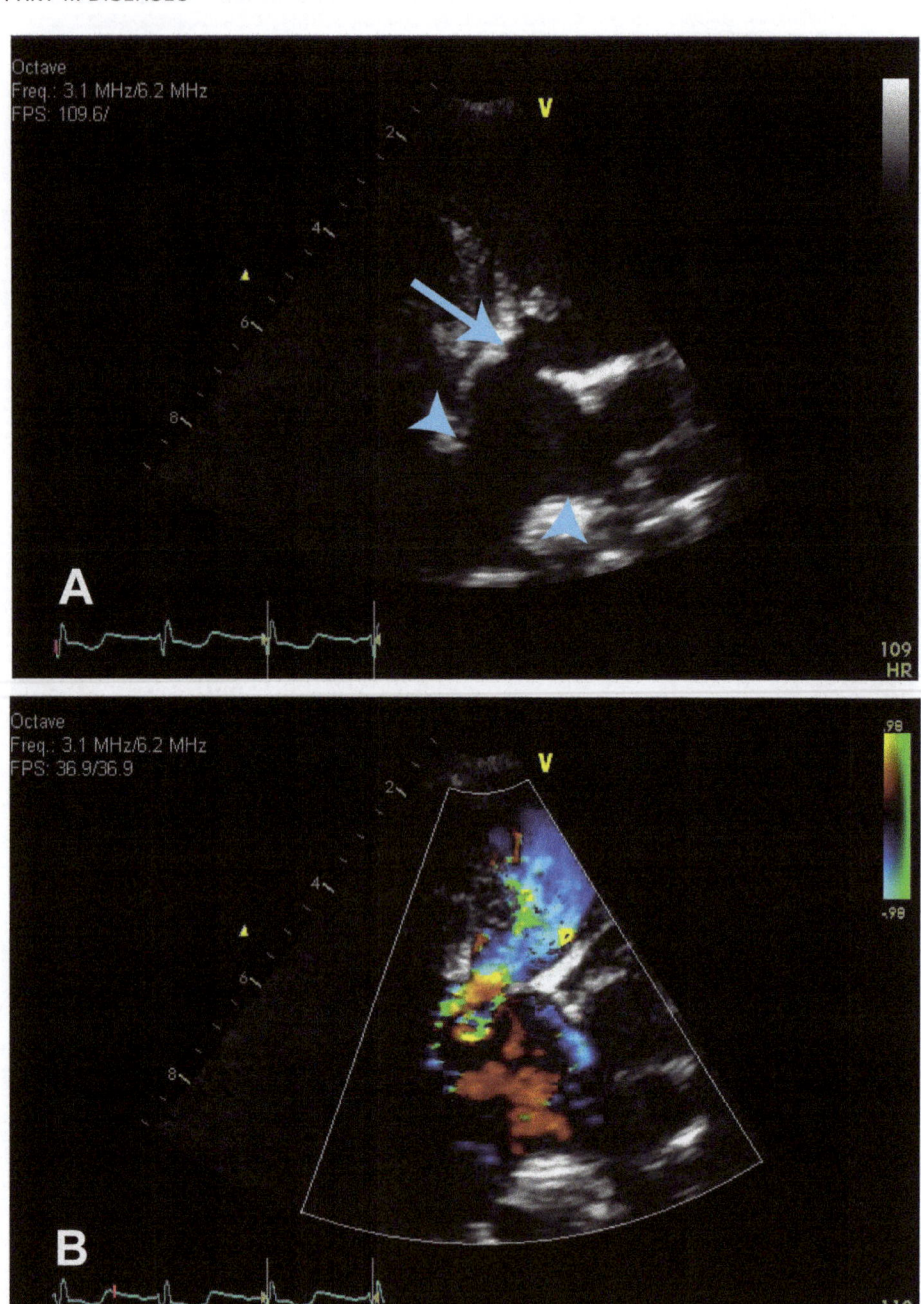

Figure 19-2. Parasternal short-axis view in a patient with APVS. Panel A shows a stenotic annulus (arrow) with an absent pulmonary valve and massively dilated branch PAs (arrowheads). Panel B with color shows increased velocity across the annulus.

19. ABSENT PULMONARY VALVE SYNDROME

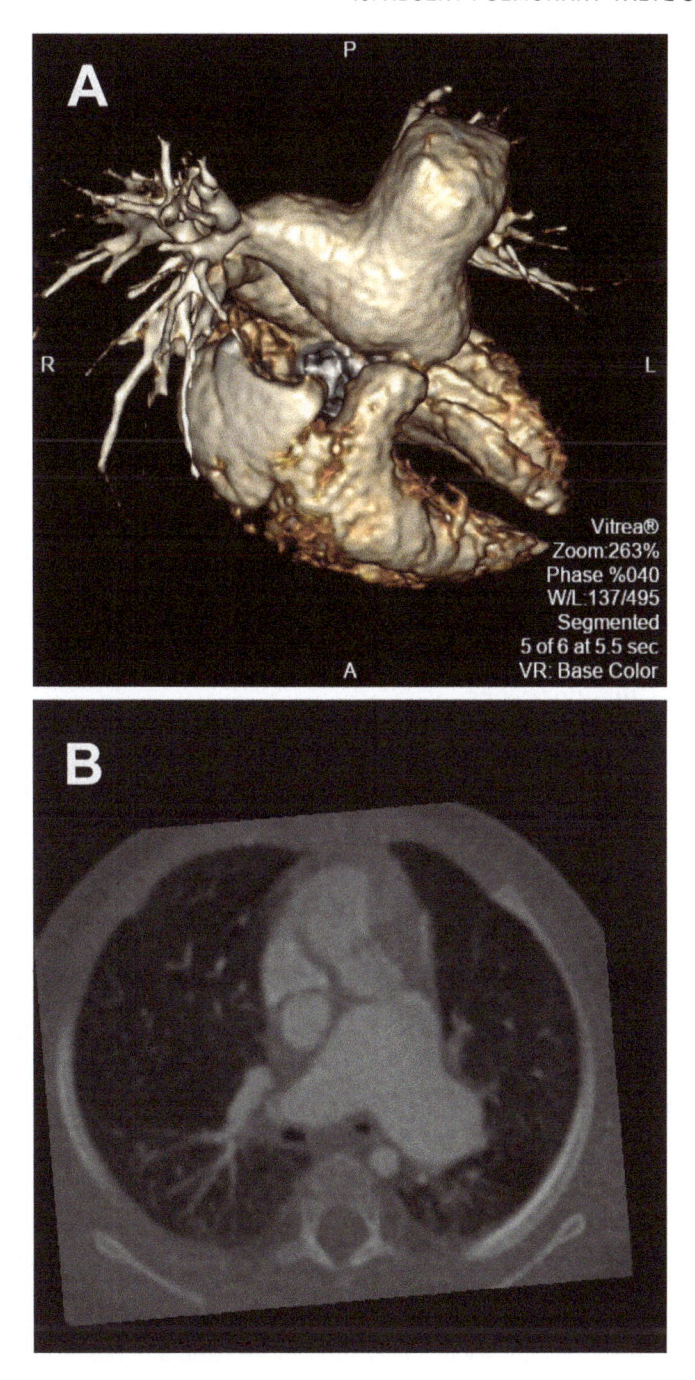

Figure 19-3. CT reconstruction of a patient with APVS (A) showing aneurysmal branch PAs. The axial cuts (B) show compression of the bronchi by the dilated branch PAs and hyperinflation of the right upper and middle lobes.

to assess the degree of PA dilation, the compression of the tracheobronchial tree, and the degree of distal airspace disease. Dynamic airway CT can help document the presence of dynamic tracheobronchomalacia in addition to the fixed compression of the airway.
- **Direct laryngoscopy and bronchoscopy (DL&B).** Used sometimes at the time of the repair to determine the degree of airway narrowing and dynamic tracheobronchomalacia.
- **Other studies.** Genetic evaluation should be undertaken in the newborn period if not accomplished prenatally. An ionized calcium should be obtained as ~20% of these children will have DiGeorge syndrome.

Indications / Timing for Intervention

The optimal timing for surgical repair of patients with APVS depends on the clinical status of the patient. Surgical repair is undertaken during the neonatal period for those patients that are ventilator-dependent due to the degree of tracheobronchial compression, or those that have significant cyanosis. Repair is delayed until later in infancy (6-12 months) in patients that are extubated in the neonatal period and have minimal or absent respiratory symptoms with adequate oxygen saturations.

Anesthetic Considerations

One of the main anesthetic concerns for these patients is the airway. Neuromuscular blockade during intubation can lead to worsening airway compression and inability to ventilate the patient. In the OR, induction is conducted with inhaled anesthetics and spontaneous breathing to determine the degree of airway obstruction prior to neuromuscular paralysis. Usually, higher airway pressures are required to maintain good oxygenation. A prolonged expiratory phase may help with ventilation.

Surgical Repair

Surgical intervention entails repair of the VSD, relief of RVOT obstruction, and reduction/plication of the branch PAs. The repair is performed using standard median sternotomy and bicaval cannulation, usually under moderate hypothermia. Working through a right atriotomy, a VSD baffle between the LV and the aorta is created with autologous pericardium. Care is taken not to injure the conduction system that travels on the posteroinferior margin of the VSD. A longitudinal incision is performed on the main PA and extended proximally into the infundibulum. Patients with APVS tend to have a long, narrow, and muscular infundibulum. As such, the incision usually extends more proximally than in patients with tetralogy of Fallot. The goal is to achieve an RVOT opening equal or larger than the expected measurement of the pulmonary valve for their BSA.

The pulmonary arterioplasty involves anterior excision and posterior plication of the branch PAs. An oval-shaped segment of tissue is excised from the anterior surface of each branch PA. The excision extends from the main pulmonary arteriotomy up to the hilum of each lung. It is useful to mark the branch PAs with fine sutures in advance in order to define the extent of the incision, since it is difficult to assess the redundant vessels once they are open and decompressed. A running sutureline is then started on the posterior wall of each branch PA, just proximal to the segmental branches, and run towards the main PA while incrementally grabbing more posterior tissue, therefore performing a posterior plication. The anterior edges are then reapproximated with running suture. It is important to measure each branch PA with a dilator to assure that the vessels are not narrowed.

Because of the relatively high PVR and airway issues, patients with APVS tend not to tolerate severe PI in the early postoperative period as well as patients with tetralogy of Fallot. It is therefore important to provide some pulmonary valve competence in the early postoperative period. In general, newborns that require surgical intervention will undergo pulmonary valve replacement with a homograft conduit. Older patients may benefit from either a pulmonary valve replacement or creation of a monocusp valve. Monocusp valves tend to provide competence in the early postoperative period but usually fail with time.

Postoperative Management / Complications

- **Respiratory compromise from airway compression.** Despite performing PA plication and relieving the tracheal and bronchial compression, tracheobronchomalacia tends to persist for a few weeks or months. Some of these patients require positive pressure ventilation for a prolonged time, sometimes with high airway pressures required and frequent airway clearing maneuvers. These patients remain at high risk for barotrauma. Ventilator strategies should be adjusted to avoid lung hyperinflation and barotrauma, if possible. It is important to evaluate the ideal ventilator settings frequently in the first postoperative days, as especially the PEEP levels required to prevent airway collapse or hyperinflation may vary. Some patients may require frequent bronchoscopy procedures to clear the airways from any additional obstruction. Patients with absent or mild respiratory symptoms can usually be extubated in the immediate postoperative period. Patients with early severe respiratory symptoms may require prolonged intubation, and a small number of them require tracheostomy.
- **RV dysfunction.** Just like patients with tetralogy of Fallot and other diseases with RVH, patients are at risk for diastolic dysfunction. Significant PI may worsen the RV dysfunction, especially in newborns. The use of a monocusp or other type of competent valve in the pulmonary position may ameliorate the volume overload of the RV. Milrinone and iNO can help with RV afterload reduction. Heart-rate control may improve RV filling in the setting of diastolic dysfunction. RV diastolic dysfunction is also responsive to volume resuscitation.
- **Arrhythmias.** Right-bundle-branch block is not uncommon in these patients due to the VSD sutureline. Other potential arrhythmias include AV delays, heart block, or JET. Temporary pacing wires are useful to help manage postoperative arrhythmias.

20 Tricuspid Atresia

Elena C. Ocampo, Carlos M. Mery

Tricuspid atresia is a type of single-ventricle CHD that is characterized by the absence of the tricuspid valve, such that there is no direct communication between the RA and the RV. An ASD with an obligate right-to-left shunt is present in all cases and is crucial for survival. Other cardiac anomalies are typically present such as a VSD, transposition of the great arteries, pulmonary atresia or hypoplasia, aortic stenosis, coarctation of the aorta, PDA and a left SVC. The RV is typically hypoplastic, the degree of which depends on the presence and size of the VSD. Other extracardiac anomalies may be present as well.

Classification
The classification of tricuspid atresia is based on the relationship of the great vessels, the presence and size of a VSD, and the amount of pulmonary blood flow:
- Type I: Normally related great arteries (~70%)
  - Ia: No VSD, pulmonary atresia
  - Ib: Small VSD, pulmonary stenosis
  - Ic: Large VSD, no pulmonary stenosis
- Type II: D-transposition of the great arteries (TGA) (~25%)
  - IIa: VSD, pulmonary atresia
  - IIb: VSD, pulmonary or subpulmonary stenosis
  - IIc: Large VSD, no pulmonary stenosis
- Type III: L-TGA (~5%)
  - IIIa: VSD, pulmonary or subpulmonary stenosis
  - IIIb: Subaortic stenosis

A useful way of remembering the subclassification for types I and II is "a" for atresia (pulmonary atresia), "b" for balanced circulation (pulmonary stenosis), and "c" for overCirculation (no pulmonary stenosis).

Pathophysiology and Clinical Presentation
Infants can present with cyanosis, CHF symptoms, or relatively asymptomatic, depending on the amount of pulmonary blood flow and the presence of systemic outflow obstruction.

Infants with decreased pulmonary blood flow (types Ia and IIa) present with cyanosis within the first 24-48 hours of life when the PDA closes. Severe cyanosis can lead to acidosis and shock. Those with unrestricted pulmonary blood flow (types Ic and IIc) present with signs of CHF when the PVR drops. A balanced circulation may be possible in patients with types Ib and IIb.

An important consideration in patients with tricuspid atresia and TGA is that the aorta arises from the hypoplastic RV and flow into the aortic valve is dependent on blood crossing the VSD to reach the aorta. Determining the size and type of VSD (muscular VSDs tend to decrease in size with time) is crucial to prevent the development of

20. TRICUSPID ATRESIA

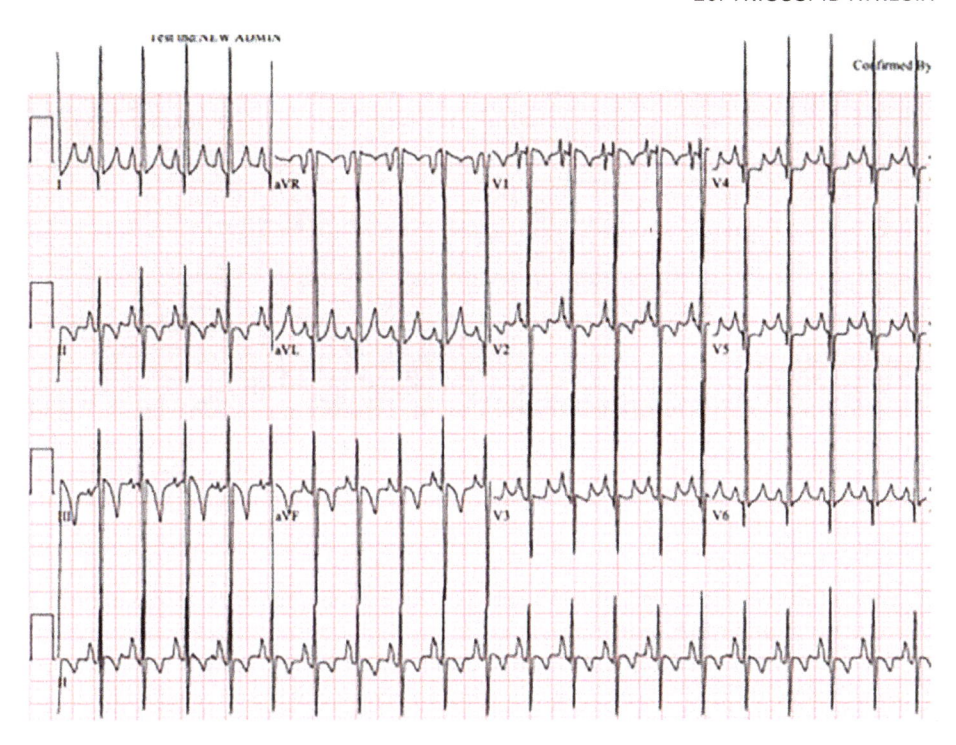

Figure 20-1. ECG on a patient with tricuspid atresia.

systemic outflow obstruction. In general, if a patient with tricuspid atresia and TGA also has an aortic coarctation and/or a hypoplastic aortic arch, it is likely that the VSD is not large enough to sustain the systemic circulation in the long term.

It is important to note that an unrestricted atrial level communication is necessary for survival, and an emergent balloon atrial septostomy may be indicated.

Diagnosis

- **CXR.** The appearance will depend on the amount of pulmonary blood flow. Patients with diminished pulmonary blood flow will have a normal or mildly enlarged cardiac silhouette with decreased pulmonary vascular markings. Patients with increased pulmonary blood flow will have cardiomegaly and pulmonary congestion.
- **ECG (Figure 20-1).** A typical ECG will show RA enlargement, left-axis deviation, and decreased RV forces with LVH.
- **Fetal echocardiogram.** Tricuspid atresia in a fetus is suspected when a hypoplastic RV is seen in a typical 4-chamber view performed routinely. A full study demonstrates the absence of inflow to the RV and a plate-like tricuspid valve. In tricuspid atresia with an intact ventricular septum, the RV and PA will be severely hypoplastic and the PDA will be small. The aorta will typically be enlarged as it carries the combined cardiac output. Other associated lesions will need to be demonstrated clearly, such as the atrial communication, VSD presence and size,

151

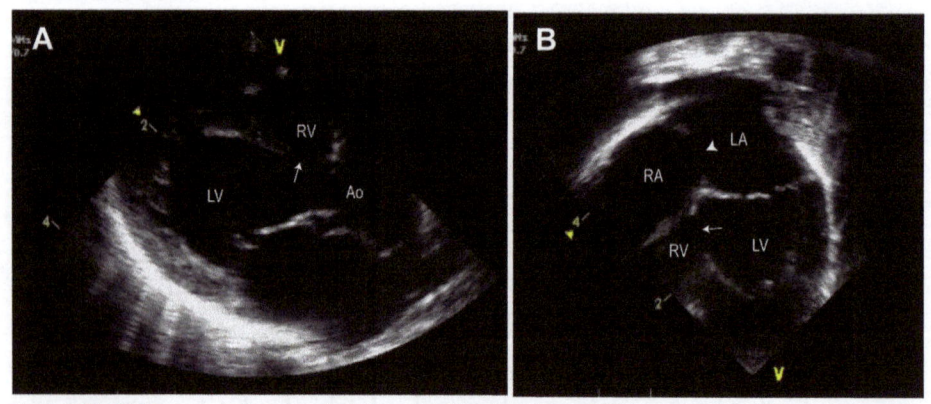

Figure 20-2. Parasternal long-axis (A) and 4-chamber (B) echocardiographic views of a patient with tricuspid atresia and normally related great vessels. There is no communication between the RA and the hypoplastic RV. A large ASD (arrowhead) and a large VSD (arrow) are visualized. Images courtesy of Dr. Josh Kailin, www.pedecho.org.

- great vessel relationship, and associated cardiac anomalies. This allows planning for delivery and need for PGE infusion.
- **Postnatal echocardiogram (Figure 20-2).** Echocardiography is the standard imaging technique for diagnosis, showing an absence of the tricuspid valve with a hypoplastic RV. The presence and size of the VSD, the semilunar valves, the relationship of the great vessels, the size of the ASD, and the presence of other cardiac defects need to be well delineated.
- **CTA.** Cross-sectional imaging is typically not required to make a diagnosis of tricuspid atresia. However, it may be useful if the anatomy of the PA, PDA, or aortic arch is unclear on echocardiography.
- **Cardiac catheterization.** Rarely needed for diagnostic purposes. It may be used in certain circumstances for PDA stenting (see Chapter 38).

Surgical Considerations

Patients with tricuspid atresia will require staged surgical palliation towards a Fontan circulation. For details of the single ventricle paradigm, timing of intervention, and surgical techniques, see Chapter 39.

The details of management of patients with tricuspid atresia will depend on the clinical presentation (Figure 20-3). Patients with increased pulmonary blood flow and CHF symptoms will require placement of a PA band (see Chapter 39) in order to protect the pulmonary vasculature prior to the second stage of palliation (bidirectional Glenn). Patients with decreased pulmonary blood flow and significant cyanosis may require administration of PGE to keep the ductus arteriosus open, followed by placement of a shunt or PDA stent (see Chapter 38) in order to provide a stable source of pulmonary blood flow prior to the second stage. Some patients will have a relatively balanced circulation or mild CHF symptoms or cyanosis. These patients can be observed closely until the second stage of palliation, which is usually performed between 4 and 6 months

20. TRICUSPID ATRESIA

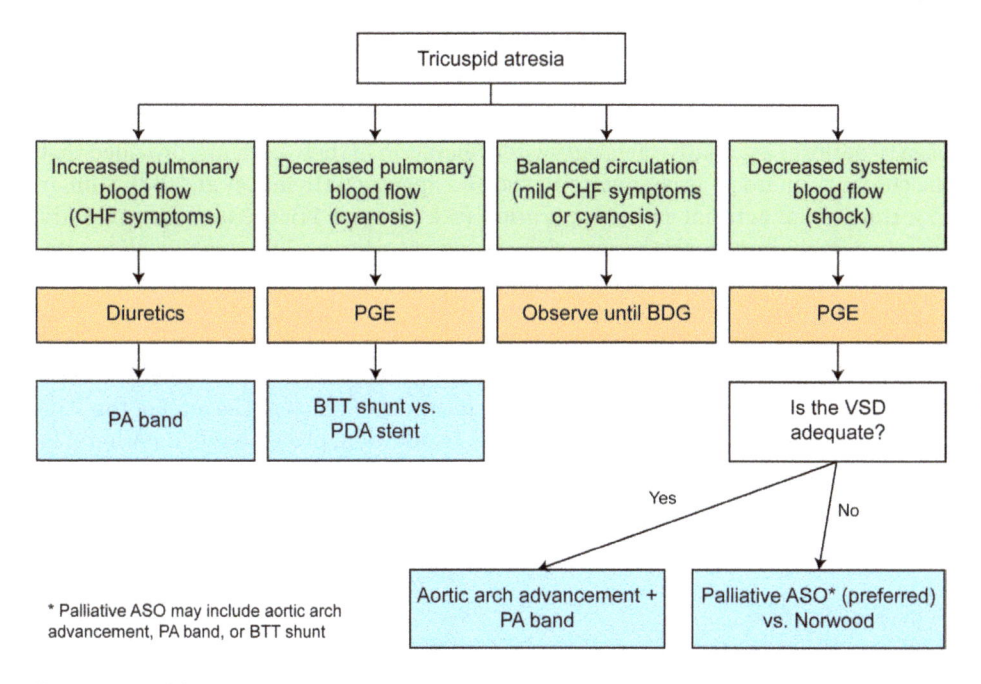

Figure 20-3. Management algorithm for patients with tricuspid atresia based on clinical presentation. ASO: arterial switch operation, BDG: bidirectional Glenn, BTT: Blalock-Taussig-Thomas, PGE: prostaglandin.

of age. However, it is not unusual for patients that start with a balanced circulation to develop significant cyanosis due to progressive closure of the VSD over the first few weeks or months of life.

Patients with tricuspid atresia and TGA pose a challenging situation. A careful assessment is necessary to decide whether the VSD (which serves as the systemic outflow tract) and the aortic arch are adequate to sustain the systemic circulation. If the arch is inadequate and the VSD is considered large enough, the patient may undergo an aortic arch reconstruction (usually an aortic arch advancement, see Chapter 25) and placement of a PA band as a first stage. It is important though not to pursue this approach if the VSD is marginal as the patient will be left with a doubly obstructed heart. A careful determination will then need to be made at the second stage to reassess the size of the VSD. Further narrowing of the VSD may dictate the creation of a Damus-Kaye-Stansel (DKS) anastomosis (anastomosing the proximal ascending aorta with the proximal PA in order to provide unimpeded cardiac outflow) at the time of the Glenn. An incorrect judgment of the VSD at this stage with oversewing of the pulmonary valve and PA at the time of the Glenn may lead to significant subaortic obstruction in the long term, a condition that is challenging to treat and with suboptimal results.

If the VSD (and therefore the systemic outflow) is deemed to be inadequate at the newborn period, there are 2 surgical options: a Norwood-type procedure and a palliative arterial switch operation. Most centers would pursue a Norwood-type strategy for these patients (see Chapter 27). However, the anteroposterior arrangement of the vessels makes a DKS anastomosis suboptimal and can lead to entrapment of the left PA by the dilated DKS with time. Therefore, the preferred strategy at TCH has been to perform a palliative arterial switch operation in these patients, provided that the coronary anatomy is conducive to such an approach (Heinle et al. 2013). Similar to a traditional arterial switch operation (see Chapter 14), the aorta and PA are switched, including translocation of the coronary arteries. This strategy aligns the LV (with the unobstructed outflow) with the aorta, and the RV (with the obstructed VSD and outflow) with the PA. Most of these patients will also require an aortic arch reconstruction. In these cases, if there is significant discrepancy between the proximal PA and the smaller ascending aorta, the ascending aorta may be enlarged with a small autologous pericardial or homograft patch. If the obstruction at the level of the VSD is not that significant, patients may require, in addition, placement of a PA band in order to further limit the pulmonary blood flow. In some other occasions, placement of an additional Blalock-Taussig-Thomas shunt (see Chapter 38) may be necessary to increase pulmonary blood flow.

Suggested Reading

Heinle JS, Carberry KE, McKenzie ED, et al. Outcomes after the palliative arterial switch operation in neonates with single-ventricle anatomy. Ann Thorac Surg 2013;95:212-218.

21 Ebstein Anomaly

Heather A. Dickerson, Stuart R. Hall, Charles D. Fraser Jr.

Ebstein anomaly is a very rare congenital heart lesion representing <1% of all CHD. It is a complex condition involving failure of tricuspid valve leaflet delamination during embryogenesis. It represents a broad continuum of morphologic derangements but the central defining feature is apical displacement of the septal leaflet of the tricuspid valve, usually associated with severe TR. Even though the septal leaflet tends to be the most involved, usually all 3 leaflets are involved to a certain extent, with the anterior leaflet being the least involved. The leaflets tend to be dysplastic, muscularized, and tethered to short chords and papillary muscles that may insert directly into the leaflets. The valve is spirally rotated with the septal and posterior leaflets displaced inferiorly into the RV. This in turn displaces the functional annulus of the valve downward, leaving a variable portion of RV on the atrial side of the valve leaflets ("atrialized" portion of the RV). The atrialized portion of the RV tends to be thin and dyskinetic, and is usually significantly dilated due to the degree of TR. This also leads to significant dilation of the true annulus of the tricuspid valve.

Pathophysiology and Clinical Presentation

In Ebstein anomaly, the degree of prograde flow across the RV is limited due to the severe TR and variable impairment of RV function. In addition, the atrialized portion of the RV tends to distend during atrial contraction, further limiting prograde flow. All of these structural abnormalities lead to massive right-heart dilation. Massive right-heart dilation can lead to in utero underdevelopment of the lungs due to lack of physical space. Patients with Ebstein anomaly will usually have an ASD that tends to shunt right to left, causing variable degrees of cyanosis.

The clinical presentation varies significantly depending on the degree of TR, degree of RA dilation, extent of atrialization of the RV, RV function, and degree of pulmonary hypoplasia. It can vary from cardiogenic shock in the neonate to an asymptomatic presentation in adulthood.

In neonates, the high PVR and the presence of a ductus arteriosus lead to a higher afterload of the RV, further limiting prograde flow. As such, neonates tend to present with variable degrees of cyanosis and heart failure.

Patients with less severe forms of the disease, or those who survive the neonatal period without intervention, may present later in life with cyanosis, decreased exercise tolerance, dyspnea on exertion, or palpitations due to arrhythmias. A systolic murmur in the left sternal border is usually heard, and there is wide splitting of the first and second heart sounds. There may be IJ distention.

Children and adults with Ebstein anomaly are at significant risk for atrial tachyarrhythmias (atrial ectopic tachycardia and atrial flutter) due to RA dilation. In addition, 15-20% of patients have accessory pathways along the tricuspid valve annulus that can lead to reentrant supraventricular tachycardia.

PART II. DISEASES

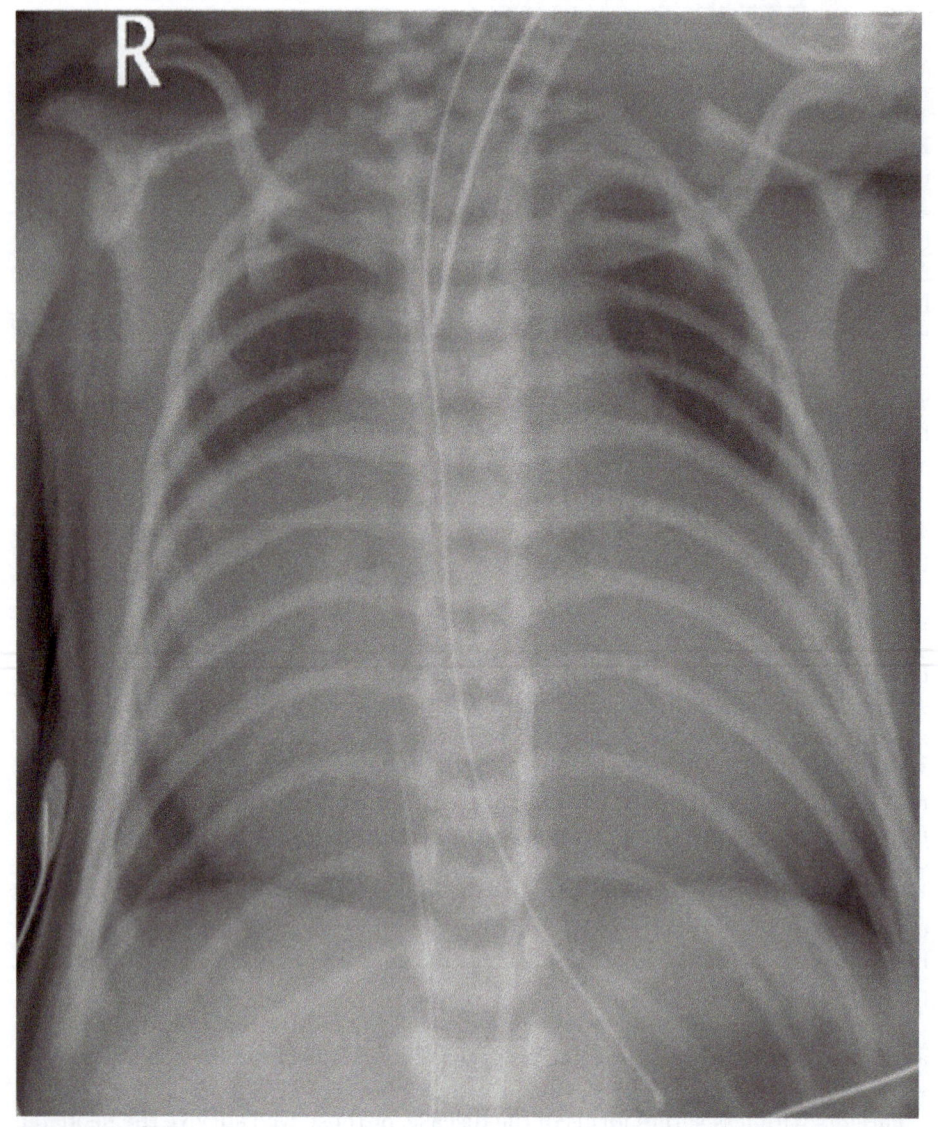

Figure 21-1. CXR in an infant with Ebstein anomaly showing massive cardiomegaly due to severe RA dilation.

Diagnosis
- **Fetal echocardiography.** The diagnosis of Ebstein anomaly is now frequently made in fetal life by identifying apical displacement of the tricuspid valve, severe TR, an atrialized RV, and RA dilation.
- **ECG.** RA enlargement and diminished RV forces. It may also show ventricular preexcitation (Delta wave) consistent with Wolff-Parkinson-White syndrome as accessory pathways are common in this disease.

21. EBSTEIN ANOMALY

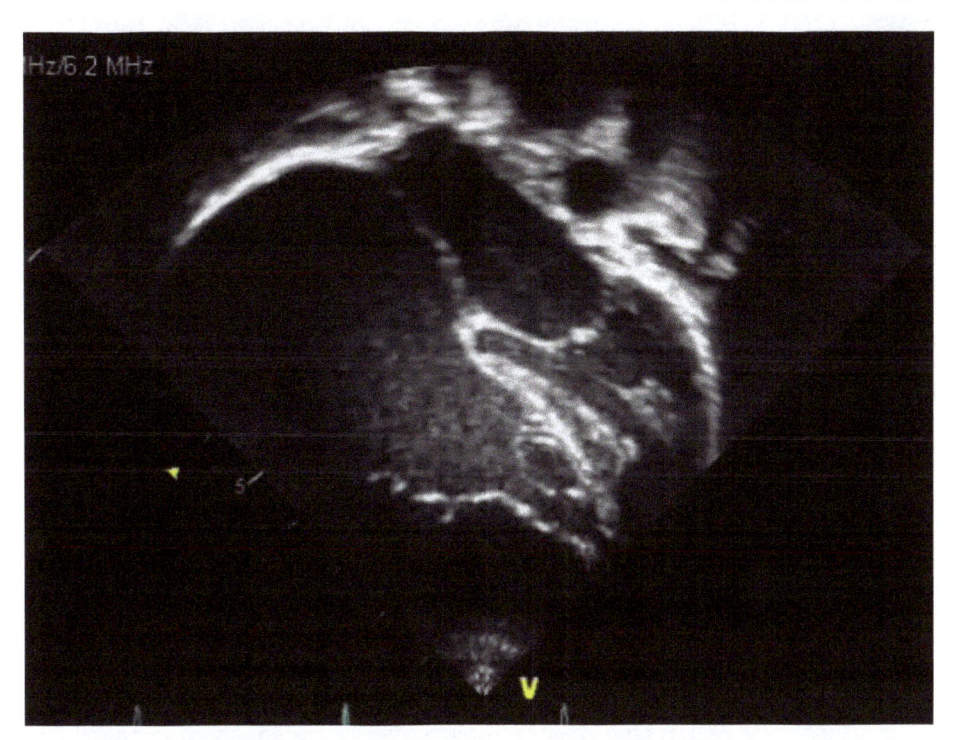

Figure 21-2. 4-chamber echocardiographic view showing significant apical displacement of the septal leaflet of the tricuspid valve compared to the mitral valve insertion in a patient with Ebstein anomaly. The image also displays RA enlargement, atrialization of the RV, and its relative hypoplasia. Image courtesy of Dr. Josh Kailin, www.pedecho.org.

- **CXR (Figure 21-1).** Severe cardiomegaly due to the severe TR and RA dilation is the pathognomonic finding on Ebstein anomaly. There are 3 cardiac lesions that present with such a significant degree of cardiomegaly: Ebstein anomaly, dilated cardiomyopathy, and a large pericardial effusion. The amount of visible lung may be significantly limited due to the degree of cardiomegaly and pulmonary hypoplasia.
- **Echocardiography.** Main diagnostic modality. The formal definition of Ebstein anomaly is apical displacement of the septal leaflet of the tricuspid valve >8 mm/m^2 (Figure 21-2). The displacement is measured compared to the level of attachment of the mitral valve annulus and indexed to BSA. It is important to define the degree of TR and the extent of atrialization of the RV (Figure 21-3). In neonates, it is imperative to evaluate the pulmonary valve for patency, since a closed pulmonary valve may be *anatomically* atretic or *functionally* atretic (Figure 21-4). Pulmonary valve patency may be predicted by observing PI but the lack of PI does not necessarily indicate anatomic pulmonary atresia. In newborns with a large PDA, there may not be prograde flow across the RVOT due to severe TR (retrograde flow) and elevated PVR.
- **Cardiac MRI.** It has become a useful adjunct in the management of older patients in recent years. It allows further assessment of RV and LV size and function.

PART II. DISEASES

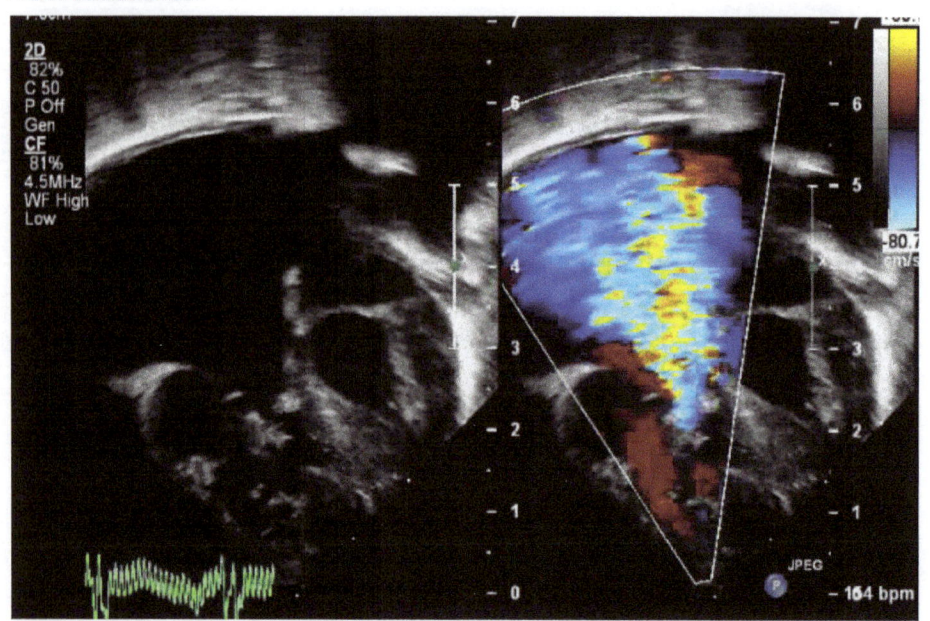

Figure 21-3. Side-by-side 4-chamber color-compare views of Ebstein anomaly with significant apical displacement of the septal leaflet of the tricuspid valve and severe TR. Image courtesy of Dr. Josh Kailin, www.pedecho.org.

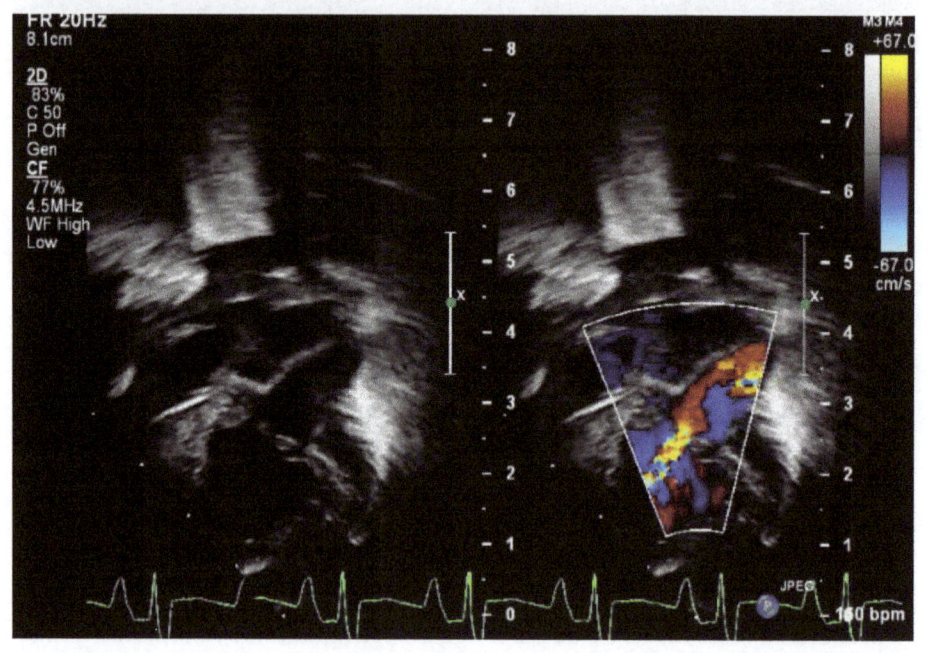

Figure 21-4. Side-by-side subcostal color-compare views of flow through the PDA and then retrograde through the pulmonary valve. This patient had functional pulmonary valve atresia due to the lack of prograde flow across the pulmonary valve, but not anatomic or true atresia, as noted by the presence of PI.

Preoperative Management

Initial treatment of critical newborns with *functional* pulmonary valve atresia is aimed at decreasing PVR with ventilation, oxygenation, and iNO. Patients require sedation and possibly neuromuscular blockade to further decrease PVR. Afterload reduction can be added if the BP is adequate to promote systemic blood flow. In patients with poor cardiac output, inotropes may need to be initiated with the known increased risk of tachyarrhythmias in these patients. In such individuals (who typically have been started on PGE at birth in the setting of a fetal diagnosis), the decision to attempt PGE weaning can be very challenging. The key question is whether the RV can generate enough force to overcome the PVR and manage the degree of TR. In many patients, it is very important for the management team to be persistent in these efforts: many patients can ultimately be weaned from PGE after failing initial attempts (and thereby avoid newborn surgery).

A unique situation in neonates occurs in the presence of significant PI. The presence of a PDA in this setting allows blood to flow through the PDA, retrograde through the incompetent pulmonary valve, then retrograde through the insufficient tricuspid valve to the RA and across the ASD (right-to-left shunting), through the left heart out to the aorta, and the back through the PDA. This "circular shunt" (Figure 21-5) can compromise both systemic and pulmonary blood flow. In these profoundly cyanotic patients, starting prostaglandins may be detrimental. The same circular shunt can occur if the pulmonary valve is atretic and is ballooned open, leading to PI.

Care of a neonate with severe Ebstein anomaly can also be complicated by lung hypoplasia due to limited in utero development. Inability to ventilate due to severe lung hypoplasia can impact survivability in these patients. Decisions to proceed with surgical intervention or possibly extracorporeal support need to take into consideration the degree of pulmonary hypoplasia. In these challenging situations, CT of the lungs may be helpful in delineating the degree of parenchymal immaturity.

Indications / Timing for Intervention

In the neonatal period, initial evaluation of oxygen saturations and cardiac output determine if any intervention is needed. Most children with Ebstein anomaly will ultimately achieve a balanced circulation with adequate systemic oxygen saturation. As per above, persistent attempts at medical management are warranted unless the infant is critically unstable. If neonates present with high PVR, a circular shunt, and compromised cardiac output, interventions are aimed at ventilating and decreasing PVR to reverse the retrograde flow through the pulmonary valve. The decision to intervene is often based on response to these therapies.

In patients with true (*anatomic*) pulmonary atresia, there will be a need to establish a source of pulmonary blood flow. This is best accomplished after the PVR has dropped, and can be in the form of a modified Blalock-Taussig-Thomas shunt (mBTTS) or a ductal stent (see Chapter 38) with or without dilation of the pulmonary valve depending on echocardiographic size. In neonates with a diminutive RV, consideration should be made of a Starnes procedure (see below). If there is a sizeable RV but the child cannot maintain a good cardiac output due to the amount of TR, consideration can be made

PART II. DISEASES

of attempting to repair the tricuspid valve. Tricuspid valve repair is also a consideration in older children with heart failure symptomatology due to severe TR (see below).

Anesthetic Considerations
Anesthetic considerations should reflect careful assessment of the patient's current status and ongoing management. A controlled, careful induction with IV narcotic and benzodiazepine can be supplemented with anesthetic vapor to minimize rapid changes in physiology. iNO, inotropes, and vasopressors should be available if not already initiated. Given the proclivity of children with Ebstein anomaly to develop tachyarrhythmias, this is one situation for which defibrillation pads may be helpful even with a first-time sternotomy.

In critical newborns presenting with low cardiac output and marginal systemic arterial oxygen saturations, anesthetic management is focused on optimizing ventilation and maintaining cardiac output. These babies may be very unstable during transport and anesthesia

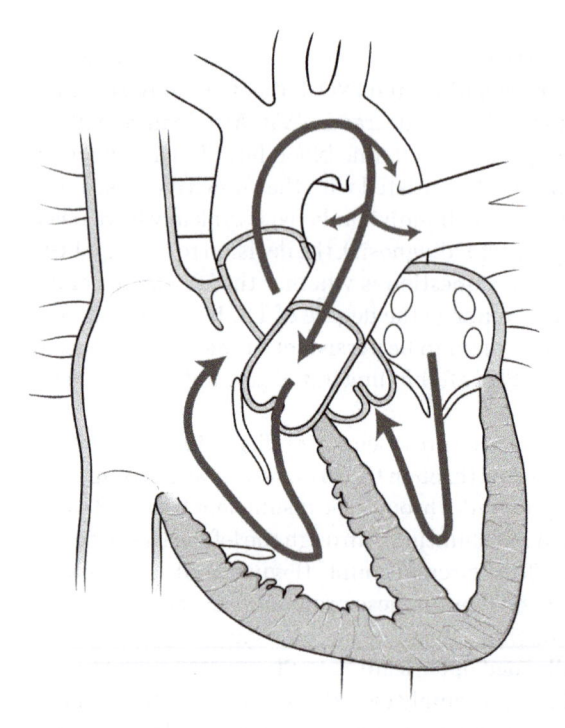

Figure 21-5. Circular shunt in Ebstein anomaly in the presence of PI and a PDA. Blood flows from the aorta, through the PDA, and then retrograde through the pulmonary valve, the tricuspid valve (severe TR), and right to left through the ASD, just to go back into the aorta. Minimal flow goes to the aorta to provide systemic output and to the branch PAs to oxygenate the blood. This results in both cyanosis and poor cardiac output.

induction. As such, it is critical to have all members of the surgical and OR team in attendance at induction.

Surgical Intervention
Timing of surgical intervention and mode of operative correction has evolved significantly over the past 2 decades as surgical techniques have improved. The primary goal of surgery for Ebstein anomaly is to improve right-heart effectiveness in generating prograde PA flow through tricuspid valve repair, reduction/elimination of nonfunctional portions of the RV (atrialized portion), partial or complete ASD closure, and where necessary, pulmonary valve replacement.

As discussed previously, newborns with symptomatic Ebstein present a challenging surgical problem and historically, operations on these babies have been associated with significant risk of mortality. The primary decision in newborns is whether or not to attempt tricuspid valve repair. In those individuals in whom the valve is deemed irreparable, RV exclusion through patch closure of the tricuspid orifice ("Starnes" operation) may be the only viable option. When this is done, it is imperative to fenestrate the patch such that the RV is able to decompress into the RA. The operation also includes an atrial septectomy and creation of an mBTTS.

Several investigators have documented encouraging results with tricuspid valve repairs in newborns, but these results are not widely consistent in the greater congenital heart surgery community. In repairing the tricuspid valve in small babies, the operation is made all the more challenging by the very delicate nature of tricuspid valve tissue in these children. As such, it has been our approach that if possible, interim palliation is offered such that tricuspid repair is offered later in childhood when the valve tissue is more substantial.

In older children and adults, the "Cone" operation as initially described and implemented by Da Silva has revolutionized surgical repair of Ebstein anomaly. The core principle of the Cone operation is to mobilize all available tricuspid valve tissue (including the portion that is not fully delaminated from the RV free wall) from its abnormal attachements, leaving only the apical support intact. The valve is separated from the abnormal tricuspid annulus, rotated in a clockwise direction and then a "cone" of valve tissue is created by suturing all the valve tissue together. The conceptual understanding of this operation is greatly facilitated by thinking of the reconstructed cone like a sort of long Hemlich valve. Once the cone is reconstructed, the atrialized portion of the RV is plicated longitudinally to create a more efficient RV cavity and to construct a new tricuspid annulus that is normally positioned. The cone is then reattached at the level of the new annulus with great care to avoid the AV node. Most surgeons then add a formal annuloplasty ring. Following reconstruction of the tricuspid valve, the ASD is either partially or completely closed, depending on the effectiveness of the reconstruction and the size of the tricuspid inlet. In patients where we are concerned about the repair, we will typically leave a fenestration in the atrial septum (4-5 mm). If there is concern that the tricuspid orifice is too small, we will add a bidirectional Glenn shunt to augment pulmonary blood flow and offload the RA.

In desperate situations where there has been a failed attempt at tricuspid repair, it may be necessary to replace the tricuspid valve. Of course, this is a problematic solution in that all available tissue prostheses will eventually degenerate and have to be replaced. This degeneration is notoriously more rapid in children. It is also critical to make every effort to prevent surgical AV block in tricuspid valve replacements and in patients where there is deficient tissue in the region of the true annulus near the AV node. As such, the prosthesis is placed well up into the body of the RA, leaving the coronary sinus below the sewing ring of the prosthesis. In recent years, with the advent of transcatheter valve replacement alternatives, the option of "valve-in-valve" replacement of degenerated prostheses may be considered.

Postoperative Management

Postoperative management is dependent on the intervention undertaken. In neonates, much of the postoperative management involves dealing with the ramifications of preoperative instability, elevated PVR, and pulmonary hypoplasia/ventilator concerns. Sedation is imperative to managing these critically ill neonates. At times, they may also require neuromuscular blockade in the initial postoperative days. In neonates who undergo an mBTTS or ductal stent, management is aimed at balancing Qp:Qs, which can be fluid as PVR drops (see Chapter 38). In those that undergo a Starnes procedure, in addition to managing Qp:Qs, there are the usual considerations involved in managing a neonate who has undergone CPB and cross-clamping, with the IV fluid, inotrope, and inflammatory considerations that this entails. Patients who undergo a tricuspid valve repair in the neonatal period will have similar considerations and will benefit from further attempts to decrease PVR and maintain cardiac output. Consideration of the patient's risk of tachyarrhythmias is important as many children have accessory pathways and irritable atria due to dilation and suture lines that lead to a higher risk of this complication. Inotropes may need to be tailored to avoid increasing arrhythmia burden by decreasing adrenergic agents.

For older patients, early extubation (ideally intraoperative) following repair mitigates the deleterious effects of positive-pressure ventilation. Inotropic support should be tailored to reduce PVR and minimize the tendency for atrial tachycardia.

> **Patients with Ebstein anomaly initially diagnosed at TCH (1995-2017)**
> Number of patients: 215
> - Neonates: 87 (40%)
> - Infants: 23 (11%)
> - Children: 69 (32%)
> - Adults: 36 (17%)
>
> Of the 87 neonates diagnosed, only 15 (17%) required surgery in the neonatal period (13 with anatomical pulmonary atresia). Of these, 9 underwent single ventricle palliation and 6 underwent biventricular repair.

Long-Term Management

Patients can remain asymptomatic if the degree of TR is mild and there is limited atrialization of the RV. Tachyarrhthymias can be the presenting sign leading to diagnosis in older children with less hemodynamically significant lesions.

All patients with Ebstein anomaly should be assessed for the presence of an accessory AV conduction pathway and it is preferred that such pathways be ablated in the electrophysiology lab prior to surgical intervention. In those rare individuals with persistent accessory pathways after attempted catheter ablation, surgical division of the pathway should be performed at the time of the tricuspid valve repair operation. In addition to tachyarrhthmias, patients with Ebstein anomaly can have progressive heart failure symptomatology due to the degree of TR. In addition to right-sided heart failure symptomatology, they can also develop LV failure due to poor interventricular interactions and septal shift secondary to right-sided volume overload. Much of the long-term care in patients with Ebstein anomaly is determined by their initial course and required surgical interventions.

22 Congenital Aortic Stenosis

Asra Khan, R. Blaine Easley, Charles D. Fraser Jr.

Congenital aortic stenosis (AS) is one of the five most common congenital heart lesions and accounts for 5-10% of all congenital heart defects. It can be classified as: valvar (70%), subvalvar (10-20%), supravalvar (5-10%), or mixed (8%) (Figure 22-1). The importance of AS is disproportionate to its incidence because it is either critical and requires emergent intervention or it is progressive and requires frequent follow-up throughout life, regardless of type of intervention. This chapter will focus on valvar AS. Subvalvar and supravalvar AS are described in Chapters 23 and 24, respectively.

Pathophysiology and Clinical Presentation

Only 2% of congenitally abnormal aortic valves develop clinically significant AS or AI by adolescence. Valvar degeneration and dysfunction of congenitally abnormal valves, however, is progressive over time and a higher percentage of patients require intervention later in life. Approximately 20% of patients have associated cardiac lesions including aortic coarctation, VSD, and PDA.

In patients with congenital AS, approximately one third will have tricuspid valves, two thirds will have bicuspid valves (true bicuspid or functionally bicuspid due to fusion of a commissure), 8% will have monocuspid valves, and rare patients will have quadricuspid valves. Long-term outcomes and response to therapy correlates with valvar morphology. The presence of a bicuspid aortic valve (which is thought to be present in as much as 4% of the general population) may also be associated with aortic root dilation and the development of an ascending aortic aneurysm ("bicuspid aortopathy"). The incidence and severity of aortic dilation does not directly correlate with the severity of AS.

Patients with severe AS (approximately 10% of patients with congenital AS) may present in the newborn period or during infancy. Severe AS is well tolerated in utero from the standpoint of cardiac output as the RV maintains adequate cardiac output through the arterial duct. However, in severe cases, LV function may be severely depressed in fetal life. The management of fetal critical AS is highly controversial and beyond the scope of this chapter, other than to note that detection of severe AS and depressed LV function should alert the postnatal management team of the potential for an unstable newborn requiring urgent attention. In postnatal life, as the PDA closes, patients may develop symptoms of low cardiac output and CHF. If the degree of stenosis is severe with depressed LV function, systemic perfusion is compromised, leading to rapidly progressive cardiogenic shock after PDA closure. Pre- and postductal saturations (differential saturations with decreased SaO_2 in the lower extremities) are useful in detecting ductal dependency. In critically ill newborns, PGE infusion to maintain or reestablish ductal patency may be a life-saving temporizing measure.

In older patients, as AS progresses, symptoms including easy fatigability and exertional fatigue occur in about 30% patients. Angina, syncope, and sudden death after exercise are rare. Patients with less severe forms of AS will initially be asymptomatic. However, AS tends to be progressive over time and close follow-up is required.

PART II. DISEASES

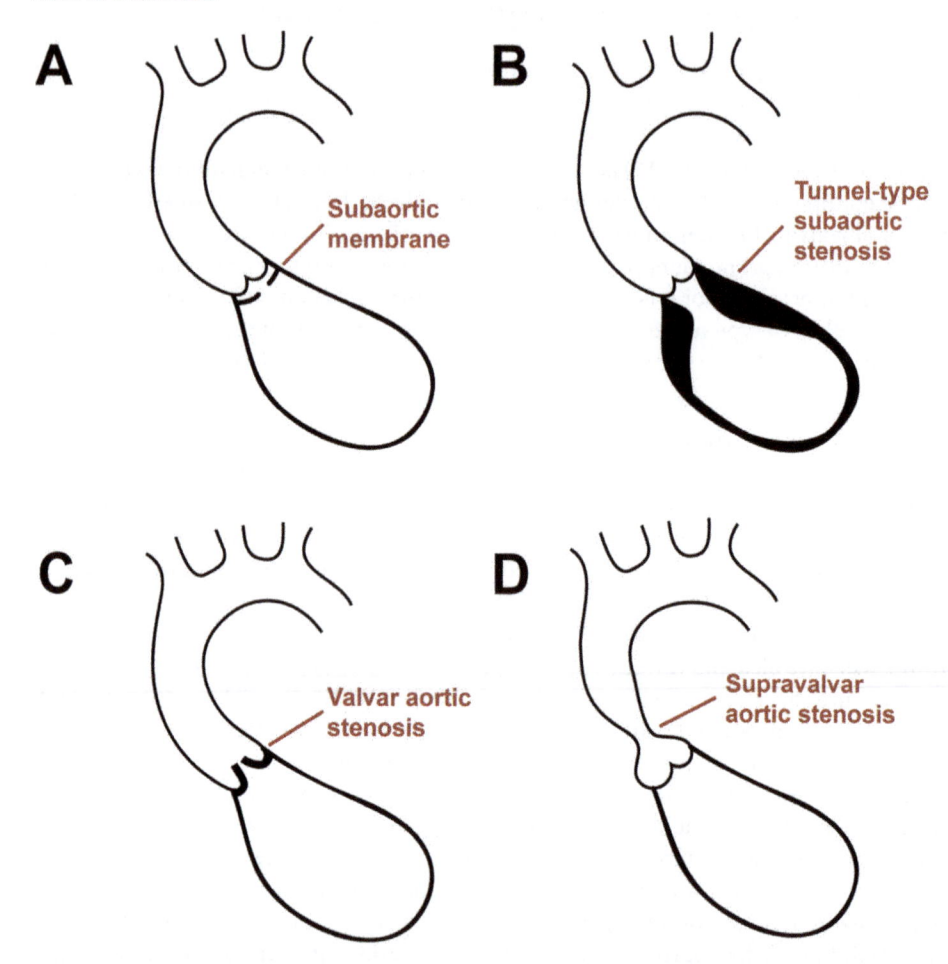

Figure 22-1. Different levels of left ventricular outflow tract obstruction including: A) fixed subaortic obstruction due to a membrane, B) diffuse tunnel-type subaortic stenosis, C) valvar aortic stenosis, and D) supravalvar aortic stenosis.

On physical exam, patients with critical AS may present in cardiogenic shock with weak pulses and mottled appearance. In general, patients with AS will have an increased apical impulse with a harsh systolic ejection murmur at the right upper sternal border radiating into both carotids. A suprasternal thrill with a systolic ejection click is consistent with valvar stenosis. A precordial thrill and an S_4 gallop may be present in severe AS.

Diagnosis
- **ECG.** LVH is often present, although the ECG may be normal even with significant AS. LVH with strain pattern (ST depression and T-wave inversion in lateral leads) at baseline or with exercise is concerning for severe AS.

22. CONGENITAL AORTIC STENOSIS

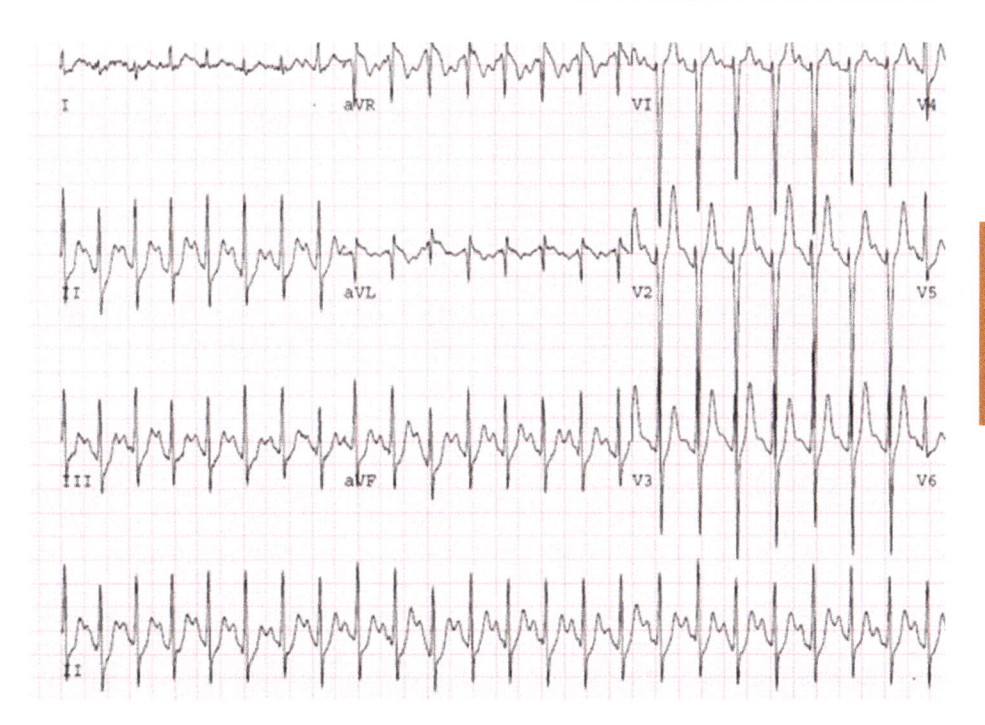

Figure 22-2. ECG showing significant ST-segment changes with exercise.

- **CXR.** Nonspecific. There may be a rounded apex, prominent aortic shadow, LA dilation, and posterior displacement on lateral views.
- **Echocardiogram.** Useful for definitive diagnosis, evaluating valvar morphology, presence of myocardial fibrosis, and associated defects. In utero fetal echocardiography may also be used to diagnose significant AS. Tachycardia, increased contractility, or cardiac output status (including anemia) may falsely increase the observed gradients across the aortic valve. Echocardiography can help define the severity of AS (Table 22-1).
- **Exercise stress test.** Useful to determine exercise capacity in moderate to severe AS. ST-segment changes with exercise are indicative of ischemia (Figure 22-2).

Medical Management

Patients with critical AS presenting as newborns in cardiogenic shock require initiation of PGE (to support the systemic circulation), intubation, inotropic support, and urgent intervention.

Patients with less severe forms of congenital AS may be followed closely. For patients with mild-moderate AS (mean gradient <30 mmHg), follow-up is recommended every 2 years. Patients with moderate-severe AS (mean gradient >30 mmHg), should be followed every year. Life-long follow-up is recommended. Antibiotic prophylaxis is currently not routinely recommended (Nishimura et al. 2014), although opinions on this issue are highly variable.

Based on ACC/AHA guidelines, patients with AS may need to be exercise-restricted as follows (Bonow et al. 2015):
- Patients with mild AS and normal maximal exercise response should not be exercise-restricted
- Patients with moderate AS can participate in low and moderate static or dynamic competitive sports if normal exercise-tolerance testing
- Asymptomatic patients with severe AS should not participate in competitive sports
- Symptomatic patients with AS should not participate in competitive sports

Indications / Timing for Intervention
AS is progressive over time and valve replacement is the ultimate therapy for most patients with significant AS. Timing for intervention and outcomes correlate with initial gradient and degree of valvar dysplasia. Balloon valvuloplasty and surgical repair may delay timing of valve replacement considerably. Many patients develop progressive AI, in both native and postintervention states.

Newborns and infants that present with critical AS and cardiogenic shock require urgent intervention in the form of aortic balloon valvuloplasty or surgical valvotomy. Asymptomatic patients are put forward for intervention when peak gradient is >50 mmHg. For patients that are symptomatic, show ischemic or repolarization ECG changes at rest or exercise, or are planning to play competitive sports or become pregnant, a peak gradient of >40 mmHg is generally used as an indication for intervention.

Catheter-Based Intervention
In many centers, balloon valvuloplasty (Figure 22-3) is the initial line of therapy for isolated valvar AS, although data are conflicting concerning the question of whether this therapy is as effective and durable as open surgical valvotomy. Freedom from reintervention after balloon dilation is approximately 50% at 10 years. Recovery is typically rapid; most patients with normal ventricular function are eligible for discharge within

Table 22-1. Severity of AS based on echocardiographic and cardiac catheterization findings.

	Peak Velocity[a]	Peak Instantaneous Gradient[a]	Mean Gradient[a]	Peak-to-peak Gradient[b]	Valve Area[c]
Mild	3 m/s	<36 mmHg	<25 mmHg	<30 mmHg	>1.5 cm^2
Moderate	3-4 m/s	36-64 mmHg	25-40 mmHg	30-50 mmHg	1-1.5 cm^2
Severe	>4 m/s	>64 mmHg	>40 mmHg	>50 mmHg	<1 cm^2

[a] By echocardiography.

[b] By cardiac catheterization.

[c] In adolescents and adults, normal valve area is 3-4 cm^2. For children, normal valve area is 2 cm^2/m^2 and severe AS is 0.6 cm^2/m^2.

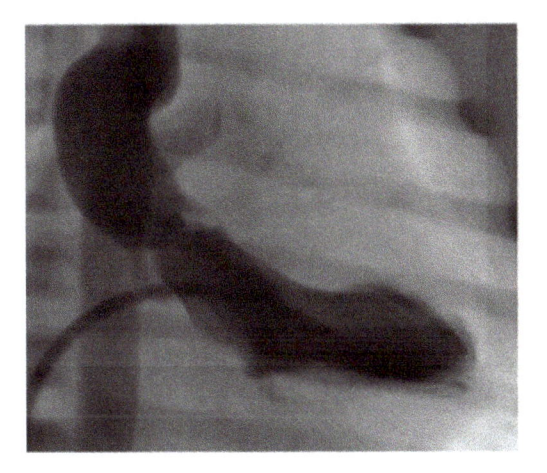

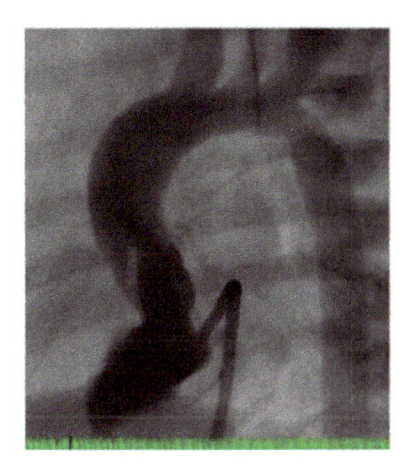

Figure 22-3. Angiogram showing a typically thickened and dysplastic aortic valve with a small effective orifice.

24 hours. Although high risk, balloon valvuloplasty may be better tolerated than surgical valvotomy in neonates with critical AS or with depressed ventricular function, and can delay surgical intervention.

Surgical Repair

Aortic Valve Repair

Open surgical valvotomy is very effective for primary AS and several series suggest this mode of treatment may be associated with superior durability and less AI when compared to balloon valvuloplasty. However, at present, balloon valvuloplasty is more frequently offered in most centers, including TCH.

Primary surgical repair is most frequently offered for patients with associated cardiac lesions, progressive AI, or recurrent AS not adequately treated with balloon valvuloplasty. Techniques for valve repair include accurate commissurotomy with leaflet debulking. In cases where leaflet tissue is limited, cusp extensions may be performed with the use of autologous pericardium or commercially available bovine pericardium. Complex aortic valve repair methodologies have been developed to address even the most malformed aortic valves, including the so-called "monocusp" valves. These techniques essentially amount to an on-table construction of a tissue valve within the patient's native aortic root and represent a formidable geometric and technical challenge. Many units have reported early success with these methods, however, these repairs do not tend to be as durable as replacement, particularly in small children (see aortic valve replacement below).

Secondary valve repair may also be considered after a previous balloon valvuloplasty. In patients undergoing balloon valvuloplasty for primary AS, the valve does not consistently tear along commissural lines; on the contrary, the leaflet is often torn not only in a radial fashion, but it may be avulsed from the annulus in a circumferential fashion. As such, reparative strategies after previous dilations are typically complex. A central limiting feature in all forms of repair for severe AS is the annular dimension. Neither balloon valvuloplasty or isolated reparative surgery can effectively overcome severe annular hypoplasia. It is imprudent for the surgeon to accept a hypoplastic annulus in performing a primary open valvotomy for AS. In this setting, AS will recur rapidly if the annulus is not dealt with appropriately (see annulus enlarging techniques below).

Aortic Valve Replacement (AVR)

The entire topic of AVR in children is complex and highly debated. Our own data (Khan et al. 2013), as well as those from other centers performing large numbers of AVRs in children, appear conclusive in demonstrating that the pulmonary autograft aortic root replacement (Ross operation) is the superior option for most children.

> **TCH experience with aortic valve repairs (1995-2011)** (Khan et al. 2013)
> Number of procedures: 97
> Median age 2.6 years (1-18 years)
> Median weight 11.6 kg (21-110 kg)
> Perioperative mortality: 2%
> 5-year freedom-from-reintervention or death:
> - Simple repair: 84%
> - Complex repair: 61%
>
> **TCH experience with aortic valve replacements (1995-2011)** (Khan et al. 2013)
> Number of procedures: 188
> Median age 8.3 years (4 days – 18 years), median weight 25.4 kg (2-109 kg):
> Types of aortic valve replacements:
> - Autograft (Ross): 68 (36%)
> - Homograft: 74 (39%)
> - Mechanical: 36 (19%)
> - Bioprosthetic: 10 (6%)
> Perioperative mortality: 3%
> 5-year freedom-from-reintervention or death:
> - Autograft (Ross): 91%
> - Homograft: 52%
> - Mechanical: 95%

Nonetheless, there are instances in which other options can and should be considered. In the setting of profound LV dysfunction, an expedient operation with limited myocardial ischemia may be better tolerated than the more lengthy and technically demanding Ross procedure. As such, viable alternatives for children include homograft aortic root replacement or mechanical AVR. The latter is less attractive in most patients due to the necessity and thereby risk of chronic anticoagulation. Homograft root replacements offer the patient the option of an active lifestyle without anticoagulation, but the implants degenerate at unpredictable rates.

The Ross operation offers the patient the option of a more durable, native semilunar valve in the aortic position. The operation is predicated on a satisfactory pulmonary valve, and we have not offered the Ross operation if we find a bicuspid pulmonary valve or multiple deep-cusp fenestrations (we have seen one case of a quadricusp pulmonary valve). The pulmonary valve complex is harvested as a muscular sleeve of the RV infundibulum. It is important to remember that the pulmonary valve does not have a fibrous "annulus" and it is therefore subject to dilation. As such, many surgeons reinforce the implanted autograft muscular apron with a Dacron® strip or some other material to "fix" the dimension of the annulus. Our opinion is that the full root method, which includes direct reimplantation of the coronary arteries is superior to the sub-coronary technique.

22. CONGENITAL AORTIC STENOSIS

In cases where the aortic annulus is hypoplastic, the Ross-Konno method is preferred to achieve an adequate annular dimension. The root enlarging portion of the operation is actually facilitated by the harvest of the autograft. Once the autograft is procured, the surgeon has a direct view of the ventricular septum, which is then incised for several millimeters to increase the annular dimension. The defect in the septum is repaired with a Dacron® or pericardial patch and the autograft is implanted appropriately.

As noted previously, patients with AS will often have a dilated ascending aorta and in some patients, it is frankly aneurysmal. In the latter setting, the ascending aorta will have to be replaced, frequently including extending the replacement up into the aortic arch ("hemi-arch" replacement) using a Dacron® tube graft. In cases of an ectatic ascending aorta, some surgeons favor an anterior aortoplasty to "tailor" the size of the ascending aorta to match the autograft, while others do not. In either case, the autograft will still have the tendency to dilate at the level of the aortic anastomosis and over time, this will lead to progressive dilation at the level of the autograft valve pillars and subsequent AI. It is therefore prudent to reinforce the anastomosis between the ascending aorta and autograft with a strip of Teflon™ felt or some other durable material.

Postoperative Management

Postoperative management of patients undergoing surgery for AS (either valve repair or replacement) is rather generic in assuring adequate preload (volume), carefully controlled afterload (to control BP in the setting of multiple aortic suturelines and to facilitate LV function), and judicious inotropic and lusotropic support. In many cases, early extubation facilitates management, but in patients who have gone into surgery with profound LV dysfunction, particularly newborns with critical AS, sedation and mechanical ventilation may be useful in reducing overall body oxygen consumption and thereby myocardial demand.

In patients with longstanding AS with associated severe LVH, the LV will often appear "hyperdynamic" after successful intervention or surgery. In these situations, volume resuscitation is paramount. As tachycardia may be poorly tolerated, the judicious addition of a short-acting intravenous beta-blocker (esmolol) may facilitate perioperative management.

Complications

Complications after both balloon valvuloplasty and open surgery for AS should be infrequent. In very small infants, vascular access may be challenging and thereby, compromise of distal perfusion when the femoral approach is used may occur. This typically is responsive to anticoagulation therapy and expectant management, although there have been rare cases of profound extremity compromise that have required surgical revascularization (in very small babies this may require the assistance of surgeons experienced in microvascular methods). In some very small babies, an open carotid artery cutdown has been used for cath access and in these cases, the carotid artery should be repaired primarily following the procedure. While rare, balloon valvuloplasty in small, critically ill newborns has been associated with aortic rupture and sudden cardiac arrest. It is therefore mandatory that the surgical team be notified and on standby when a critical newborn is taken for an urgent or emergent balloon valvuloplasty, where emergent surgery or ECMO support may be needed.

Complications after surgery should also be infrequent, but may be significant. For the Ross operation, the autograft must be harvested from the RV infundibulum and as such, the left main, LAD, and first septal perforating coronary arteries may be at risk. Furthermore, in performing the root replacement, the coronary ostia must be reimplanted into the autograft root. These considerations all emphasize the need for careful ongoing assessment for the potential of myocardial ischemia in the perioperative period.

Other potential surgical complications include failure of the valvuloplasty or autograft (persistent AS or AI), recurrent AS, complete AV block, myocardial dysfunction, and bleeding, to name a few. All patients face the lifetime risk of need of repeat surgical or catheter intervention and thereby require a consistent and longitudinal follow-up management plan.

Suggested Readings

Bonow RO, Nishimura RA, Thompson PD, et al. Eligibility and disqualification recommendations for competitive athletes with cardiovascular abnormalities: Task Force 5: Valvular heart disease. Circulation 2015;132:e292-e297.

Khan MS, Samayoa AX, Chen DW, et al. Contemporary experience with surgical treatment of aortic valve disease in children. J Thorac Cardiovasc Surg 2013;146:512-521.

Morales DL, Carberry KE, Balentine C, et al. Selective application of the pediatric Ross procedure minimizes autograft failure. Congenit Heart Dis 2008;3:404-410.

Nishimura RA, Otto CM, Bonow RO, et al. 2014 AHA/ACC guideline for the management of patients with valvular heart disease. J Thorac Cardiovasc Surg 2014;148:e1-e132.

23 Subaortic Stenosis

William Buck Kyle, Antonio G. Cabrera, Carlos M. Mery

Subaortic stenosis (SAS) makes up a relatively small portion of all CHD but it can be one of the most vexing problems faced by providers because no consensus exists to guide management in a large subset of these patients. While SAS can occur in association with other cardiac lesions (e.g., malalignment VSD, hypertrophic cardiomyopathy), this chapter focuses on SAS in an otherwise normal heart.

Pathophysiology and Clinical Presentation

SAS is usually classified into discrete (i.e., "subaortic membrane") and tunnel-type SAS. The former is much more common and is characterized by a partially or completely circumferential fibrous ridge in the LVOT. Tunnel-type SAS describes a long (1-3 cm) segment of circumferential fibromuscular narrowing of the LVOT that may be associated with hypoplasia of the aortic valve annulus.

The pathophysiology of SAS is unclear. However, it is believed that the turbulence and shear stress caused by abnormal flow patterns incite an inflammatory reaction that is felt to be responsible for occurrence and progression of disease. An acute angulation of the LVOT or associated anomalies (e.g., VSD) may be partly responsible for the turbulent flow. It is also possible that some patients may be more prone to develop fibrosis and scarring, increasing the incidence and recurrence of SAS. The fibrous membrane that develops as a consequence of the fibrotic reaction tends to grow (worsening the stenosis) and attach to surrounding structures including the mitral and aortic valves (causing AI).

In children, progression is associated with higher gradient at diagnosis (mean gradient >30 mmHg), aortic valve thickening at diagnosis, shorter distance from the membrane to the aortic valve, and membrane attachment to the mitral valve. In addition to stenosis, some degree of AI may be present, likely the result of the membrane encroaching on the valve or the effect of a high-velocity turbulent jet damaging the valve over time. Long-term preservation of the aortic valve is an important consideration when determining management. LVH, initially a compensatory response to decrease wall stress, becomes pathologic over time and can lead to heart failure.

Patients with SAS are usually young (<10 years old) and asymptomatic. A murmur is the most common reason for patients to seek medical attention. It is typically a harsh, high-frequency, crescendo-decrescendo murmur (without a click) at the left midsternal border that radiates to the carotids. An early diastolic decrescendo murmur indicates AI. An S_4 gallop would suggest severe obstruction and diastolic dysfunction. Even with severe obstruction, symptoms are rare in children. They include decreased endurance, chest pain, and presyncope or syncope.

PART II. DISEASES

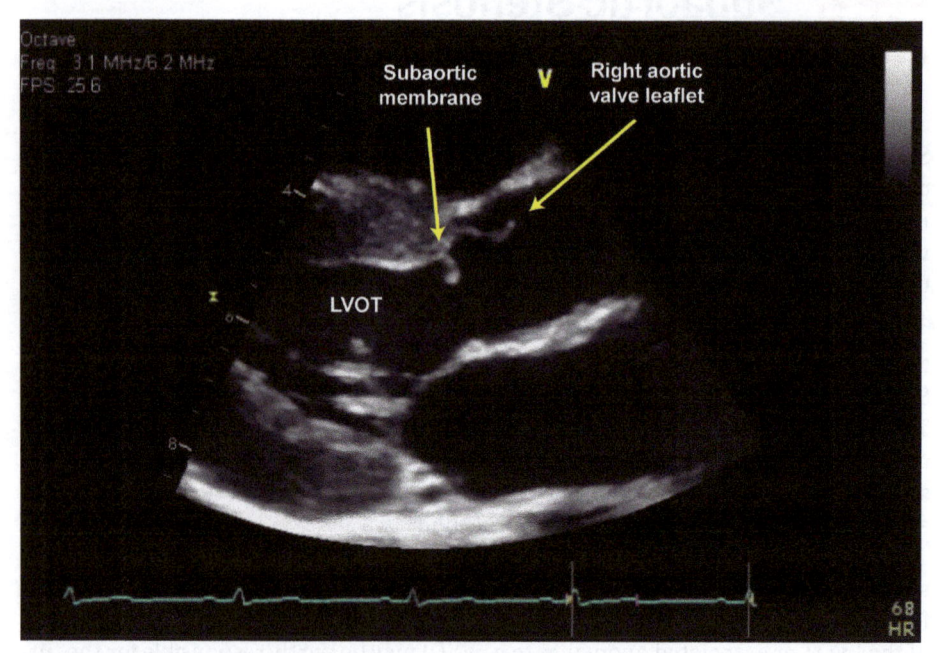

Figure 23-1. Parasternal long-axis echocardiographic image of a discrete subaortic membrane. Image courtesy of Dr. Josh Kailin, www.pedecho.org.

Diagnosis

- **ECG.** The degree of LVH correlates poorly with the degree of obstruction. ST depression in lateral leads represents significant myocardial strain or ischemia regardless of the gradient, and is a potential indication for surgery.
- **CXR.** Usually normal.
- **Echocardiography (Figure 23-1).** In discrete SAS, parasternal long-axis demonstrates a ridge extending from the septum into the LVOT. One should look closely for a corresponding tissue ledge arising from the anterior leaflet of the mitral valve. In tunnel-type SAS, the LVOT will appear diffusely narrow. Aliasing of the color Doppler signal in this view reveals the level of obstruction and can demonstrate AI. Parasternal short-axis 2D view demonstrates the aortic valve architecture and leaflet mobility (sometimes limited by an encroaching membrane), and color will localize the insufficiency. Anterior images in the apical view disclose the location and extent of the obstruction, and the angle of interrogation with color Doppler from this view is favorable in estimating the degree of obstruction and insufficiency. The subcostal view adds to the findings from the apical view and often provides even better resolution in both 2D and color. The importance of slow, complete sweeps through the LVOT cannot be overstated with careful characterization of the LVOT, membrane, and mitral and aortic valves with 2D, color, and spectral Doppler. The suprasternal view often produces the highest measured velocities and should be performed routinely. When choosing an echocardiographic probe, a PEDOF (Pulsed

Echo DOppler Flow-velocity meter) probe will provide the most accurate velocity. When determining the severity of obstruction, one must be careful to consider the angle of interrogation as well as confounding lesions (VSD, contamination from MR). The mean gradient is felt to most closely approximate the catheter gradient in this lesion, and this value should be trended over time.
- **Exercise stress testing (EST).** Indicated when considering participation in competitive sports.
- **Cardiac catheterization.** Can measure the gradient with great accuracy and is sometimes used to confirm or supplant echocardiographic estimations, particularly when imaging is poor or intervention is being considered. However, most patients do not require catheterization prior to intervention.

Indications / Timing of Intervention

SAS is often progressive in children (less so in adults), but the rate of progression is highly variable. At least annual visits and echocardiograms are warranted to monitor for progression; more often when progression occurs. Patients with symptoms (ischemic chest pain or decreased exercise performance), severe obstruction, or LV dysfunction should be referred for surgical intervention. At TCH, patients with AI, especially if progressive, are usually considered for intervention in order to avoid further injury of the aortic valve. The optimal timing of surgery for asymptomatic patients without AI is controversial. It has been suggested that a mean gradient of 30 mmHg or peak gradient of 40 mmHg is a reasonable indication for intervention. However, no consensus recommendation exists, and one should carefully consider the decision on a case-by-case basis.

When an athlete is considering highly static or dynamic competitive sports participation, eligibility guidelines will factor into the decision-making process, as would EST results. Desire for pregnancy influences management in females of childbearing age. It is the recurrence rate of these membranes (up to 20%) and need for reoperation (15%) that necessitate a thoughtful approach.

Surgical Repair

The procedure is performed via median sternotomy and under CPB with aorto-bicaval cannulation. After cardioplegic arrest and venting of the left heart via the atrial septum or the right upper pulmonary vein, an oblique aortotomy is performed. The aortic valve is carefully retracted to examine the LVOT. The extent of involvement of the subaortic membrane is usually more extensive than appreciated on echocardiography (Booth et al. 2010), and it is common for the membrane to involve one or more leaflets of the aortic valve.

The resection is started by incising the membrane in the LVOT, at a level below the nadir of the right coronary cusp. The area rightward of this site contains the conduction tissue and should be addressed carefully. Depending on the thickness of the ventricular septum and the LVOT angle, the incision may extend for a few millimeters into the muscular septum as there is a suggestion that performing a myectomy at the time of SAS resection may reduce recurrence by rectifying the LVOT angle. Resection of the membrane is then continued leftward towards the mitral valve. Additional muscular septum may be excised just anterior to the mitral valve. The membrane is then peeled off the mitral valve and, carefully, off the area near the conduction system. When the membrane involves the aortic valve, it is peeled off with care not to injure the valve. Some membranes are intimately attached to the valve and peeling the membrane may be challenging.

> **TCH experience on subaortic stenosis (1995-2018)**
> (Binsalamah et al. 2019)
> Number of patients: 84
> Median age: 6.6 years
> 5-year freedom from reintervention: 87%

If the SAS is more diffuse or tunnel-like, a more extensive resection into the body of the ventricle or an alternative surgical strategy (e.g., modified Konno operation or Ross-Konno operation if the aortic valve annulus is small) may be required.

Postoperative Management

Patients are usually extubated in the OR or shortly thereafter. Postoperative management of patients with SAS is focused on limiting the hyperdynamic response after SAS resection. Patients may have significant LVH and diastolic dysfunction. As such, an esmolol infusion may be beneficial to reduce heart rate in some patients. A left-bundle-branch block may be present if the subaortic resection involved an extensive septal myectomy. If present, there may be some additional systolic dysfunction.

Complications

SAS resection is usually a low-morbidity operation. However, potential complications include the creation of a VSD from an extensive myectomy (which should be identified and repaired at the time of surgery) and the presence of complete heart block from injury to the AV conduction system. Heart block may be temporary but if normal conduction is not recovered by postoperative day 10, a pacemaker may be indicated (see Chapter 75).

Long-Term Follow-Up

The incidence of reintervention after SAS resection at TCH is approximately 15%. As such, relatively close follow-up after surgical intervention is mandatory. Risk factors for membrane recurrence are an increased peak gradient at the time of diagnosis (>60 mmHg), membrane involvement of the aortic valve, a short distance between the membrane and the valve, and early age at diagnosis. Performing a myectomy at the time of SAS resection seems to be protective for development of recurrence. Data are mixed as to whether early intervention curbs the progression of AI, in particular for patients with more advanced degrees of insufficiency.

Suggested Readings

Binsalamah ZM, Spigel ZA, Zhu H, et al. Risk factors for reoperation after isolated subaortic membrane resection. Presented at the 55th Annual Meeting of the Society of Thoracic Surgeons, San Diego, CA, 2019.

Booth JH, Bryant R, Powers SC, et al. Transthoracic echocardiography does not reliably predict involvement of the aortic valve in patients with a discrete subaortic shelf. Cardiol Young 2010;20:284-289.

Ezon DS. Fixed subaortic stenosis: a clinical dilemma for clinicians and patients. Congenit Heart Dis 2013;8:450-456.

24 Supravalvar Aortic Stenosis

Lisa C. D'Alessandro, Antonio G. Cabrera, Zhe Amy Fang, Carlos M. Mery

Supravalvar aortic stenosis (SVAS) is an LVOT lesion that poses unique challenges and can be part of a more diffuse arteriopathy syndrome.

Pathophysiology and Clinical Presentation

SVAS is the characteristic congenital heart lesion of elastin deficiency, secondary to deletion of one copy of the ELN gene as part of Williams syndrome or to mutations in ELN (non-syndromic SVAS). Elastin deficiency primarily affects the large arteries resulting in medial thickening and luminal narrowing. SVAS is therefore often seen in the context of diffuse arteriopathy. Associated cardiovascular lesions are common and include valvar and supravalvar pulmonary stenosis, branch PA stenosis, aortic arch hypoplasia and coarctation, and mitral valve prolapse. SVAS is also commonly associated with coronary artery ostial stenosis, which may be secondary to tethering of the aortic valve leaflets at the narrow sinotubular junction. Anatomically, SVAS is classically categorized as membranous type, hourglass type, or diffuse hypoplasia; the later two are seen in elastin deficiency. From a surgical standpoint, SVAS is classified as isolated or as part of a diffuse arteriopathy.

Timing of presentation is dependent upon the severity of the obstruction and the presence of associated cardiovascular lesions. Most individuals with SVAS are asymptomatic at presentation and are evaluated due to findings on examination (e.g., dysmorphic features, heart murmur). In Williams syndrome, moderate to severe obstruction is more likely to progress, but the majority of individuals are stable over time. Individuals with Williams syndrome are less likely to require intervention compared to those with non-Williams SVAS (i.e., due to ELN mutations or other as-of-yet undefined causes); the reasons for this are not yet delineated.

Like other LVOT lesions, SVAS results in a harsh systolic ejection murmur with carotid radiation and a suprasternal notch thrill. One potentially distinguishing examination finding is a difference in BP (greater than approximately 18 mmHg) between the right and left arms, which is hypothesized to arise secondary to the Coanda effect (streaming of blood along a boundary wall).

Diagnosis

- **ECG.** May show LVH or BVH depending on the age of presentation and severity of the lesion.
- **CXR.** May suggest LVH or BVH.
- **Echocardiography.** Mainstay of diagnosis. Complete characterization includes 2D measurements of the sinotubular junction, color Doppler across the stenosis, and assessment of the maximal spectral Doppler velocity. The peak instantaneous gradient calculated from the maximal velocity overestimates the peak-to-peak gradient by cardiac catheterization; the mean gradient should therefore also be reported. The aortic valve annulus size and aortic morphology are also important

for surgical planning. Assessment for associated cardiovascular lesions is essential. Importantly, coronary ostial stenosis cannot be excluded by echocardiography.
- **CTA and MRI.** Primarily used as adjunct imaging modalities for assessment of the coronary arteries and detection of distal stenoses in diffuse arteriopathy. The abdomen is often included to assess for midaortic syndrome and stenosis of the aortic branches, particularly renal artery stenosis. Cross-sectional imaging is also useful to assess the branch PAs.
- **Genetic evaluation.** Should be performed at diagnosis, including family history and assessment of dysmorphic features and extracardiac anomalies, in order to direct genetic testing (i.e., chromosomal microarray to assess for Williams syndrome, elastin gene sequencing with deletion/duplication analysis to assess for nonsyndromic SVAS).

Indications / Timing of Intervention

The treatment of SVAS is surgical. Since the degree of stenosis may be progressive, especially in patients with moderate or severe SVAS, and there is commonly coronary involvement, patients are put forward for surgery earlier than patients with subvalvar or valvar AS. In general, a peak-to-peak gradient or a mean gradient of 50 mmHg is an indication for surgical intervention. Patients with lower gradients may benefit from surgical intervention if there is evidence of coronary ischemia at rest or during exercise. Isolated branch PS may be addressed by balloon angioplasty in the cardiac catheterization lab unless the stenosis is diffuse.

Anesthetic Considerations

Patients with SVAS are at high risk for myocardial ischemia, especially during induction of anesthesia. The hemodynamic goals are to avoid tachycardia and maintain adequate coronary perfusion pressure. It is imperative to have adequate preload, maintain SVR, and avoid hypotension. The combination of tachycardia and hypotension can lead to rapid hemodynamic deterioration in an already tenuous oxygen supply and demand situation. The combination of LVH and coronary obstruction puts patients at high risk for cardiac arrest, especially during induction, and make CPR less effective. For this reason, it is customary at TCH for the surgeon and the perfusionist to be available in the OR during induction.

Medications that increase heart rate (e.g., atropine, glycopyrrolate, ketamine), or decrease SVR (e.g., propofol, volatile anesthetics) should be used with caution. It is common to administer vasopressors during induction to keep an adequate SVR. It is important to note that the degree of SVAS does not correlate with the severity of coronary obstruction. Patients with mild-to-moderate SVAS can have significant coronary obstruction. Branch PA stenosis and RVOT obstruction can also lead to RVH and RV dysfunction. It is thus imperative to avoid increases in PVR with adequate ventilation and oxygenation.

After repair, patients with SVAS tend to do well. It is important to avoid wide swings

PART II. DISEASES

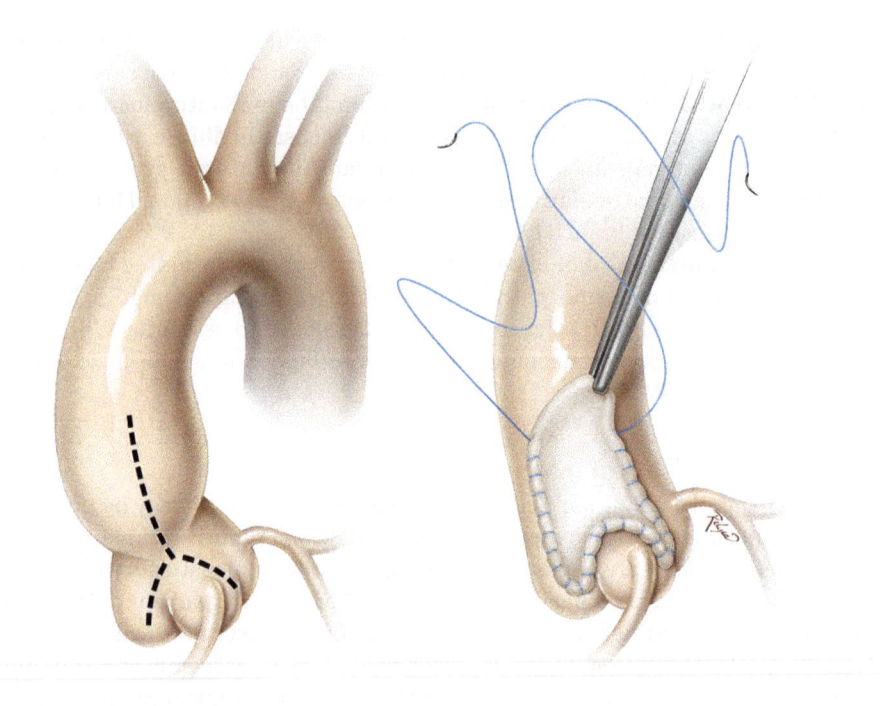

Figure 24-1. Surgical repair of SVAS with the Doty-patch technique. An inverted "Y" incision is created across the area of stenosis and an autologous pericardial pantaloon patch is used to enlarge the aortic root.

in BP. Other anesthetic considerations for patients with SVAS associated with Williams syndrome include hypertension and potential renal dysfunction.

Surgical Repair

The procedure may be performed using standard aorto-bicaval cannulation. However, the aorta in these patients tends to be thick and difficult to cannulate. A reasonable alternative is to suture a Gore-Tex® graft into the innominate artery for arterial cannulation. This also leaves more room on the ascending aorta to perform the repair. Myocardial protection in these patients may be challenging due to coronary obstruction and the degree of LVH.

The preferred repair at TCH is the Doty (pantaloon) patch aortoplasty (Figure 24-1). After cardioplegic arrest and venting of the left heart, a longitudinal incision is performed on the ascending aorta and carefully extended proximally up to the sinotubular junction, just above the right/non-coronary commissure. This is the usually the area where the thick fibrous ring creates the worst obstruction. The incision is then extended as a "Y" with one limb into the nadir of the right coronary cusp, between the right coronary and the left/right coronary commissure, and the other limb into the nadir of the non-coronary cusp. All dimensions of the "Y" incision are carefully measured, in particular the length between the apex of the incision on the distal ascending aorta and the bifurcation site of the "Y" at the sinotubular junction. Leaving this length too long will allow the anterior aspect of the aortic valve to fall down and may create significant AI or torsion of the right coronary artery.

It is not unusual to have fibrous tissue involve the ostia of the coronary arteries, in particular the left coronary, thus creating a "hood". The fibrous tissue at the sinotubular junction is shaved and the fibrous hood excised from the coronary ostia. A pantaloon-type, short, and wide patch of glutaraldehyde-treated pericardium is then used to reconstruct the aortic root and ascending aorta, therefore enlarging the sinotubular junction.

In some patients, the extent of SVAS may be more diffuse and extend into the arch and brachiocephalic vessels. These patients will require more extensive and/or separate patch aortoplasties. If there is significant stenosis of the central branch PAs, it may be addressed at the time of surgery with homograft or autologous pericardial patches.

Postoperative Management

Postoperative management of patients with SVAS is focused on the following tenets:

- **Preservation of coronary perfusion pressure.** Preoperatively, the coronary arteries are perfused at higher diastolic pressures. If the coronaries are of small caliber and have been unroofed, systemic hypertension may not be necessary, but if they are small and there is a history of ventricular arrhythmias, a combination of epinephrine at doses not higher than 0.05 mcg/kg/min and low-dose vasopressin (no more than 0.03 U/kg/hr) may be helpful given the abnormal coronary wall elasticity.
- **Adequate ventricular performance.** RV or LV dysfunction may be present due to coronary insufficiency from RVH or LVH, and/or prolonged cross-clamp time from more extensive repairs. Given the degree of LVH and poor LV compliance, there will be more significant changes in ventricular filling pressures at small changes in volume. One should aim for the lowest filling pressures to achieve normal hemodynamics. Inotropes may be used, if needed, to increase BP and perfusion. Significant ventricular unloading with diuretics could easily precipitate hypotension. Diuresis should be conservative.
- **Identification and treatment of arrhythmias.** Ectopic atrial rhythms are infrequent but could be secondary to elevated ventricular filling pressures and more than moderate mitral or tricuspid valve regurgitation. Ventricular arrhythmias should increase suspicion for coronary ischemia and ventricular dysfunction.

Complications

Some potential complications after repair of supravalvar AS include:

- **Development of AI.** Failure to achieve an adequate geometry of the aortic root and ascending aorta during repair may distort the aortic valve and condition the development of AI. This complication should be noted and corrected in the OR.
- **Coronary insufficiency.** Adequate myocardial protection is imperative during

repair to avoid myocardial dysfunction. In addition, an inadequate repair may cause torsion of the coronary arteries.

Long-Term Follow-Up

Individuals with SVAS require lifelong follow-up as they may develop arterial stenoses in other locations or recurrence of SVAS following intervention. Additionally, they are at risk for hypertension secondary to stenotic lesions, vascular stiffness, or renal involvement. Hypertension can be difficult to manage and may require a multidisciplinary approach. Nonsyndromic SVAS secondary to ELN mutation is an autosomal dominant condition and therefore families should be counseled that an affected individual has a 50% chance of passing the trait to their offspring.

25 Aortic Coarctation and Interrupted Aortic Arch

Keila N. Lopez, Sebastian C. Tume, Stuart R. Hall, Aimee Liou, S. Kristen Sexson Tejtel, Carlos M. Mery

Coarctation of the aorta (CoA), aortic arch hypoplasia, and interrupted aortic arch (IAA) are congenital conditions where a portion of the aorta (not including the aortic valve) measure small for BSA or a segment of the arch is atretic or missing. These lesions can present in the newborn period, childhood, and more rarely, in the adult period. Timing of presentation is dependent on the severity of the lesion (degree and extent of arch narrowing) as well as the presence of a PDA and aortopulmonary collaterals. Arch lesions may also be accompanied by other left-sided obstructive lesions including an abnormal aortic valve, mitral valve, or LV. For multilevel left-heart hypoplasia, see Chapter 26.

The aortic arch is usually divided into different segments (Figure 25-1):
- **Proximal arch:** between the innominate artery and left carotid artery
- **Distal arch:** between the left carotid artery and the left subclavian artery
- **Isthmus:** between the left subclavian artery and the ductus arteriosus or ligamentum arteriosum

The dimensions of each of the aortic arch segments are important to define the clinical presentation and management of patients with aortic arch hypoplasia. Focal CoA classically presents with significant narrowing at the level of the isthmus.

IAA is classified into 3 types depending on the aortic arch segment involved with the interruption:
- **Type A:** the interruption is distal to the left subclavian artery
- **Type B:** the interruption is between the left common carotid artery and the left subclavian artery
- **Type C:** the interruption is between the innominate artery and the left common carotid artery

Pathophysiology and Clinical Presentation

Fetal

Mild aortic arch lesions are often difficult to detect in utero, and may only be detected postnatally, after the PDA closes. On the contrary, if there is significant ascending, transverse, or isthmus arch narrowing, there will be retrograde flow in the aortic arch, which can be detected on fetal echocardiogram.

IAA can also be detected in utero, when a fetal echocardiogram reveals a lack of communication between parts of the transverse and descending aorta. However, the type of interruption may be difficult to determine depending on the size, position, and gestational age of the fetus.

Regardless of severity, there are typically minimal clinical fetal manifestations of arch obstruction in utero due to the patency of the PDA. However, it is critical to determine which arch lesions will be severe or critical (such as the case in IAA), as it will help

PART II. DISEASES

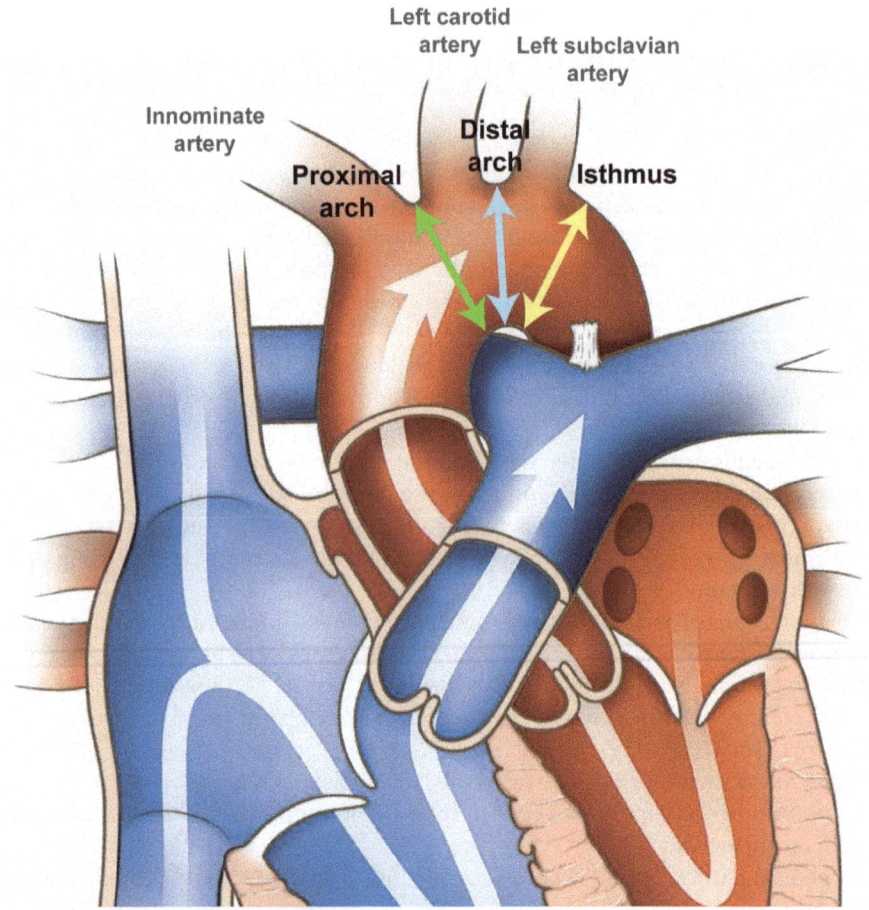

Figure 25-1. Aortic arch segments.

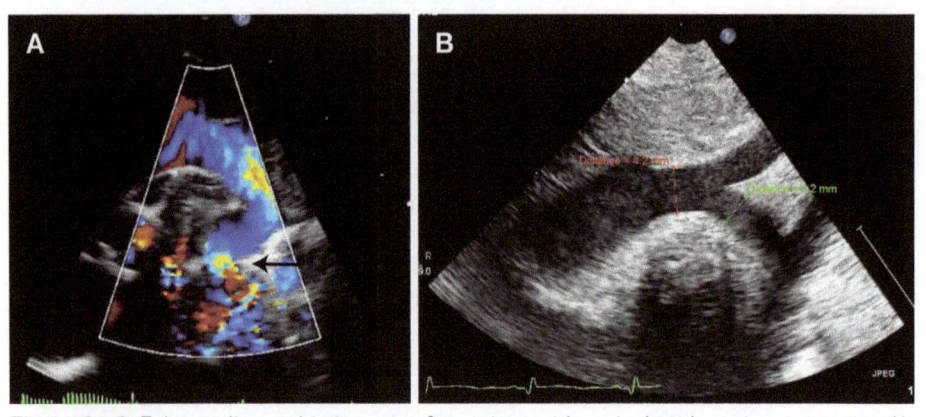

Figure 25-2. Echocardiographic images of a patient with an isolated aortic coarctation (A, arrow) and a patient with a hypoplastic aortic arch (B).

182

25. AORTIC COARCTATION AND INTERRUPTED AORTIC ARCH

Aortic Arch Watch
(patients with mild to moderate suspicion for coarctation of the aorta)

Where should the baby go?

```
Fetal Center patient identified as having possible coarctation of the aorta
Born at term without major associated congenital anomalies
               │
               ▼
In Delivery Room:
Easily palpate pulses, RR and HR
within expected limits?
   │Yes                    │No
   ▼                       ▼
May go to WT NICU     To WT NICU level 4
No lines placed       Obtain emergent echo
No standard lactates  Notify cardiologist
   │                  Have PGE available
   ▼
On admission:
Obtain VS, four-extremity
BPs, palpate pulses, place PIV
   │
   ▼
Easily palpate pulses?
No significant upper-to-lower     ── No ──►
extremity BP gradient*?
Normal RR (<60) and HR (<170)?
   │Yes
   ▼
Remain in WT NICU
- Q 3 hour RR, HR, and pulses (with feeds)
- Q 6 hour four-extremity BPs
- Consult Cardiology               ── No ──► WT NICU level 4
- Obtain an echo by 8 hours of age            Start PGE
   │
   ▼
No hemodynamically significant aortic     NO COARCTATION per Cardiology
arch obstruction per cardiology?          MBU or discharge
   │Maybe       │Yes                      No follow-up
   ▼           ▼
PDA open but  PDA closed? ── Yes ──► MILD COARCTATION per Cardiology
arch                                  MBU or discharge
questionable    │No                   Follow-up in 2-4 weeeks
   │           ▼
   ▼      Monitor as per Cardiology ──► SMALL PDA, NO ARCH GRADIENT
Monitor in NICU                          Discharge and follow-up in 1-2 weks

                                         MOD-LARGE PDA
                                         Continue monitoring
```

* BP gradient >20 mmHg

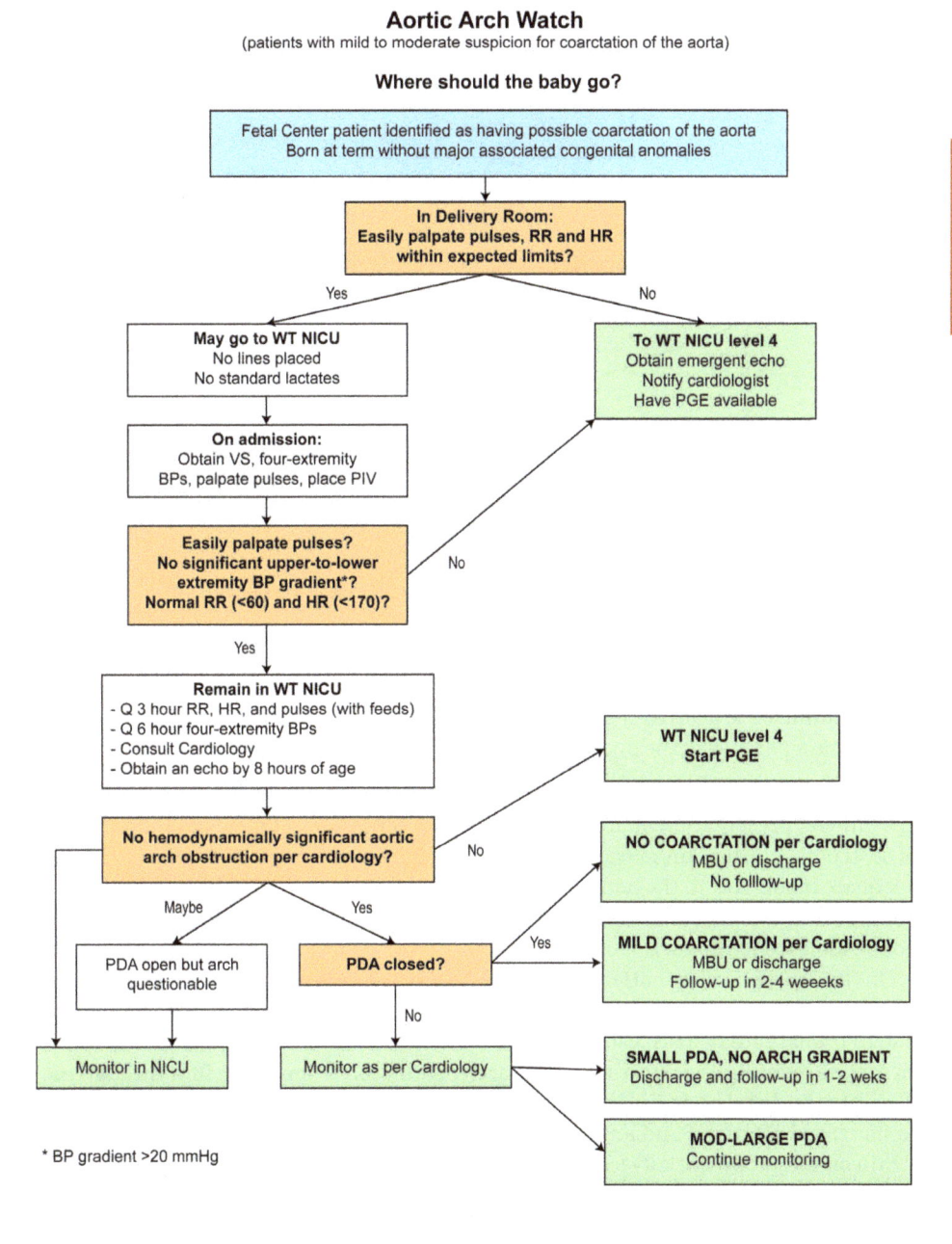

Figure 25-3. "Arch-watch" protocol at TCH. BP: blood pressure, HR: heart rate, MBU: Mother and Baby Unit, NICU: Neonatal Intensive Care Unit, PDA: patent ductus arteriosus, PGE: prostaglandin E, PIV: peripheral intravenous line, RR: respiratory rate, VS: vital signs, WT: West Tower.

183

PART II. DISEASES

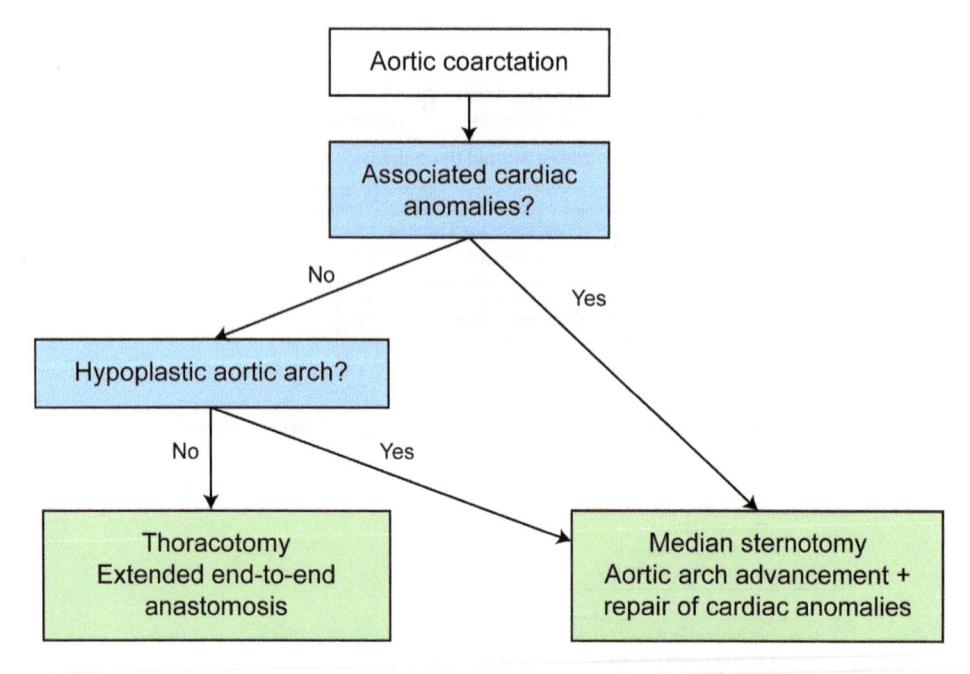

Figure 25-4. Algorithm for management of CoA and hypoplastic aortic arch in newborns and infants.

dictate immediate postnatal care including location of delivery and initiation of PGE to maintain patency of the ductus.

Neonatal

The clinical presentation of aortic arch lesions after birth will depend on the degree of obstruction. Mild CoA may not present in the neonatal period, as it typically allows adequate blood flow to the body, making it clinically less obvious. Often, these milder lesions are discovered and/or become clinically apparent during childhood (see Childhood/Adolescence below).

On the contrary, most patients with severe CoA and IAA tend to present in the first 24-72 hours after birth as the PDA closes, unless PGE is started immediately after birth due to prenatal diagnosis. Closure of the PDA can result in significant narrowing of either one or multiple parts of the aortic arch in addition to impeding flow through the PDA into the distal body. Furthermore, the neonatal myocardium is uniquely sensitive to increased afterload and any significant narrowing of the arch can cause a severe strain on the LV, potentially leading to LV dysfunction.

Early in the course of PDA closure (often first 12-24 hours), it may be noted that femoral and pedal pulses are diminished, or that patients have a BP gradient difference between upper and lower extremities. Compromise to blood flow distal to the PDA may not be very clinically obvious at this point. If detected later in the neonatal course (after 24-72 hours), patients may have severe compromise of blood flow distal to the

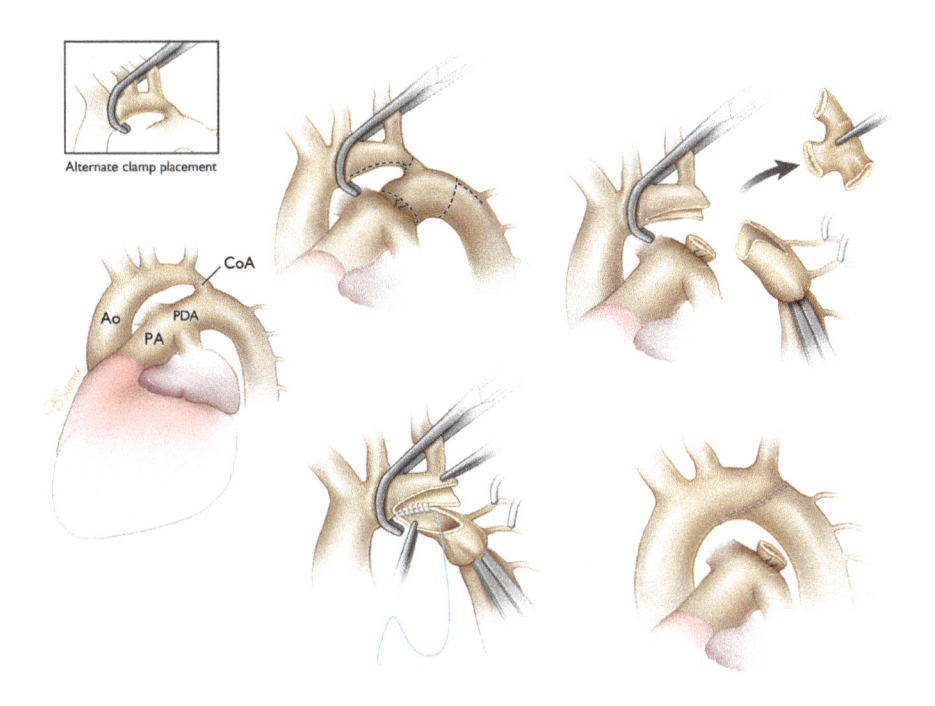

25. AORTIC COARCTATION AND INTERRUPTED AORTIC ARCH

Figure 25-5. Coarctectomy and extended end-to-end anastomosis repair of CoA. The aortic arch, brachiocephalic vessels, descending aorta, and ductus arteriosus / ligamentum arteriosum are fully mobilized. The intercostal vessels / collaterals are controlled with fine tourniquets. A Castaneda clamp is used to clamp the left subclavian artery and the aortic arch. An angled or straight clamp is placed on the descending aorta. The ductus arteriosus is divided and the coarctation segment with all ductal tissue is removed. The proximal incision is extended into the undersurface of the aortic arch. The distal incision is extended posteriorly. A large anastomosis is created between the descending aorta and the aortic arch with polypropelene suture (7-0 for newborns). The clamps are released.

area of narrowing or PDA, and they may present with poor feeding, tachypnea, lethargy, irritability, and cardiogenic shock with acidosis and multisystem organ failure within the first week of life.

Childhood / Adolescence
Aortic arch obstructive lesions that present in childhood and adolescence are typically less severe and there is time for collateral flow to develop to deliver blood to the lower body despite obstruction in the aortic arch. These lesions can also develop as a result of aortic injury due to trauma or inflammatory processes.

Otherwise asymptomatic patients may present with a murmur or during evaluation for hypertension. Patients may also present with frequent headaches and stomach aches that are worse with activity. On examination, they will have decreased or delayed

PART II. DISEASES

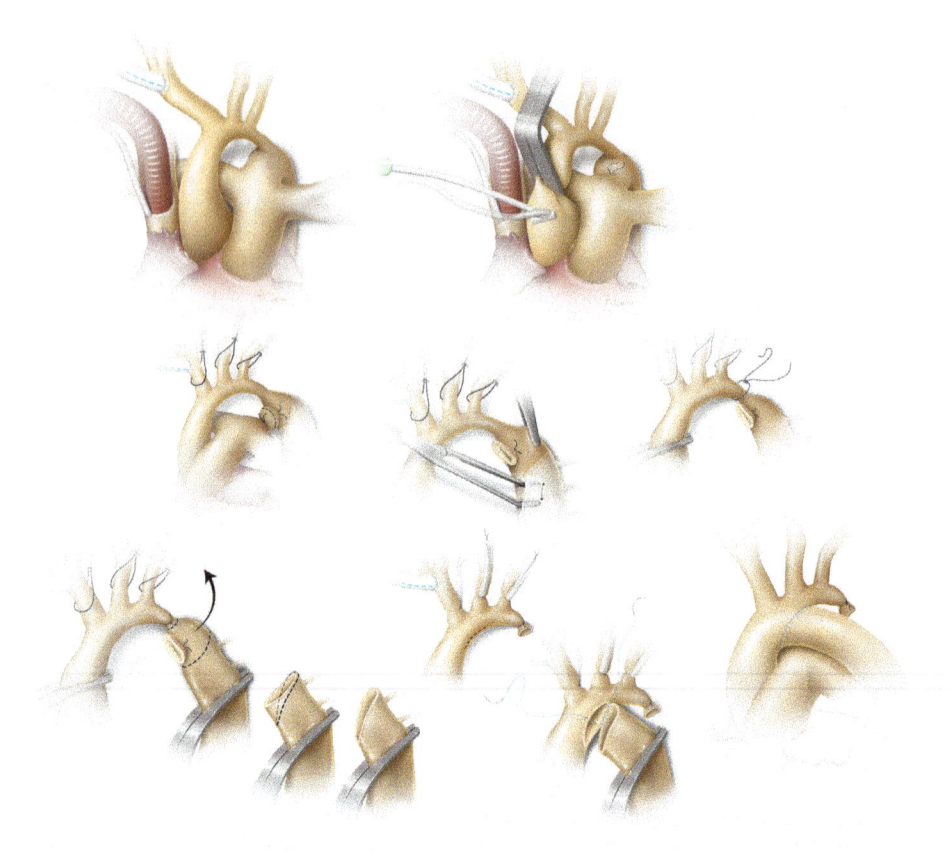

Figure 25-6. Aortic arch advancement for repair of aortic arch hypoplasia in newborns and infants. CPB is instituted through a graft on the innominate artery and bicaval cannulation. The aortic arch, brachiocephalic vessels, and the descending aorta are widely mobilized as distal as possible to allow adequate mobility. After division of the ductus arteriosus / ligamentum arteriosum, the isthmus is divided and sutured closed. All ductal tissue is removed and the descending aorta is spatulated. An incision is made on the proximal aortic arch and an end-to-side anastomosis is performed between the descending aorta and the arch. It is important to properly align the anastomosis to avoid torsion of the ascending aorta with resultant obstruction.

pulses, though the amount of decrease or delay depends on the amount of collateral vessel flow that has developed over the duration of the obstruction. These patients will also have a significant systolic BP gradient (>20 mmHg) on 4-extremity BP. A systolic murmur that persists into diastole may be heard in the left paravertebral area and represents flow across the area of obstruction. Continuous murmurs may also be heard due to flow through large collateral vessels. Presentation at this age is typically not associated with poor cardiac function or cardiovascular collapse.

25. AORTIC COARCTATION AND INTERRUPTED AORTIC ARCH

Sliding Arch Aortoplasty

Patch Aortoplasty

Interposition Graft

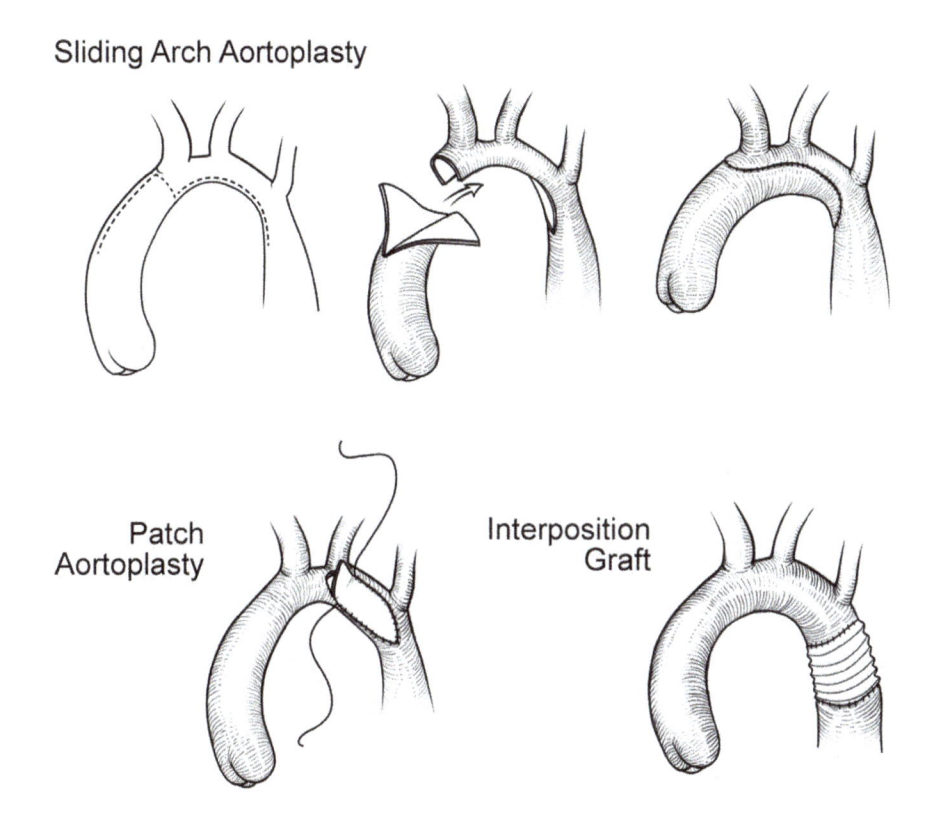

Figure 25-7. Alternative surgical approaches for aortic arch reconstruction. The sliding arch aortoplasty is an all-autologous repair in which a tongue of ascending aorta is used to enlarge the aortic arch. If all-autologous repairs are not possible, a patch aortoplasty or an interposition graft placement may be used.

Diagnosis
- **Fetal echocardiogram.**
  - *Mild CoA.* There can be subtle signs on fetal echocardiogram that suggest a possible CoA (often mild) ex utero, including persistent color flow in the area of the mild arch narrowing, and borderline or mildly small measurements of the aortic arch for gestational age by 2D. Presence or severity of a potentially mild CoA in these cases cannot be fully realized until postnatal assessment, as the PDA closes and BP gradients and femoral/pedal pulses can be assessed.
  - *Severe CoA, moderate-to-severe tubular hypoplasia, and IAA.* These lesions can be detected in utero by fetal echocardiogram. In the case of severe CoA and moderate-to-severe tubular arch hypoplasia, arch 2D measurements are typically small for gestational age and retrograde flow is noted in the narrowed aortic arch by color and pulse-wave Doppler. Arch sidedness is able to be determined

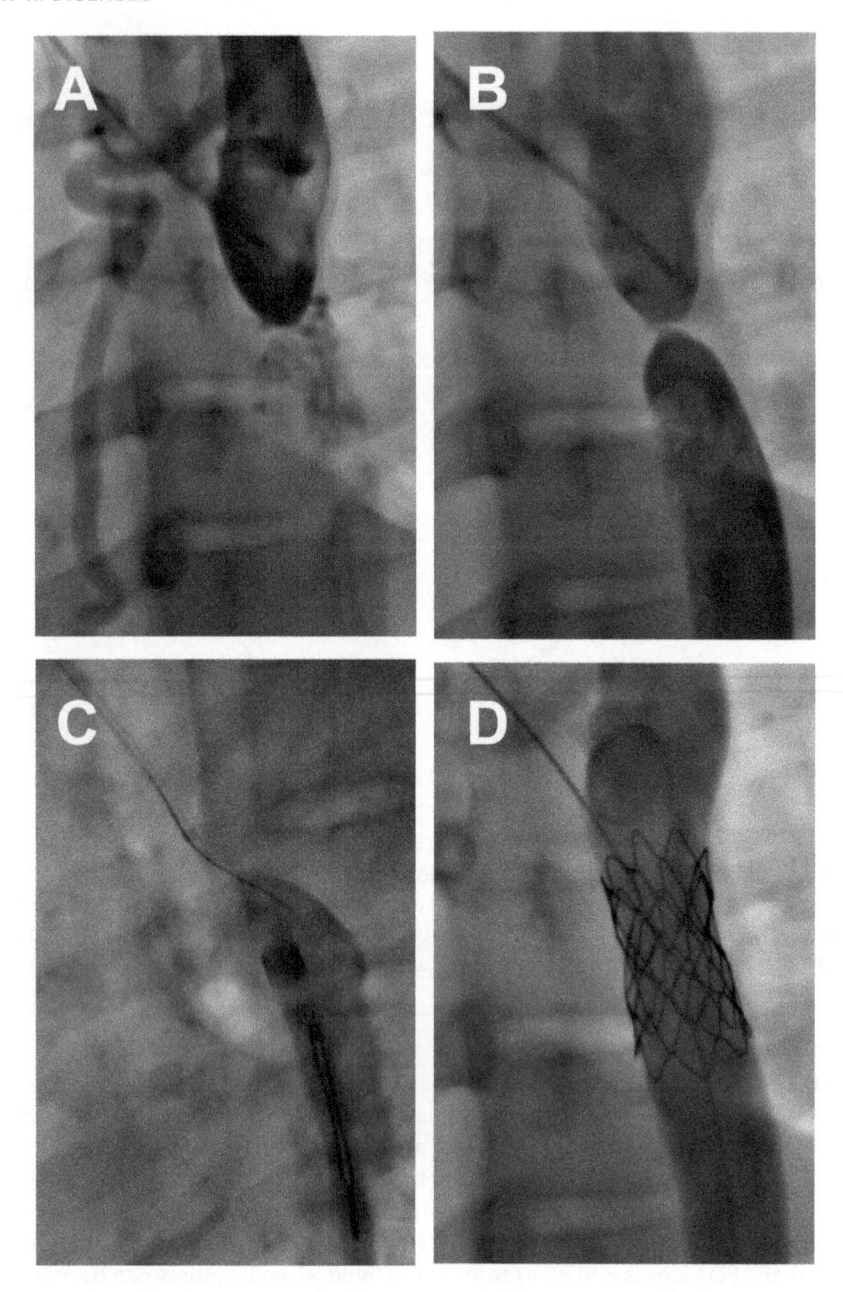

Figure 25-8. Angiograms of a patient with near atresia of the aorta at the level of CoA. A) Note extensive arterial collateral vessels typical in severe aortic obstruction. B) Simultaneous injections are performed above and below the obstruction demonstrating the severity of the CoA. C) A wire is passed through the narrowed segment, to be snared from below. D) Angiography after placement of a covered stent demonstrating normal caliber of the treated area.

in most cases. In the case of an IAA, the ascending aorta typically takes a very linear course superiorly and does not connect with the descending aorta, which arises from a large PDA. It can be very challenging to determine arch sidedness prenatally in a patient with IAA.
- **Pulse oximetry.** Unlike other cyanotic congenital heart lesions that present in the neonatal period, pulse oximetry screening cannot accurately detect CoA (whether mild or severe). However, in the setting of IAA, pulse oximetry screening can detect differential cyanosis (higher SaO_2 levels in the arms than in the legs).
- **CXR.** In the neonatal period, CXR is not very helpful for diagnosis of a CoA, although it may help with determination of arch sidedness. In the childhood/adolescent period, where a CoA may have been present for some time and aortopulmonary collaterals exist, CXR may demonstrate proximal rib notching along the sternal border. Additionally, with later presentation, one may see the "3" sign where there is indentation in one portion of the aorta where the localized narrowing exists.
- **ECG.** In the childhood/adolescent period there may be LV hypertrophy.
- **Echocardiogram (Figure 25-2).** Mainstay of diagnosis. Evaluation should include arch sidedness, arch branching, and measurements of the ascending aorta, proximal and distal transverse aortic arch, and aortic isthmus. A complete evaluation of the aortic arch must be performed. The primary goal is to define the site and extent of obstruction with additional focus on evaluation of function, myocardial changes, and other coexistent lesions (e.g., bicuspid aortic valve, small left-heart structures, VSD). Multiple views must be obtained to provide adequate definition. Retrograde flow may be noted in the narrowed aortic arch by color and pulse-wave Doppler if there is a PDA or if there are collaterals supplying flow in retrograde fashion to a portion of the transverse aortic arch. Color-Doppler echocardiography can show increased turbulence at the site of narrowing and spectral Doppler can show increased velocity of flow through the area. The abdominal aorta should be evaluated to determine if there is flow continuation throughout the cardiac cycle. Reduced or delayed systolic amplitude with flow that continues into diastole would be concerning for aortic arch obstruction. Additional images should be obtained to evaluate cardiac function and provide function estimates. One can also ascertain injury to the myocardium by looking for echobrightness suggestive of endocardial fibroelastosis. In older patients, the arch may not be well seen and alternative imaging modalities may be necessary.
- **CTA/MRI.** May be useful in cases where the degree of arch narrowing is unclear, arch sidedness cannot be determined, or arch anatomy cannot be fully delineated by echocardiogram (as is often in the case in late presenting CoA with several aortopulmonary collaterals). In patients with IAA and unclear anatomy on echocardiogram, CTA/MRI may be helpful in identifying the type of interruption, distance between the proximal and distal segments, and other defects that may interfere with surgical planning (including anomalous subclavian arteries and arch sidedness).
- **Genetics.** Arch anomalies may be associated with genetic abnormalities, such as DiGeorge syndrome. For details on genetic testing, see Chapter 50.

Indications/Timing of Intervention

In some situations, it is unclear whether a newborn will develop a significant CoA upon closure of the PDA. In those cases, the patient may be placed on an "arch watch". The purpose of this "arch watch" is to closely monitor hemodynamic and anatomic parameters as the PDA is allowed to close off PGE. If upon PDA closure, the patient develops a significant CoA, PGE is started and the patient is referred for surgical intervention. The "arch watch" protocol at TCH is shown in Figure 25-3.

The presence of a severe CoA and/or aortic arch hypoplasia that is dependent on PGE to keep the PDA open is an indication for intervention. Similarly, the diagnosis of IAA warrants intervention in the newborn period.

Patients that present in cardiogenic shock a few days or weeks after birth due to closure of the PDA are started on PGE in an attempt to reopen the PDA and/or relax the ductal tissue of the isthmus and relieve the obstruction. If PGE is successful in reestablishing blood flow to the lower body, the patient is medically stabilized for a few days to allow end-organ function recovery prior to surgical intervention. If administration of PGE is unsuccessful in reestablishing adequate blood flow, the patient is taken emergently to the OR for intervention.

Patients that present beyond the newborn period with milder forms of CoA still benefit from intervention in order to decrease the risks associated with long-standing hypertension. However, intervention (cath or surgical) can be performed in a more elective fashion.

Anesthetic Considerations

The anesthetic management of patients with COA is straightforward, particularly in neonates. It is customary to have the ability to monitor BP both proximal and distal to the CoA, either with a right-radial arterial line and a BP cuff on the lower extremity or a right-radial arterial line with an umbilical or femoral arterial line. Be cognizant of the arch anatomy and the possibility of an aberrant right subclavian origin (which will interfere with assessment of proximal aortic pressures). Discuss the surgical approach and the need for invasive arterial pressure distal to the CoA with the surgeon: in very small infants or infants with Down syndrome, the risk may outweigh the benefit.

For CoA repair via left thoracotomy, patients can be allowed to cool during the initial dissection, with core temperatures reaching the 34-35 °C range. Small infants may cool passively in the room, while a larger patient might need more active cooling measures. Likewise, as patients become larger, specialized airway techniques can be used as tolerated to isolate the ipsilateral lung. There is not generally an indication for TEE in CoA repair via thoracotomy.

Surgical Repair

The ideal type of surgical repair depends on the anatomy of each particular patient (Figure 25-4). In general, an all-autologous repair is favored, avoiding the use of patch or graft material. If the proximal aortic arch is adequate in size, the procedure is performed through a left thoracotomy. On the contrary, if the proximal arch is small and there

> **CoA repair via left thoracotomy (1995-2013)** (Mery et al. 2015)
> - Median number of procedures done per year: 18 (0-26)
> - Median age at surgery: 2 months
> - Median hospital length of stay: 7 days (2-194 days)
> - Perioperative mortality: 1%
> - Reintervention rate (median follow-up 6 years): 4%
>
> **Aortic arch advancement (1995-2012)** (Mery et al. 2014)
> - Median number of procedures per year: 14 (0-30)
> - Median age at surgery: 14 days
> - Vocal cord dysfunction on routine laryngoscopy: 38%
> - Clinical vocal cord residual dysfunction at last follow-up: <1%
> - Median hospital length of stay: 16 days (5-235 days)
> - Perioperative mortality: 1%
> - Reintervention rate (median follow-up 6 years): 3%

is concern that addressing the arch through a left thoracotomy would leave a more proximal gradient, or if there are concomitant intracardiac lesions to be addressed, the procedure is performed through a median sternotomy using CPB. In general, for neonates and infants, the proximal arch size in centimeters should be equal or greater than the weight in kilograms of the patient plus 1. For example, a 3.5-kg newborn is expected to have a proximal arch that measures at least 4.5 cm.

Coarctation Repair Via Left Thoracotomy

The procedure is performed using a serratus-sparing left posterolateral thoracotomy through the third or fourth intercostal space. The descending aorta, aortic arch (up to the innominate artery), and ductus arteriosus/ligamentum arteriosum are completely dissected with care not to injure the vagus and recurrent laryngeal neves (RLN) (the RLN wraps around the ductus arteriosus/ligamentum arteriosum) or the intercostal vessels and collaterals that may be quite prominent in this disease. 100 Units/kg of heparin are administered 2-3 minutes prior to clamping.

For newborns and young children, the coarctectomy and extended end-to-end anastomosis (Figure 25-5) is the surgical technique of choice for repair of CoA. In older children and adults, the decreased elasticity of tissues will preclude using this technique. In those cases, other techniques such as simple end-to-end anastomosis, patch aortoplasty, or placement of an interposition graft may be needed.

Aortic Arch Reconstruction Via Median Sternotomy

In cases of aortic arch hypoplasia or intracardiac anomalies, the procedures are performed through a median sternotomy under CPB. These procedures are usually performed using antegrade cerebral perfusion through a Gore-Tex® graft (3 or 3.5 mm for newborns) that is sutured to the innominate artery after administration of 100 Units/kg of heparin. Bicaval cannulation is commonly used. After institution of CPB, the patient is cooled down to 18 °C and the aortic arch, ductus arteriosus/ligamentum arteriosum, and descending aorta are completely dissected. Once the goal temperature is reached, an aortic cross-clamp is placed and antegrade cardioplegia administered. The RA is opened and the left heart is vented through the atrial septum.

The procedure of choice for newborns and infants is the aortic arch advancement (Figure 25-6) which entails an end-to-side anastomosis between the descending aorta and the proximal aortic arch. This technique is not used in older patients due to the lack of mobility of the tissues. In those patients, alternative techniques include the sliding arch aortoplasty, patch aortoplasty, or placement of an interposition graft (Figure 25-7).

IAA

In addition to arch interruption, patients with IAA usually have a posterior malalignment VSD and a hypoplastic aortic annulus. However, in the majority of patients, the aortic valve annulus is sufficient to support the systemic circulation (~5 mm in a 3 kg newborn). The surgical repair is performed in the newborn period and entails an aortic arch advancement, resection of the posteriorly malaligned ventricular septum causing subaortic obstruction, and transatrial VSD repair with an autologous pericardial patch. The distance between the ascending aorta and the descending aorta after ductal tissue resection in these patients can be quite significant. As such, in order to reduce tension, it may be useful in some patients to perform a posterior direct anastomosis between the ascending and descending aortas and place an anterior patch of glutaraldehyde-treated pericardium or homograft.

Catheter-Based Intervention

Catheter-based techniques serve an important role in the treatment of children of all ages with aortic obstruction (Figure 25-8). In general, intervention is indicated when the pressure gradient is >20 mmHg. It is also indicated in patients with gradient <20 mmHg in the setting of significant collaterals, univentricular heart, or ventricular dysfunction.

Balloon Angioplasty

Balloon angioplasty involves dilation of the CoA, and is effective in providing relief of obstruction. However, in the native CoA, recurrence of obstruction can occur, especially in younger patients (<6 months), and reintervention can be required. In postoperative recurrent CoA (i.e., after repair for CoA, IAA, or hypoplastic left heart syndrome with a Norwood procedure), relief of obstruction is more durable than in native CoA, and balloon angioplasty is the therapy of choice. Balloon angioplasty is also helpful in providing early relief of aortic obstruction for young infants who have other associated congenital heart lesions, depressed ventricular function, severe MR, or low cardiac output and who will benefit from delay of surgery.

Balloon-Expandable Bare-Metal Stents

Balloon-expandable bare-metal stents provide for safe, more effective, and more durable relief of aortic obstruction than standard balloon angioplasty. They are employed when standard balloon angioplasty does not achieve a durable result, as may happen in cases of intraprocedural vessel recoil or rapid recurrence after standard balloon angioplasty. Smaller pediatric patients who receive stents will undergo reintervention for dilation of the stent as they grow. All efforts are made to adhere to the tenet of implanting stents that are capable of being expanded to adult size.

Stenting is frequently avoided in infants and small children, in whom small vessel size may preclude easily implanting stents with potential to reach adult size. Exceptions to this can occur when individual clinical factors render implantation of smaller stents necessary (e.g., surgery undesirable in a small patient with recurrent CoA, intimal flap raised during angioplasty). In such cases, these smaller stents may later be overdilated to the point of intentional fracture to keep up with somatic growth. The stented area is then restented with a stent that has adult-size potential.

For lesions near the head-and-neck vessels, open-cell stents can be used. Open-cell stents that are by necessity implanted near or across the orifice of a branch vessel allow for selective dilation of the cell adjacent to the vessel orifice, such that flow through the orifice remains completely unobstructed.

Covered Stents
Covered stents are composed of a metal stent covered with fabric or graft material such as polytetrafluoroethylene (PTFE). Covered stents are used more frequently in patients that are at higher risk for aortic wall injury, including older pediatric and adolescent/adult patients with severe CoA/near-interruption of the aorta. They may also be used in patients who have already developed evidence of aortic wall injury (e.g., pseudoaneurysm). The covering serves to seal off the affected or potentially injured area. An additional benefit of the covering is the prevention of neointimal ingrowth.

Postprocedural Management
Approach to postoperative care depends on the procedure performed. In general, appropriate support of end-organ perfusion, control of hypertension, and early diagnosis of any postoperative complications are the most important goals.

Patients following catheter interventions are admitted to CICU for observation overnight focusing primarily on management of hypertension and puncture site complications. Compression safeguards remain in place and must be passively deflated every 2 hours and removed to ensure appropriate extremity perfusion. The extremity used for arterial access must be frequently assessed for signs of bleeding and poor perfusion. In cases of compromised extremity perfusion, anticoagulation therapy with heparin or enoxaparin should be immediately initiated. If poorly responsive to intervention, Doppler study of the vessels should be completed to document the location and degree of obstruction. Any compromise in perfusion leading to loss of pulses or change in color and appearance must be treated as an emergency. Vascular surgery should be involved immediately. Other rare but reported complications related to catheterization include pneumothorax and retroperitoneal bleeding.

Surgical repair through thoracotomy involves an incision through several muscular layers as well as physical compression of the lung to achieve visualization. Postoperative management is focused around close neurologic monitoring, tight BP control, symptoms of lung contusion, bleeding, and management of pain.

Postoperative hypertension warrants aggressive treatment to avoid anastomotic bleeding and is usually multifactorial. The early catecholamine storm-related hypertension is treated with agents such as nitroprusside sodium or nicardipine. In older children, esmolol drip or intermittent labetalol should be considered. Additional therapy with long-term agents such as enalapril or captopril may be initiated on postoperative days 1-2 to address the elevated renin levels reported in this patient population. Renal perfusion and function should be satisfactory before initiating these agents.

Pain is also a significant and common contributor to postoperative hypertension, particularly in patients undergoing a left thoracotomy. We recommend the use of nonsedating agents such as IV acetaminophen, and patient-controlled analgesia. Other agents to consider include dexmedetomidine drip during the first postoperative night and ketorolac for older children (>1 year) provided the platelet count and renal function are satisfactory.

The management of patients that undergo aortic arch repair through a median sternotomy is similar to other patients undergoing CPB. Older children are commonly extubated in the OR unless other surgical repairs accompany the repair. Newborns and infants usually return from the OR intubated. Once hemodynamic stability is observed within the first 6-12 hours, the patients are progressed to extubation. Attention should focus around symptoms of upper-airway obstruction as manipulation of RLN may lead to temporary paresis or injury. RLN injury commonly presents as stridor or even significant upper-airway obstruction; evaluation is warranted by ENT.

Complications

Surgical Repair

The main complications after surgical repair of CoA and hypoplasia of the aortic arch include:

- **Injury to the RLN.** If routine laryngoscopy is performed, approximately 25-30% of patients undergoing repair through a median sternotomy will have left vocal cord paresis due to stretching of the nerve during dissection (Dewan et al. 2012). The vast majority of these patients will recover vocal cord function within a few weeks. However, newborns with RLN injury may exhibit swallowing difficulties and may need thickened formula or nasoenteral feeds until recovery.
- **Chylothorax.** The disruption of lymphatic channels in the thorax, in particular during repairs using a left thoracotomy, may lead to a chylothorax (see Chapter 77).
- **Postcoarctectomy syndrome.** Thought to be a reperfusion reaction of the organs below the prior CoA and is commonly accompanied by abdominal tenderness, feeding intolerance, and leukocytosis at 2-3 days following repair. Appropriate BP control helps prevent these symptoms in the majority of patients.
- **Left mainstem bronchus compression.** Aortic arch reconstruction reduces the window between the ascending and descending aorta, potentially causing compression of the left mainstem bronchus. However, it is very rare for bronchial compression to be significant (<1%).

Catheter-Based Treatment

Aortic wall injury can occur in catheter-based interventions. This may take the form of early or late pseudoaneurysm formation or dissection; both can be treated with transcatheter techniques. Stent embolization may occur intraprocedurally or in the immediate postcatheterization period. Stent fracture can occur late and results in recurrence of obstruction; this is treated with restenting.

Patients undergoing balloon angioplasty will by definition sustain some degree of intimal tear; such therapeutic tears can sometimes be visualized on angiography. These tears are intrinsic to the treatment strategy and as such, are not considered a complication, but rather as evidence of efficacy.

Long-Term Follow-Up
Repair of aortic arch obstruction is not without long-term risk. Lifelong follow-up with clinical exam and echocardiographic imaging is needed to continue to monitor and treat issues as they arise. Potential long-term complications include:
- **Hypertension.** The long-term development of hypertension or exercise-induced hypertension in patients after aortic arch repair is high, likely related to an abnormal wall structure causing increased stiffness and poor compliance. The patients more likely to develop postintervention hypertension are those with preintervention hypertension, although most patients will develop hypertension whether or not they had preexisting hypertension. A normal BP in the physician's office does not rule out hypertension as a significant portion of those with normal BP in the clinic will have elevated BP on ambulatory or exercise evaluation. Exercise-induced hypertension is a predictor for developing hypertension in the future. Many who develop hypertension will be resistant to treatment and require multiple medications to control or improve their BP.
- **Recurrent aortic arch obstruction.** Recurrent arch obstruction requires lifelong monitoring. Echocardiogram, MRI, and CTA may be used to evaluate for recurrent obstruction and help define need for reintervention. The incidence of recurrent arch obstruction at TCH after repair through a left thoracotomy or a median sternotomy is approximately 3-4% at a median follow-up of 6 years.
- **Aortic arch aneurysm/dissection.** Aortic arch aneruysms may develop mainly in patients that have undergone arch repairs using patch aortoplasty or subclavian flaps.
- **Premature coronary artery disease.** Patients with aortic arch intervention are at higher risk of developing premature coronary artery disease. Abnormal flow dynamics in muscularized arteries can lead to a high atherosclerotic potential. Additionally, due to abnormal flow dynamics in these patients, there is an increase in LV pressure that can result in LV hypertrophy. Continued evaluation of cardiac hypertrophy and function is important.

Suggested Readings
Dewan K, Cephus C, Owczarzak V, et al. Incidence and implication of vocal ford paresis following neonatal cardiac surgery. Laryngoscopy 2012;122:2781-5.

Feltes TC, Bacha E, Beekman RH 3rd, et al. Indications for cardiac catheterization and intervention in pediatric cardiac disease. Circulation 2011;123:2607-2652.

McKenzie ED, Klysik M, Morales DL, et al. Ascending sliding arch aortoplasty: a novel technique for repair of arch hypoplasia. Ann Thorac Surg 2011;91:805-810.

Mery CM, Guzmán-Pruneda FA, Trost JG Jr, et al. Contemporary results of aortic coarctation repair through left thoracotomy. Ann Thorac Surg 2015;100:1039-1046.

Mery CM, Guzmán-Pruneda FA, Carberry KE, et al. Aortic arch advancement for aortic coarctation and hypoplastic arch in neonates and infants. Ann Thorac Surg 2014;98:625-633.

Mery CM, Khan MS, Guzmán-Pruneda FA, et al. Contemporary results of surgical repair of recurrent aortic arch obstruction. Ann Thorac Surg 2014;98:133-140.

Qureshi AM, McElhinney DB, Lock JE, et al. Acute and intermediate outcomes, and evaluation of injury to the aortic wall, as based on 15 years experience of implanting stents to treat aortic coarctation. Cardiol Young. 2007;17:307-318.

Richter AL, Ongkasuwan J, Ocampo EC. Long-term follow-up of vocal cord movement impairment and feeding after neonatal cardiac surgery. Int J Pediatr Otorhinolaryngol 2016;83:211-214.

26 Multilevel Left-Heart Hypoplasia

Shaine A. Morris, Erin A. Gottlieb, Carlos M. Mery

Multilevel left-heart hypoplasia (LHH) is a heterogeneous entity that involves variable underdevelopment of the mitral valve, LV, aortic valve, ascending aorta, and aortic arch. It exists within a wide spectrum that spans from hypoplastic left heart syndrome (HLHS) to mild hypoplasia of left-sided structures. The optimal management strategy for patients with a "borderline left heart" in the middle of the spectrum (i.e., single ventricle palliation [SVP] vs. biventricular repair [BVR]) is difficult to decide.

Pathophysiology and Clinical Presentation

This group of lesions, if not diagnosed prenatally, typically present in the first week of life as the PDA closes. They may present with shock (poor perfusion, tachycardia, weak pulses). Alternatively, they may be diagnosed earlier with more subtle findings such as a murmur when there is AS or a VSD, low postductal oxygen saturations on newborn pulse oximetry screening, a cardiac gallop in cases of AS, or differential pulses or BP gradient in the case of aortic coarctation. While LHH is often described as a single disease on a continuum, most lesions present as one of 3 distinct patterns, and each of these patterns likely has a different etiology of left heart hypoplasia.

Pattern 1: HLHS with Absent LV Cavity

In contrast with other forms of LHH that present with borderline left-heart structures, this pattern only presents as HLHS. In this pattern, the LV is thought to never have formed. This is the most common mechanism of mitral atresia/aortic atresia HLHS and is more thoroughly discussed in Chapter 27.

- No visible LV cavity, or only a slit-like 1-3 mm LV
- No endocardial fibroelastosis (EFE)
- Mitral atresia and aortic atresia
- Severe hypoplasia of the ascending aorta and proximal arch with more generous distal arch measurements from ductal flow filling the aortic arch retrograde throughout gestation

Pattern 2: History of Fetal AS

After a relatively normal development of the heart in utero, AS and EFE rapidly develop and the LV becomes dilated and dysfunctional. The LV and ascending aorta undergo growth arrest and are ultimately hypoplastic at birth. This postnatal presentation is highly variable, depending when the AS developed. In its most severe form, it results in HLHS (most often mitral stenosis/aortic atresia). The etiology of this pattern is unknown but is postulated to be either a primary aortic valve or myocardial disorder.

- Globular, non-apex-forming, and severely dysfunctional LV
- EFE
- Mitral stenosis with abnormal mitral valve architecture or mitral atresia
- Severe aortic valve stenosis or atresia
- The arch is typically hypoplastic

PART II. DISEASES

Pattern 3: The Long Skinny LV with Arch Hypoplasia/Coarctation
This pattern is sometimes called the "long, skinny pattern" or "hypoplastic left-heart complex" (HLHC). This is also sometimes referred as a "Shone-complex variant", although this a misnomer, as Shone complex describes a unique subset of these cases with supravalvar mitral ring, parachute mitral valve, subaortic stenosis, and coarctation. The postnatal presentation is highly variable. The etiology of this pattern is unknown but it is postulated to be secondary to restricted inflow to the mitral valve and LV in utero.
- Apex-forming or near apex-forming LV that appears compressed with normal systolic function
- No EFE
- Mitral annular hypoplasia and aortic annular hypoplasia with no discrete valvar stenosis and laminar flow
- Moderate-to-severe transverse aortic arch hypoplasia with coarctation of the aorta

Approach to Management
In cases of LHH, the goal is to perform a BVR whenever possible. However, BVR is not performed when it is anticipated that patients will struggle significantly or may need a takedown back to SVP. Some patients qualify for fetal intervention to make them better BVR candidates. Postnatally, the final decision is made after echocardiographic imaging, clinical presentation, and in cases in which SVP is strongly being considered, intracardiac exploration.

Fetal Imaging and Intervention
All patients with a fetal diagnosis of LHH considered to be borderline are followed closely and counseled for a range of possible postnatal outcomes, including SVP. Some families are offered fetal intervention to make their fetus a better BVR candidate at birth. For pattern 2 (fetal AS), fetuses generally between 20 and 30 weeks gestation may be offered fetal aortic valvuloplasty if 1) the anatomic features are predicted to result in HLHS at birth and 2) aortic valvuloplasty still has the potential to stop LV-growth arrest and to improve LV function. For fetuses with pattern 3 LHH (HLHC) who are suspected to need SVP, mothers may be offered chronic maternal hyperoxygenation as part of an ongoing trial to determine if this therapy can help grow the left heart and improve neurodevelopmental outcomes.

Echocardiography
At birth, all patients are started on PGE and echocardiography is performed. Close attention is paid to LV morphology and function, mitral valve morphology, and Z-scores of all left-sided structures. When determining what treatment course to take, the type of LHH pattern (2 or 3) is seriously considered. Patients with pattern 2 LHH often have significant diastolic dysfunction and high left ventricular end-diastolic pressures that often do not improve tremendously over time. A variety of scores have been developed in the past for this pattern like the Rhodes score (Rhodes et al. 1991) to evaluate their candidacy for biventricular repair. These scores may be used in concert with clinical assessment and surgical assessment to determine treatment.

For pattern 3 LHH, most developed scores do not apply well. In fact, if they are used, many patients would be categorized as needing SVP who would actually tolerate BVR. In pattern 3 LHH, the LV has much better postnatal growth potential, and echocardiographic measures may underestimate annular sizes due to RV compression. The large majority of these patients can successfully tolerate a BVR, even with severely hypoplastic mitral valve annuli by echocardiography. In cases in which the mitral valve or LV appear too small to undergo BVR, it may be best to try to wait at least a week after birth before intervention to reassess by echocardiography. Often, the mitral valve annulus will measure larger, the LV will be larger, and the atrial septal gradient will be lower on the second echocardiogram due to improved LV filling and improved diastolic function. This may allow for more reassurance in proceeding with a BVR. Preoperative assessment with MRI to measure flow in the ascending aorta may also be helpful to evaluate the capacity of the left-heart structures to deliver systemic cardiac output.

Surgical Considerations

One of the most important decisions that has to be made is whether the patient is suitable for a BVR or requires SVP. This complex decision involves careful analysis of all data including echocardiography and clinical status. However, echocardiographic measurements tend to underestimate the dimensions of left-heart structures in some patients due to compression by a dilated RV. As such, relying solely on echocardiographic measurements is poised to place some patients in the SVP pathway that could potentially have been adequate for BVR.

Typically, patients with LHH at TCH are not placed on a SVP pathway without an intracardiac exploration of the left heart. Intracardiac exploration includes assessment of the mitral valve size, morphology of the mitral leaflets, mitral subvalvar apparatus, size of the LV, and in some situations, size of the aortic valve. Valve size is determined based on the largest Hegar dilator that the valve easily accepts. In general, neonates with a mitral valve diameter <8 mm and an abnormal subvalvar apparatus appear to benefit from SVP. An aortic valve annulus ≥5 mm in a newborn appears to be adequate to support the systemic circulation without intervention.

In some situations, an intraoperative hemodynamic assessment is performed by temporarily occluding the PDA (thus eliminating left-to-right shunting) and assessing changes in hemodynamics, including LAP. A decrease in LAP with an increase in systemic pressure is encouraging for a BVR. In patients with a large VSD, the adequacy of the LVOT may be better assessed by placing a temporary PA band while performing a TEE.

These strategies have allowed us to offer BVR to the large majority of patients with LHH. In a recent study of 42 patients at TCH with true borderline left-heart structures, 35 (83%) patients underwent BVR (Mery et al. 2017).

The type of surgical intervention needed for patients with borderline left-heart structures is variable and depends on the specifics of each particular patient. Most patients will have some degree of involvement of the aortic arch requiring intervention to the arch early in life. The type of intervention – aortic arch reconstruction via median sternotomy (70%) vs. repair of aortic coarctation via left thoracotomy (30%) (see Chapter 25) – depends on the morphology of the aortic arch and the need to address any intracardiac anomalies at the time. Other interventions that may be required at the index operation, besides intracardiac exploration and aortic arch reconstruction, include VSD closure, aortic valvotomy, subaortic resection, mitral valvuloplasty, aortic root replacement, or in patients with an inadequate left heart, a Norwood-type operation. Reoperations to the mitral or aortic valves later in life are common in patients undergoing BVR.

Anesthetic and Postoperative Considerations

The anesthetic management of the patient with LHH requires flexibility and good communication with the surgical team. Preoperatively, a discussion should take place regarding the need for intraoperative hemodynamic assessment and how intraoperative findings will dictate the surgical plan. The location and plan for invasive arterial pressure monitoring line placement should also be discussed; a right-radial arterial line is often preferred during aortic arch advancement to guide antegrade cerebral perfusion, and simultaneous pressure monitoring in the lower body (umbilical or femoral artery) can be helpful during coarctation repair. Extra transducers and pressure monitoring cables should be available for direct pressure monitoring.

If an intraoperative decision is made to proceed with a BVR, one must recognize that although it is a BVR, the left heart is still not normal. The LV is small and noncompliant, and diastolic dysfunction is an issue. An LAP monitoring line is often placed to guide management, especially intravascular volume management intraoperatively and postoperatively. Careful attention to the LAP can prevent volume overload and the pulmonary edema that can quickly develop in a patient with a small, noncompliant LV.

It is also essential to recognize that the valves may not be normal after CPB. In the neonatal period and in early infancy, the goal is often to repair the valve, as prosthetic valve options are severely limited. Patients may have mitral or aortic stenosis or regurgitation after CPB. Hemodynamic goals for these valvar lesions still apply.

With diastolic dysfunction and potential mitral and/or aortic stenosis, heart rate and rhythm should be monitored closely. A shortened diastole that comes with significant tachycardia limits filling, especially in a patient with a noncompliant ventricle or mitral stenosis. Likewise, dysrhythmias can be poorly tolerated, as the contribution of the atrial contraction to filling is substantial in these conditions.

Pulmonary hypertension due to preexisting LA hypertension can also be an issue perioperatively. Even after the repair of the left-sided valves, the propensity for pulmonary hypertension still exists. Care should be taken to provide a deep plane of anesthesia and to avoid hypercarbia, hypoxemia, and acidosis. Administration of milrinone or iNO should be considered to reduce PVR further.

Suggested Readings

Lara DA, Morris SA, Maskatia SA, et al. Pilot study of maternal hyperoxygenation and effect on aortic and mitral valve annular dimensions in fetuses with left heart hypoplasia. Ultrasound Obstet Gynecol 2016;48:365-372.

Mery CM, Nieto RM, De Leon LE, et al. The role of echocardiography and intracardiac exploration in the evaluation of candidacy for biventricular repair in patients with borderline left heart structures. Ann Thorac Surg 2017;103:853-861.

Moon-Grady AJ, Morris SA, Belfort M, et al. International Fetal Cardiac Intervention Registry: A Worldwide Collaborative Description and Preliminary Outcomes. J Am Coll Cardiol 2015;66(4):388-399.

Rhodes LA, Colan SD, Perry SB, et al. Predictors of survival in neonates with critical aortic stenosis. Circulation 1991;84:2325-2335.

27 Hypoplastic Left Heart Syndrome

Judith A. Becker, Nancy S. Ghanayem, Ashraf Resheidat, Carlos M. Mery

Hypoplastic left heart syndrome (HLHS) describes varying degrees of underdevelopment of the left-sided heart structures that cannot independently support the systemic circulation (Figure 27-1). It is most commonly classified based on whether the aortic and mitral valves are atretic or stenotic into 4 types: aortic atresia/mitral atresia, aortic stenosis/mitral stenosis, aortic atresia/mitral stenosis, and aortic stenosis/mitral atresia. The most common variant of HLHS is aortic atresia, which results in significant hypoplasia of the ascending aorta and aortic arch. Patients with mitral stenosis/aortic atresia may have associated coronary fistulas, akin to the development of fistulas in patients with pulmonary atresia and intact ventricular septum (see Chapter 18).

Even though HLHS accounts for only 1-4% of all CHD, it causes one-fourth of all cardiac deaths in the first week of life and ~15% of deaths from CHD in the first month of life. There are no known genetic abnormalities linked to HLHS but it occurs more commonly in males. Most patients are born at term and rarely have other noncardiac anomalies. It is unusual to have structural brain malformations but approximately 20-25% of patients will have some preoperative MRI evidence of brain injury indicating varying degrees of immaturity of the brain.

Pathophysiology and Clinical Presentation

In HLHS, the LV is not functional, so the pulmonary venous return must be routed to the RA through a stretched PFO or an ASD. Systemic and pulmonary venous return mix in the right side of the heart. The RV then provides cardiac output to both the systemic and pulmonary circulations in a parallel fashion. Blood flows from the RV to the main PA, which provides flow to the lungs, and through the PDA to the descending aorta, brachiocephalic vessels, and coronary arteries (particularly in the case of aortic atresia). Ductal patency and an unrestrictive interatrial communication are thus crucial for survival in these neonates.

A majority of patients with HLHS are now diagnosed prenatally. This allows adequate family counseling, arranging for delivery in a tertiary care center, and immediate administration of PGE after birth to maintain ductal patency. At birth, most neonates have a balanced circulation. On exam, they tend to be warm and well perfused, but with some degree of cyanosis. On auscultation, they will have a single S_2 sound. Neonates with a restrictive interatrial communication will develop intense cyanosis/hypoxemia and respiratory distress from pulmonary venous congestion that is unresponsive to conventional medical management. If ductal patency is not maintained (e.g., patients with no prenatal diagnosis of HLHS), patients will develop poor systemic perfusion with signs of cardiogenic shock including lethargy, cool extremities, diminished pulses, hypotension, respiratory distress, and metabolic acidosis with end-organ ischemia.

The relationship between the amount of blood flow to the lungs (Qp) and the systemic circulation (Qs) depends on a delicate balance between PVR and SVR. After birth, as the PVR drops, an eventual imbalance in the parallel circulation will result in an increase

PART II. DISEASES

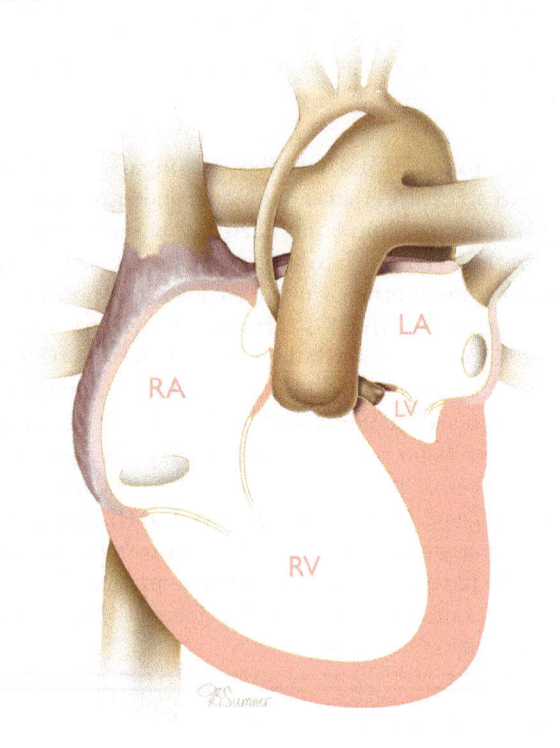

Figure 27-1. Anatomy of HLHS with a hypoplastic LV, a stenotic or atretic mitral valve, and a stenotic or atretic aortic valve. The ascending aorta is usually significantly hypoplastic and there are varying degrees of aortic arch hypoplasia. A large PDA and an unrestrictive ASD are important for survival.

in pulmonary blood flow through the PDA. Over the span of a few days, patients will start developing pulmonary overcirculation (Qp>Qs), leading to the development of CHF symptoms (i.e., tachypnea, diaphoresis, failure to thrive, pulmonary congestion) and reduced systemic circulation.

Diagnosis
- **ECG.** Classically shows RA enlargement and RV hypertrophy.
- **CXR.** Can reveal cardiomegaly and as the patient becomes overcirculated, it will show signs of pulmonary congestion.
- **Echocardiography.** Mainstay of diagnosis. It is important to show the anatomic details, interatrial communication, ductal patency, RV function, degree of TR, and pulmonary venous drainage.
- **CTA and cardiac catheterization.** Rarely used. However, in patients with mitral stenosis and aortic atresia, CTA and/or catheterization may be indicated to rule out the presence of significant coronary fistulas.

27. HYPOPLASTIC LEFT HEART SYNDROME

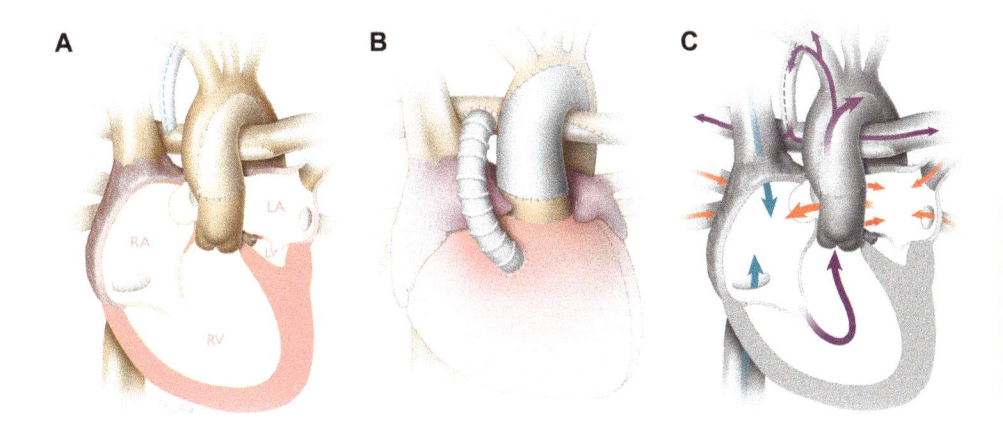

Figure 27-2. Norwood procedure. A) Norwood procedure with an mBTTS from the right subclavian artery to the right PA. B) Norwood procedure with an RV-PA conduit brought to the right of the aorta (Brawn modification). C) Hemodynamic flows after a Norwood procedure.

Preoperative Management

The primary goal of the management of the HLHS patient is to optimize systemic oxygen delivery and organ perfusion.

Immediately after delivery, arterial and venous access are obtained (UAC and UVC) in the delivery room. A PGE infusion (0.01-0.1 mcg/kg/min) is started to maintain systemic perfusion. An echocardiogram is necessary to rule out the presence of a restrictive interatrial communication. If there is significant restriction, the patient may need to undergo a balloon atrial septostomy (BAS). These patients usually need to wait for several days after the BAS to allow for resolution of organ dysfunction (from severe hypoxia) prior to any surgical palliation. Patients with mild restriction at the atrial level and no clinical embarrassment are better left alone as a BAS can otherwise lead to more overcirculation.

The preoperative management of the patient entails optimizing the balance between Qp and Qs. An excess of one will lead to compromise of the other. A few days after birth and while on PGE, the patient will develop pulmonary overcirculation with an increase in SaO_2 and pulmonary congestion. If left untreated, it can lead to systemic hypoperfusion, resulting in coronary ischemia and end-organ dysfunction. This may lead to mesenteric ischemia (necrotizing enterocolitis), acute kidney injury, and cerebral hypoxic-ischemic injury. The medical management goals thus include limiting Qp. This is partly achieved by avoiding pulmonary vasodilators like oxygen or respiratory alkalosis. Noninvasive ventilation to increase PVR can also be used. Diuretics can be used to decrease pulmonary congestion as the resulting tachypnea may lead to respiratory alkalosis. Careful use of systemic vasodilators (such as sodium nitroprusside infusion or milrinone) can also be utilized to reduce Qp and improve Qs. Eventually,

PART II. DISEASES

if not taken for surgical palliation, these patients may become unstable and require intubation and mechanical ventilation.

Indications for intubation include apnea or severe respiratory distress, significant metabolic acidosis, significant pulmonary overcirculation, or end-organ dysfunction such as myocardial dysfunction. The ventilation management should target blood gases to limit pulmonary blood flow: $PaCO_2$ 35-45 mmHg, pH 7.35-7.40, FiO_2 21%, PEEP 4-5. The goal SaO_2 should be 75-85% (since this indicates close to a 1:1 Qp:Qs with this physiology), and the hemoglobin should be maintained at 14-16 g/dL.

At TCH, all neonates requiring cardiac surgical intervention undergo a brain MRI prior to surgery (see Chapter 52).

Anesthetic Considerations

The principles of intraoperative management of these patients remain the same – to maintain "balanced" systemic and pulmonary circulations. Standard anesthetic and cardiac monitors, NIRS, and transcranial Doppler (TCD) are routinely used. TEE is typically not used.

Intravenous induction is performed using synthetic opioids (fentanyl). Inhaled anesthetics are kept to a minimum or avoided prior to initiating CPB since they can significantly affect the patient's hemodynamics. The preferred route of intubation is nasotracheal. Immediately after intubation, the FiO_2 is reduced to 21%, if possible, to avoid overcirculation. The ventilator management strategy should be the same as mentioned above, with target $PaCO_2$ 35-45 mmHg, pH 7.35-7.40, FiO_2 21%, and PEEP 4-5 cmH_2O. The goal SaO_2 should be 75-85%, although it tends to be difficult to achieve due to the degree of overcirculation. Blended nitrogen, which was previously used on these patients, is not used anymore at TCH due to safety reasons.

A right-radial arterial line is useful with titration of CPB flows once antegrade cerebral perfusion (ACP) is initiated. A femoral arterial line or UAC is generally also placed to allow for monitoring of distal perfusion on CPB and adequate reads on the post-CPB period, since the radial artery is prone to spasm. In addition, if a right modified Blalock-Taussig-Thomas shunt (mBTTS) shunt is placed on the right subclavian artery, the reads from the arterial line may be falsely lower due to runoff into the pulmonary circulation. A femoral central line is routinely placed for CVP monitoring and infusion of medications during and after the procedure. The patient may require inotropic or vasopressor support prior to initiating CPB in order to maintain stable hemodynamics. Having the surgeon snare the right PA during initial dissection can also improve hemodynamics by reducing Qp. An initial dose of 100 Units/kg of heparin is administered prior to suturing the graft on the innominate/subclavian artery for ACP, and an additional 400 Units/kg of heparin are administered prior to initiating CPB.

During CPB, the patient is cooled down to 18 °C and vasodilators (e.g., phentolamine – an alpha-receptor blocking agent) are used to allow maximum organ perfusion while cooling. Baseline TCD measurements (measured through the anterior fontanel) and bilateral NIRS are established prior to ACP. CPB flows on ACP are titrated based on right-radial MAP, TCD, and NIRS.

Patients will require inotropic support to separate from CPB. Support usually includes an epinephrine infusion and a calcium-chloride infusion. Nitroprusside is used to counteract elevated BP. Platelets and cryoprecipitate are used to help stop bleeding after administration of protamine. The same principles in balancing Qp and Qs are used in the immediate post-CPB and postoperative periods.

Surgical Palliation

The diagnosis of HLHS is on itself an indication for surgical intervention. The surgical paradigm of HLHS has evolved significantly over the last few decades. The goal is to achieve a Fontan circulation through a staged approach that involves 3 operations: the Norwood procedure (performed at the newborn stage), the bidirectional Glenn (performed at 4-6 months of age), and the completion Fontan (usually performed between 3 and 5 years of age). For details of the bidirectional Glenn and the Fontan completion, please see Chapter 39. Long-term effects and management of the Fontan circulation can be found on Chapter 47.

The goals of the Norwood procedure (Figure 27-2) are: 1) to create an unobstructed outflow to the systemic circulation, 2) to allow unimpeded drainage of the pulmonary circulation, 3) to provide a stable source of pulmonary blood flow, and 4) to provide a reliable source of coronary blood flow. These goals are achieved by amalgamating the ascending aorta and the proximal PA (Damus-Kaye-Stansel [DKS] anastomosis), reconstructing the aortic arch, performing an atrial septectomy, and creating an mBTTS or placing an RV to PA conduit (Sano modification). Both mBTTS and RV-PA conduits are used at TCH. Patients that undergo an RV-PA conduit tend to have better hemodynamics postoperatively due to the lack of diastolic runoff seen in patients with mBTTS. Diastolic runoff causes the diastolic BP to be lower, potentially leading to coronary ischemia. On the contrary, it is more common for patients with RV-PA conduits to develop stenoses of the PA branches, potentially requiring intervention.

The Norwood procedure is performed via a median sternotomy. Due to the sometimes diminutive size of the ascending aorta, it is customary to mark with fine sutures the location where the ascending aorta kisses with the proximal PA to later facilitate the DKS anastomosis. It is sometimes useful to partially snare the right PA with a fine tourniquet at this time in order to improve hemodynamics by reducing overcirculation (the FiO_2 is increased as needed). The PDA and the brachiocephalic vessels are dissected and a 3.5 mm Gore-Tex® graft is sutured to the distal innominate artery/proximal right subclavian artery. If an mBTTS is expected, an effort is made to place the graft as far distal as possible on the subclavian artery since this graft would serve as the shunt (see Chapter 38). Particular care is taken not to injure the right recurrent laryngeal nerve that travels around the subclavian artery since temporary dysfunction of the left recurrent laryngeal nerve is not uncommon due to the dissection of the aortic arch and descending aorta.

CPB is instituted via the innominate/subclavian graft and a single venous cannula in the RA. The PDA is ligated with a 5-0 Prolene pursestring. The patient is cooled down to 18 °C. While cooling, the aortic arch, brachiocephalic vessels, PDA, and descending aorta are completely dissected. The PA may be divided at this time and the distal orifice closed, or partially closed, with or without a patch, depending on the plans for

PART II. DISEASES

sourcing of pulmonary blood flow. It is important to dissect well the PA branches, in particular if an RV-to-PA conduit is expected to be placed. At this time, a decellularized homograft patch is prepared.

Once the goal temperature is reached, the head is packed on ice, the brachiocephalic vessels and descending aorta are controlled with fine tourniquets and CPB flows are reduced and stopped, thus initiating a short period of deep hypothermic circulatory arrest. Cardioplegia is administered through a sideport on the arterial limb of the circuit, therefore administering the cardioplegia through the innominate/subclavian graft and into the dimininutive ascending aorta. Future cardioplegia doses (every 20 minutes throughout the cross-clamp period) will be administered directly once the ascending aorta is open. After the initial cardioplegia dose is administered, the venous cannula is removed from the RA and working through the cannulation site, an atrial septectomy is performed. The venous cannula is replaced and a period of ACP is initiated through the innominate/subclavian artery graft. Flows are titrated using a combination of transcranial Doppler, NIRS, and right-radial arterial line pressure monitoring, and are usually between 30% and 40% of full CPB flows (see Chapter 6).

The PDA is divided and the aorta is opened longitudinally from the marking stitch on the proximal ascending aorta all the way to the descending aorta, past the insertion of the ductus arteriosus. The isthmus is divided and all ductal tissue is excised unless the left subclavian artery originates from the ductus arteriosus, in which case a small amount of posterior wall may need to be left in place. A posterior half-circumference anastomosis is performed between the descending aorta and the isthmus, the ascending aorta and the PA are anastomosed with fine sutures, and the remaining of the ascending aorta/aortic arch are reconstructed with the previously prepared homograft patch. After the aorta is reconstructed, all tourniquets around the brachiocephalic vessels are released, full-flow CPB is reinstituted, and the patient is rewarmed.

If an *RV-to-PA conduit* will be placed, a ringed Gore-Tex® graft is cut flush with one of the rings and "dunked" into the RV prior to finishing the aortic reconstruction. Usually, 2 rings are completely dunked into the RV and the third one is left flush outside of the RV. The graft is secured to the RV surface with a pursestring and a few interrupted stitches. In general, a 5 mm ringed graft is used for patients <3 kg and a 6 mm graft for those >3 kg. The graft may be brought to the left of the aorta (conventional Sano) or to the right side (Brawn modification). If an *mBTTS* will be used, the arterial limb of the circuit is changed to a cannula inserted into the reconstructed aorta, the previously placed graft on the subclavian artery is trimmed, and an anastomosis is performed between the graft and the right PA.

A peritoneal dialysis catheter is routinely placed on all patients undergoing the Norwood procedure and temporary atrial pacing wires are also usually placed. If the patient's hemodynamics and oxygen saturations are adequate, there is no bleeding, and there are no other concerns, the chest is routinely closed.

Other Management Strategies

There are several risk factors that significantly increase the risk of performing a Norwood operation. Some of these factors include prematurity, low-birth weight (<2.5 kg),

RV dysfunction, and significant TR. Even though a Norwood procedure is almost always used at TCH for palliation of HLHS, some high-risk patients may benefit from alternative strategies on a case-by-case basis.

> **Recent TCH Norwood experience (2017-2018)**
> Number of Norwood procedures: 57 (49 primary, 8 after prior biventricular repair or hybrid)
> Patients discharged home between first and second stages: 60%
> Survival to second stage (bidirectional Glenn): 96%
> 1-year overall survival: 93%
> 1-year transplant-free survival: 89%

The *hybrid approach* to HLHS has been used in some programs as an alternative to the Norwood operation. In general, this approach is not favored at TCH except in conditions where the risk of a Norwood operation may be prohibitive. The goals of the hybrid approach are the same as those of the Norwood operation (unobstructed systemic outflow, unimpeded pulmonary venous return, a stable source of pulmonary blood flow, and a reliable source of coronary blood flow) but achieved in a different way. The hybrid procedure consists of placement of bilateral PA bands, a BAS, and either placement of a PDA stent or continuation of PGE to maintain ductal patency ("chemical" hybrid). Patients with no prograde flow across the aortic valve that undergo placement of a PDA stent need to be closely monitored for development of a "retrograde arch malperfusion", i.e., obstruction of the aortic arch at the level of the stent obstructing retrograde flow into the arch, brachiocephalic vessels, and coronary arteries.

Listing for *neonatal heart transplantation* is another strategy that can be used on high-risk patients with HLHS. However, due to the overall shortage of organ donors, this strategy is fraught with risk and thus reserved for very particular circumstances. Due to the risk of overcirculation, it is not unusual to proceed with placement of bilateral PA bands or a hybrid approach as a bridge to transplantation.

Comfort care is a strategy that may be used by some families in cases in which the risk of palliation is prohibitively high. However, this is a strategy rarely used nowadays.

Postoperative Management

The postoperative management of patients after the Norwood procedure follows some of the same guidelines described for the preoperative and intraoperative management. Overall, the goal is to maintain adequate system oxygen delivery and organ perfusion by allowing a careful balance of pulmonary and systemic circulations (Qp:Qs).

Hemodynamics and oxygen saturations are carefully monitored. Patients usually arrive to the CICU with a combination of inotropes including low-dose epinephrine and calcium. Milrinone may be started in the OR or is sometimes added in the CICU. Patients with an RV-to-PA conduit tend to have better diastolic BP than those with an mBTTS due to the lack of diastolic runoff. As such, some patients with mBTTS may require addition of vasopressin in order to improve the diastolic BP and thus coronary perfusion. See Chapter 38 for different clinical postoperative scenarios and recommended interventions in postoperative patients with a shunted circulation, scenarios that are directly applicable to patients after a Norwood operation.

Mechanical ventilation is slowly weaned with the goal of extubating patients within the first 24-48 hours. However, some patients, especially those that were intubated preoperatively, may require a longer intubation. Peritoneal dialysis is routinely started on the day of surgery and continued until the patient mobilizes fluids and urine output increases, usually within the first few days. Prophylactic heparin at 6 U/kg/hr is started 6 hours after surgery if there is no bleeding. It is then converted to aspirin once the patient starts taking PO.

Enteral feeds via nasogastric tube are slowly started if the patient is expected to be intubated for a longer period of time. Otherwise, they are slowly advanced once the patient is extubated. It is not unusual for patients after a Norwood procedure to have some degree of feeding intolerance, likely due to the marginal gut circulation. This mandates slow progression of feeds as per protocol (see Chapter 58). In general, feedings are not fortified beyond 24 kcal/oz in patients after a Norwood procedure.

For details regarding requirements for transfer from CICU to the ward, interstage management, discharge planning, and home monitoring, see Chapter 39.

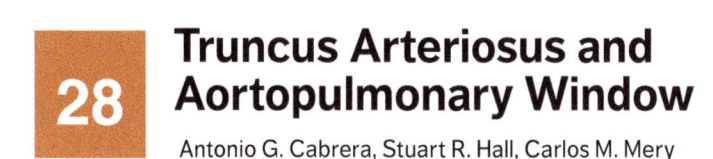

28 Truncus Arteriosus and Aortopulmonary Window

Antonio G. Cabrera, Stuart R. Hall, Carlos M. Mery

Truncus arteriousus is a rare congenital heart anomaly comprised of a single origin of 3 vascular structures: the aorta, the PAs, and the coronary arteries (Figure 28-1). An aortopulmonary (AP) window is a proximal communication between the aorta and PA, with separate origins of both vessels, due to an incomplete division of the common arterial trunk (Figure 28-2). Even though both lesions share some common characteristics, in truncus arteriosus there is only one semilunar valve and one arterial trunk, contrary to an AP window, where there are two. The truncal valve is usually tricuspid, although it may also be quadricuspid or bicuspid.

As is the case with other conotruncal abnormalities, truncus arteriosus is associated with DiGeorge syndrome. AP window may also be associated with other extracardiac anomalies such as the VACTERL association (vertebral anomalies, imperforate anus, cardiac anomalies, tracheoesophageal fistula, renal anomalies, and limb abnormalities).

Classification

The most commonly used classification of truncus arteriosus is the classification of Collet and Edwards (Figure 28-1):
- **I:** A single PA arises from the common trunk and divides into 2 PA branches
- **II:** Two separate posterior or posterolateral PA branches arise from the common trunk
- **III:** Two lateral PA branches arise from the common trunk
- **IV:** The PA branches arise from the descending aorta (hemitruncus). This class is no longer used as it is more appropriately classified as pulmonary atresia with VSD and major aortopulmonary collaterals (see Chapter 17).

Most patients with truncus arteriosus present with what is called "type one-and-a-half" since both branch PAs arise very close to each other.

An alternative classification is the Van Praagh classification in which A1 is equivalent to type I, A2 combines types II and III, A3 describes a single origin of a PA from the truncus with a collateral or PDA perfusing the other PA, and A4 is truncus arteriosus with an interrupted aortic arch.

A more recent classification by the STS divides truncus it into either aortic or pulmonary dominance. Most cases are characterized by aortic dominance with a large ascending aorta and aortic arch, and smaller PA branches arising from the trunk. In pulmonary-dominant truncus, the ascending aorta is hypoplastic and the descending aorta is supplied by the PDA. Truncus arteriosus with interrupted aortic arch is an example of pulmonary dominance.

Pathophysiology and Clinical Presentation

Both truncus arteriosus and AP window are characterized by a significant left-to-right shunt resulting in overcirculation. The degree of overcirculation in patients with an AP window is obviously dependent on the size of the defect.

PART II. DISEASES

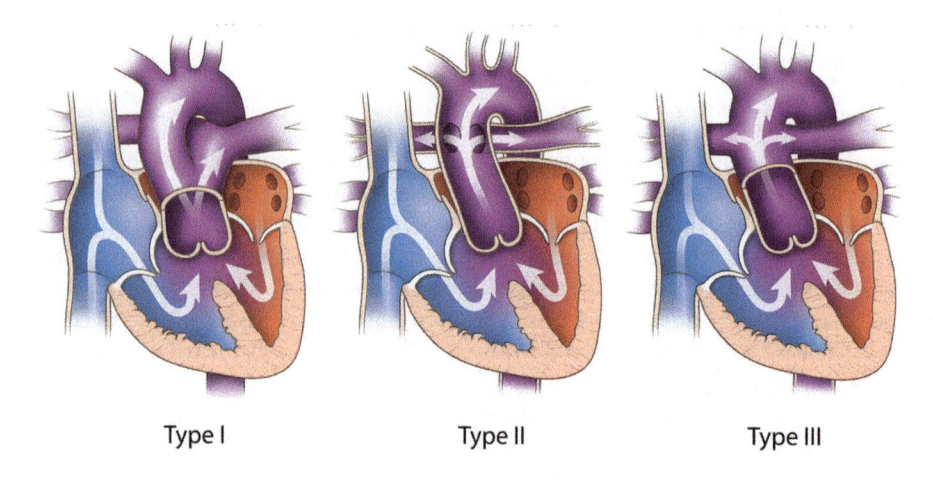

Type I   Type II   Type III

Figure 28-1. Collet and Edwards classification of truncus arteriosus (see text for details).

Patients with truncus arteriosus or a large AP window will present with tachypnea and pulmonary edema shortly after birth. The pulmonary overcirculation and CHF symptoms worsen as the PVR decreases with time. If the lesion is associated with aortic arch obstruction, shock and cyanosis may be presenting signs. Patients with a small AP window may present later in life and this lesion may be missed in the presence of other lesions such as tetralogy of Fallot, VSDs, and PDA.

If the lesion is not repaired, PVR will slowly increase and lead to irreversible pulmonary vascular changes (Eisenmenger syndrome). As a result, the shunt will decrease with time and once the PVR is significantly higher, it will reverse and become a right-to-left shunt with resulting cyanosis.

On physical exam, the child will be tachycardic and tachypneic. Grunting can be present due to pulmonary circulation and pulmonary edema. The precordium is hyperactive. Patients with truncus arteriosus will have a single S_2 and a systolic ejection click. Patients with an AP window will have a continuous mid frequency murmur, similar to a PDA. When presenting late, these patients may present with a single S_2 due to elevated PA pressure and early P_2 closure.

Diagnosis
- **CXR (Figure 28-3).** Cardiomegaly with pulmonary edema and pulmonary hyperinflation.
- **ECG.** Right-axis deviation. There can be biventricular hypertrophy with non-specific ST-T wave changes. In cases of coronary artery insufficiency, ST-segment depression may be present.
- **Echocardiogram (Figure 28-4).** Important features to assess in patients with truncus arteriosus include the truncal valve, VSD, coronary arteries, and associated anomalies, including the aortic arch. Because the combined ventricular output is going through the single truncal valve, there will be increased velocity across

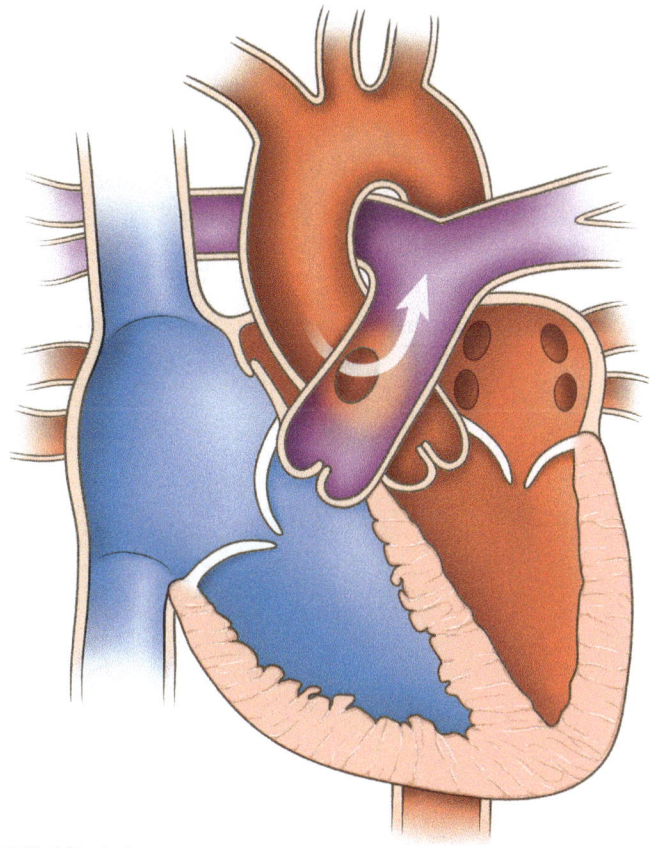

Figure 28-2. AP window.

it. Velocities higher than 3-3.5 m/s should increase suspicion for truncal valve stenosis. Imaging in patients with AP window should be focused on the location of the window and associated cardiac defects, such as tetralogy of Fallot, subaortic stenosis, and PDA.
- **CTA.** Usually not necessary for patients with truncus arteriosus. However, it can be useful if the anatomy is not completely resolved with echocardiogram. It may also be useful for patients with AP window to assess the location and extent of the window, and help with surgical planning.
- **Cardiac catheterization.** Not usually necessary for diagnosis except in cases with late presentation to evaluate PVR and operability.

Indications / Timing of Intervention
A diagnosis of truncus arteriosus or AP window is an indication for surgical intervention. The prognosis of patients with unrepaired truncus arteriosus is dismal due to the severity of CHF symptoms and the rapid development of pulmonary vascular

PART II. DISEASES

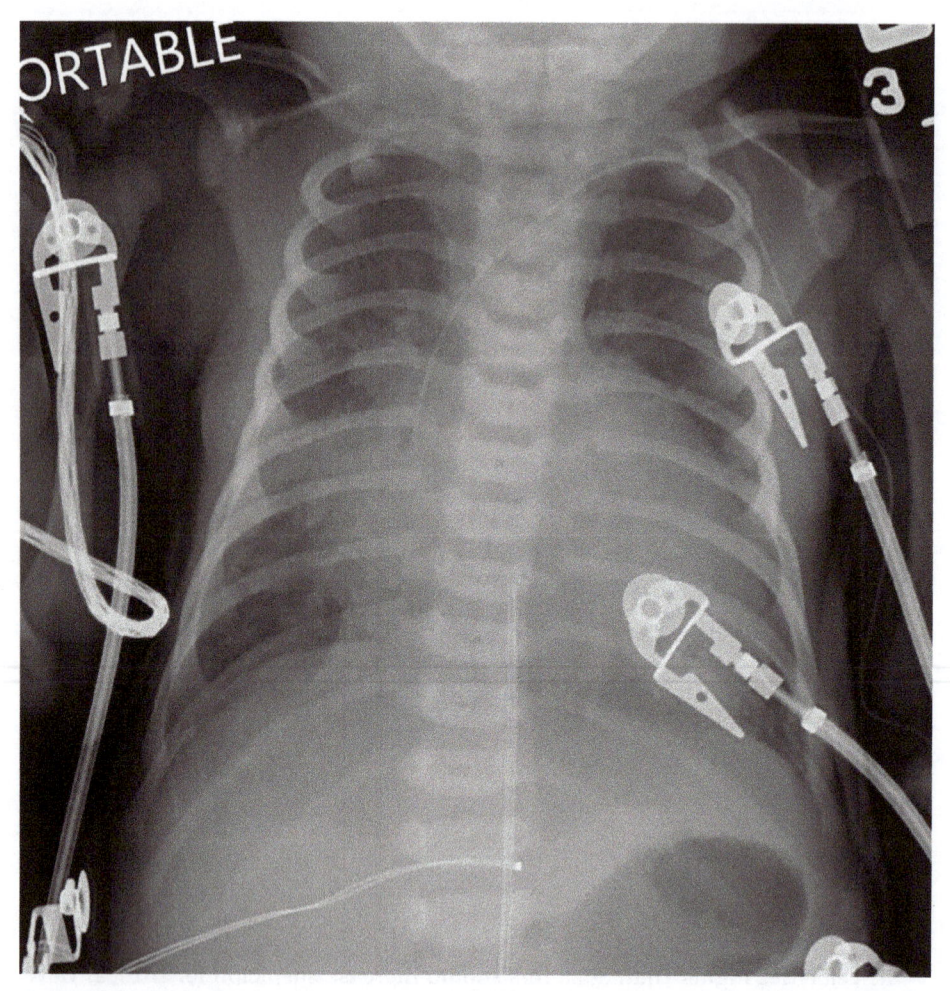

Figure 28-3. CXR of a patient with truncus arteriosus showing significant cardiomegaly, pulmonary congestion, and a narrow mediastinum due to the lack of thymus from DiGeorge syndrome.

disease. In addition, delaying surgical intervention does not provide any advantage for the repair. As such, patients with truncus arteriosus are repaired during the newborn period. Similarly, patients with AP window should be intervened upon at the time of diagnosis unless the window is small, in which case an elective repair can be offered.

Anesthetic Considerations
The chief consideration for the anesthetic management of these patients is to balance the pulmonary and systemic circulations. PVR is usually orders of magnitude lower than SVR, making these patients at best suffer from pulmonary overcirculation or at worst coronary ischemia. Invasive arterial pressure monitoring can help guide a slow,

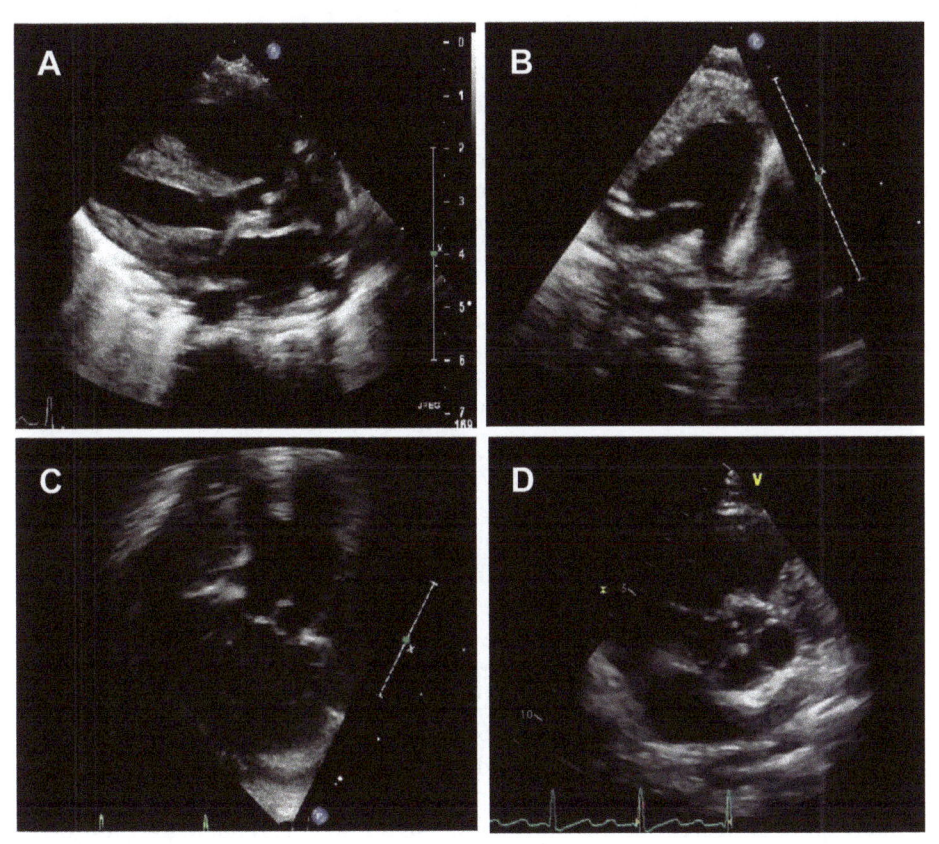

Figure 28-4. Echocardiograms of patients with truncus arteriosus. A) Parasternal long-axis view showing a thickened and dysplastic truncal valve overriding a VSD. B) Suprasternal-notch view of a patient with truncus arteriosus type I demonstrating the origin of the MPA and branch PAs from the common trunk. C) Apical view demonstrating the common arterial trunk as well as the MPA segment arising from the ascending trunk. D) Parasternal-short axis view showing a quadricuspid truncal valve en-face. Images courtesy of Dr. Josh Kailin, www.pedecho.org.

controlled induction. Ventilation management should target keeping the PVR elevated: room air with gentle hypoventilation and hypercarbia. Subatmospheric oxygen (FiO$_2$ 18%) has been used historically but is not currently an accepted management strategy. ST-segment analysis and diastolic BP need to be closely monitored for any signs of ischemia. Vasoconstriction in the form of vasopressin can help keep diastolic BP in a comfortable range with the caveat that increasing SVR will decrease the systemic circulation. Once the sternum is open, the surgeon can snare the branch PAs to create a temporary "banded" circulation, improving systemic cardiac output and allowing greater latitude in increasing inspired oxygen. Assessment of the function, PVR, and SVR post-CPB can help guide decisions regarding what combination of pharmacologic therapies will best support the patient.

PART II. DISEASES

Surgical Repair

Truncus Arteriosus

The goal of the surgical repair of truncus arteriosus is to separate the PAs from the common trunk, repair the VSD by creating a baffle between the LV and the truncal valve, and establish continuity between the RV and the PAs with a valved conduit. The procedure is performed via median sternotomy with CPB, aorto-bicaval cannulation, and mild-moderate hypothermia. The PA branches are snared after initiation of CPB to avoid runoff into the lungs.

After cardioplegic arrest, the PA or branch PAs are separated from the common trunk. Depending on the anatomy, this may be achieved by transecting the common trunk and leaving a rim of aortic tissue around the PAs or harvesting the PAs as a button while visualizing the anatomy through an anterior aortic incision. It is important to recognize the relationship between the PAs and both the coronary arteries and the aortic valve in order to avoid injury, as they may be in close proximity. The truncal valve should be inspected and repaired if necessary. Truncal valve repair is challenging but there are different surgical techniques that can be used for this purpose. The coronary arteries are also inspected and may require intervention (e.g., unroofing in the case of intramural coronaries).

If the common trunk is transected, the aortic root and the distal ascending aorta are reanastomosed (an autologous pericardial patch may be necessary). If the PAs are harvested as a button, the defect is usually repaired with an autologous pericardial patch in order to avoid distortion of the coronary arteries and aortic valve.

A right ventriculotomy is performed and the VSD is closed toward the truncal valve with a piece of glutaraldehyde-treated autologous pericardium using either a series of interrupted pledgeted sutures or a continuous sutureline. A homograft RV-to-PA conduit is then placed. Due to the location of the ventriculotomy, the conduit tends to sit directly behind the sternum and may thus be smaller than the conduit used for other repairs.

Both an LA line and a peritoneal dialysis catheter are placed routinely. It is not customary to leave an open atrial communication in these patients.

In the case of a truncus arteriosus with an interrupted aortic arch, arterial cannulation is achieved using a graft sutured to the innominate artery (for the upper body) and a second cannula inserted into the PDA. The aortic arch is reconstructed using an aortic arch advancement technique (see Chapter 25). The rest of the procedure is performed as described for isolated truncus arteriosus.

AP Window

The surgical management of an AP window depends on the size and location of the window. In general, aortic cannulation is achieved on the distal ascending aorta or aortic arch. If the AP window is very distal, it may require placement of a graft on the innominate artery and performing the repair using antegrade cerebral perfusion (see Chapter 6). AP windows are usually repaired by dividing the window and closing each vessel with a patch of autologous pericardium to prevent distortion. However, each case should be individualized to the particular anatomic characteristics.

Postoperative Management

General Management
- **Fluids.** 25% maintenance with D5%/0.45% NS is standard. Careful attention should be paid to managing the patient with the barely necessary preload. Unnecessary preload may produce increases in myocardial wall stress and lead to further ventricular dysfunction and hypotension. In cases involving arch repair, the ischemic time may have been longer, thus potentially prolonging the period of possible postoperative LCOS.
- **Analgesia and sedation.** Analgesics and sedatives are adjusted for patient's comfort. For analgesia, a fentanyl infusion is used. Scheduled acetaminophen q6h (enteral, rectal, or IV) is used as an adjuvant. Sedation is achieved with a combination of dexmedetomidine and midazolam as a drip.
- **Vasoactive drugs.** Most patients will arrive from the OR on milrinone 0.25-0.75 mcg/kg/min, epinephrine 0.02-0.05 mcg/kg/min, and calcium chloride 5-15 mg/kg/hr (especially if suspected DiGeorge). Hypotension should be primary managed with inotropes when the LA pressure is higher than 10 mmHg.
- **Mechanical ventilation.** Patients are usually ventilated on SIMV-VC with pressure support, Vt 8-10 mL/kg and PEEP 5-7 cmH$_2$O, aiming for a pH of 7.35-7.45 and a SaO$_2$ >95%.

> **Truncus arteriosus repair (1995-2016)**
> Number of repairs: 99
> Median age at surgery: 17 days (4 days – 2.6 years)
> Median ICU length of stay: 10 days (3-74 days)
> Median hospital length of stay: 18 days (5-42 days)
> Perioperative mortality: 8%
> Mechanical circulatory support: none
>
> **Aortopulmonary window repairs (1996-2016)**
> Number of repairs: 26
> Median age at surgery: 22 days (6 days – 3 years)
> Median hospital length of stay: 13 days (4-60 days)
> Perioperative mortality: 4%
> Mechanical circulatory support: none

What to Expect in the First 24 Hours Postoperatively
The postoperative management is mainly directed to address possible LV and RV dysfunction from prolonged CPB time and pulmonary hypertension. If there is preoperative coronary insufficiency and there was coronary unroofing, there may be further systolic and diastolic dysfunction. Pulmonary hypertension should be managed with iNO and decreasing oxygen consumption with sedation and intermittent muscle relaxation.
- **Ventilation.** Transitioning from the OR, the lungs will be significantly improved from the preoperative period secondary to continuous ultrafiltration. There may be mild pulmonary hemorrhage that should managed with PEEP 5-10 cmH$_2$O.
- **Fluids.** Even to slightly negative. Peritoneal dialysis is instituted on arrival to the CICU. If additional fluids/colloids are needed, one should carefully titrate small-volume boluses (1-5 mL/kg/dose), not to exceed LAP >12 mmHg.
- **Nutrition.** Should write for TPN the day after surgery. If DiGeorge syndrome is suspected or confirmed, there may be oropharyngeal dysfunction and OT should be consulted before starting feeds (see Chapter 58).

Complications

- **LCOS.** Primarily treated with inotropes. A combination of low-dose epinephrine and standard-dose milrinone.
- **Pulmonary hypertension.** It should be managed initially with iNO and potentially other advanced therapies (see Chapter 79).
- **Chylothorax.** May be secondary to a combination of pulmonary hypertension, RV dysfunction, and PA branch stenosis. Also, patients with DiGeorge syndrome have a higher incidence of chylothorax. For management of chylothorax see Chapter 77.
- **Mechanical circulatory support.** The use of mechanical support is rare after truncus arteriosus repair, except when there is significant preoperative ischemia with severe ventricular dysfunction.
- **PA branch stenosis.** Due to the size of the truncal root, the right PA may be compressed behind the reconstructed truncal root. This possible complication should be monitored using echocardiography.

Long-Term Follow-Up

Close follow-up of patients with truncus arteriosus and routine echocardiographic surveillance is mandatory. Long-term prognosis will be partly determined by the status of the truncal valve. Patients with truncal valve insufficiency, in particular those that underwent truncal valve repair during the initial operation, are at high risk of requiring truncal valve replacement in the future. Most patients will require RV-PA conduit replacement in the first 3-5 years of life. Larger conduits placed at future operations tend to have a longer longevity.

29 Vascular Rings

Iki Adachi, M. Regina Lantin Hermoso, Siddharth P. Jadhav, Lisa Caplan

Vascular rings are a group of aortic arch anomalies (occasionally involving the PA) that can result in tracheoesophageal compression. By definition, true ("complete") vascular rings consist of vascular structures that entirely surround the trachea and the esophagus. The 2 most common variants are the double aortic arch and the right aortic arch with aberrant left subclavian artery (arising from a diverticulum of Kommerell) and a left ligamentum arteriosum (or ductus arteriosus, if patent) (Figure 29-1). Other potential causes of vascular tracheobronchial compression such as innominate artery syndrome (anterior compression of the trachea by the innominate artery) and PA sling (origin of the left PA from the right PA and subsequent course between the trachea and esophagus, Figure 29-1, C) are not truly vascular rings but are sometimes called "incomplete" vascular rings. PA slings may be associated with complete tracheal rings causing further tracheal obstruction.

Pathophysiology, Clinical Presentation, and Associated Abnormalities

Vascular rings occur when there is abnormal persistence or regression of the various components of the embryonic totipotential arch. The location and severity of tracheo-esophageal compression determines the timing of presentation. With the exception of critical airway obstruction, symptoms are rare in neonates. Those with a double aortic arch may present earlier, during the first year of life. Many patients are asymptomatic, but over time may develop stridor, cough, increasing distress with intercurrent respiratory illnesses, and reflux or dysphagia with the introduction of solids in the diet. Some children may be noted to favor nonsolid foodstuff. Dysphagia is more common in older children and adolescents.

Vascular rings may be associated with cardiac anomalies such as tetralogy of Fallot, VSD, and coarctation of the aorta. Noncardiac anomalies include tracheoesophageal fistulae, and cleft lip and palate. Children with DiGeorge and Down syndromes have a higher incidence of vascular rings.

Diagnosis

- **Fetal echocardiogram.** Color Doppler imaging may reveal vascular structures around the trachea during cephalad transducer sweeps from a three-vessel view.
- **CXR (Figure 29-2).** May be shown as right aortic arch indentation on the distal trachea and anterior bowing of trachea on lateral view due to the retroesophageal vessel (aberrant subclavian artery).
- **Barium esophagram (Figure 29-3).** Not necessary but may show a posterior indentation on the esophagus from an aberrant subclavian artery or anterior indentation from a pulmonary sling.
- **CTA/MRI (Figure 29-4).** Definitive diagnosis of vascular ring requires a CTA or MRI. CTA is the preferred modality due to fast acquisition times without the need

PART II. DISEASES

for sedation, superior resolution, and superior airway information compared to MRI. It allows for detailed 3D reconstructions and characterization of the type of vascular ring that assist with surgical planning. The differentiation of a right aortic arch with aberrant left subclavian artery from a double aortic arch with an atretic left arch can be challenging (Adachi et al. 2011).

Indications/Timing for Intervention

The presence of a vascular ring alone is not necessarily an indication for operation. In general, intervention is warranted if the patient has symptoms attributable to the vascular ring (dysphagia or airway obstruction) and characteristic imaging studies (e.g., esophagram or CTA). Intervention may be considered for asymptomatic patients that show significant compression on imaging studies since the risk of intervention is relatively low. It is important to rule out the presence of significant cardiac anomalies necessitating intracardiac repair. A left aortic arch with an aberrant right

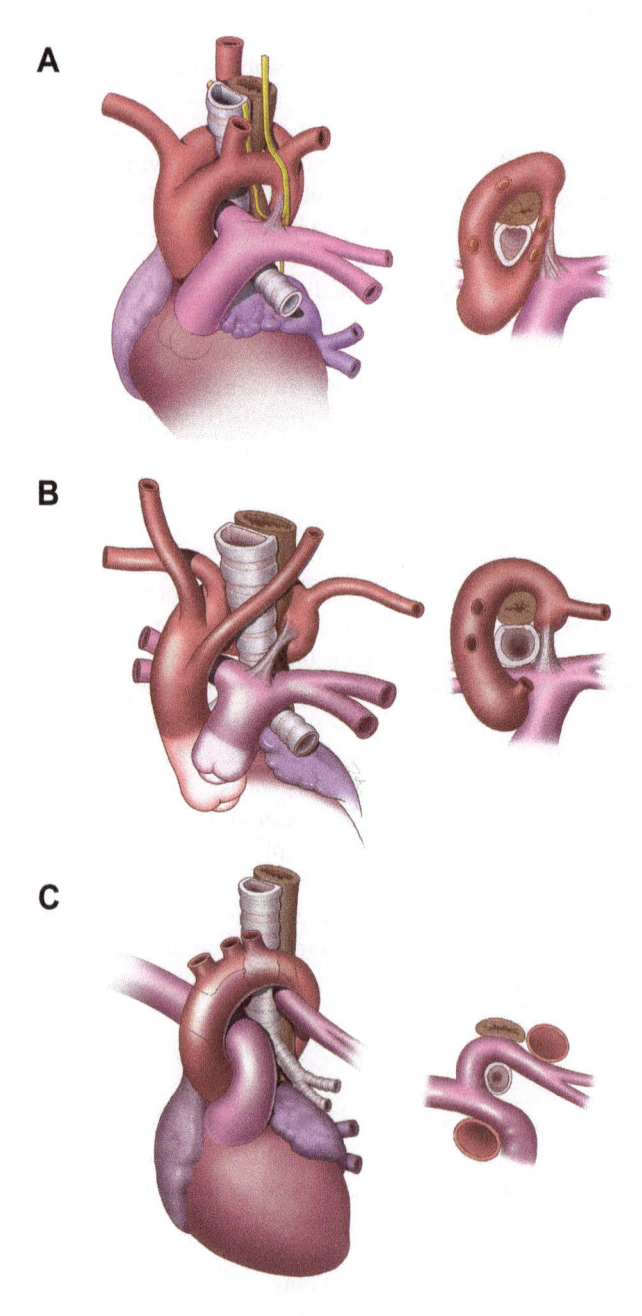

Figure 29-1. Vascular rings and other vascular causes of tracheobronchial compression. A) Double aortic arch. B) Right aortic arch with aberrant left subclavian artery and left ligamentum arteriosum. C) Left PA sling.

29. VASCULAR RINGS

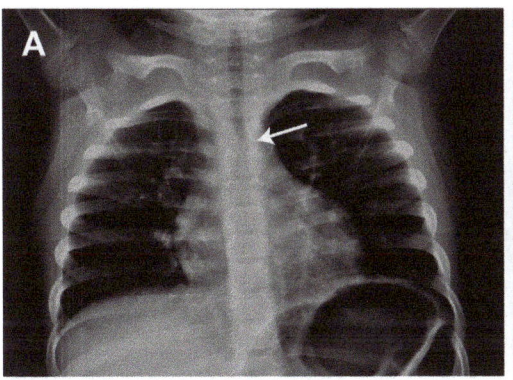

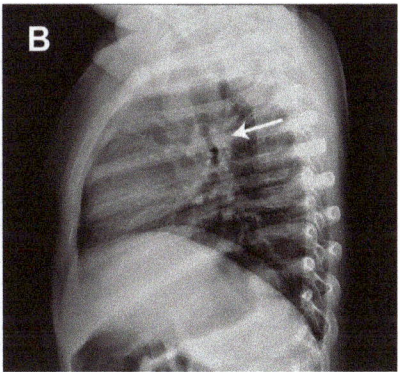

Figure 29-2. Anteroposterior (A) and lateral (B) views of a CXR of a patient with a vascular ring (right aortic arch with aberrant left subclavian artery), showing tracheal compression (arrow).

subclavian artery (i.e., dysphagia lusoria) is not a vascular ring and very rarely (if ever) requires intervention.

Surgical Repair
The type of surgical intervention depends on the type of vascular ring. Most procedures are performed through a left posterolateral thoracotomy through the 4th intercostal space. The goal of the operation is to completely relieve the tracheoesophageal compression. Patients may benefit from a direct laryngoscopy and bronchoscopy (DL&B) by ENT at the beginning of the procedure and sometimes a flexible bronchoscopy at the end to confirm relief of tracheobronchial compression. The surgical procedures for the two most common types of complete rings are:
- **Right aortic arch with aberrant left subclavian artery.** The left ligamentum arteriosum (between the origin of the left subclavian artery and the left PA) is divided, therefore releasing the ring. The descending aorta may be fixed posteriorly to the spine (i.e., aortopexy) to increase the space clearance. If there is a large diverticulum of Kommerell at the base of the left subclavian artery or if simple division of the ligamentum fails to create a wide-enough space, the diverticulum is excised and the left subclavian artery is translocated to the left carotid artery (Figure 29-5).
- **Double aortic arch.** The atretic or smallest portion of the double arch (most commonly the posterior left arch, just distal to the origin of the left subclavian artery) is divided and oversewn. It is important to also divide the ligamentum arteriosum that travels from this portion of the arch to the left PA in order not to leave a residual ring.

A circumflex aortic arch (an aortic arch that travels on one side of the trachea, crosses behind the trachea and esophagus, and descends on the other side) poses a difficult challenge. Patients with a right aortic arch, aberrant left subclavian artery, and a circumflex arch (left descending aorta) may benefit from a simple repair of the vascular ring (division of the left ligamentum arteriosum and translocation of the left

PART II. DISEASES

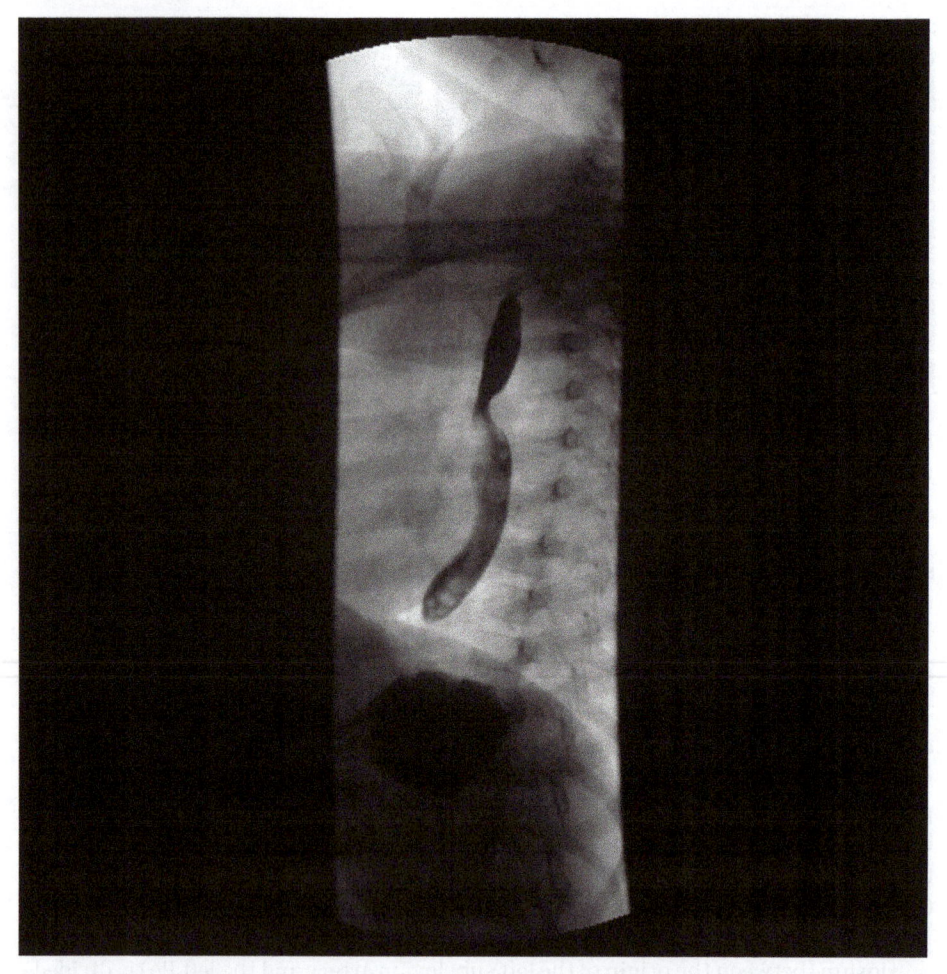

Figure 29-3. Esophagram of a patient with a vascular ring (right aortic arch with aberrant left subclavian artery) showing posterior indentation of the esophagus.

subclavian artery to the left carotid artery). In some instances, patients may require a more complicated procedure (e.g., aortic uncrossing procedure) through a median sternotomy (Backer et al. 2016).

Anesthetic Considerations
Preoperatively, anesthetic management should begin with a thorough chart review of radiologic images defining the anatomy of the vascular ring. Clear communication is needed between the surgical and anesthetic teams with regards to lung isolation, regional anesthesia, and invasive monitoring lines, as occlusion of blood vessels are likely included in the surgical plan. Most children will not be large enough to accommodate double-lumen tubes for lung isolation. However, there are other alternative

29. VASCULAR RINGS

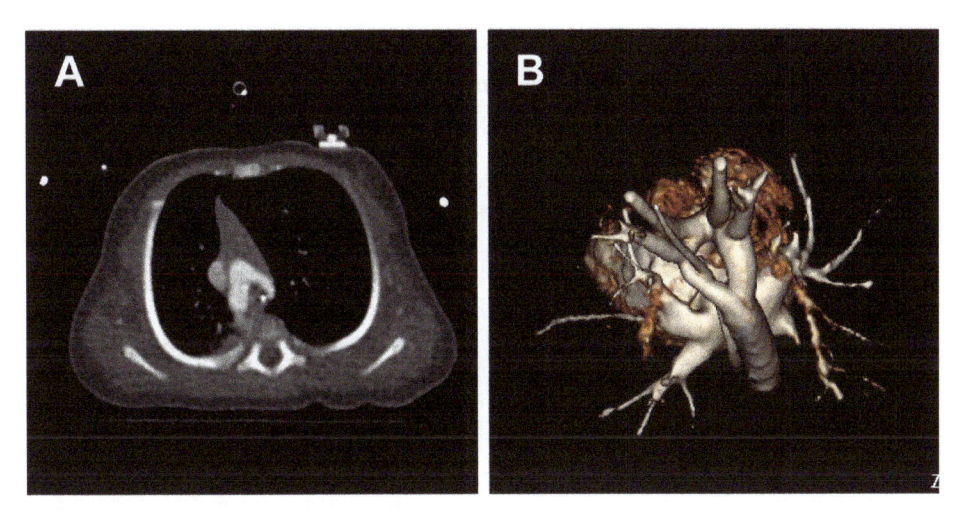

Figure 29-4. CTA of a patient with a double aortic arch with axial cuts (A) and 3D reconstruction (B). The right arch is dominant, compared to the left arch.

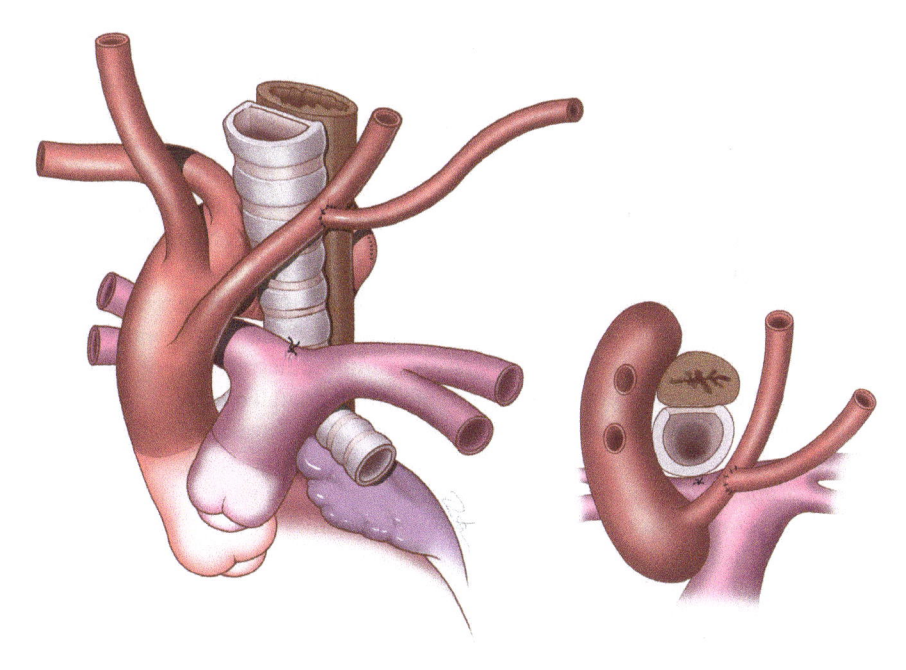

Figure 29-5. Surgical repair of a right aortic arch with an aberrant left subclavian artery, left ligamentum arteriosum, and a prominent diverticulum of Kommerell consisting of division of the ligamentum, excision of the diverticulum, and translocation of the left subclavian artery to the left carotid artery.

221

> **TCH experience with vascular rings (1996-2018)**
> (Binsalamah et al. 2019)
> Number of patients: 148
> Median age: 1 year (interquartile range 0.4-5.2 years)
> Median weight: 12.8 kg (interquartile range: 7.5-26.5 kg)
> Types of ring:
> - Double aortic arch: 72 (49%)
> - Right aortic arch with aberrant left subclavian artery: 69 (47%)
> - Others: 7 (5%)
>
> Perioperative mortality: 0
> Complications:
> - Chylothorax: 12%
> - Vocal cord paresis: 1 (<1%)

techniques for pediatric lung isolation (Hammer et al. 1999), including the use of bronchial blockers and right-mainstem intubation.

Tracheal compression by the vascular ring seldom precludes endotracheal tube placement or easy bag-mask ventilation during inhalational induction. However, the use of orogastric or nasogastric tubes is discouraged, especially in patients with tight vascular rings, to avoid esophageal perforation. If adequate analgesia is obtained, early extubation may be considered, as cardiac dysfunction and bleeding are rarely encountered in this surgery.

Postoperative Management

- **Fluids.** 100% maintenance with D5%/0.45% NS is standard. Large volume fluid resuscitation is seldom necessary.
- **Analgesia and sedation.** The use of regional anesthesia, including intercostal and paravertebral peripheral nerve blocks and thoracic epidurals, may be utilized for supplemental postoperative pain control. The Acute Pain Service will assist with co-managing analgesia if a catheter is placed. A PCA with continuous and intermittent opioid dosing is commonly utilized with scheduled adjunctives such as acetaminophen and ketorolac. Adequate analgesia is key to enable adequate airway clearance.
- **Mechanical ventilation.** Most patients are extubated in the OR, or considered for expedited extubation, if otherwise hemodynamically stable. Postoperative stridor, typically treated with steroids, is relatively common. Retractions or "seal-bark" cough may be present due to residual tracheobronchomalacia. Depending on the level of residual bronchomalacia, patients may need non-invasive positive mechanical ventilation (NIMV) after extubation. In some instances, even mild residual tracheobronchomalacia in association with postsurgical chest wall pain may need NIMV temporarily. Steroids may play a role when there is secondary inflammation.
- **Nutrition.** Clear fluids can be started 4 hours postextubation if the patient is otherwise hemodynamically stable. This may be advanced to a regular diet in the absence of postoperative dysphagia. Chest tubes should be monitored for chylous output, particularly when fat-containing food is introduced.

Complications
- **Neuropathy.** The vagus, recurrent laryngeal, and phrenic nerves are close to the area of surgical dissection. The recurrent laryngeal nerve may be particularly prone to injury, often times transient.
- **Chylothorax.** Complication due to the presence of large lymphatic nodes and channels in the area.

Suggested Readings

Adachi I, Krishnamurthy R, Morales DL. A double aortic arch mimicking a right aortic arch with an aberrant subclavian artery. J Vasc Surg 2011;54:1151-1153.

Backer CL, Mongé MC, Popescu AR, et al. Vascular rings. Semin Pediatr Surg 2016;25:165-175.

Binsalamah ZM, Ibarra C, John R, et al. Contemporary mid-term outcomes in pediatric patients undergoing vascular ring repair. Presented at the 55th Annual Meeting of the Society of Thoracic Surgeons, San Diego, CA, 2019.

Hammer GB, Fitzmaurice BG, Brodsky JB. Methods for single-lung ventilation in pediatric patients. Anesth Analg 1999;89:1426-1429.

Ramos-Duran L, Nance JW, Schoepf UJ, et al. Developmental aortic arch anomalies in infants and children assessed with CT Angiography AJR Am J Roentgenol 2012;198:W466–W474.

30 Anomalous Left Coronary Artery from the Pulmonary Artery

Antonio G. Cabrera, Stuart R. Hall, Charles D. Fraser Jr.

Anomalous origin of the left coronary artery from the pulmonary artery (ALCAPA) is a congenital coronary abnormality associated with high infant mortality and adult sudden cardiac death. In ALCAPA, the left coronary artery arises from variable locations in the PA system.

Pathophysiology and Clinical Presentation

In ALCAPA, as the PVR decreases after birth, the resistance in the coronary arterial system becomes higher than in the pulmonary circulation and the blood flow in the anomalous coronary artery reverses, causing primarily a left-to-right shunt. This coronary steal in the absence of adequate collateralization results in severe myocardial ischemia and dysfunction, classically within a few weeks to months of life.

ALCAPA is characterized by chronically ischemic hypocontractile, yet potentially salvageable myocardium. The variable equilibrium between timing of closure of the ductus arteriosus, pulmonary hypertension, and the speed of development of preexisting collateral circulation between the right and left coronary arteries define the extent of myocardial necrosis and scarring of the LV. If left uncorrected, the mortality is very high. Extensive collateral arteries may enable some patients to survive beyond infancy. However, chronic hypoperfusion causes subendocardial ischemia and later fibrosis, increasing the risk of sudden death secondary to ventricular arrhythmias. There are some rare situations of advanced-age patients presenting with ALCAPA.

When presenting in infancy (most common), the history will be significant for crying during feeds (angina on exertion), diaphoresis, and tachypnea with intermittent grunting – this is a distinctive constellation of symptomatology known as Bland-White-Garland syndrome. As ischemia progresses, feeding sessions will be more brief (infant becomes a "snacker") and pallor, fatigue, and grunting become prominent. When there is good collateralization, symptoms might be more subtle with failure to thrive being a typical clinical presentation.

On physical exam, the child is typically tachycardic and tachypneic. Grunting may be present with angina or when there is established pulmonary edema from poor ventricular function and high LAP +/- MR. The precordium is hypoactive. The second heart sound may be narrowly split from elevated PA pressures and sometimes there could be a single S_2. There is usually a gallop (S_3) and at times an S_4 (atrial kick on a poorly compliant LV).

Diagnosis

- **CXR (Figure 30-1).** Cardiomegaly with pulmonary edema and pulmonary hyperinflation are typical findings.
- **ECG (Figure 30-2).** Atrial enlargement (LA or biatrial). Abnormal (deep and wide) Q waves in leads I and aVL tend to be a classic finding. Nonspecific ST-T wave changes.

30. ANOMALOUS LEFT CORONARY ARTERY FROM THE PULMONARY ARTERY

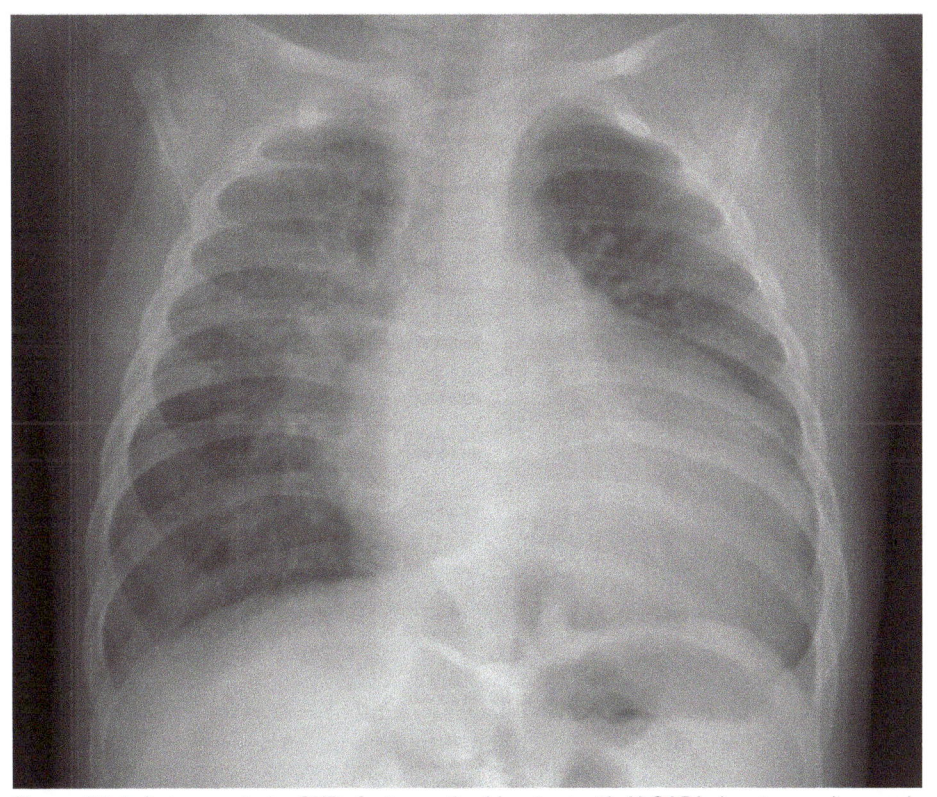

Figure 30-1. Anteroposterior CXR of a 5-month-old patient with ALCAPA showing cardiomegaly with LV dilation and bilateral pulmonary edema.

- **Echocardiogram (Figure 30-3).** Surface echocardiography is the primary diagnostic mode. The most important feature includes a severely depressed global LV function with MR. The LV endocardium will often appear echo bright with profound depression of contractility (ejection fraction <10%). The left coronary artery is found to arise from the main PA trunk in most cases and the ostial location is highly variable (sometimes at higher/more distal positions). Systolic and diastolic flow from the suspected anomalous coronary into the PA is pathognomonic. It is important to note that the 2D appearance of the left main coronary artery in relationship to the leftward facing aortic sinus can be very misleading and *appear* to connect to the aorta. We have seen cases in which experienced echocardiographers believe the left main coronary originates from the aorta, *but they are unable to demonstrate prograde flow by color Doppler in the coronary.* This is a situation that mandates another diagnostic study.
- **Cardiac CTA.** A properly conducted contrast CTA of the coronaries is an important diagnostic adjunct in suspected cases where the echocardiogram is insufficient or incomplete at showing the defect and there is high clinical suspicion.
- **Cardiac catheterization.** Catheterization is rarely necessary for diagnosis. This

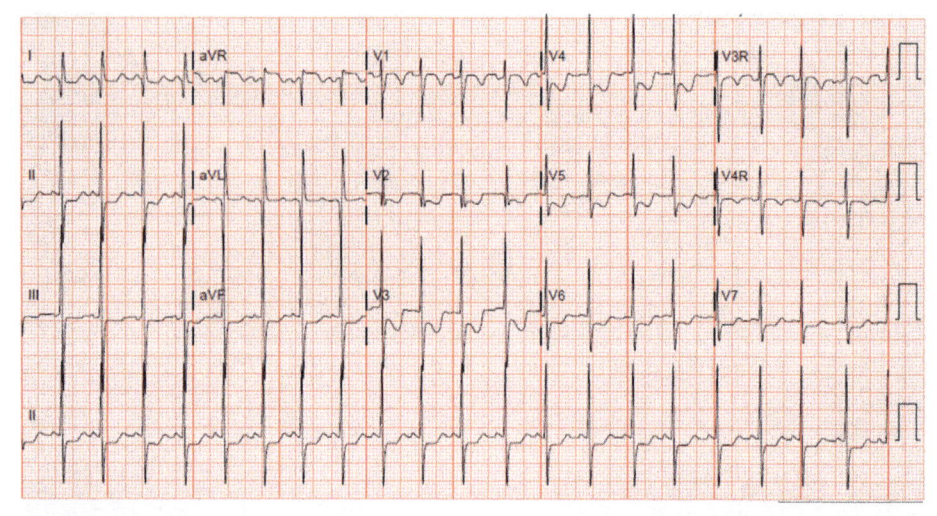

Figure 30-2. ECG of a patient with ALCAPA showing deep and broad Q waves in I and aVL (pathognomonic of ALCAPA). In addition, there is significant ST-segment depression in precordial leads.

---

may be helpful in patients in which a CTA cannot be obtained or the diagnosis remains equivocal and there is high clinical suspicion. Catheterization may be very dangerous in patients with profound ventricular dysfunction and a highly irritable myocardium. Coronary angiography is the only goal of catheterization in these cases.

Indications / Timing for Intervention
The diagnosis of ALCAPA is an indication for surgical intervention. Surgical intervention should be performed once the diagnosis is obtained.

Preoperative Management
Preoperatively, these infants may present in a warm/cold + wet state. Not all patients will need inotropes, but likely all will need diuresis to decrease the pulmonary symptoms from pulmonary edema and congestion. One should stay away from pure vasoconstricting agents, as they are likely to increase afterload and deteriorate function further. Noninvasive ventilation with HFNC or CPAP should be considered.

Anesthetic Considerations
The main goals of the pre-CPB period are to maintain myocardial perfusion without increasing oxygen consumption or drastically reducing BP. If the patient is not intubated, the process of intubation may represent a high risk for cardiac arrest. One should be prepared for emergent initiation of CPB, with a primed and ready CPB circuit and the surgeon present for induction. Induction is usually incremental, with titrated doses of

30. ANOMALOUS LEFT CORONARY ARTERY FROM THE PULMONARY ARTERY

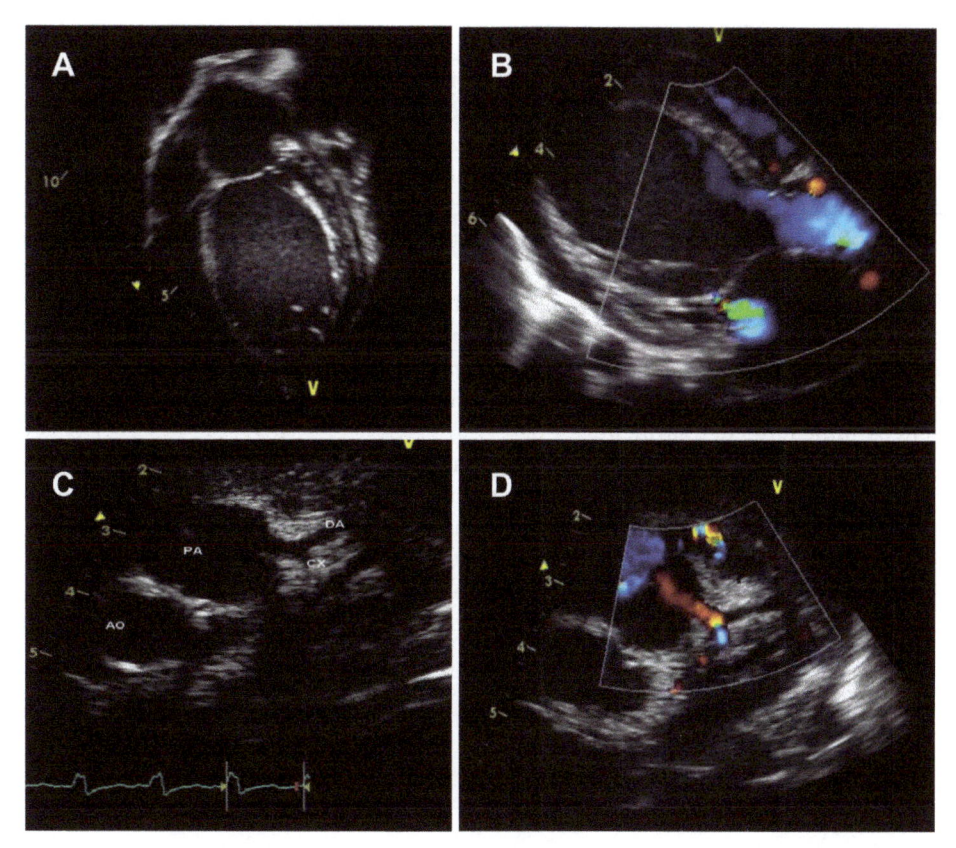

Figure 30-3. Echocardiograms of patients with ALCAPA. The apical 4-chamber (A) and parasternal long-axis (B) views show a severely dilated and globular LV with secondary MR. Of note, this can be easily misdiagnosed as dilated cardiomyopathy. A 2D parasternal short-axis view (C) demonstrates the takeoff of the anomalous left coronary from the PA. A color Doppler image (D) shows reverse flow from the left coronary artery into the PA. Ao: Aorta, CX: Circumflex coronary, DA: Anterior descending coronary, PA: Pulmonary artery. Images courtesy of Dr. Josh Kailin, www.pedecho.org.

anxiolytic and narcotic with or without small doses of anesthetic vapor. Arterial access should be obtained as quickly as feasible to facilitate close hemodynamic monitoring. Remember that while it is important to maintain normal oxygen saturation, maneuvers which decrease PVR should be avoided in order to keep (left) coronary perfusion pressure as high as possible.

Post-CPB, even with the "revascularization" of the left system, myocardial function does not usually immediately improve. Inotropic agents (milrinone/epinephrine) at moderate doses are often needed to maintain good cardiac output. While afterload reduction might be desirable, it is not uncommon to need vasoconstriction to maintain an adequate BP. Discuss with the surgeon the need or desire for an agent like nitroglycerin, if tolerated, to promote dilation of the reimplanted coronary.

PART II. DISEASES

Surgical Repair

Direct aortic reimplantation (Figure 30-4) or creation of an intrapulmonary baffle (Figure 30-5) when coronary translocation is not feasible (rarely) have been the primary modes of repair in the recent era. Primary ligation has been virtually abandoned as it is well established that even in the setting of profound LV dysfunction, establishing a two-coronary system by whatever means confers a survival advantage over simple ligation. Preservation of the two-coronary system leads to recovery of LV function and long-term survival rates greater than 80% or better in patients with profound heart failure at presentation. Historical operations including left subclavian artery "turn-down" and coronary artery bypass grafting are now almost never indicated. MR from LV dilation, mitral annular dilatation, or papillary muscle ischemia and secondary dysfunction may also occur in ALCAPA patients and may require the consideration of concomitant surgical treatment.

Intraoperative management of these patients must be a highly choreographed scenario. The anesthesiologist will be alerted to the very precarious nature of the patient's condition and as such, will avoid techniques that increase myocardial demand or lower systemic BP precipitously. *All members of the surgical team must be in the OR during the induction of anesthesia and early preparation of the patient.* This includes the perfusion

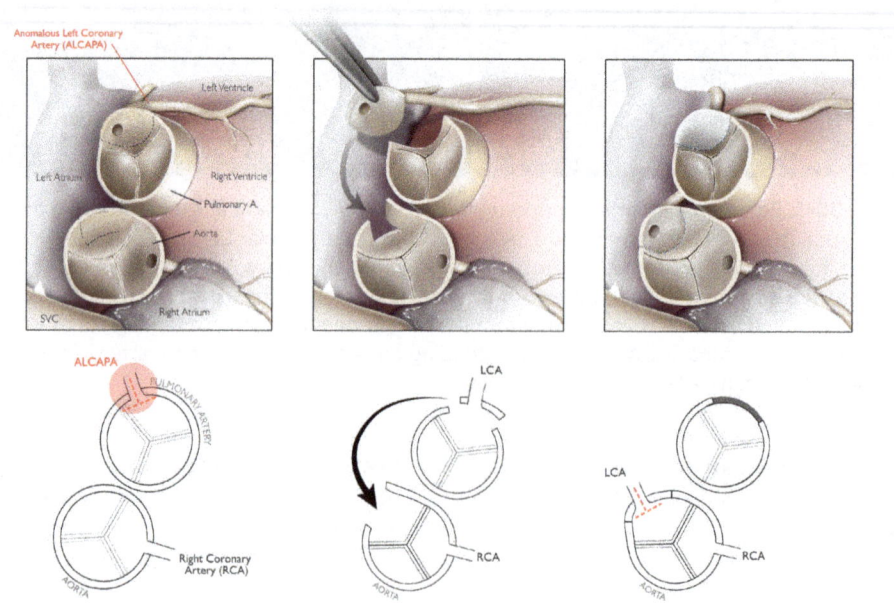

Figure 30-4. Translocation of a left coronary artery arising from the left posterior sinus of the PA. A generous button is harvested around the coronary artery, the coronary artery is widely mobilized, a trapdoor incision is created in the optimal location of the aortic root, and the button is reimplanted avoiding any torsion of the vessel. The PA defect is reconstructed with an autologous pericardial patch.

team who should be prepared for the urgent institution of CPB in critical situations. During sternal entry, the surgeon and assistants must be extremely careful in avoiding unnecessary manipulation of the heart. These hearts may be extremely irritable and even a minimal brush of the heart can induced intractable dysrhythmias or even ventricular fibrillation, a scenario that may require urgent initiation of CPB.

> **TCH experience with ALCAPA repair (1996-2011)** (Cabrera et al. 2015)
> Number of patients: 34
> Median age at surgery: 5 months (3 days – 39 years)
> Median ICU length of stay: 7 days (1-26 days)
> Median hospital length of stay: 16 days (3-540 days)
> Perioperative mortality: 0
> Postoperative mechanical circulatory support: 0

We have favored separate vena caval cannulation and moderate hypothermia (nasopharyngeal temperature of ~30-32 °C). After initiating CPB, the pulmonary vasculature is completely decompressed leading to further coronary steal. It is critical for the surgeon to gain circumferential control of either the main or branch PAs *distal* to the anomalous coronary ostium such that the PA may be occluded after initiating bypass. This also facilitates the effectiveness of antegrade, aortic root cardioplegia. After the heart is arrested, the main PA is strategically opened anteriorly at or just proximal to the bifurcation. The location of the anomalous ostium is then visualized. One should note that the ostium may originate from anywhere on the main or proximal branch PAs. Given the extensive and very successful experience congenital heart surgeons have with the arterial switch operation for transposition of the great arteries, coronary artery translocation to the ascending aorta is performed now in almost all newborn and infant cases. As patients get older, and particularly in rare adult cases, the coronary ostium is not as elastic and translocation may be inappropriate. This decision has to be made on a case-by-case basis. Our experience has been that in small children, all ostial locations, including an anterior and leftward location of the coronary, are amenable to translocation to the aorta (Figure 30-4). The surgeon should mobilize the ostium as a very liberal "button" of PA wall. In posteriorly located ostia, this may include taking down the posterior pulmonary valve commissure. The coronary is then mobilized to optimize the translocation with minimal traction and avoidance of axial torsion. The location for translocation to the aorta is selected on the basis of the best available geometric location; this is not necessarily the true leftward-facing aortic sinus in all cases. We have used an appropriately oriented "trapdoor" flap incision in the aorta to facilitate the coronary anastomosis, which is accomplished with a running, non-absorbable suture. In some cases, surgeons have used a small, anterior patch (typically autologous pericardium) to augment the reconstructed neo-ostium, although we have not found this to be necessary. It is very important to reconstruct the PA sinus defect with a generous pericardial patch, again much as one would do with an arterial switch operation, prior to removing the aortic cross-clamp.

In cases where coronary ostial translocation is not believed to be feasible, an intrapulmonary tunnel (as originally described by Takeuchi and colleagues) may be constructed across the back wall of the PA (Figure 30-5). Options for tunnel construction include a native anterior flap of PA wall or some form of prosthetic material. A neo-ostium is

PART II. DISEASES

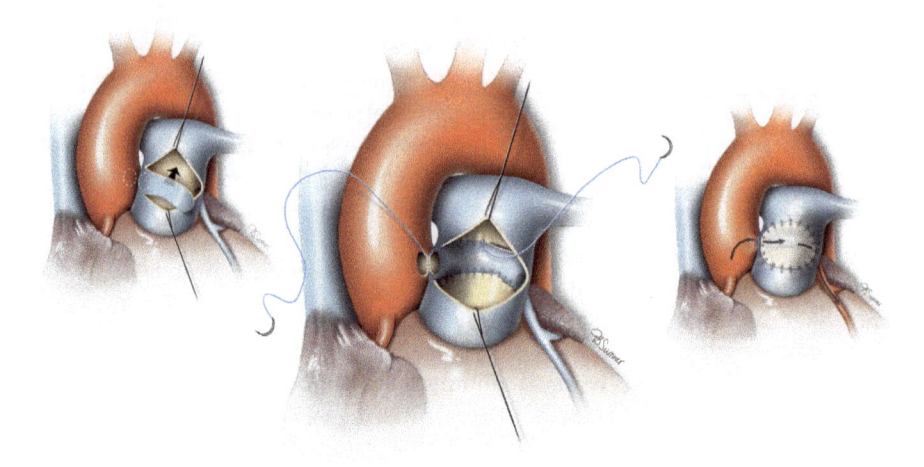

Figure 30-5. Takeuchi repair for ALCAPA. A baffle is created inside of the PA with either an anterior flap of PA tissue or other type of material, and an aortopulmonary window is created to redirect the flow from the aorta, through the intrapulmonary baffle, and into the left coronary artery. The anterior PA segment is reconstructed with a generous patch.

constructed which essentially amounts to the creation of an aortopulmonary window. It is critical to liberally augment the anterior PA wall deficit with pericardium or some other patch. Failure to do so has been associated with a high incidence of supravalvar PS in patients undergoing this operation.

Deciding whether or not to intervene on important MR at the index coronary artery operation can be very challenging. In patients with profound ventricular dysfunction, the additional obligate myocardial ischemic time required for mitral valve repair/annuloplasty may be critical. As such, our approach has been that in patients with massively dilated LV with MR in the setting of profound LV dysfunction, we have not proceeded with mitral repair. Our belief has been, and this has been born out in our complete avoidance of postoperative mechanical circulatory support, is that with improved myocardial performance, the MR may improve. Alternatively, persistent important MR may be dealt with at a subsequent operation, at a time when LV function is improved.

Despite being compromised, these patients are for the most part managing an adequate cardiac output when they come into the OR. It is our belief that we should, through diligent attention to myocardial protection, be able to get the patient through the operation without needing a VAD or ECMO. In the setting of refractory heart failure or inability to wean from CPB, we would likely favor a temporary LVAD (left atrium to ascending aorta) over ECMO.

Although rare, some patients will present with ALCAPA late in life. We have seen several adult patients with ALCAPA and massive right-to-left coronary collateralization who have normal LV function. In general, we have still favored operating to create a two-coronary system in such individuals, although this may be a difficult and controversial decision.

Postoperative Management

The postoperative management is mainly directed to address LV systolic dysfunction, early identification of arrhythmias, and transitioning from IV vasoactive medications to oral decongestive therapies (i.e., angiotensin converting enzyme-inhibitors, beta-blockers, diuretics).

General Management
- **Fluids.** 25% or less maintenance with D5%/0.45% NS is standard. Careful attention should be paid to manage the patient with the minimal necessary preload. Unnecessary preload may worsen myocardial wall stress and lead to further ventricular dysfunction and hypotension. An LA line will facilitate adjudication of intracardiac filling.
- **Analgesia and sedation.** Analgesics and sedatives are adjusted for patient's comfort. For analgesia, a fentanyl infusion is used with scheduled acetaminophen (enteral, rectal, or IV) as an adjuvant. Sedation is achieved with a combination of dexmedetomidine (both intubated and extubated patients) and/or benzodiazepines. Midazolam as a drip is preferred, as significant shifts in afterload or BP may produce instability.
- **Vasoactive drugs.** Most patients will arrive from the OR on a milrinone infusion 0.25-0.75 mcg/kg/min and an epinephrine infusion 0.02-0.05 mcg/kg/min. Hypotension should be primarily managed with inotropes when LV filling pressure (LAP) is >5-10 mmHg.
- **Mechanical ventilation.** Patients are usually ventilated on SIMV-VC with pressure support, Vt 8-10 mL/kg and PEEP 5-7 cmH$_2$O, aiming for a pH of 7.35-7.45 and SaO$_2$ >95%. Postoperative ALCAPA patients are expected to be extubated when their pulmonary edema has improved. Ventricular dysfunction takes weeks to months to show measurable echocardiographic improvement. Extubation should not be delayed as long as the patients are managing an adequate systemic cardiac output. Active preload reduction with diuretics before extubation tends to attenuate the effects of significant MR.

What to Expect in the First 24 Hours Postoperatively
- **Vasoactive drugs.** Probably reasonable to manage milrinone and low-dose epinephrine (<0.03 mcg/kg/min) through extubation to support the LV, as extubation will lead to an increase in transmural pressure and consequently higher afterload.
- **Ventilation.** Transitioning from the OR, the lungs will be significantly improved from the preoperative period secondary to continuous ultrafiltration. There may still be some lung injury from pulmonary edema as the LV end-diastolic pressure is unlikely to change significantly in the immediate postoperative period.
- **Fluids.** Even to slightly negative. If a peritoneal dialysis catheter is present, it should be used from the day of surgery.
- **Nutrition.** If considering to extubate within 24 hrs, it is not necessary to write for TPN. If longer periods of mechanical ventilation are anticipated, full TPN should be ordered. Oral feeds should be reinstated once successfully extubated.

Complications
The most common postoperative complications after ALCAPA repair are:
- **LCOS.** Primarily treated with inotropes. A combination of low-dose epinephrine and standard-dose milrinone. High inotrope doses increase the likelihood of arrhythmias.
- **Arrhythmias.** The incidence of arryhthmias after ALCAPA repair at TCH is 9%. Any arrhythmia (atrial tachycardia or ventricular tachycardia), should be treated promptly and should raise the clinical suspicion of deterioration in ventricular function or worsening MR.
- **Mechanical circulatory support.** Although other institutions have used pre- and/or postoperative mechanical circulatory support, at TCH we have been able to recover all of these patients without mechanical assistance.

Long-Term Follow-Up
Despite excellent LV recovery and long-term survival rates after ALCAPA repair, follow-up complications such as persistent MR, late-onset CHF, and coronary arterial stenosis may necessitate reinterventions, including heart transplantation. As such, long-term follow-up with appropriate diagnostic testing (including provocative testing for ischemia later in life) is paramount.

Outpatient management of patients after ALCAPA repair requires ongoing assessment of systolic and diastolic ventricular function. Conventional methods have largely relied on echocardiographic parameters such as shortening fraction or ejection fraction. Myocardial strain has been a useful tool in detecting myocardial dysfunction to identify subclinical dysfunction before the echocardiogram can detect meaningful differences in ejection or shortening fraction.

Suggested Reading
Cabrera AG, Chen DW, Pignatelli RH, et al. Outcomes of anomalous left coronary artery from pulmonary artery repair: beyond normal function. Ann Thorac Surg 2015;99:1342-1347.

31 Congenital Coronary Anomalies

Silvana Molossi, S. Kristen Sexson Tejtel, Prakash M. Masand,
Athar M. Qureshi, Carlos M. Mery

Congenital coronary anomalies are a heterogeneous group of abnormalities with variable clinical presentation. This chapter will focus on anomalous aortic origin of a coronary artery (AAOCA) and myocardial bridges (MB). For anomalous left coronary artery from the PA (ALCAPA) see Chapter 30.

AAOCA is an abnormality of the origin or course of a coronary artery that arises from the aorta (Figure 31-1). Its prevalence is unclear, but likely between 0.2% and 0.9%. MB is a segment of a coronary artery that travels within the myocardium instead of having a normal epicardial course. The prevalence of MB is estimated to be approximately 25% and, thus many times is considered a normal variant.

An increasing number of children and adolescents are being diagnosed with AAOCA or MB following routine athletic preparticipation screening, presence of a murmur, or an abnormal ECG. Due to multiple controversies on risk stratification and incomplete understanding of the natural history of these conditions, the Coronary Anomalies Program (CAP) was developed at TCH in December 2012. Since its inception, over 250 patients have been evaluated and managed as part of the program.

Pathophysiology and Clinical Presentation

AAOCA

AAOCA is the second most common cause of sudden cardiac death (SCD), especially when the anomalous coronary originates from the opposite sinus of Valsalva and takes an *interarterial* (coronary travels between the great vessel) or *intramural* (proximal segment of the coronary travels within the wall of the aorta prior to exiting into the mediastinum) course. However, the pathophysiological mechanisms that predispose to SCD are not fully understood. It appears that age and anatomy play an important role in the development of symptoms, signs of myocardial ischemia, and/or SCD. Reports of SCD in children younger than 10 years of age are uncommon, with most events appearing to affect individuals between 10 and 30 years of age. Moreover, despite anomalous right coronary artery (ARCA) being approximately 4-6 times more prevalent than anomalous left coronary artery (ALCA), ALCA is associated with 85% of SCDs related to AAOCA and, hence, a more lethal condition than ARCA.

Occlusion and/or compression of the anomalous vessel during exercise may lead to reduced perfusion with myocardial ischemia and subsequent ventricular arrhythmia. However, it is unknown why an athlete can exercise intensely for several years with no symptoms until the sentinel event occurs. Several mechanisms have been proposed, including compression of the intramural segment of the coronary during vigorous exercise, compression of the interarterial segment between the aorta and the PA, and ostial abnormalities including an acute-angle takeoff, a slit-like ostium that may collapse with aortic expansion, or frank ostial stenosis. The intercoronary pillar (a thickening of the wall of the aorta that extends cranially from the intercoronary commissure of the aortic

PART II. DISEASES

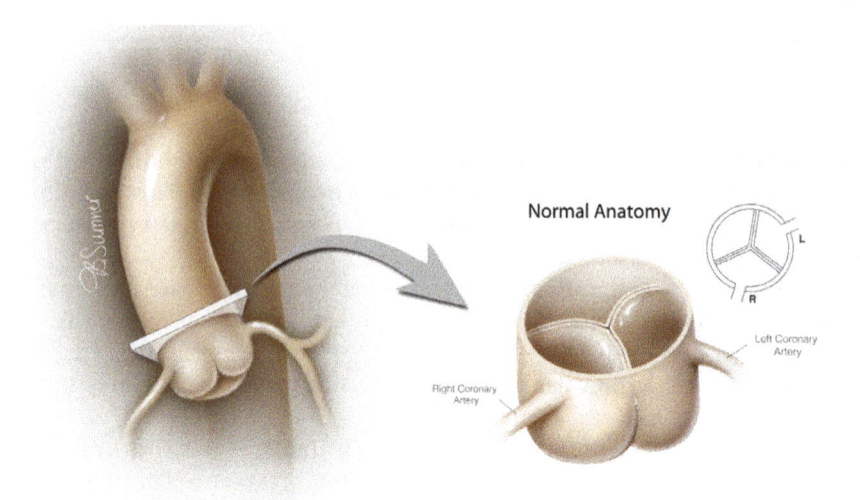

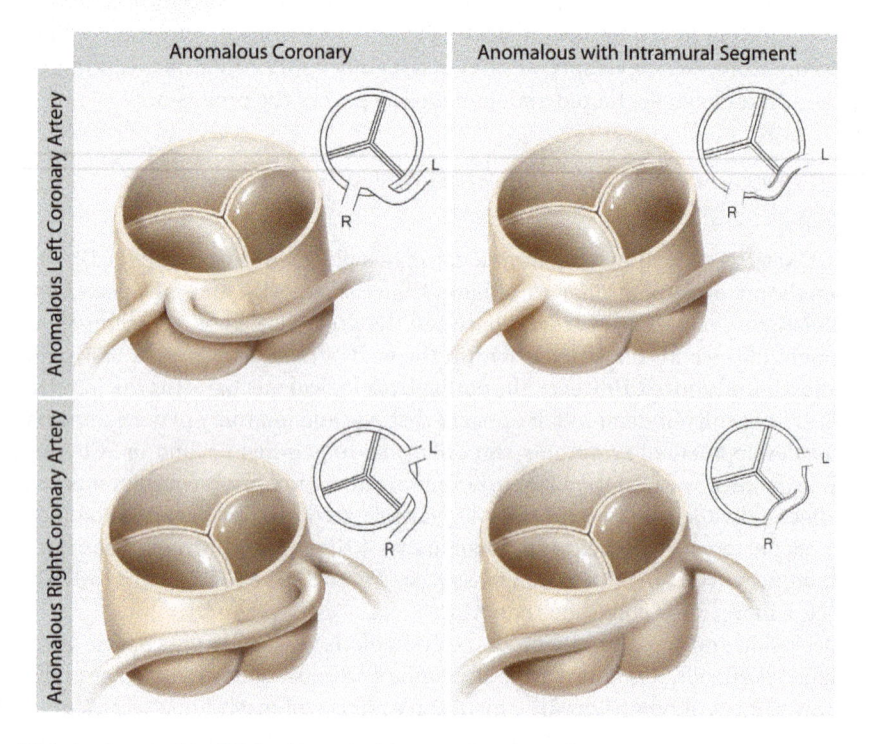

Figure 31-1. Anatomy of AAOCA with and without an intramural segment.

valve up to the sinotubular junction) may play a significant role by compressing the anomalous coronary that travels behind it, as it can be quite thick in some patients. The clinical presentation of AAOCA is variable. Symptoms are usually not present in half of the patients, and an episode of aborted SCD might be the initial event in a few.

31. CONGENITAL CORONARY ANOMALIES

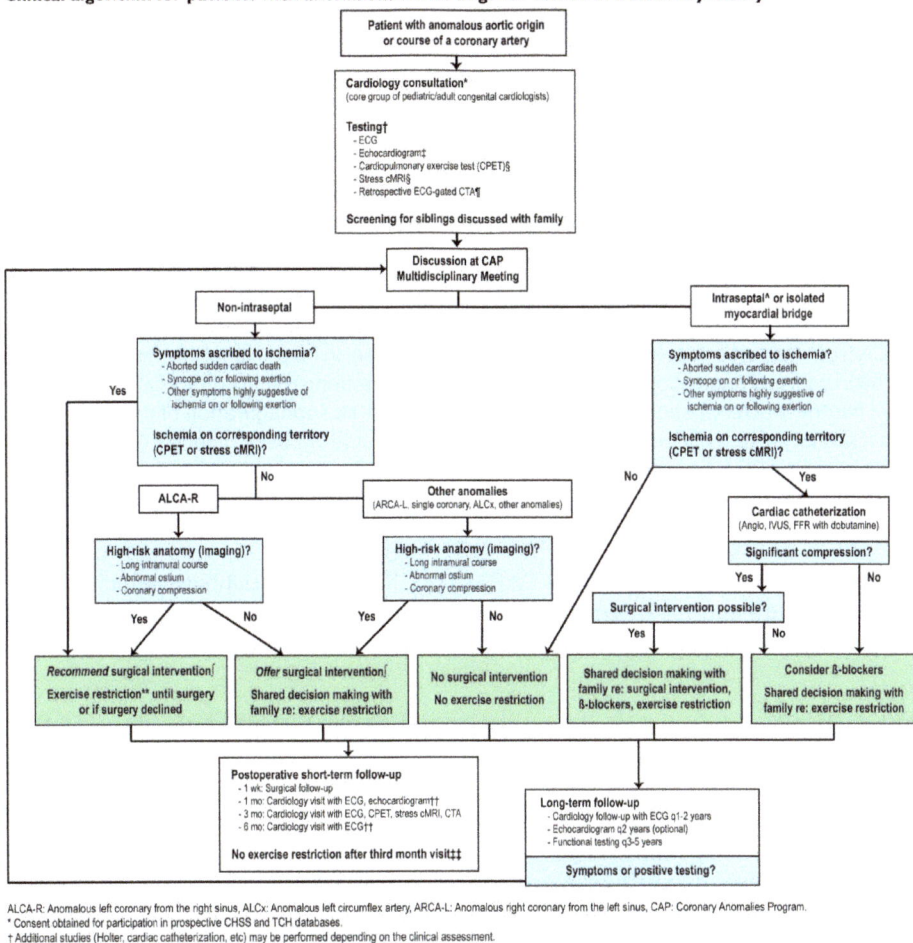

Clinical algorithm for patients with anomalous aortic origin or course of a coronary artery

```
Patient with anomalous aortic origin
or course of a coronary artery
            │
            ▼
Cardiology consultation^
(core group of pediatric/adult congenital cardiologists)

Testing†
  - ECG
  - Echocardiogram‡
  - Cardiopulmonary exercise test (CPET)§
  - Stress cMRI§
  - Retrospective ECG-gated CTA¶

Screening for siblings discussed with family
            │
            ▼
Discussion at CAP
Multidisciplinary Meeting
       /              \
  Non-intraseptal    Intraseptal^ or isolated
                     myocardial bridge
```

Non-intraseptal branch:
- Symptoms ascribed to ischemia?
  - Aborted sudden cardiac death
  - Syncope on or following exertion
  - Other symptoms highly suggestive of ischemia on or following exertion
- Ischemia on corresponding territory (CPET or stress cMRI)?
  - Yes → ALCA-R / Other anomalies (ARCA-L, single coronary, ALCx, other anomalies)
  - No → High-risk anomaly (imaging)? (Long intramural course, Abnormal ostium, Coronary compression)
    - Yes (ALCA-R): **Recommend** surgical intervention∫ — Exercise restriction** until surgery or if surgery declined
    - No: Offer surgical intervention∫ — Shared decision making with family re: exercise restriction
    - Yes (Other): Offer surgical intervention∫ — Shared decision making with family re: exercise restriction
    - No: No surgical intervention — No exercise restriction

Intraseptal branch:
- Symptoms ascribed to ischemia?
  - Aborted sudden cardiac death
  - Syncope on or following exertion
  - Other symptoms highly suggestive of ischemia on or following exertion
- Ischemia on corresponding territory (CPET or stress cMRI)?
  - Yes → Cardiac catheterization (Angio, IVUS, FFR with dobutamine) → Significant compression?
    - Yes → Surgical intervention possible?
      - Yes → Shared decision making with family re: surgical intervention, β-blockers, exercise restriction
      - No → Consider β-blockers — Shared decision making with family re: exercise restriction
    - No → Consider β-blockers — Shared decision making with family re: exercise restriction

Postoperative short-term follow-up
  - 1 wk: Surgical follow-up
  - 1 mo: Cardiology visit with ECG, echocardiogram††
  - 3 mo: Cardiology visit with ECG, CPET, stress cMRI, CTA
  - 6 mo: Cardiology visit with ECG††

No exercise restriction after third month visit‡‡

Long-term follow-up
  - Cardiology follow-up with ECG q1-2 years
  - Echocardiogram q2 years (optional)
  - Functional testing q3-5 years

Symptoms or positive testing?

ALCA-R: Anomalous left coronary from the right sinus, ALCx: Anomalous left circumflex artery, ARCA-L: Anomalous right coronary from the left sinus, CAP: Coronary Anomalies Program.
* Consent obtained for participation in prospective CHSS and TCH databases.
† Additional studies (Holter, cardiac catheterization, etc) may be performed depending on the clinical assessment.
‡ External echocardiograms do not need to be repeated if the study is deemed appropriate.
§ CPET or stress cMRI not necessary on patients that present with aborted sudden cardiac death. These studies may be deferred in young patients.
¶ An external CTA may be used if able to upload the images and the study provides all necessary information to make a decision. CTA should be deferred in patients <8 years unless clinical concerns.
^ An intraseptal coronary is an an abnormal vessel (usually a left coronary arising from the right sinus) that travels posteriorly into the septum below the level of the pulmonary valve.
∫ Unroofing if significant intramural segment, neo-ostium creation or coronary translocation if intramural segment behind a commissure, coronary translocation if short or no intramural segment. Surgical intervention will be offered for patients between 10 and 35 years of age. Other patients will be considered on a case-by-case basis. Aspirin will be administered for 3 months after surgery.
** Restriction from participation in all competitive sports and in exercise with moderate or high dynamic component (>40% maximal oxygen uptake - e.g., soccer, tennis, swimming, basketball, American football). (Mitchell et al, JACC 2005; 1364-7).
†† Patient may be seen by outside primary cardiologist.
‡‡ Postoperative patients will be cleared for exercise and competitive sports based on findings at the third month postoperative visit including results of CPET, stress cMRI, and CTA.

Figure 31-2. Current algorithm for diagnosis and management of patients with AAOCA and intramyocardial coronaries at TCH.

The other half of patients may present with chest pain, palpitations, shortness of breath, dizziness or syncope, during or immediately following exertion. These symptoms are quite common in the outpatient pediatric cardiology practice and this young population is the one at risk for SCD, making the validation of symptoms as it relates to the the diagnosis even more complex. Not infrequently, symptoms may be attributed to bronchospasm from asthma rather than a manifestation of myocardial ischemia. In a

PART II. DISEASES

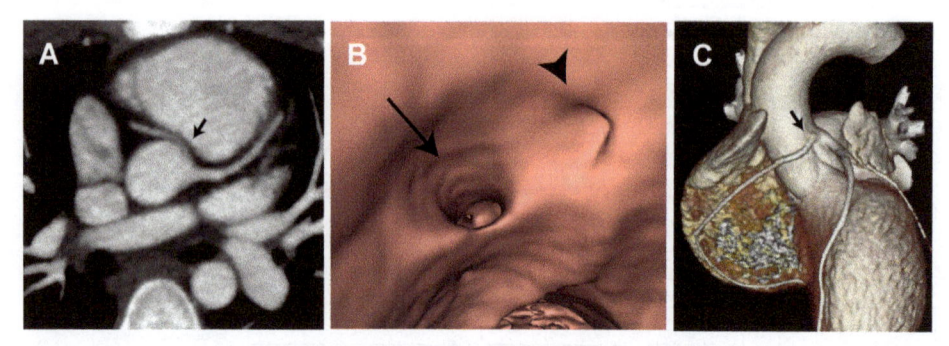

Figure 31-3. CTA in patients with AAOCA. A) Axial image in a 15-year-old demonstrating an ARCA from the left sinus, with narrow caliber of the vessel in its proximal interarterial course (arrow). B) Virtual angioscopy view showing a normal-appearing round configuration of the left main coronary artery ostium (arrow) and an elliptical, slit-like configuration of the anomalous right coronary artery ostium (arrowhead). C) Coronal volume-rendered image from a coronary CTA showing ARCA from the left sinus (arrow), with the anomalous coronary coursing just above the intercoronary commissure.

recent analysis of patients from the CAP at TCH, half of the patients were incidentally diagnosed, with another quarter presenting with symptoms on exertion, and 4 out of 163 patients presenting with aborted SCD.

MB

Although MB can be considered a normal variant, clinical manifestations vary widely. It has been suggested that myocardial bridges surrounding the coronary can compress and twist the vessel, therefore compromising flow. The functional significance may relate to the length and depth of the segment embedded in the myocardium, and the presence of more than one bridged segment.

The large majority of MB are asymptomatic. However, patients may manifest angina or angina-like symptoms, including exertional chest pain, exertional dyspnea, syncope, troponin leak, ventricular arrhythmia, myocardial infarction, and SCD.

Intraseptal Coronaries

Some patients may have a complex coronary anatomy in which an ALCA arises from the right sinus of Valsalva or from a single right coronary artery and dives into the ventricular septum within the RVOT. The coronary travels in an intramyocardial/intraseptal fashion for a variable length prior to becoming epicardial. Even though many patients with this anatomy are asymptomatic, patients can have significant coronary compression and symptomatology.

Diagnosis

Figure 31-2 shows our most recent CAP algorithm for workup and management of patients with coronary anomalies. All patients are evaluated by a specialized group

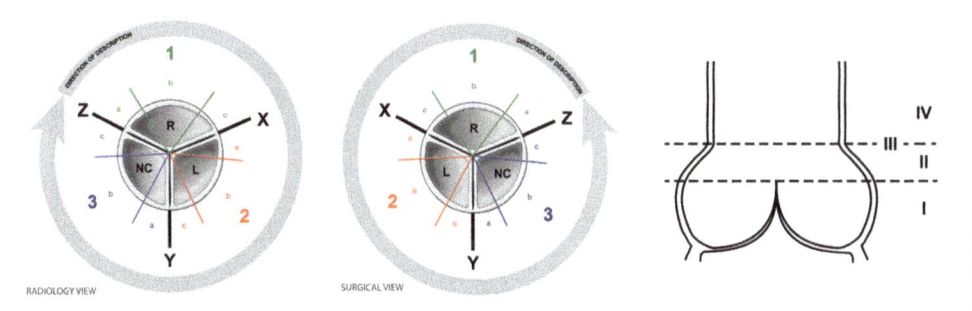

Figure 31-4. Topographic map for description of coronary ostia. The left panels describe the location of the coronary ostia based on the radiologic or surgical views. The right panel allows description of the height of the ostium (I: centrally located, II: above the aortic valve commissures but below the sinotubular junction, III: at the sinotubular junction, IV: above the sinotubular junction).

of cardiologists and undergo a standardized workup. Their data is then discussed at dedicated multidisciplinary meetings of the CAP.
- **ECG.** In the absence of ischemia, the resting ECG will be normal.
- **Echocardiogram.** May suspect AAOCA and in experienced hands, may be diagnostic. Its role is limited in MB. It is important to document ventricular function, the presence of intracardiac shunting, and other cardiac abnormalities.
- **Exercise stress test (EST).** An EST with measurement of MVO_2 is performed in all patients. Although the EST is normal in most (even those that might later present with SCD), it may disclose inducible myocardial ischemia. A positive EST is helpful for risk stratification although a normal EST does not rule out a high-risk lesion.
- **CTA (Figure 31-3).** Retrospective ECG-gated CTA provides excellent spatial resolution and is routinely used for noninvasive evaluation of coronary anatomy in children at TCH. Images are then postprocessed using a 3D workstation. Most studies are performed without the use of pharmacologic agents but beta-blockers may be needed when evaluating coronary ostial issues in patients less than 4-5 years of age. The use of new-generation scanners has significantly decreased the amount of ionizing radiation administered (approximately 2-5 mSv). The CTA report is standardized and includes information about the location of all coronaries, the presence of interarterial or intramural portions (and their length), ostial morphology and relationship, and coronary course including the relation to the intercoronary commissure or pillar. A standardized topography map is used to determine the location of the ostia (Figure 31-4).
- **Stress cardiac MRI (CMR).** Due to its excellent sensitivity and specificity to demonstrate the presence of myocardial ischemia, CMR has substituted nuclear perfusion imaging as the test of choice for functional imaging at TCH. The study is performed using dobutamine, which increases myocardial contractility while decreasing SVR, therefore mimicking exercise physiology. The perfusion sequences

PART II. DISEASES

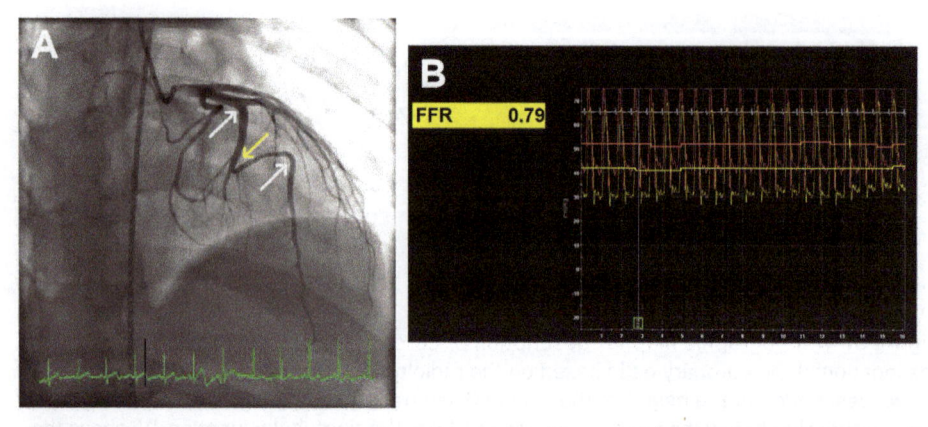

Figure 31-5. A) Left coronary artery angiogram in a 15-year-old with a long intramyocardial course of the mid left anterior descending (LAD) (corresponding to the coronary segment between white arrows) with a V- shaped hypoplastic intramyocardial segment of the LAD (yellow arrow). The fractional flow reserve (FFR) decreased from a baseline value of 0.92 to 0.79 with dobutamine infusion (B).

are performed at rest and at peak stress, with IV injection of gadolinium, to assess myocardial perfusion abnormalities and myocardial scarring.
- **Cardiac catheterization.** Cardiac catheterization may be indicated in: 1) patients in whom the coronary anatomy is not well defined with noninvasive testing, 2) patients with MB with symptoms or equivocal noninvasive testing, or 3) postoperative patients with symptoms or equivocal noninvasive testing. Coronary angiography, fractional flow reserve (FFR) testing, and intravascular ultrasound (IVUS) are performed. FFR (the ratio of pressure distal to the lesion to the pressure proximal to the lesion) is performed with the administration of intravenous adenosine (140 mcg/kg/min for 3 min) and/or dobutamine (20-40 mcg/kg/min) to achieve a heart rate of at least 75% of the predicted peak exercise heart rate. A positive FFR is considered to be <0.80 with provocative testing (Figure 31-5).

Indications / Timing for Intervention

Indications for intervention in AAOCA and MB are controversial. In general, indications depend on the type of anomaly identified and the presence of symptoms concerning for ischemia (i.e., chest pain or syncope upon or immediately following exertion), troponin leak, and/or evidence of ischemia on myocardial functional studies (i.e., EST, nuclear perfusion test [no longer used at TCH], stress CMR) (Figure 31-2). Additionally, the age of the patient will influence decision making. It is rare to entertain intervention in patients <10 years of age given the rarity of SCD, although intervention may be indicated if there is evidence of ischemia.

Due to the controversies surrounding the indications for intervention in AAOCA and the anxiety associated with this diagnosis, a long discussion with the family is of utmost importance. Patients with symptoms or evidence of ischemia are recommended surgical intervention. Most asymptomatic patients with ARCA do not require intervention due to the low risk of SCD. However, surgical intervention may be offered for patients with significant ostial stenosis or hypoplasia, or a long intramural segment (>5 mm) with a narrowed caliber of the vessel. Due to the higher risk of SCD, intervention is usually offered to patients with ALCA from the opposite sinus. It is unclear whether patients with ALCA and no intramural segment should undergo surgical intervention; a discussion with the family is important. An anterior and prepulmonic ALCA is likely a benign variant and no intervention is required. Anomalous circumflex coronaries are also considered normal variants unless there is evidence of ischemia.

For patients with MB or intramyocardial coronaries, intervention is considered whenever there is evidence of ischemia on cardiac catheterization with FFR measurement. If surgical intervention is considered high risk, medical management with beta-blockers or calcium-channel blockers may be considered.

Strategies for intervention should always be the result of shared decision-making among all involved in the care of the patient, including the cardiologist, the surgeon, and the family. Surgical intervention may be considered or offered if there are enough concerns to impose exercise restrictions in patients with these anomalies. There are several concerns recommending exercise restriction to patients, including the difficulty of children and adolescents have adhering to such recommendation, the possibility of SCD occurring at rest or with minimal activity, the psychological and emotional consequences of restricting exercise in a child or adolescent, and the known health consequences of not exercising. As such, it is rare for exercise restriction to be recommended as a strategy at TCH.

Surgical Repair

AAOCA

Preoperative TEE is performed prior to surgical intervention to rule out the presence of an intracardiac shunt (e.g., PFO) that needs to be repaired at the time of surgery. The procedures are performed via median sternotomy and under CPB using aorto-bicaval cannulation. After cardioplegic arrest and left-heart venting through either the pulmonary vein or the atrial septum, an oblique aortotomy is performed and the coronary anatomy is inspected. Documentation of the location of the ostia (Figure 31-4) and length of intramurality is critical.

Surgical unroofing of the anomalous coronary artery is the treatment of choice at TCH for patients with a long intramural segment that travels above the level of the intercoronary commissure (Figure 31-6). The wall between the coronary artery and the aortic lumen is excised and the intimas of the aortic wall and the coronary are attached with a series of fine interrupted sutures in order to evert the edges, increase the coronary lumen, and exclude the aortic-wall fatty tissue from the circulation. By unroofing a long intramural segment, the ostium is augmented and in essence moved to the correct sinus, away from the intercoronary pillar. Unroofing of a short intramural segment may augment the size of the ostium but fail to reposition the ostium away from the intercoronary pillar, potentially causing persistent narrowing of the coronary as it travels behind the intercoronary pillar. In these cases, or in patients where the

PART II. DISEASES

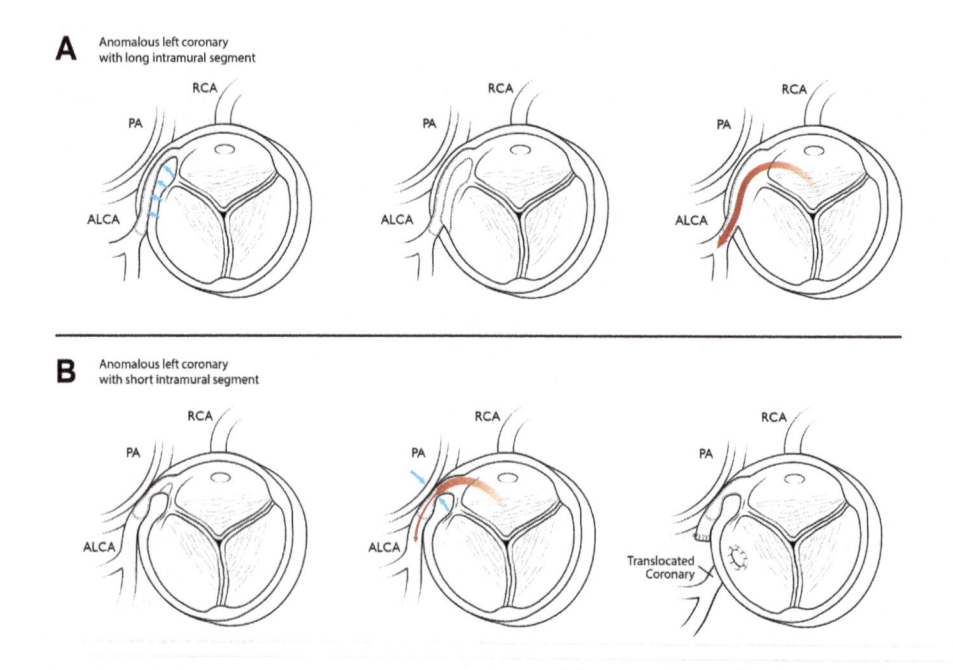

Figure 31-6. Surgical management of patients with AAOCA. A) Patient with AAOCA and a long intramural segment. By unroofing a long intramural segment, the coronary ostium is enlarged and the ostium is moved to the correct sinus and away from the thick intercoronary pillar, resulting in an unobstructed coronary ostium. B) Patient with AAOCA and a short intramural segment. Unroofing of a short segment may improve the size of the ostium but the anomalous coronary may continue to arise from the incorrect sinus and/or in close relationship with the thick intercoronary pillar, which can continue to compress the anomalous coronary. In this scenario, a coronary translocation may provide a better surgical alternative.

intramural segment travels below the level of the aortic valve, a *coronary translocation* may be a better alternative (Figure 31-6). It is important to note that different than coronary translocation in an arterial switch operation, in AAOCA, the anomalous vessel is transected as it comes out of the aortic wall (without an aortic button) and sutured circumferentially to the correct sinus. The long-term consequences of a circumferential anastomosis on a small coronary artery are unclear.

Other surgical procedures that may be used for AAOCA include the *creation of a neoostium* in the correct sinus for patients with a very long intramural segment traveling below the level of the aortic valve, and *anterior or lateral pulmonary translocation* PA (which has not been used at TCH) to theoretically prevent the compression of the interarterial segment of the coronary by the PA. Figure 31-7 shows an algorithm indicating how the optimal surgical procedure is chosen at TCH.

31. CONGENITAL CORONARY ANOMALIES

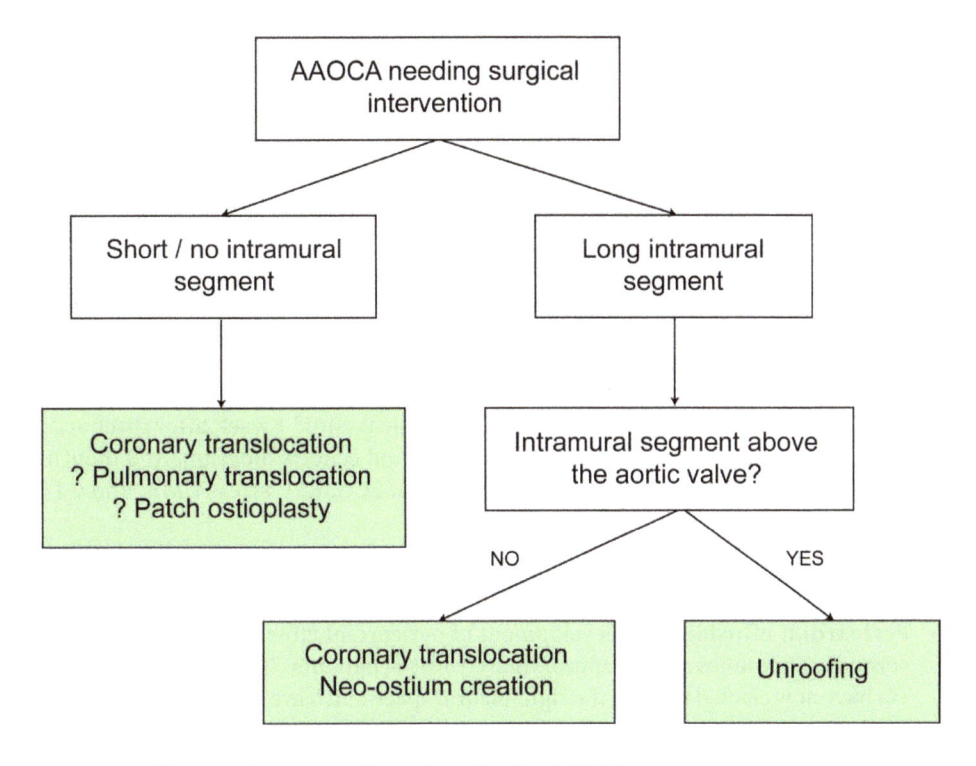

Figure 31-7. Surgical decision-making algorithm for AAOCA.

MB
The management of MBs is also performed under CPB and with cardioplegic arrest and venting of the left heart. It is important to study the anatomy of the MB and its relationship with the different coronary branches on CTA and/or cardiac catheterization to aid with intraoperative identification of the MB. Once the MB is identified, the myocardium above the coronary artery is carefully incised until the intramyocardial coronary is completely unroofed.

Intraseptal Coronaries
The surgical management of intraseptal coronaries is difficult due to their anatomy. Some proposed surgical interventions include: 1) unroofing the intramyocardial segment behind the pulmonary valve; 2) excising the pulmonary root (similar to what is performed during the Ross procedure), unroofing the myocardium above the coronary, and reimplanting the pulmonary root into the RVOT below the level of the coronary; and 3) opening the RVOT transversely, unroofing the myocardium above the coronary, and reconstructing the defect with a patch.

Postoperative Management

Patients are generally extubated in the OR and then transferred to the CICU. No inotropes are usually required for these patients. An ECG is obtained on arrival and on postoperative day 1. Approximately 70-80% of patients will have diffuse ST changes consistent with early repolarization. Classic changes involve elevation of the J point and diffuse scooping of the ST segments. As long as the changes are diffuse and consistent with early repolarization ("pericarditis"), no intervention is required. Localized ST changes, in particular related to the region of the involved coronary, should be investigated.

Patients are typically transferred to the acute floor on postoperative day 1. Low-dose aspirin is started and continued for 3 months to avoid thrombi formation in the area of surgical manipulation (tacking sutures). Patients are discharged once the chest tubes are out and discharge studies (echocardiogram and CXR) are performed, usually 4-7 days postoperatively. Patients are seen in surgical clinic 1 week after discharge, and then by the cardiologist at 1 month with ECG and echocardiogram. At 3 months postoperatively, patients undergo echocardiogram, ECG, EST, stress CMR, and CTA to assess the results after surgery.

Complications

- **Pericardial effusion.** The development of pericardial effusions after surgery for coronary anomalies affects approximately 10% of patients. The etiology is unclear. We have now elected to open the right pleural space and leave the pericardium open on these patients to avoid the development of significant effusions.
- **Coronary ischemia.** Ischemia is very rare but should be entertained if there are localized ECG changes or wall-motion abnormalities on echocardiography.

Long-Term Follow-Up

All patients evaluated are followed up for life. Patients are generally seen with a clinical visit and an ECG every year. For surgical patients, myocardial functional studies are performed at 3-5 years after surgery to reevaluate potential long-term effects of the surgical procedure. Long-term follow-up for patients with AAOCA is critical to eventually define the optimal management for these patients.

Suggested Readings

Agrawal H, Mery CM, Krishnamurthy R, Molossi S. Anatomic types of anomalous aortic origin of a coronary artery: A pictorial summary. Congenit Heart Dis 2017;12:603-606.

Agrawal H, Molossi S, Alam M, et al. Anomalous coronary arteries and myocardial bridges: Risk stratification in children using novel cardiac catheterization techniques. Pediatr Cardiol 2017;38:624-630.

Agrawal H, Qureshi AM, Alam M, et al. Anomalous aortic origin of a coronary artery with an intraseptal course: novel techniques in hemodynamic assessment. BMJ Case Rep 2018;pii:bcr-2018-225707.

Doan TT, Wilkinson JC, Agrawal H, et al. Instantaneous wave-free ratio (iFR) correlates with fractional flow reserve (FFR) assessment of coronary artery stenoses and myocardial bridges in children. J Invasive Cardiol 2020;32:176-179.

Doan TT, Zea-Vera R, Agrawal H, et al. Myocardial ischemia in children with anomalous aortic origin of a coronary artery with intraseptal course. Circ Cardiovasc Interv 2020; 13(3):e008375. doi: 10.1161/CIRCINTERVENTIONS.119.008375. Epub 2020 Feb 27.

Mery CM, De Leon L, Molossi S, et al. Outcomes of surgical intervention for anomalous aortic origin of a coronary artery: A large contemporary prospective cohort study. J Thorac Cardiovasc Surg 2018;155:305-319.

Mery CM, Lopez KN, Molossi S, et al. Decision analysis to define the optimal management of athletes with anomalous aortic origin of a coronary artery. J Thorac Cardiovasc Surg 2016;152:1366-1375.

Molossi S, Agrawal H. Clinical evaluation of anomalous aortic origin of a coronary artery (AAOCA). Congenit Heart Dis 2017;12:607-609.

Molossi S, Agrawal H, Mery CM, et al. Outcomes in anomalous aortic origin of a coronary artery following a prospective standardized approach. Circ Cardiovasc Interv 2020;13: e008445. doi: 10.1161/CIRCINTERVENTIONS.119.008445. Epub 2020 Feb 13.

Qureshi A, Agrawal H. Catheter-based anatomic and functional assessment in anomalous aortic origin of a coronary artery, myocardial bridges and Kawasaki disease. Congenit Heart Dis 2017;12:615-618.

32 Myocarditis and Cardiomyopathy

Susan W. Denfield, Jack F. Price, Iki Adachi

Myocarditis

Myocarditis is an inflammatory disease of the myocardium most commonly caused by cardiotropic viruses, most of which have no specific antiviral therapies. Therapies are largely supportive to try to allow the myocardium to recover while supported either pharmacologically or with mechanical circulatory support. Making the diagnosis of myocarditis is difficult because viral syndromes are very common in children and it can be difficult to determine whether a child presenting with a viral prodrome or ongoing viral illness and heart failure actually has an acute process or has had a subclinical longer-standing cardiomyopathy (typically dilated cardiomyopathy [DCM]) that has been "tipped over the edge" by the increased stress and metabolic demands of an intercurrent infectious illness.

Diagnosis

Laboratory studies that are typically ordered include sedimentation rate (ESR), C-reactive protein (CRP), CBC with differential, troponins and cardiotropic viral PCRs of the blood, nasal washing and/or tracheal aspirate, if intubated. Viral PCRs are preferred over viral serologies. Electrolytes, BUN, creatinine, lactate, LFTs, amylase, and lipase are checked to estimate the degree of end-organ compromise. Brain natiuretic peptide is also measured. Significantly elevated ESR, CRP, troponins, and a positive PCR favor a diagnosis of myocarditis over DCM.

In myocarditis, the ECG often demonstrates ST- and T-wave changes that mimic ischemia (Figure 32-1). Very low voltages may be seen. DCM more typically demonstrates LVH with nonspecific ST changes, T-wave inversion, or a strain pattern.

The echocardiogram demonstrates varying degrees of dysfunction, but often the LV function is severely depressed. A more normal LV end-diastolic dimension with severe dysfunction favors myocarditis while a severely dilated thin-walled LV favors DCM.

Cardiac MRI (CMR) has become a frequently used tool to assess for evidence of cardiac inflammation; scarring would suggest a more long-standing process. However, CMR often requires anesthesia, the risk of which often outweighs the benefit in a critically ill child with severe cardiac dysfunction. Findings often do not change therapy, further reducing the risk-benefit ratio.

Endomyocardial biopsy is the gold standard for the diagnosis of myocarditis, however it also carries significant risks, including anesthesia in a critically ill child. Sampling error reduces the reliability of this test since the histopathologic changes of myocarditis can be patchy and absent in the samples taken. Similar to CMR, findings often do not change therapy.

Treatment

Therapy is largely supportive. If a virus is found that has specific antiviral therapy, the antiviral agent should be used. Diuretics, inotropes, and vasopressor support are titrated per cardiorespiratory status. While milrinone (if BP is adequate) and/or epinephrine

32. MYOCARDITIS AND CARDIOMYOPATHY

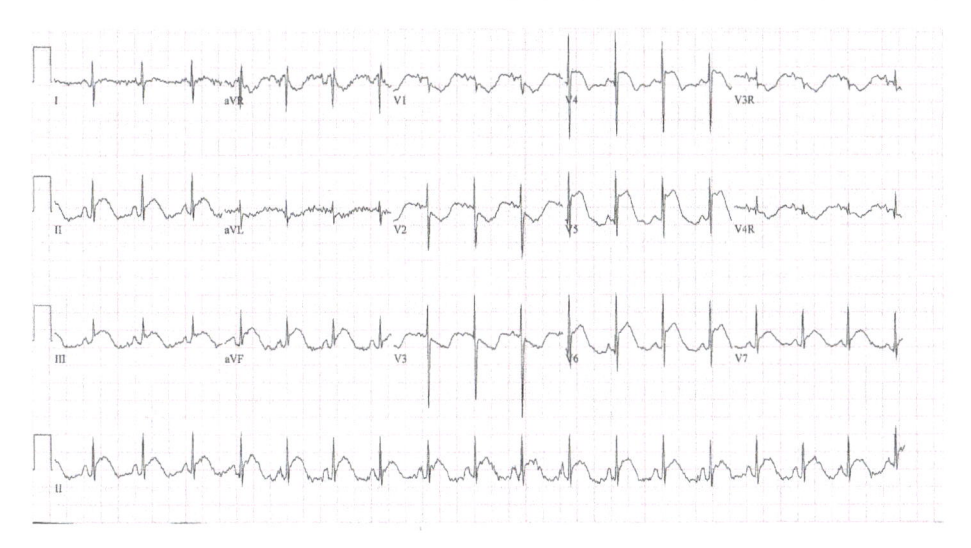

Figure 32-1. ECG from a patient with myocarditis demonstrating marked ST-segment elevation in the inferior leads and V4 to V7 with "tombstoning", most classically shown in leads V5 and V6. ST-segment depression is seen in aVR, aVL, and V1 to V3.

are commonly used, other institutions commonly use other agents. Ventilatory support is often needed and can help with cardiac support to some extent.

The use of IV immunoglobulin (IVIG) and other immunomodulating drugs has had mixed results in a variety of study types. In patients with a preponderance of evidence suggesting myocarditis, as opposed to acutely decompensated DCM, IVIG is used. We reserve corticosteroids for those with "tombstoning" ST segments on ECG.

In patients who continue to decline despite maximal medical therapy with poor oxygenation, ECMO with an LA vent or atrial septostomy may be needed. If the pulmonary status is not severely compromised, a temporary left ventricular assist device (LVAD) is preferred due to better LV decompression, which is important to promote LV recovery. If there is no, or very limited myocardial recovery, the patient may need to be transitioned to long-term LVAD support to await cardiac transplantation.

Outcomes
Those with a fulminant presentation frequently are the most likely to recover with aggressive early support. Freedom from death and transplant varies widely in reports from 50 to 90%, with about 75-80% being a reasonable statistic to quote.

Dilated Cardiomyopathy (DCM)
DCM is a disease of the heart muscle characterized by an enlarged LV chamber and in most cases, impaired systolic function. It is the most common form of cardiomyopathy in children in the US. Symptoms of heart failure may progress to end-stage disease necessitating mechanical circulatory support (MCS) as a bridge to transplant.

Diagnosis

The most common time of diagnosis of DCM is infancy. Signs of heart failure are typically present, including hepatomegaly, gallop rhythm, failure to gain weight, diaphoresis while feeding, tachypnea, and retractions. In older children, symptoms may include abdominal pain, vomiting, fatigue, dyspnea with exertion, and orthopnea. CXR usually reveals cardiomegaly and less commonly, pulmonary vascular congestion and/or pleural effusions. The ECG often demonstrates LVH and nonspecific ST-segment abnormalities. Sinus tachycardia is common. A fixed tachycardia should be investigated for possible tachycardia-induced cardiomyopathy, as this is a potentially reversible cause. Conduction disturbances may occur. Echocardiography reveals a dilated LV with depressed systolic function, with or without MR.

Causes

Most cases are "idiopathic", as a cause usually is not determined. Metabolic causes/inborn errors of metabolism and malformation syndromes should be assessed for, particularly in infants. Neuromuscular diseases should be excluded. Other etiologies include familial or genetic mutations and possible infectious or inflammatory diseases. Genetic testing is recommended.

Treatment

When presenting with decompensated heart failure, the primary therapeutic goals are alleviation of symptoms and correction of hemodynamic derangements. IV diuretics are usually necessary and effective for treating congestion. Inotropic agents such as milrinone and epinephrine are useful for treating low cardiac output. Once symptoms are relieved and fluid balance restored, oral therapies are initiated. If tolerated, most outpatients should be treated with a beta-blocker (carvedilol or long-acting metoprolol), angiotensin-converting enzyme (ACE) inhibitor and an aldosterone antagonist (spironolactone). If symptoms cannot be controlled and there is evidence of progressive end-organ damage, MCS should be considered. Temporary LV support can be transitioned to a long-term LVAD for those without evidence of ventricular recovery. Long-term RV mechanical support is seldom necessary.

Outcome

Survival after diagnosis of DCM varies widely. For all causes of DCM, 5-year freedom from death or transplantation is about 50%.

Hypertrophic Cardiomyopathy (HCM)

HCM is the second most common form of cardiomyopathy in children. It is characterized by abnormally thick ventricular walls, usually with preserved or hyperdynamic systolic function. Restrictive physiology may develop in some and a "burned-out dilated" form in a small subset. HCM is the most common cause of sudden cardiac death in young athletes in the US.

Diagnosis

The signs and symptoms of HCM may be subtle or nonexistent. Symptoms may include fatigue, dyspnea with exertion, chest pain, palpitations, and lightheadedness. Sudden death may be the first symptom, with diagnosis at autopsy. Findings on examination may include a parasternal heave, systolic ejection murmur that increases with Valsalva maneuver, and an extra heart sound. The ECG usually demonstrates LVH with or without a strain pattern. CXR may reveal a normal or minimally enlarged cardiac silhouette. On echocardiogram, asymmetric septal hypertrophy is frequently present, with or without obstruction in the LVOT. The RV is typically spared, but may be hypertrophied. Gene testing should be considered in new cases of HCM, especially when another family member is affected. Exercise testing is suggested in new cases of HCM if the resting peak instantaneous gradient is <50 mmHg for risk profile assessment for sudden death (e.g., abnormal BP response to exercise).

Causes
Most cases of HCM are likely attributable to gene mutations in sarcomeric proteins. First-degree relatives should undergo screening with echocardiography as HCM may be familial. If a gene has been identified in the proband, family members should be offered gene testing. Other etiologies include metabolic disorders and genetic syndromes, which are more commonly diagnosed in infancy, and neuromuscular disorders.

Treatment
There is no medical therapy for HCM that will result in remodeling of the ventricular myocardium. Treatment of HCM is focused on relief of symptoms and includes beta-blockers or calcium-channel blockers. These patients are restricted from physical education and sports. Patients who remain symptomatic with severe LVOT obstruction usually benefit from surgical myectomy. Those at increased risk of sudden death should be considered for implantation of a cardioverter-defibrillator for primary prevention. Patients considered at greater risk include those with a first-degree relative who died suddenly, documented ventricular tachycardia, syncope, and severe ventricular hypertrophy. MCS and cardiac transplantation are not usually needed in HCM, however those with refractory life-threatening arrhythmias, progressive restrictive physiology, "burned-out" forms, or other refractory symptoms may benefit from transplant.

LV Noncompaction Cardiomyopathy (LVNC)
LVNC is a less common form of cardiomyopathy and is characterized by a hypertrabeculated spongy appearance of the LV more commonly than the RV. It can manifest in dilated, hypertrophic, and restrictive forms. Treatment is based on the phenotype. These patients are also arrhythmia-, clot-, and stroke-prone, requiring vigilance for those morbidities with initiation of antithrombotic therapies, particularly in the dilated and restrictive phenotypes. Antiarrhythmic therapies, including consideration of an implantable cardioverter defibrillator, may be necessary in some at-risk patients.

Restrictive Cardiomyopathy (RCM)
RCM results in severe diastolic dysfunction with limited cardiac filling leading to low cardiac output and eventual pulmonary hypertension. There are no good medical therapies for RCM. Treatment consists of judicious use of diuretics for overt systemic or

pulmonary venous congestion and aspirin or other anticoagulant to prevent thrombosis. Prognosis is poor; within 3 years of diagnosis approximately 50% have died or undergone cardiac transplantation. Early consideration and listing for cardiac transplantation is advised as these patients are difficult to support pharmacologically and mechanically once they become critically ill.

Arrhythmogenic Right-Ventricular Cardiomyopathy (ARVC)
ARVC typically presents in late adolescents or young adults with symptoms related to ventricular arrhythmias, preceding overt cardiomyopathy. However, in early childhood, it may present as a dilated form of cardiomyopathy with a higher ventricular tachycardia burden than is typically seen in childhood DCM. Features of RCM may also be present. Treatment is directed towards arrhythmia control and the cardiac phenotype, using standard heart failure therapies.

33 Infective Endocarditis

Claire E. Bocchini, Thomas J. Seery, Carlos M. Mery

Infective endocarditis (IE) is a rare, but important diagnosis to consider in children with a predisposing cardiac lesion or history of cardiac surgery. Targeted prolonged IV antibiotics are the mainstay of therapy, with aggressive early surgery intervention being warranted in certain situations.

Pathophysiology

Turbulent blood flow from cardiac lesions results in injury to the endocardial surface and subsequent thrombus formation. The injured endocardial surface and thrombus become infected secondary to transient bacteremia, which occurs routinely in otherwise healthy children. Noncardiac complications from IE occur as a result of either embolic or immune-mediated phenomena.

Although a variety of microorganisms can cause IE, Gram-positive bacteria are by far the most common. Streptococcal species, especially Viridans-group Streptococci, are the most common bacteria identified in children with CHD. *Staphylococcus aureus* is also an important cause of IE in children with and without CHD, and frequently results in a more fulminant clinical presentation. Other organisms that cause IE include HACEK organisms (*Haemophilus* species, *Aggregatibacter* species, *Cardiobacteria hominis*, *Eikenella corrodens*, and *Kingella kingae*). More unusual pathogens include *Bartonella* species, *Coxiella burnetti*, *Brucella* species, and *Mycoplasma* species. IE can also be caused by *Candida* species, particularly in infants.

Table 33-1. Microorganisms identified in 67 children with IE at TCH, 2011-2016

Microorganism	CHD patients N=51	Non-CHD patients N=16	p-value
Staphylococci species	9 (18%)	8 (50%)	
Methicillin-resistant *S. aureus*	0	6	
Methicillin-susceptible *S. aureus*	7	1	<0.01
Coagulase-negative Staphylococcus	2	1	
Streptococci species	28 (55%)	6 (38%)	
Viridans-group Streptococci	24	2	
Gemella spp.	1	1	
Granulicatella adiacens	1	1	<0.05
Streptococcus pneumoniae	1	1	
Group A/G Streptococcus	1	1	
HACEK species	6 (12%)	1 (6%)	
Haemophilus spp.	3	1	
Aggregatibacter spp.	2	0	NS
Cardiobacteria hominis	1	0	
Other	2 (4%)	1 (6%)	
Neisseria gonorrhoeae	0	1	
Enterococcus faecalis	1	0	NS
Candida tropicalis	1	0	

Table 33-2. AHA Guidelines for the Prevention of Infective Endocarditis (Wilson et al. 2007)

Cardiac conditions warranting antibiotic prophylaxis prior to dental procedures (involving manipulation of gingival tissue or perforation of the oral mucosa) *or* surgical procedures involving infected skin or musculoskeletal tissue

- Prosthetic cardiac valve, prosthetic material used for cardiac valve repair
- Previous occurrence of IE
- Certain types of CHD
   - Unrepaired cyanotic CHD, including palliative shunts and conduits
   - Completely repaired CHD with prosthetic material or device (placed by surgery or interventional cath) during the initial 6 months postprocedure
   - Repaired CHD with residual defects at the site or adjacent to the site of a prosthetic patch or prosthetic device
- Cardiac transplantation recipients who develop cardiac valvulopathy
 	
Prophylaxis is not indicated:
- Prior to dental radiographs, routine anesthetic injections through noninfected tissue, placement or removal of orthodontic appliances, shedding of deciduous teeth, and bleeding from trauma to the lips or oral mucosa.
- Prior to genitourinary or GI tract procedures, including diagnostic endoscopy

Table 33-1 shows the microorganisms identified in our patient population based on a recent review of cases at TCH from 2011 to 2016.

Prevention

The most important step in the management of IE is prevention. For this reason, any patient with a history of CHD must adhere to vigilant dental hygiene and routine dental visits. The 2007 AHA Guidelines for the Prevention of Infective Endocarditis (Table 33-2) were designed to ensure appropriate use of antibiotic prophylaxis in certain high-risk groups while minimizing unnecessary use in those for whom the risk does not warrant prophylaxis.

Clinical Presentation and Diagnosis

The clinical presentation of IE in children with CHD is variable, and depends on a number of factors such as the microorganism involved, the degree of local cardiac disease, and whether noncardiac embolic or immune-mediated complications are present. Children with IE typically have either a subacute or acute clinical presentation.

Children with *subacute* IE can present with long-standing (weeks to months) low-grade fever and nonspecific somatic complaints including fatigue, weakness, myalgias, arthralgias, weight loss, night sweats, rigors, and exercise intolerance. Subacute IE is more likely to be associated with immune-mediated noncardiac complications, such as glomerulonephritis, Roth spots, and Osler nodes, although these findings are less common in children compared with adults. Children with Viridans-group Streptococci typically have a more subacute presentation. In addition, infections associated with the bovine jugular RV-PA valved conduits have also been described as having a more indolent, subacute presentation.

In contrast, children with *acute* IE usually have more severe symptoms and can

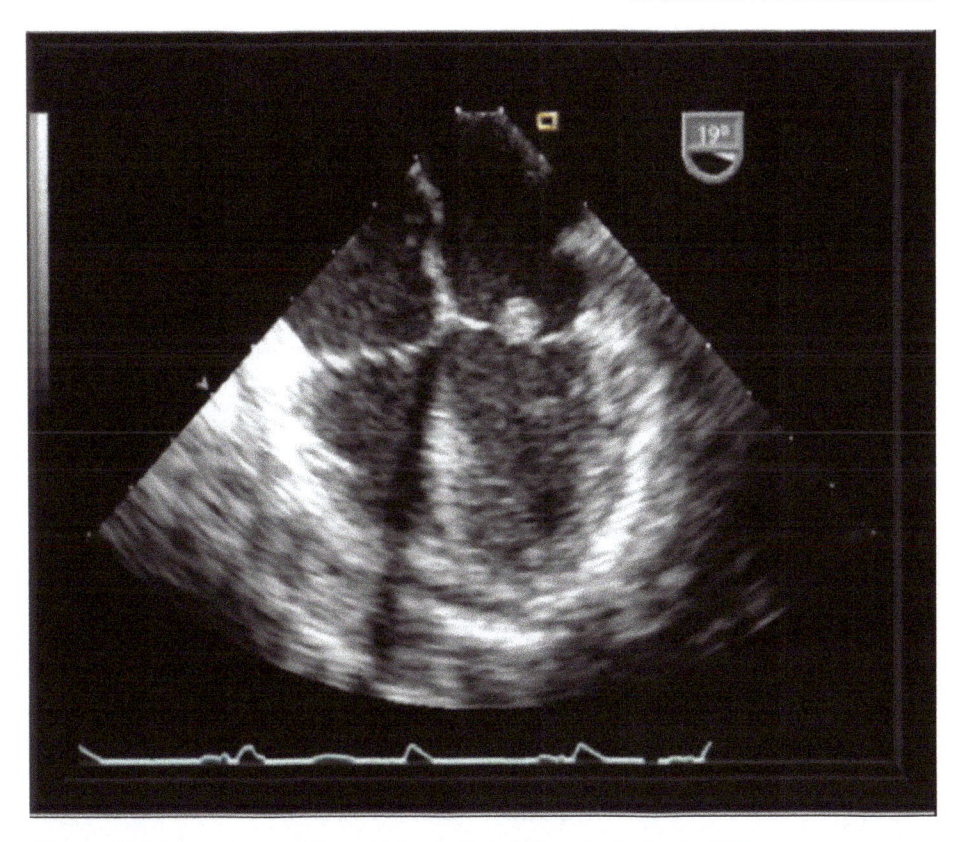

Figure 33-1. Large mass on the anterior leaflet of the mitral valve by TEE.

experience a rapid clinical deterioration requiring emergent intensive care interventions. Symptoms include high fevers, tachycardia, and overall ill appearance. These infections are associated with more aggressive local disease in the heart (including larger vegetations) as well as noncardiac embolic disease, which can result in stroke/neurologic injury, pulmonary embolism/pneumonia, osteomyelitis, kidney injury, and GI injury. Organisms that are associated with an acute presentation of IE and large vegetations include *S. aureus*, *Streptococcus pneumoniae*, and fungal pathogens.

The modified Duke criteria (Table 33-3) are used for diagnosis of IE. Clinical signs are supplemented by imaging with echocardiography (Figure 33-1, Figure 33-2, and Figure 33-3) or CT (Figure 33-4).

For children who are clinically stable, every attempt should be made to obtain 3 sets of blood cultures prior to the initiation of antimicrobial therapy (over 24-48 hours). To maximize blood culture sensitivity, it is essential that each blood culture bottle is inoculated with the appropriate blood volume based on patient weight. Blood-culture sets should include aerobic and anaerobic cultures when clinically feasible.

For children who are more seriously ill, 3 sets of blood cultures from 3 separate

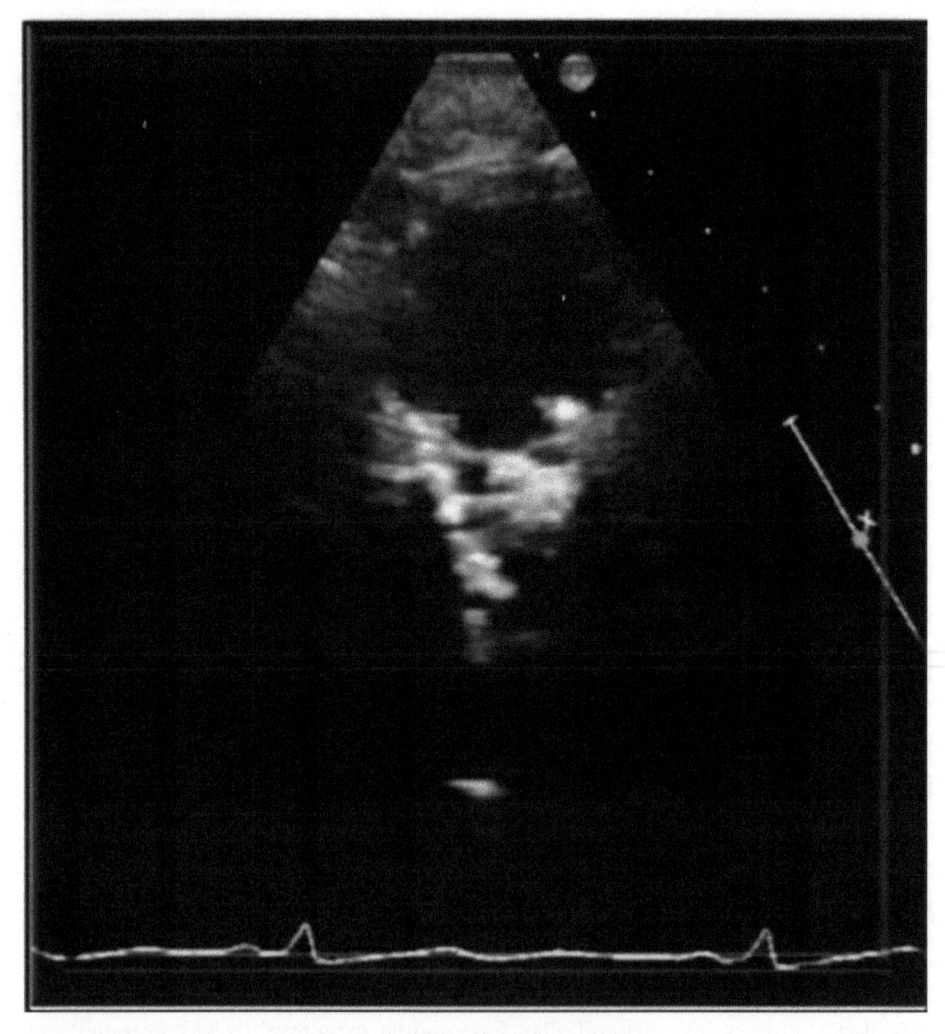

Figure 33-2. Vegetation within a bovine jugular RV-PA conduit.

venipuncture sites should be obtained as soon as clinically feasible (within an hour) and empirical antibiotic therapy should be started as soon as possible.

All patients with suspected IE should also receive an echocardiogram. In children, TTE is usually adequate, but in older children or in children who are overweight, TEE may be required. TEE may also be prefered in children with grafts/conduits or suspected aortic valve lesions.

At TCH, children undergoing evaluation for IE may also undergo head imaging (CT or MRI with contrast) and chest/abdominal imaging (high-resolution CT of the chest, abdominal CT with contrast, or abdominal ultrasound) to evaluate for septic emboli. Ophthalmology may be consulted to complete a funduscopic exam looking for Roth spots. Laboratory evaluation may include complete blood count with differential (CBC

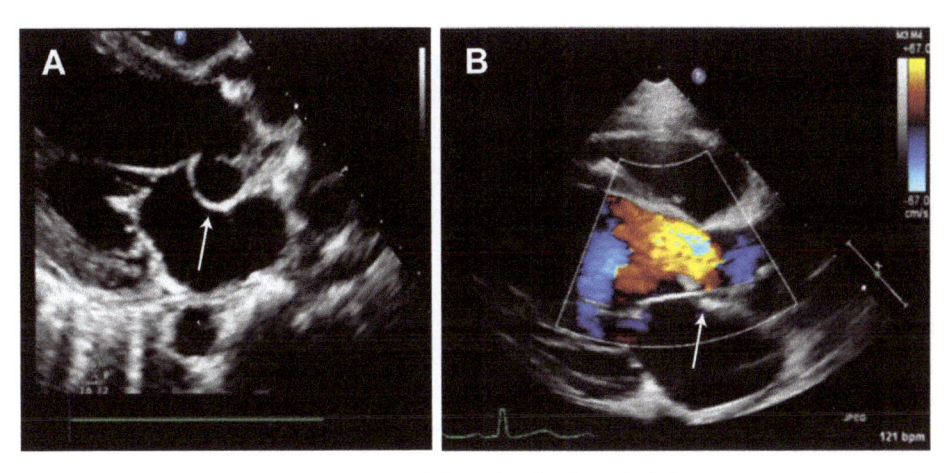

Figure 33-3. Parasternal long axis view (2D and color Doppler) demonstrating a periaortic root abscess. (arrow) with severe AI. Images courtesy of Dr. Josh Kailin, www.pedecho.org.

with differential), C-reactive protein (CRP), erythrocyte sedimentation rate (ESR), rheumatoid factor, complement levels, and urine analysis.

Children who require surgical management should also have diagnostic specimens sent from the OR. Vegetations and other infected material should be sent for aerobic, anaerobic, fungal, and possibly mycobacterial cultures. In addition, newer techniques such as broad-range bacterial (16S rRNA) and fungal (28S rRNA) PCR should be considered, especially if preliminary culture results are negative.

Medical Management

Children with IE typically require a prolonged course of IV antibiotic therapy. Antibiotic choice, dosage, and duration depends on the microorganism responsible for the infection as well as whether the infection involves prosthetic material. Updated recommendations for medical management of IE were published in 2015 (Baddour et al. 2015). Most children with IE will require placement of a PICC for long-term access to complete their antibiotic therapy. Placement of PICC lines should be delayed until the patient has had 48-72 hours of negative blood cultures.

Children receiving prolonged antibiotic therapy for IE should be closely monitored. At TCH, weekly blood work typically includes CBC with differential, CRP, and ESR. Kidney function should also be monitored 1 or more times per week depending on the risk of nephrotoxicity from the antibiotic regimen. In addition, children who are receiving therapy with aminoglycosides (and possibly vancomycin) should have troughs checked weekly.

Indications / Timing for Intervention

IE carries a significant mortality risk and the extent of disease is usually underappreciated by imaging. As such, early surgical intervention is generally favored at TCH.

Table 33-3. Modified Duke criteria for diagnosis of IE (Li et al. 2000).

Modified Duke Criteria for Diagnosis of IE	
Major criteria	Minor criteria
1. Positive blood culture for IE 　A) Typical microorganism consistent with IE from ≥2 blood cultures: 　　- Viridans strep, Strep bovis, or HACEK group 　　　or 　　- Community-acquired Staph aureus or enterococci, in the absence of a primary focus 　B) Microorganisms consistent with IE from persistently positive blood cultures, defined as: 　　- 2 positive cultures of blood samples drawn >12 h apart 　　　or 　　- All of 3 or a majority of ≥4 blood cultures (irrespective of the timing) 　　　or 　　- 1 positive blood culture for Coxiella burnetti or antiphase-I Immunoglobulin G antibody titer >1:800 2. Evidence of endocardial involvement 　A) Positive echocardiogram 　　- Oscillating intracardiac mass on valve or supporting structures, in the path of regurgitant jets (Figure 33-1), or on implanted material (Figure 33-2) in the absence of an alternative anatomic explanation 　　　or 　　- Abscess (Figure 33-3) 　　　or 　　- New partial dehiscence of a prosthetic valve 　B) New valvar regurgitation	1. Predisposing heart condition or IV drug use 2. Fever ≥38°C 3. Vascular phenomena 　• Janeway lesions 　• Intracranial hemorrhage 　• Conjunctival hemorrhages 　• Septic pulmonary infarcts 　• Major arterial emboli 　• Mycotic aneurysm 4. Immunologic phenomena 　• Osler nodes 　• Roth spots 　• Glomerulonephritis 　• Rheumatoid factor 5. Positive blood cx not meeting major criteria Definite IE Pathological criteria 　- Culture positive vegetation / abscess 　　　or 　- Vegetation / abscess confirmed by history showing active endocarditis Clinical criteria 　- 2 major criteria 　　　or 　- 1 major + 3 minor criteria 　　　or 　- 5 minor criteria Possible IE Findings consistent with IE that fall short of "definite" but not "rejected"

Early surgery should be considered in patients with CHF or severe valve involvement, suspicion of periannular involvement or abscess, left-sided vegetations at risk for embolization (>1 cm, mobile) especially if evidence of a previous systemic emboli, virulent organisms (*S. aureus* or fungi), presence of heart block (usually indicating invasion into the conduction system between the aortic and tricuspid valves), prosthetic valve endocarditis, previous endocarditis, or poor response to antimicrobial therapy.

A difficult question is the optimal timing of intervention in patients with IE and a stroke from embolization. There are no adequate studies to address the risk of hemorrhagic conversion of a stroke with the heparinization needed for CPB. In general,

33. INFECTIVE ENDOCARDITIS

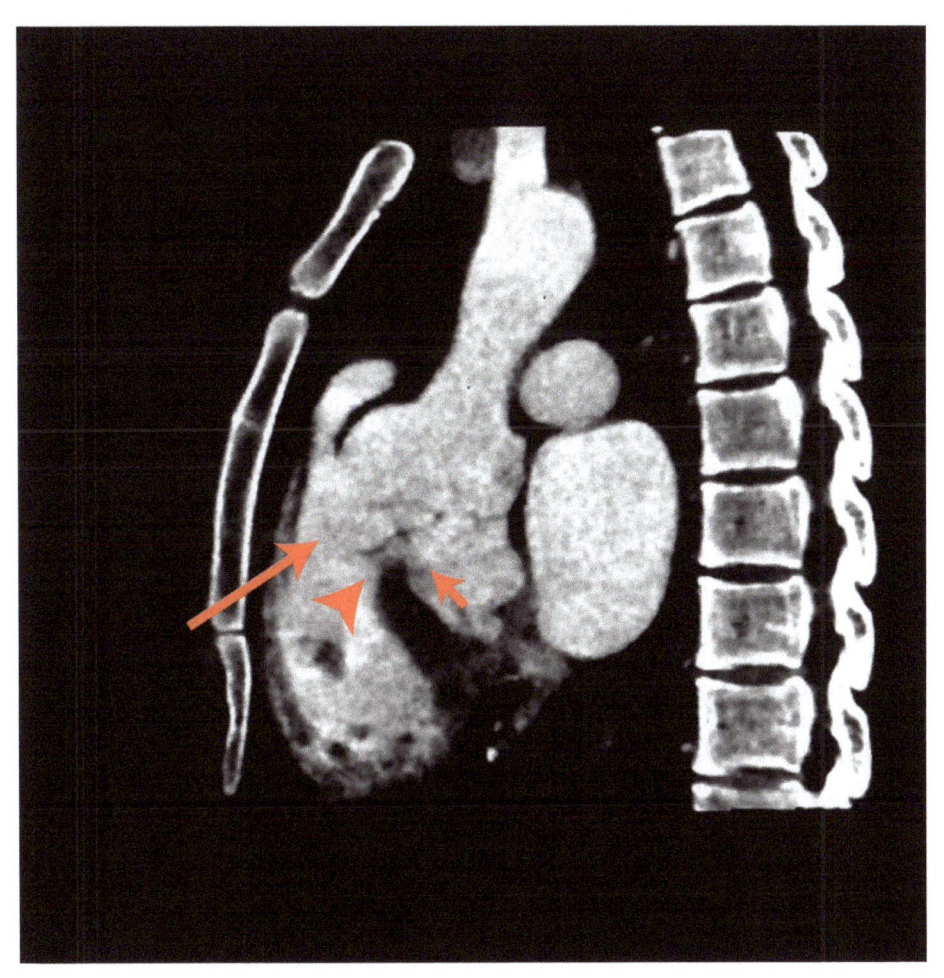

Figure 33-4. CT on a patient with a doubly-committed juxta-arterial VSD, mitral and aortic valve endocarditis, and severe AI. Images show a prolapsing right coronary leaflet (long arrow) through the VSD (arrowhead) and irregular masses consistent with vegetations on the ventricular side of the aortic valve leaflets (short arrow).

patients with a small stroke and a significant indication for early intervention should undergo surgical intervention. In patients with a large ischemic stroke and no evidence of hemorrhage, surgery may be delayed for 2-4 weeks, if possible. Similarly, for stable patients with intracerebral hemorrhage, surgery should be delayed for 4 weeks, if possible. However, the clinical status of the patient may mandate early surgical intervention regardless of the presence of a stroke or intracerebral hemorrhage. In these cases, surgery is performed with the understanding that the risk of neurologic deterioration is likely higher than if delay was possible.

Surgical Intervention

Surgical treatment is individualized for each particular patient based on anatomy and extent of infection. Surgical intervention for IE is best described as two separate processes: *debridement* and *reconstruction*. Debridement involves removal of all infected tissue and should be the main priority of surgical intervention. This may entail partial or complete removal of valve leaflets, debridement of valve annuli or aortic wall, removal of subvalvar chordal apparatus for mitral or tricuspid valves, etc. Once all tissue is debrided, reconstruction proceeds. Patch material, in particular autologous pericardium, is used to repair small or moderate defects in valve tissue, VSDs, defects on the free wall of the atria or ventricles, or the aortic root. Some particular scenarios include:

- **Aortic valve endocarditis.** If the infection is confined to a small portion of an aortic valve leaflet, especially in children, the defect may be reconstructed with autologous pericardium. However, it is not uncommon to have significant involvement of the aortic valve or aortic root, precluding an adequate and durable reconstruction. In those cases, aortic valve replacement should be entertained. Aortic homograft valves are favored, although replacement with a bioprosthetic or mechanical prosthesis may be appropriate in older children or adults with no involvement of the aortic root. If the aortic root is partially involved, it may be reconstructed with a patch to allow placement of a prosthesis. Alternatively, the patient may undergo an aortic root replacement with an aortic homograft. A Ross procedure may be a possible alternative although in many cases the long cross-clamp period due to the added debridement may preclude it at this time.
- **Mitral valve endocarditis.** Reconstruction of the mitral valve may be feasible, especially if the process is confined to part of one leaflet. Excised mitral chords may be treated by different techniques such as chordal transfer, artificial chords, or leaflet anchoring to surrounding leaflet tissue, depending on the situation. It is important to assess the integrity of the AV junction. If compromised, the area may need placement of a patch prior to replacing the valve. If needed, the valve is usually replaced with a mechanical prosthesis although placement of a bioprosthesis is also an option.
- **Tricuspid valve endocarditis.** It is extremely rare to have to replace the tricuspid valve, especially in children. Reconstruction may include patch material and other surgical techniques. Some degree of tricuspid regurgitation is usually well tolerated.

Statistics

In a recent 15-year retrospective review conducted at TCH involving 76 cases of IE, 46 (61%) patients required surgical intervention within 6 weeks of diagnosis (Shamszad et al. 2016). Median age at presentation was 8.3 years. The main organisms involved were *S. aureus* (24%), *Streptococcus* (22%), and coagulase-negative *Staphylococcus* (10%). Among surgical patients, median interval to surgery was 3 days. There was 1 perioperative mortality on a patient that had a significant stroke from a previous embolus. Of the 38 patients with native-valve involvement that underwent surgery, 50% had valve repairs and 50% had valve replacements:

- 12 aortic (8 aortic homograft, 3 Ross, 1 bioprosthetic)

- 5 mitral (4 mechanical)
- 2 pulmonary

Suggested Readings

Baddour LM, Wilson WR, Bayer AS, et al. Infective endocarditis in adults: Diagnosis, antimicrobial therapy, and management of complications: A Scientific Statement for Healthcare Professionals from the American Heart Association. Circulation 2015;132:1435-1486.

Li JS, Sexton DJ, Mick N, et al. Proposed modifications to the Duke criteria for the diagnosis of infective endocarditis. Clin Infect Dis 2000;30:633-638.

Mery CM, Guzmán-Pruneda FA, De León LE, et al. Risk factors for development of endocarditis and reintervention in patients undergoing right ventricle to pulmonary artery valved conduit placement. J Thorac Cardiovasc Surg 2016;151:432-439.

Shamszad P, Khan MS, Rossano JW, et al. Early surgical therapy of infective endocarditis in children: a 15-year experience. J Thorac Cardiovasc Surg 2013;146:506-511.

Wilson W, Taubert KA, Gewtiz M, et al. Prevention of infective endocarditis: guidelines from the American Heart Association. Circulation 2007;116:1736-1754.

34 Arrhythmias

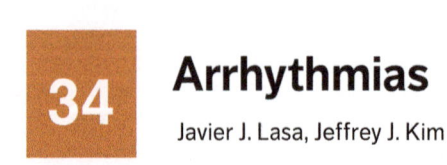

Javier J. Lasa, Jeffrey J. Kim

Arrhythmias are defined as abnormalities of electrical conduction and rhythm of the heart and encompass a broad range of congenital and acquired disease states. Although relatively rare in the general pediatric population, arrhythmias can lead to significant morbidity and mortality, especially when occurring during the postoperative care of children with CHD. Figure 34-1 and Figure 34-2 provide algorithms for the diagnosis of narrow- and wide-complex tachyarrhythmias, respectively.

Sinus-Rhythm Abnormalities

Sinus rhythm occurs when electrical impulses originating in the sinoatrial node (SA node) propagate throughout the atria and coalesce at the center of the heart in the AV node before continuing via the bundle of His and Purkinje fibers to the individual right/left ventricular bundles. These electrical impulses are most commonly translated into an ECG as the P-Q-R-S-T wave forms. The waveforms provide a visual depiction of the SA nodal/atrial impulse (P wave) and subsequent ventricular depolarization (Q-R-S waves) and repolarization (T wave) activity.

Rhythm that occurs in a sinus fashion but is faster than established upper limits of normal for age is labeled *sinus tachycardia*. It often occurs in response to stress or painful stimuli, fever, anemia, hypovolemia, high catecholamine state, or medications. Treatment is directed at the underlying cause. Conversely, slow heart rates below the lower limits of heart rate for age are labeled *sinus bradycardia* and are usually benign and without hemodynamic significance. Sinus bradycardia can be observed during sleep but also occur in conditions of high vagal tone, hypothermia, hypotension, hypoxemia, acidosis, drugs, electrolyte abnormalities, or increased intracranial pressure. Treatment, if needed, is usually focused on addressing the underlying cause. Patients with certain forms of CHD, including heterotaxy syndrome, may be more prone to bradycardia that may indeed be clinically significant.

Sinus node dysfunction (also known as sick-sinus syndrome) may also present with slow heart rates frequently alternating with periods of tachycardia and is most commonly due to secondary causes such as cardiac surgery, infection (myocarditis), trauma, ischemia, or cardioactive drugs rather than a primary arrhythmia. In symptomatic cases, permanent pacemaker implantation may be needed for definitive therapy.

Absent SA node activity may contribute to the development of *junctional rhythm*, a condition characterized by QRS complexes that have an identical morphology to that of sinus rhythm but lack preceding P waves. Pacing the atrium at 10-20 bpm above the junctional rate demonstrates normal AV nodal conduction, restores AV synchrony, and leads to improvement in stroke volume and cardiac output.

Conduction Abnormalities

Abnormal AV conduction occurs when transmission of the normal SA node impulses is delayed or blocked due to an abnormality in the conduction system, specifically of the

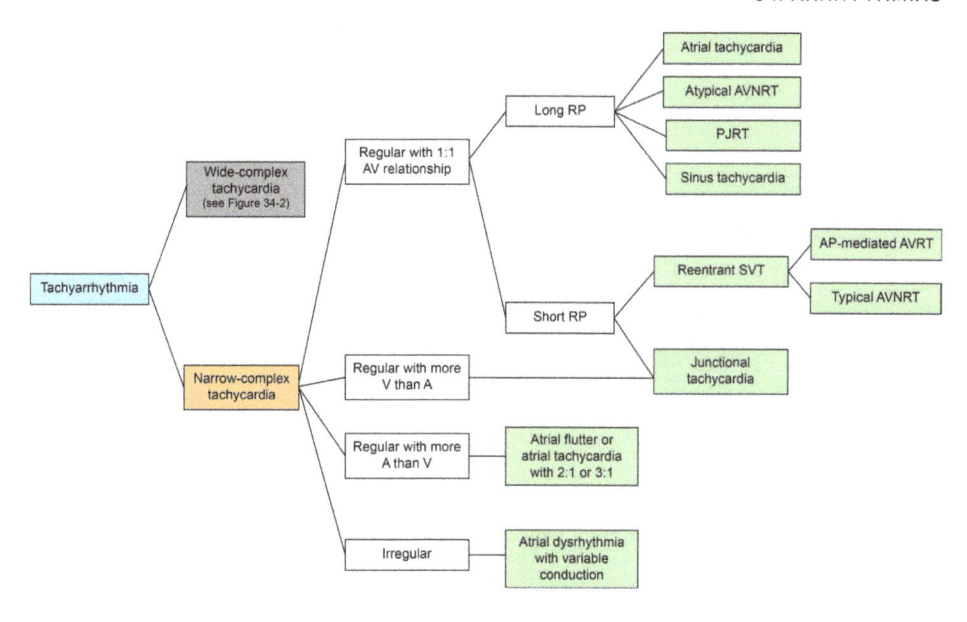

Figure 34-1. Diagnostic algorithm for narrow-complex tachyarrhythmias. PJRT: Permanent junctional reciprocating tachycardia.

AV node or His-Purkinje system. AV conduction deficits are covered in Chapter 75 and only briefly mentioned here.

First-degree AV block results in stable prolongation of the PR interval above the upper limits of normal for age and heart rate and is a result of an abnormal delay in conduction through the AV node. This is typically a benign phenomenon.

Second-degree AV block results from intermittent failure of AV conduction and is categorized into two common forms: Mobitz type I (Wenckebach phenomenon) and Mobitz type II. Type I second-degree AV block occurs at the level of the AV node yielding progressive lengthening of the PR interval until it fails to conduct the atrial impulse to the ventricle. Type II second-degree AV block occurs below the level of the bundle of His and is defined as the sudden loss of AV conduction occurring after normal sinus rhythm (no evidence of PR-interval prolongation). Although less common than type I, type-II second-degree block is a more serious form of AV conduction disorder in which progression to complete heart block with hemodynamic compromise is more likely. Higher grade forms of second-degree AV block occur when two successive P waves fail to be followed by QRS complexes.

Third-degree (complete) AV block is defined as complete interruption of atrial impulse transmission resulting in atrial and ventricular activity that is independent of each other (AV dissociation). Surface ECG morphology will show regular P waves at a rate appropriate for age but with independent QRS complexes occurring at regular and slower rates than the atrial rate (junctional escape). Congenital complete heart block occurs in 1/20,000 live births in association with structural heart disease (e.g.,

PART II. DISEASES

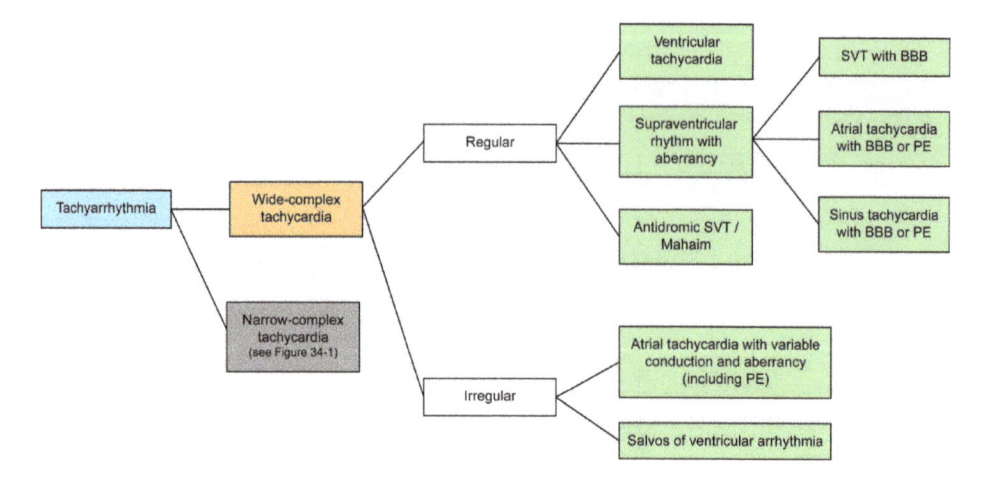

Figure 34-2. Diagnostic algorithm for wide-complex tachyarrhythmias. BBB: Bundle branch block, PE: Preexcitation.

L-transposition of the great vessels, heterotaxy syndrome with polysplenia/left atrial isomerism) or associated with maternal collagen vascular abnormalities (e.g., systemic lupus erythematosus, Sjögren syndrome). Postoperative surgical AV block may occur after some types of cardiac operations. Over 60% of patients usually recover normal conduction within the first 10 postoperative days. Permanent cardiac pacing is indicated for patients without recovery after 7 to 10 days postoperatively.

Supraventricular Arrhythmias

Premature atrial contractions (PAC) are relatively common in infants and small children and represent a benign phenomenon. Each QRS complex is preceded by a P wave that may have a normal axis or suggest an axis directed from outside the SA node.

Supraventricular tachycardia (SVT) represents the most common arrhythmia occurring in the pediatric population and is commonly divided into 2 main categories: reentrant and automatic. Both forms of SVT are characterized by a narrow or baseline QRS-complex morphology and can occur in structurally normal hearts as well as in various forms of CHD. Evaluation includes a 15-lead ECG and a continuous rhythm strip to evaluate onset, termination, and response to medications like adenosine or pacing maneuvers. Figure 34-1 displays a common diagnostic algorithm for classification of narrow-complex tachycardias, including SVT.

Common forms of narrow-complex tachycardias seen in infancy as well as adolescence include *atrioventricular reentrant tachycardia* (AVRT) and *atrioventricular nodal reentrant tachycardia* (AVNRT). AVRT is the most common type of SVT encountered in infancy/childhood and results from electrical signals crossing an accessory pathway of conduction tissue between the atria and ventricles. A cycle of conduction propagating normally down the AV node but returning to the atria via the accessory pathway creates the reentrant circuit which can be terminated with vagal maneuvers, adenosine, or, in cases of poor perfusion and hemodynamic compromise, synchronized cardioversion (0.5-1 Joule/kg). Surface ECG will usually demonstrate P waves immediately after QRS complexes or within the ST segment or T wave (i.e., short RP tachycardia). AVNRT occurs most commonly in adolescents and young adults and is characterized by a similar reentrant circuit that occurs primarily within the AV node. Surface ECG makes discerning P waves difficult as they are often buried within the QRS complex. The management strategy for AVNRT is similar to AVRT.

Narrow complex tachycardias that result from automatic foci of electrical activity (e.g., *ectopic atrial tachycardia* [EAT], *multifocal atrial tachycardia* [MAT]) do not respond to electrical cardioversion and generally require pharmacologic therapies in addition to the avoidance of sympathetic stimulants like fever, pain/agitation, inotropic agents, and the correction of electrolyte imbalances.

Junctional ectopic tachycardia (JET) is a narrow-complex tachycardia that can occur with AV dissociation. Narrow QRS complexes occur at a rate faster than P waves due to an automatic focus of electrical activity within the AV node or junction. This arrhythmia often occurs in the perioperative setting as a result of cardiac manipulation and dissection around the RA. The distinction from accelerated junctional rhythm is based on heart rate (typically greater than 160 or 170 bpm) and hemodynamic status of the patient. When occurring in the postoperative period, JET is usually transient and self-limited, lasting from 24 to 72 hours but can result in hemodynamic instability, significant morbidity, and may contribute to mortality. Management is usually multimodal with focus on minimizing stimulation to the patient, avoidance of hyperthermia, use of antiarrhythmic medications, and temporary atrial pacing to overdrive the junctional rate. The use of ECMO should also be considered as a rescue modality for cases of JET refractory to conventional therapies.

Atrial fibrillation and *atrial flutter* are both less common in the general pediatric population yet are more often encountered in patients with CHD. Both conditions may benefit from the use of adenosine as a diagnostic maneuver to uncover underlying atrial activity (flutter waves vs. irregularly irregular atrial activity). Acute management of atrial fibrillation in the hemodynamically stable patient should focus on ventricular rate control and determination of underlying etiology. Normal sinus rhythm may also be restored with synchronized cardioversion after an appropriate evaluation for intracardiac thrombus. Synchronized cardioversion can also terminate atrial flutter, although atrial overdrive pacing can be utilized successfully as well.

Ventricular Arrhythmias

Premature ventricular contractions (PVC) result in early- and wide-QRS complexes without preceding P waves due to early activation of ventricular myocardium from an ectopic focus. In the patient with a structurally normal heart, PVCs of a single QRS morphology (uniform) without associated symptoms are generally considered benign. PVCs may have more significance if they are multifocal, occur in very high frequency, occur with symptoms of syncope, are accompanied by a family history of sudden death, or are associated with underlying heart disease.

Ventricular tachycardia (VT) is defined as 3 or more PVCs in series at a heart rate

PART II. DISEASES

>120 bpm in adults or more than 20% greater than the preceding sinus rate. The acute onset of VT may be due to hypoxia, acidosis, electrolyte/metabolic derangements, or in the context of depressed myocardial function, poor hemodynamics, prior surgical interventions, myocardial tumors, cardiomyopathies, myocarditis, acute injury (trauma), and primary channelopathies. Polymorphic VT in the form of "torsades de pointes" manifests as both positive and negative oscillations of the QRS complex around an isoelectric baseline. Polymorphic VT can be secondary to drug therapy, myocardial ischemia, neurologic injury, or may occur in long-QT syndrome. Cardioversion of torsades de pointes should be performed in sustained cases, although there is risk of degradation to ventricular fibrillation (VF). Magnesium sulfate should be administered as first line therapy.

Ventricular fibrillation (VF) results from asynchronous ventricular depolarizations that create chaotic and ineffective muscle contractions and loss of cardiac output. Immediate attention to the hemodynamic status of a patient is essential to the care of patients with VT and/or VF. CPR should be instituted in the unstable patient while cardiodefibrillator pads are placed in preparation for cardioversion/defibrillation (2-4 Joules/kg). Pharmacologic therapies including amiodarone and lidocaine may be indicated for the patient with stable VT or as part of the management of pulseless VT/VF as per the Pediatric Advanced Life Support algorithm (AHA guidelines).

Suggested Reading

Valdes SO, Kim JJ, Miller-Hance WC. Arrhythmias: Diagnosis and management. In: Andropoulos DB, Stayer S, Mossad EB, Miller-Hance WC (eds). Anesthesia for Congenital Heart Disease. 3rd ed. John Wiley and Sons; 2015.

35 Inherited Arrhythmia Syndromes

Christina Y. Miyake, Santiago O. Valdes, Jeffrey J. Kim

Inherited primary arrhythmia syndromes include long-QT syndrome, catecholaminergic polymorphic ventricular tachycardia, and Brugada syndrome. These syndromes are most commonly caused by single-gene mutations. Genetic alterations can also result in primary cardiomyopathy disorders that can be associated with arrhythmias. Cardiomyopathies include arrhythmogenic cardiomyopathy, hypertrophic and dilated cardiomyopathy, and LV noncompaction. Genetic results aid in diagnosis, can help guide counseling and in certain diseases, can guide management of patients.

Patients with suspected primary inheritable arrhythmia syndromes or patients with a history of aborted cardiac arrest should undergo thorough evaluation including clinical history, ECG, echocardiogram, and a 3-generational pedigree. Patients with suspected or potential Brugada syndrome should undergo a modified Brugada ECG and ECGs should be obtained during any fever. Workup and genetic testing should be guided by the Electrophysiology Team.

Long-QT Syndrome

This syndrome is a genetic condition most commonly caused by heterozygous mutations in cardiac potassium- (*KCNQ1*, *KCNH2*) or sodium-channel (*SCN5A*) genes. These mutations result in delayed repolarization and risk of a specific form of ventricular tachycardia called torsade de pointes.

Management of patients with known long-QT syndrome or those with marked QT prolongation include:
- Patients should be monitored.
- Avoid all QT-prolonging drugs (refer to crediblemeds.org) particularly in patients with long-QT syndrome.
- In patients with QT prolongation without known long-QT syndrome, the risks and benefits of QT prolonging drugs need to be weighed.
- If a QT-prolonging drug must be administered (e.g., cancer treatment), the ECG and QTc must be followed during initiation of the medication and when the steady-state level of the drug is reached. If the QTc exceeds 480 msec, the drug should be held and cardiology consulted.
- Continue beta-blocker therapy while admitted.
- Maintain electrolytes in the normal range, particularly potassium, calcium, and magnesium. Hypokalemia, hypocalcemia, and hypomagnesemia can exacerbate arrhythmias.
- In case of torsade de pointes, give magnesium 25-50 mg/kg IV, esmolol, and defibrillation if necessary. Avoid any antiarrhythmic that can prolong the QTc such as amiodarone and sotalol.

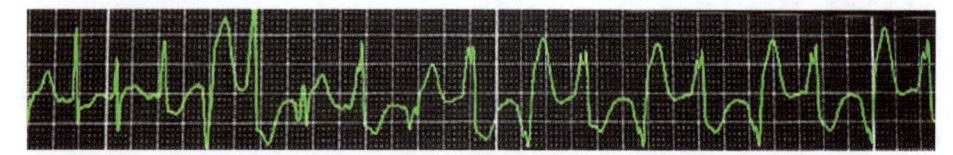

Figure 35-1. Bidirectional ventricular tachycardia seen on patient bedside monitor. This pattern is pathognomonic for CPVT when seen only during adrenergic stimulation.

Catecholaminergic Polymorphic Ventricular Tachycardia (CPVT)

CPVT is most commonly caused by heterozygous mutations in the cardiac ryanodine receptor (*RYR2*) gene although there is a rare form caused by homozygous mutations in *CASQ2*. These genes are responsible for calcium handling in the cardiac cell. Adrenergic stimulation (such as exertion or emotional stress/anxiety) results in abnormal calcium release during diastole, which triggers life-threatening ventricular arrhythmias. Arrhythmias include polymorphic and bidirectional ventricular tachycardia (Figure 35-1) as well as ventricular fibrillation. Atrial arrhythmias are also common. Both supraventricular and ventricular arrhythmias only occur under adrenergic stimulation. In the hospital setting, this may include agitating or causing pain to the child during routine care (e.g., blood draws, peripheral IV placement).

Although CPVT is rare, the mortality rate is the highest of all inherited arrhythmia disorders with a risk of cardiac event occurring in up to 30-50% by the age of 30 years. The most common age at presentation is 8-12 years and thus any child with exertional or emotional syncope should be evaluated for possible CPVT.

Treatment of patients with CPVT include:
- Make efforts to minimize catecholamine surges including painful stimuli during routine care, if possible. Avoid adrenergic inotropes or boluses such as epinephrine, if possible.
- Monitor for ventricular ectopy, couplets, or bidirectional ventricular tachycardia with stimulation (this can be diagnostic if seen in patients in whom the diagnosis is not yet known).
- Treat acute ventricular arrhythmias with esmolol and sedation, if needed. Oral nadolol or flecainide can also be used to prevent arrhythmmias during adrenergic stimulation.

Brugada Syndrome

Brugada syndrome results in ventricular arrhythmias most commonly triggered by sleep, fever, overheating, large meals, or specific medications. The most common age at presentation is 20-40 years and the most common presentation is death during sleep. Children, and even infants, can be affected at an early age. In children, arrhythmias are commonly seen during fever. Male patients are most likely to be affected. The most common genetic mutation is a heterozygous loss of function mutation in the *SCN5A* gene. Treatment of these patients include:

35. INHERITED ARRHYTHMIA SYNDROMES

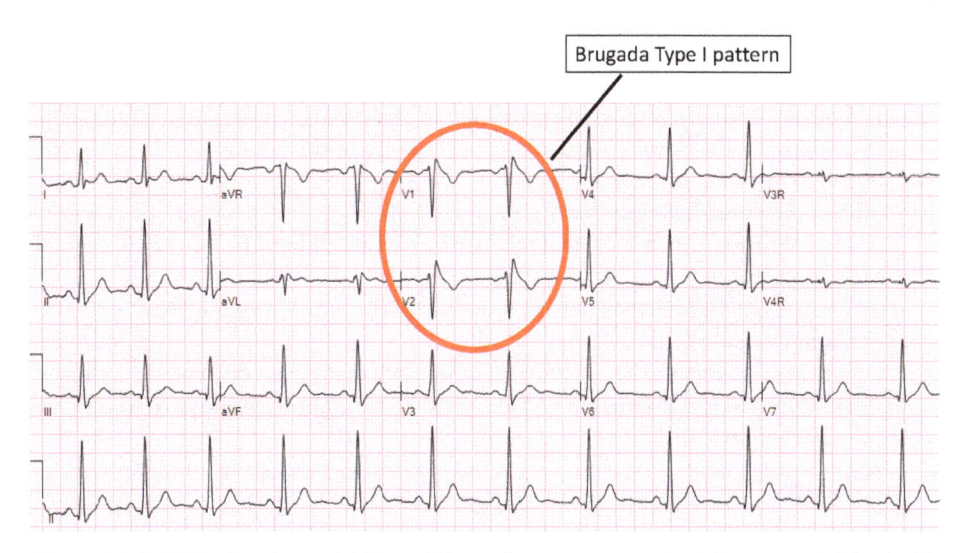

Figure 35-2. ECG of patient with Type-I Brugada pattern seen in right precordial leads (V1 and V2). There is ST elevation with T-wave inversion. This pattern can come and go and, in children, is most commonly brought out during a fever.

- Aggressively treat fever with antipyretics and avoid overheating (such as Bair Hugger™).
- Avoid Brugada-provoking drugs (refer to brugadadrugs.org), including diphenhyrdramine (Benadryl®), fexofenadine (Allegra®), amiodarone, amitriptyline, clomipramine, desipramine, lithium, loxapine, nortriptyline, oxcarbazepine, trifluoperazine, bupivacaine, procaine, propofol, disopyramide, lidocaine, propranolol, verapamil, vernakalant, bupropion, carbamazepine, clothiapine, cyamemazine, dosulepine, doxepine, fluoxetine, fluvoxamine, imipramine, lamotrigine, maprotiline, paroxetine, perphenazine, phenytoin, thioridazine. ketamine, tramadol, demenhydrinate, diphenhydramine, edrophonium, indapamide, and metoclopramide.
- Diagnosis is made by presence of a type-I Brugada pattern on ECG (Figure 35-2). This pattern can come and go and a normal ECG does not rule out disease. A specific modified-Brugada ECG protocol should be performed. ECG obtained during fever can help.
- In case of ventricular tachycardia, treatment options include isoproterenol or esmolol. If recalcitrant, sedation and intubation are recommended.

Workup for Cardiac Arrest

In cases of cardiac arrest, a complete workup should be performed. An ECG should be obtained to look for prolongation of the QTc, Brugada changes, abnormal repolarization pattern (such as inverted T waves in the right precordial leads [V1-V3] in an adolescent), and ischemia. A Brugada protocol ECG should be performed. Because the QTc is often prolonged after an arrest, multiple ECGs are recommended to follow ECG changes over time.

An echocardiogram should be performed to evaluate hypertrophic/dilated cardiomyopathy, LV noncompaction, coronary anomalies, and pulmonary hypertension. The echocardiogram should also include protocols to evaluate the RV for arrhythmogenic cardiomyopathy, which must include measurements of the RV outflow tract in the parasternal long and short axis.

Some additional considerations are:
- A history of drowning in a patient who can swim should warrant investigation of long-QT syndrome.
- A thorough patient history with exact details of the arrest and 3-generation pedigree should be obtained.
- All rhythm strips from the arrest should be reviewed. If an automated external defibrillator (AED) was used, the AED should be brought with the patient and the rhythm strips reviewed.
- An electrophysiology consult is warranted for further evaluation and for potential genetic testing, particularly if a definitive cause is not identified.

36 Kawasaki Disease

S. Kristen Sexson Tejtel, Carolyn A. Altman

While an acute systemic vasculitis, Kawasaki Disease (KD) morbidity and mortality is related to the development of coronary artery aneurysms. Coronary aneurysms can occur in up to 25% of those who are not treated within the first 10 days of illness, so prompt recognition and appropriate therapy are essential.

The definitive etiology of KD is unknown. However, the current prevailing theory is that there is an inciting trigger (possibly a viral or bacterial infection, or exposure to some environmental agent) that provokes an autoimmune response in genetically susceptible individuals. The most common age for children to have KD is between 2 and 8 years, although cases in children as young as 1 month and as old as 18 years have been reported.

Clinical Presentation and Diagnosis

In 2017, the AHA published the updated Scientific Statement on the Diagnosis, Treatment, and Long-Term Management of Kawasaki Disease (McCrindle et al. 2017). This statement provides much of the foundation for the care outlined in this chapter. The diagnosis of KD is based on clinical criteria.

Table 36-1 lists the criteria for diagnosis of complete and incomplete KD. For patients who do not meet the criteria for complete KD, incomplete (sometimes referred to as atypical) KD should be considered. Incomplete KD occurs more frequently in very young infants, or those at the older age of the spectrum.

Signs, Symptoms, and Other Infections

Concurrent viral respiratory infections can occur in complete or incomplete KD and do not exclude a diagnosis of KD. If a patient has exudative pharyngitis or exudative conjunctivitis, however, KD is very unlikely. KD can occur in patients with group-A streptococcal infection. KD should be considered if the patient has some principal features of KD, and fever uncharacteristically persists after treatment with appropriate antibiotic therapy. KD should also be considered in infants or children with prolonged fever and unexplained or culture negative shock, or cervical adenitis unresponsive to antibiotic therapy.

While not considered one of the 5 principal clinical features, marked irritability is a hallmark of the ill KD patient. Many other nonspecific symptoms can occur, including but not limited to abdominal pain, vomiting, diarrhea, jaundice, arthralgias, arthritis, or aseptic meningitis. Hydrops of the gallbladder can be seen as well.

KD Shock Syndrome

KD shock should be suspected in patients requiring fluid boluses or inotropic support and those with hypotension and tachycardia in excess of that expected for the degree of fever, presence of a gallop, or hepatomegaly. Decreased ventricular function will usually be demonstrated on echocardiogram. KD shock patients typically have prolonged clinical and laboratory findings of inflammation. They are more prone to be resistant

Table 36-1. Diagnostic criteria for complete and incomplete KD (McCrindle et al. 2017)

Complete KD

Diagnosis of complete KD is made if ≥5 days of fever (counting the day of fever onset as the first day of fever) and at least 4 of the following principal clinical features:
• Bilateral bulbar nonexudative conjunctivitis
• Rash (maculopapular, diffuse erythroderma, or erythema multiforme-like)
• Oral mucous membrane changes (strawberry tongue, dry, cracked lips, erythema of mouth, lips, pharynx)
• Extremity changes
   - Hand and foot erythema and edema (may be painful)
   - Periungual finger and toe desquamation (occurs in subacute phase, 2-3 weeks after fever onset)
• Cervical lymphadenopathy (>1.5 cm, typically unilateral)
The diagnosis of KD can be made on the 4th day of fever if ≥4 of these features are present, particularly if the patient has redness and swelling of the hands and feet. It is important to note that the principal clinical features, aside from fever, may not and often do not occur simultaneously or continuously and thus may only be elicited by thorough history of observations by a parent, pediatrician, or other care provider.

Incomplete KD

Children with fever for ≥5 days with 2-3 principal clinical features can be diagnosed with incomplete KD on the basis of supportive labs and/or a positive echocardiogram. In infants <6 months of age with fever for ≥7 days and irritability, KD should be considered even the absence of any other clinical features.
• **Supportive laboratory criteria.** Elevated acute-phase reactants (erythrocyte sedimentation rate [ESR] ≥40 mm/hr and C-reactive protein [CRP] ≥3 mg/dl) *and* 3 or more of the following:
   - Anemia for age
   - Platelet count ≥450,000 after the 7th day of fever
   - Hypoalbuminemia of ≥3 g/dL
   - Elevated ALT
   - WBC >15,000 /uL
   - Sterile pyuria: urine with ≥10 WBC/hpf
• **Echocardiographic criteria**
   - Coronary dilation: Z-score of LAD or right coronary artery ≥2.5
   - Coronary artery aneurysm
   - ≥3 other suggestive features
      ▪ Decreased LV function
      ▪ MR
      ▪ Pericardial effusion
      ▪ Z-scores in LAD or right coronary artery ≥2 but <2.5

to intravenous immunoglobulin (IVIG) and exhibit a higher risk for coronary changes. Echocardiography to assess ventricular function in this scenario is important prior to beginning treatment with IVIG to help determine if the rate of infusion should be decreased.

Table 36-2. Recommended labs for workup and follow-up of KD patients

Recommended labs
• Initial labs: CBC with differential, liver panel, C-reactive protein (CRP), erythrocyte sedimentation rate (ESR), D-dimer, basic metabolic panel, and urinalysis. • Repeat inflammatory markers (CRP, D-dimer, CBC) are recommended prior to discharge in uncomplicated cases to ensure expected improvement and to help determine need for additional therapy. Caveats: ESR will be high for 4-6 weeks post-IVIG and should then not be used to assess for improvement. Platelet counts will be expected to rise after the 7th day and through the 14th day of illness. • Repeat labs early and often if the course is complicated or not standard. • Repeat labs ~1 week from discharge may be necessary if labs are abnormal at discharge. • If lab abnormalities persist after 1 week, discuss with Rheumatology.

Management

The management of patients with KD requires a comprehensive and multidisciplinary approach during workup and follow-up of patients. This approach includes a combination of labs, imaging studies, medications, consultations, and follow-up plan.

Table 36-2 lists recommended labs during workup and follow-up of patients with KD. A baseline ECG should be obtained during the acute illness in the hospital. Subsequently, ECGs will be obtained depending on clinical course. For those with severe or complex coronary involvement, ECGs should be routinely obtained as coronary ischemia or infarct in KD can be silent.

The goal of therapy during the acute phase is to reduce inflammation, thus reducing arterial damage and thrombus formation.

Medications in Uncomplicated KD

IVIG (2 g/kg over 10-12 hours) is the first line therapy for KD and should be administered as soon as the diagnosis is made. It can be administered before an echocardiogram is performed if the patient fulfills clinical criteria. However, even with treatment within the first 10 days of fever, 20% will develop coronary artery changes and a smaller number will still develop aneurysms.

Medium-dose (30-50 mg/kg) or high-dose (80-100 mg/kg) *aspirin* is given until the patient is afebrile for 48 hours. Data does not favor either high or medium dosing for prevention of aneurysms. Subsequently, aspirin dosage is changed to low dose for antiplatelet effect (3-5 mg/kg/day once a day). Low-dose aspirin is continued for 6-8 weeks in uncomplicated cases with an echocardiogram at the end of the subacute phase. Aspirin is continued on if there is significant coronary artery dilation or aneurysms.

Medications in Complicated KD

Clopidogrel (Plavix®) may be considered as an adjunctive antiplatelet agent if platelet count exceeds 1,000,000 /mcL, if there is coronary dilation of ≥6 but <8 mm, if complex coronary artery disease at particularly high risk of stasis and thrombosis, if there is nonocclusive coronary thrombus, or if the individual is an aspirin nonresponder.

Anticoagulation is initiated in the presence of giant aneurysms (≥8 mm or ≥10 Z-scores). *Enoxaparin* (Lovenox®) is the agent of choice to ensure the most stable and consistent levels of anticoagulation, as there is some evidence to suggest that there is improved coronary remodeling with enoxaparin compared to warfarin. It is important to maintain therapeutic anti-factor Xa levels of 0.8-1.0 IU/mL.

After the second year of illness, patients requiring long-term anticoagulation (i.e., if persistent giant aneurysms or history of thrombosis) will be transitioned to *warfarin*, with a target INR of 2-3.

Additional anti-inflammatory agents (e.g., methylprednisolone, infliximab, etanercept, anakinra, and cyclosporine) will be considered by the Rheumatology service if:
- Recurrent or persistent fevers 36 hours after IVIG completed (a second round of IVIG may also be employed in this situation)
- Ongoing or uptrending markers of inflammation or persistent signs of clinical illness (the primary clinical features or irritability)
- High-risk for development of severe coronary artery disease
- Significant coronary dilation or aneurysms on initial echocardiogram (Z score >4 or size >6 mm)

Statins are considered for use in KD patients >6 years (and younger ages currently under investigation) with severe coronary disease due to their pleotropic (non-lipid lowering) anti-inflammatory properties and positive effects on arterial endothelial function.

Beta-blockers may be employed in those with coronary stenosis, ischemia, or infarction.

Tissue plasminogen activator (tPA) could be considered in consultation with hematology adult cardiology, the cardiac catheterization team, and the ICU in the presence of total or near total coronary artery occlusion, or evidence of significant ischemia (elevated troponin, ST segment changes, segmental function changes).

Echocardiographic Recommendations

Echocardiography provides essential diagnostic information and its findings will often guide therapy in KD patients (Figure 36-1). Multiple views are important to assess the coronaries thoroughly for evolution of dilation or aneurysms, or presence of thrombus. Sedation should be considered in these irritable infants and toddlers, to obtain the high-quality and complete studies necessary. The following are recommended guidelines during diagnosis and management of these patients:
- An initial echocardiogram should be performed within 24 hours of diagnosis. If the patient meets clinical KD criteria, there is no need to delay treatment while waiting for the echocardiogram.
- If the patient responds to IVIG:
  - Schedule the second echocardiogram with a cardiology clinic visit for 14 days after the onset of fever (this marks the beginning of the subacute phase).
  - Schedule the third echocardiogram with a cardiology clinic visit within 6-8 weeks from the onset of fever (this marks the end of the subacute phase and the beginning of the convalescent phase).
- If the patient does not respond to IVIG and requires additional therapy, the patient will require a subsequent echocardiogram within a few days and prior to discharge.
- If the patient has significant coronary abnormalities including aneurysms or dilation >4 Z-scores:

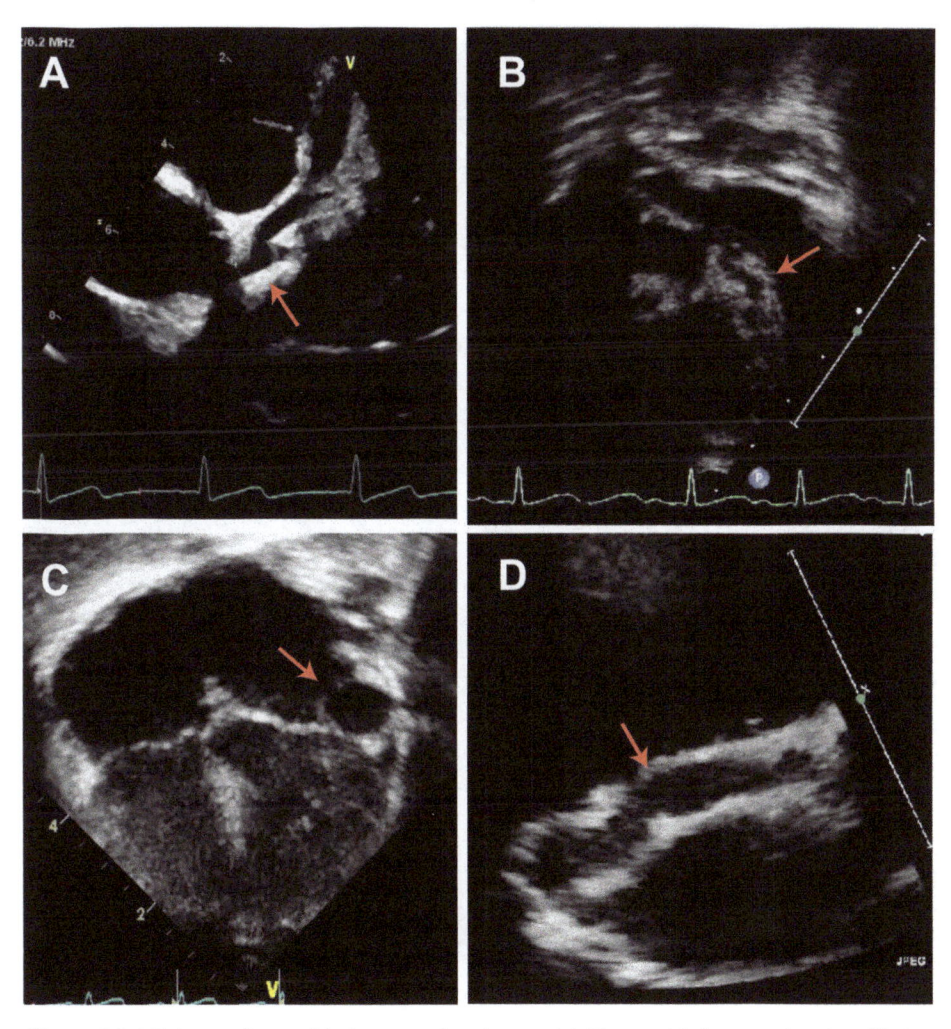

Figure 36-1. Echocardiographic images of patients with Kawasaki disease showing dilation of the proximal left anterior descending artery (A, arrow), mid left anterior descending artery (B, arrow), circumflex artery (C, arrow), and right coronary artery (D, arrow).

- While coronaries may be rapidly expanding, repeat echocardiogram every 2-4 days as guided by Cardiology consult until evidence for coronary artery stabilization and downtrending evidence of inflammation, as well as improvement or resolution of irritability and principal clinical features.
- For those with giant aneurysms, obtain twice weekly echocardiograms as surveillance for thrombus until coronary size is stabilized. Subsequently, these patients require weekly echocardiographic surveillance for at least 1 month, then biweekly for at least another month, monthly for up to 3 months, then at

PART II. DISEASES

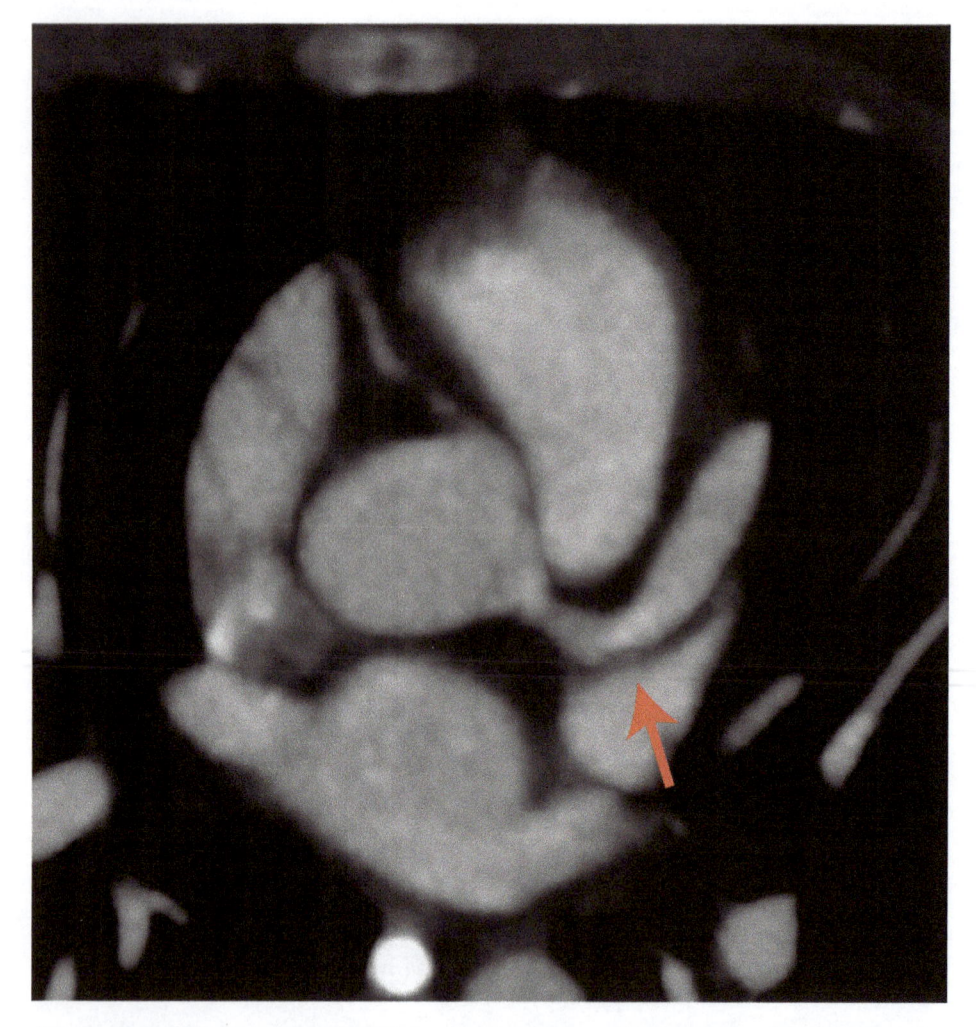

Figure 36-2. CTA of a patient with KD showing significant proximal dilation of the left coronary artery (arrow).

least every 3 months throughout the first year. Color Doppler is essential in the assessment of flow in the coronaries in these patients.

Additional Studies
CTA provides valuable information about the entire coronary distribution (Figure 36-2). Initial CTA is considered in patients with significant proximal coronary involvement. The CTA may also be expanded to include investigation of chest, abdomen, and pelvis to assess for other vascular involvement. Subsequent CTAs are obtained under the guidance of the cardiologist for those with severe or complex coronary artery involvement to assess for changes in coronary size or evolution of coronary stenosis or thrombosis. *Cardiac MRI* is used to assess for perfusion imaging and myocardial scarring in patients

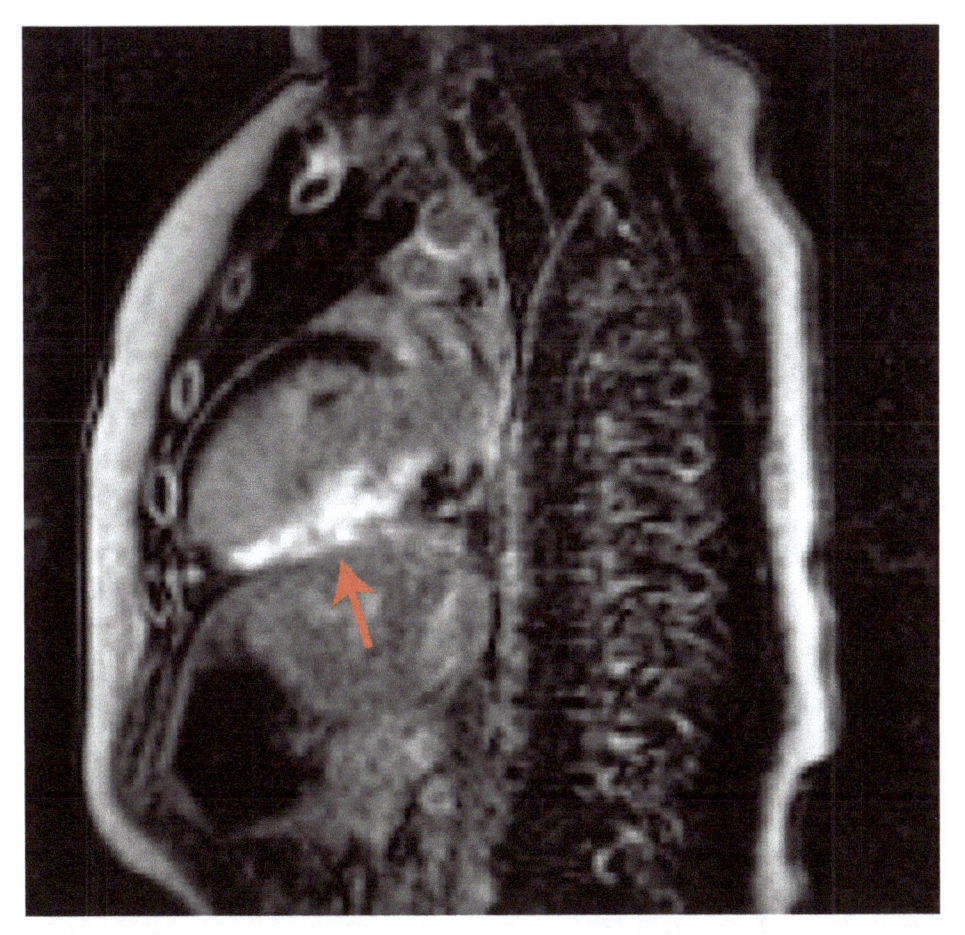

Figure 36-3. Cardiac MRI with late Gadolinium enhancement on a patient with KD showing a diffuse inferior LV infarct (arrow).

being followed with persistent or history of previous significant dilation or aneurysms. Pharmacologic stress MRI may be used to assess for inducible myocardial ischemia (Figure 36-3).

Once a child is old enough to cooperate, *nuclear or echocardiographic stress tests* can be added as additional methods of assessing at-risk myocardium or scarring. These have the benefit of being "real exercise" and thus demonstrating a more physiologic response. The need for *invasive angiography* (Figure 36-4) is guided by symptoms suggestive of ischemia or the findings of ischemia or significant coronary stenosis on CTA, MRI, or other stress tests. Cath is still better than any other imaging test to assess collateral supply. Assessment of functional flow reserve (FFR) can help determine hemodynamic significance of coronary stenoses.

Hospital Consults

Cardiology should be consulted in the following scenarios:

PART II. DISEASES

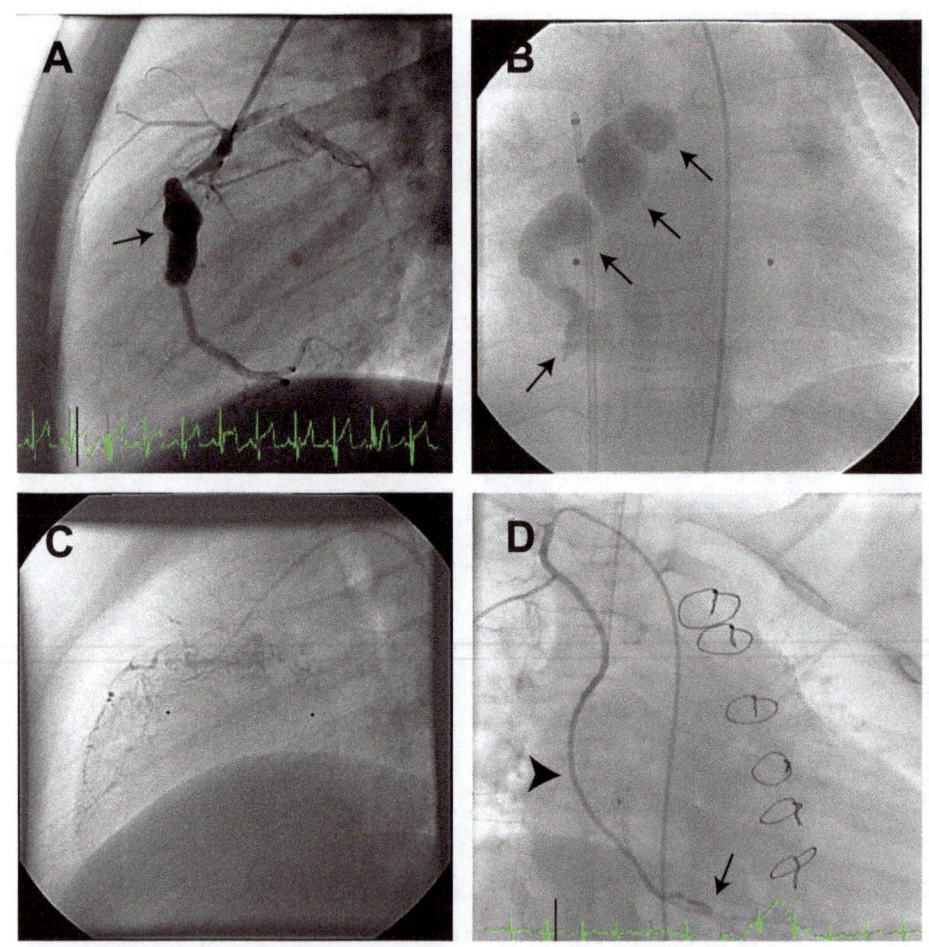

Figure 36-4. Cardiac catheterization images in patients with KD. A) Patient with a large aneurysm of the right coronary artery (arrow). B) Patient with complex aneurysms of the right coronary artery (arrows). C) Patient with occluded right coronary artery and multiple collateral vessels around the area of obstruction. D) Patent right internal mammary coronary bypass graft (arrowhead) providing supply to the distal right coronary circulation (arrow).

- All children with KD or suspicion of KD <1 year of age
- Abnormalities noted on initial or subsequent echocardiograms (including coronary artery dilation or aneurysm, thrombus, ventricular dysfunction or change in function, pericardial effusion, valvulitis)
- Concern regarding echocardiographic read
- Prolonged fever (≥10 days on presentation)
- Atypical clinical course (e.g., recurrence or persistence of fever, repeat dose of IVIG, use of adjunctive anti-inflammatory therapy)
- Help with diagnosis or treatment questions including if enoxaparin or clopidogrel is needed

Table 36-3. Important family counseling tips for patients with KD

Family counseling tips
• Coronary artery disease can worsen over the first 8 weeks of illness – a normal first echocardiogram does not ensure normal coronaries throughout the course of the disease.
• Children CAN get KD again, usually in the first 2 years after initial diagnosis.
• Siblings are at a slightly increased risk of getting KD as are children of parents who have had KD.
• Follow-up with Cardiology is at least childhood-long but infrequent if the coronary arteries are normal throughout.
• Signs and symptoms of KD typically do not occur simultaneously. Therefore, patients are frequently seen by healthcare providers several times prior to obtaining the diagnosis.
• There is a slight increase in risk of autoimmune/inflammatory disease in adults who have had KD.

- KD shock syndrome

Other consulting services may include Rheumatology (for infants <6 months of age, an atypical clinical course, prolonged fever on presentation, KD shock syndrome, or significant coronary abnormalities), Hematology (to help with anticoagulation), and Infectious Disease.

Follow-Up

All patients are seen in the Cardiology clinic within 1-2 weeks after hospital discharge (depending upon clinical course and coronary involvement), 6-8 weeks after initial fevers, and then at least at 1 year from onset of illness. KD patients with history of persistent or regressed aneurysms require continued follow-up indefinitely. Table 36-3 lists some important family counseling tips.

It is important to track the largest diameters of coronary dilation or aneurysm and corresponding Z-scores, as these have important implications for long-term outcomes. Patients with KD and moderate or larger aneurysms/dilation are at risk for a continued vasculopathy ongoing for years. This can lead to coronary stenosis, thrombosis, ischemia, infarct, ventricular dysfunction, arrhythmias, and need for eventual intervention.

Long-term prognosis for those who never develop aneurysms or significant dilation, and for those with aneurysms/dilation that have regressed significantly or resolved, is generally excellent.

In all cases, providers must engage in regular counseling on healthy lifestyle, including maintaining a healthy weight, normal BP, a healthy diet, and normal cholesterol levels to avoid other risk factors for coronary artery disease. Avoidance of tobacco product use and participation in regular active play or exercise are also essential.

Intervention is generally restricted to those with documented ischemia or at-risk myocardium by FFR or stress imaging, or those with coronary stenoses and concerning symptoms for ischemia. Coronary bypass grafting with an internal mammary artery can provide long-term benefit in children as young as 2 years of age. However, this depends upon having an adequate size distal target for the bypass anastomosis. Catheter based intervention, including ballooning or stenting of narrowings, may rarely be considered when vessels are not amenable to bypass or other intervention in the post-KD setting. However, need for frequent reintervention should be expected. KD patients may also develop collateral flow around or through thrombosed vessels and significantly contribute to myocardial perfusion.

Suggested Readings

Giglia TM, Massicotte MP, Tweddell JS, et al. Prevention and treatment of thrombosis in pediastric and congenital heart disease: A scientific statement from the AHA. Circulation 2013;128:2622-2703.

Manlihot C, Brnadao LR, Somji Z, et al. Long-term anticoagulation in Kawasaki disease: initial use of low molecular weight heparin is a viable option for patients with severe coronary artery abnormalities. Pediatr Cardiol 2010;31:834-842.

McCrindle BW, Rowley AH, Newburger JW, et al. Diagnosis, Treatment, and Long-Term Management of Kawasaki Disease: A Scientific Statement for Health Professionals From the American Heart Association. Circulation. 2017;135:e927-e999.

37 Pericarditis

Alan F. Riley, Aimee Liou

The pericardium provides a physical barrier for neoplastic or infectious processes, limits acute myocardial distension, and likely aides diastolic coupling of the ventricles. Normally lubricated with a small amount of lymphatic fluid, the pericardial space includes the cardiac mass and extends to enclose the proximal great vessels (ascending aorta to transverse aortic arch and PAs just beyond the bifurcation), the SVC proximal to the azygous vein, the proximal aspect of the IVC, and the proximal pulmonary veins. The pericardium is susceptible to infectious and autoimmune-mediated inflammation from a wide variety of etiologies and there can also be associated myocardial irritation and/or inflammation. Pericardial inflammation can result in fluid accumulating in the pericardial space, resulting in a pericardial effusion.

Accumulation of pericardial fluid can increase the pressure within the pericardial sac, which is insignificant in normal conditions. The pericardial sac can slowly distend over prolonged periods of time to accommodate chronic fluid buildup, but with acute accumulation, the pericardial sac may act as a noncompliant structure resulting in rapid rise of the pericardial pressures. In the early stages, rising pericardial pressure can intermittently exceed intracardiac pressures during cardiac-chamber pressure nadirs of the cardiac cycle, resulting in transient chamber collapse. In true tamponade, elevated pericardial pressures ultimately overcome and equalize all intracardiac chamber pressures, precipitating cardiovascular collapse.

Clinical Presentation

Pericarditis typically presents with insidious onset of substernal chest pain, which can radiate to the left upper back. Classically, the pain is worsened by lying flat and can be alleviated with elevation in bed or leaning forward. Fever and sinus tachycardia are common on presentation; fever severity and patterns are often related to etiology (see below) and can aid in differential diagnosis for the underlying process. A friction rub can be present on physical examination and distant heart sounds should raise suspicion for pericardial effusion.

Diagnosis

- **ECG.** Diffuse ST-segment elevations with associated PR depressions are often seen. Typically, the ST-segment changes are not segmental, which, if present, should raise concern for coronary artery disease, especially if they follow a coronary distribution pattern and there is an underlying risk factor for early coronary artery disease.
- **Labs.** Cardiac enzymes can be mildly elevated due to direct irritation or they can be markedly elevated if there is associated myocarditis.
- **CXR.** Cardiomegaly may or may not be present depending if there is associated pericardial effusion.
- **Echocardiography.** Echocardiography can identify an associated pericardial

effusion, but assessment for pericardial inflammation or "echo-brightness" is unreliable.

Pericardial Effusion and Tamponade

Depending on the etiology, pericarditis can be associated with a pericardial effusion, which may or may not be hemodynamically significant. Patients may present with tachycardia and dyspnea in cases of tamponade or impending tamponade, but an abnormal CXR with enlargement of the cardiac silhouette may be the first concerning clinical sign.

Even though tamponade is a clinical diagnosis, risk stratification for tamponade or impending hemodynamic compromise can be aided with careful transthoracic 2D and Doppler imaging. One should evaluate for cardiac chamber collapse during specific periods of the cardiac cycle (i.e., RA collapse during ventricular systole and/or RV collapse during ventricular diastole). Doppler imaging can identify excessive respiratory variability of cardiac stroke volume, which can be seen in early tamponade. The most consistently available flow pattern for interrogation of this phenomenon is the mitral valve inflow velocity. A >30% inspiratory decrease of mitral valve A-wave inflow velocity is suggestive of impaired LV filling and early tamponade. Excessive variability of the aortic valve outflow velocity (>10% inspiratory decrease) and tricuspid valve inflow (>50-70% inspiratory increase) can also be used to support the diagnosis. Importantly, however, diagnosis of early tamponade must be made at the bedside based upon clinical factors including history, heart rate trends, respiratory status, BP measurements (preferably via an arterial line), and physical examination. Unexplained tachycardia is usually one of the most sensitive clinical signs of impending tamponade physiology. However, caution should be employed using this sign in isolation, particularly when pathologic sinus node dysfunction could be present, either intrinsic or medication-induced.

Differential Diagnosis

Identification of etiology is important to help determine medical and interventional management strategies. *Idiopathic* pericarditis (and associated pericardial effusion) is believed to be the most common etiology in the developed world with a presumed viral cause and, generally, a benign self-limiting course. Clinical history of low-grade fever, nontoxic appearance, and a benign course resolving over several days are supportive of an idiopathic or virally mediated etiology; preceding or concurrent respiratory or GI illness may also be present. If idiopathic or virally mediated pericarditis is clinically suspected, only limited diagnostic evaluation is typically needed beyond basic labs (i.e., CBC, electrolytes, renal function, and inflammatory markers). Echocardiography should be obtained to assess for associated pericardial effusion.

High fevers, markedly elevated WBC, and/or toxic presentation should raise suspicions for other specific etiologies, such as *bacterial pericarditis, autoimmune disorder* or *associated malignancy.* Diagnostic evaluation for systemic processes should be broadened in these situations and be based on clinical history and physical exam findings.

Bacterial pericarditis is secondary to either direct extension of thoracic and/or pulmonary infections or due to bacteremia. It is often associated with septic shock.

A bacterial etiology for pericarditis should be considered in the setting of high fevers, ill presentation, or markedly elevated WBC. *S. aureus* is the most common etiology.

Prolonged or recurrent episodes of pericarditis should prompt evaluation for systemic autoimmune disease. Pericardial fluid sampling for diagnostic purposes, in the absence of other indications, may be helpful in persistent or recurrent cases, but is often unrevealing. A history of malignancy should also prompt pericardial fluid sampling to rule out malignant pericarditis.

Delayed presentation of pericarditis and/or pericardial effusion following recent pericardial injury, such as cardiac surgery, lead placement, or chest wall trauma, should raise clinical suspicion for *postcardiotomy syndrome*.

Treatment

Management of pericarditis is largely dictated by underlying mechanism and treatment of systemic autoimmune or infectious disease, if present. For most cases of presumed viral or idiopathic pericarditis, nonsteroidal anti-inflammatory drugs (NSAIDs), and possibly colchicine, help decrease the intensity and duration of symptoms. Systemic steroids for the initial bout of idiopathic pericarditis should be avoided as they may be associated with increased risk of recurrence. Management of recurrent pericarditis can be challenging and rheumatology consultation can be beneficial. Reevaluation for an identifiable underlying etiology should also be performed. Again, steroids should be avoided as best possible during initial recurrences, but they may be eventually required for symptom control in recalcitrant cases. Newer immunomodulators, such as Anakinra (Interleukin-1 receptor antagonist), have shown possible utility in early studies treating recurrent idiopathic pericarditis or cases which are steroid resistant. Associated pericardial effusions may resolve with appropriate medical therapy but may persist despite it. Indications to intervene procedurally, via percutaneous drainage with or without drain placement, or via surgical approach, include clinical tamponade and the need to obtain a sample of the effusion for diagnostic purposes.

Intubation and positive pressure ventilation are generally to be avoided in the setting of clinical tamponade, as the resultant increase in intrathoracic pressure can further hinder cardiac filling and thus precipitate cardiovascular collapse. Aggressive diuresis is likewise to be avoided in the setting of tamponade. Administration of intravenous fluid may be necessary in order to ensure adequate preload.

Antibiotics are the mainstay of treatment for bacterial pericarditis. Infectious disease consultation can help narrow antibiotic treatment, which is typically prolonged over several weeks. Bacterial pericarditis is often associated with hemodynamically active pericardial effusion or tamponade prompting intervention. However, all pericardial effusions should be drained if bacterial etiology is confirmed or strongly suspected in order to reduce the long-term risks of constrictive pericarditis. Purulent pericardial fluid can often occlude minimally invasive tubing and surgical drainage may be needed.

Constrictive Pericarditis

Constrictive pericarditis is a delayed serious complication of pericarditis, usually from an infectious etiology. Globally, tuberculosis is most often associated with constrictive pericarditis, but any infectious, usually bacterial, etiology can result in the pericardial thickening and scarring which leads to the development of constrictive physiology. Primarily, diastole is affected as the stiff pericardium impairs cardiac filling, but intrinsic myocardial diastolic and systolic function remain intact. Patients can present with exercise intolerance initially and then progress to signs of right-heart failure with hepatosplenomegaly, ascites, and protein-losing enteropathy.

Constrictive pericarditis can be detected by TTE, which can show marked respiratory variation of mitral and tricuspid inflow in the absence of a pericardial effusion. Additionally, the presence of septal bounce where the interventricular septum quickly shifts leftward with diastolic RV filling, usually during inspiration, should raise clinical suspicion for constrictive pericardial physiology when it accompanies the typical clinical scenario. Again, ventricular systolic and diastolic echocardiographic parameters are usually normal. CT scan or MRI can reveal pericardial thickening or calcifications. Cardiac catheterization typically shows near-equalization of atrial pressures and the ventricular end-diastolic pressures. This near-equalization should persist with a fluid challenge. The presence of constrictive pericardial physiology, when associated with symptoms, should prompt surgical pericardial stripping, as it can be an effective treatment.

III. Special Considerations

38 Aortopulmonary Shunts and Ductal Stents

Alexia B. Santos, Athar M. Qureshi, Carlos M. Mery, Lara S. Shekerdemian

Aortopulmonary shunts and PDA stents are important tools for the palliation of patients with CHD. They are mainly used to augment or maintain a stable source of pulmonary blood flow as part of the palliation strategy in patients with single-ventricle physiology or to postpone a definitive biventricular repair in patients with comorbidities or those in which further somatic growth would allow for a better repair. They can also be used to promote growth of the branch PAs in some patients by augmenting flow (e.g., patients with ductal-origin of the PA or those with pulmonary atresia, VSD, and major aortopulmonary collaterals). Additionally, PDA stents are selectively used as part of a hybrid palliation in patients with hypoplastic left heart syndrome.

The selection between PDA stents and different types of aortopulmonary shunts depends on the particular clinical situation of the patient and is beyond the scope of this chapter.

Aortopulmonary Shunts

Since the original description of the classic shunt by Blalock and Taussig, multiple different types shunts between the systemic and pulmonary circulations have been devised. Some of these shunts include:

- **Classic Blalock-Taussig-Thomas shunt (BTTS).** The subclavian artery is transected and then sutured directly into the PA to increase pulmonary blood flow. This shunt is rarely used currently but may be useful in patients in which growth of the subclavian artery (and the shunt) is necessary (e.g., patients with no plans for future palliation). BP measurement on an extremity that has undergone a classic BTTS will obviously be inaccurate.
- **Modified Blalock-Taussig-Thomas shunt (mBTTS).** See below.
- **Mee shunt (or Melbourne shunt).** Used for patients with pulmonary atresia, VSD, and major aortopulmonary collaterals with diminutive PAs. The main PA is disconnected from the heart and anastomosed on and end-to-side fashion to the ascending aorta in order to promote growth of the branch PAs and allow for future reconstruction. This procedure can be performed through a median sternotomy or a left thoracotomy.
- **Waterston-Cooley shunt.** Anastomosis between the ascending aorta and the right PA. Rarely used currently.
- **Potts shunt.** Anastomosis between the descending aorta and the left PA. Rarely used but has been recently applied to patients with refractory pulmonary hypertension to decompress the pulmonary circulation.

The shunt that is most commonly used currently is the mBTTS. This shunt involves placing a Gore-Tex® tube from the innominate or subclavian artery to one of the branch PAs. The amount of flow through an mBTTS is critical since it determines the degree of overcirculation or cyanosis that the patient will experience. This flow is a complex interplay of multiple factors including the size and length of the shunt, the location

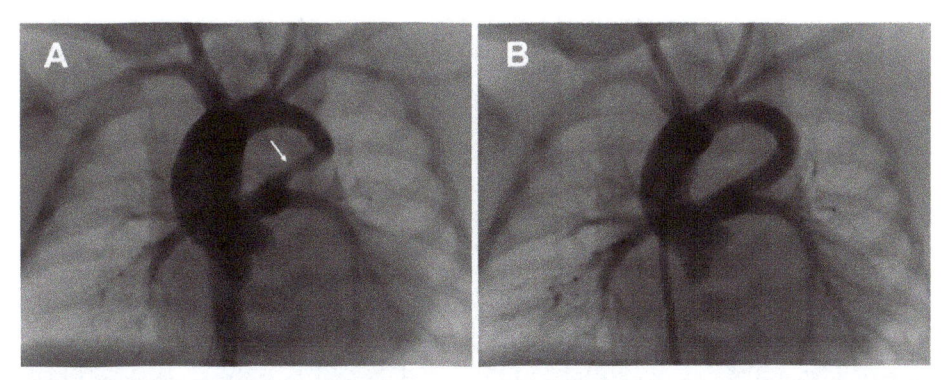

Figure 38-1. Angiogram in a neonate with tetralogy of Fallot, right aortic arch, and cyanosis. A) A PDA can be seen arising from the left innominate artery with constriction (arrow). B) After stent placement, a widely patent PDA is seen.

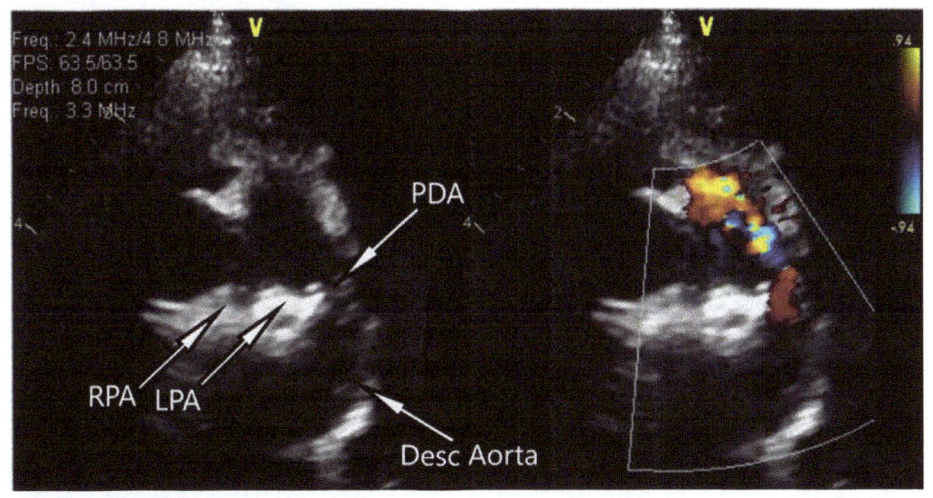

Figure 38-2. High-parasternal color-compare short-axis echocardiographic view ("3-finger view") demonstrating a small PDA.

of takeoff from the systemic circulation, and the difference between systemic and pulmonary vascular resistances.

An mBTTS can be performed either through a median sternotomy or a posterolateral thoracotomy. A clear understanding of the aortic arch anatomy (i.e., arch sidedness, brachiocephalic branching pattern, PDA sidedness) and PA anatomy is critical to plan the operation. On patients with usual anatomy, we have favored performing the procedure via a right posterolateral thoracotomy. Using this technique, the shunt is placed into the distal right subclavian artery (lateral to the recurrent laryngeal nerve), which serves as the restrictor to flow. This allows placement of a larger shunt (usually a 4 mm Gore-Tex® graft in a newborn) that will last longer into infancy as the subclavian artery slowly increases in size. In addition, it decreases the likelihood of overcirculation by

PART III. SPECIAL CONSIDERATIONS

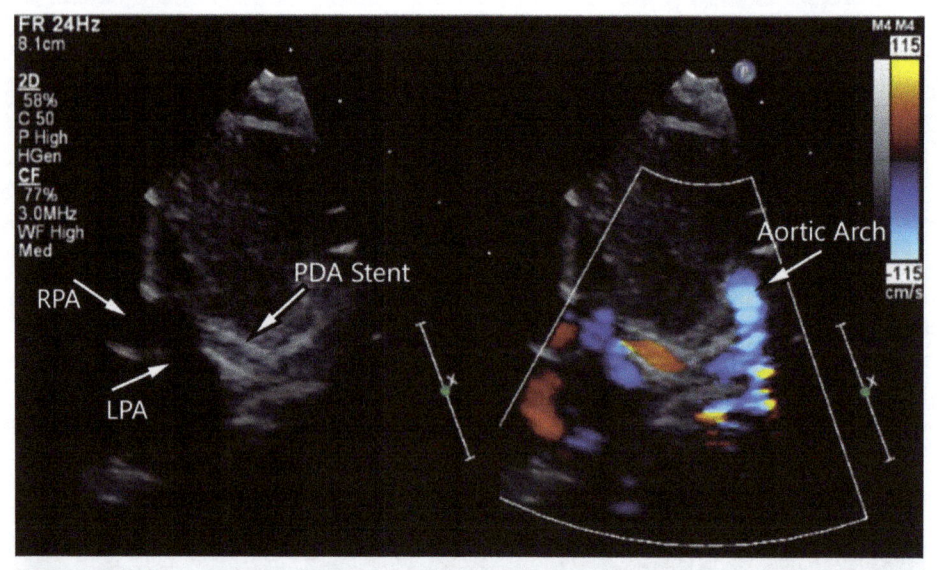

Figure 38-3. Echocardiographic image with color-compare showing a patent PDA stent.

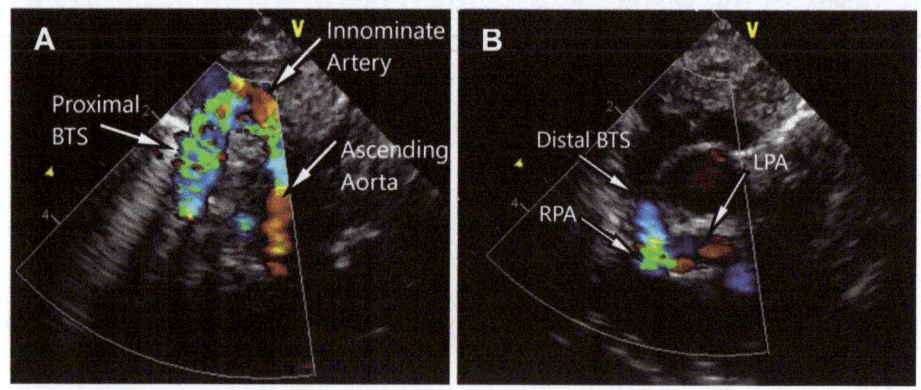

Figure 38-4. Echocardiographic suprasternal notch view showing the proximal (A) and distal (B) ends of a patent mBTTS.

allowing the subclavian artery to modulate the flow. The sidedness of the thoracotomy (right or left) is mainly determined by the location of the PDA (right thoracotomy for a left-sided PDA and left thoracotomy for a right-sided PDA) in order to allow the PDA to provide blood supply to the contralateral lung during the procedure. The PDA is then allowed to close spontaneously after the procedure.

In patients with unusual anatomy or those requiring other procedures, the shunt is created via a median sternotomy. Even when performed through a sternotomy, every attempt is made to place the shunt as far distal into the subclavian artery as possible in order to modulate flow. When performing the procedure via a median sternotomy, a 3.5 mm Gore-Tex® graft is usually used.

Table 38-1. Clinical postoperative scenarios and recommended interventions.

Clinical Scenario	Possible Etiology	Interventions
High SaO$_2$ (>95%) and early markers of low systemic output (falling NIRS, metabolic acidosis, rising lactate)	Excessive pulmonary blood flow with or without systemic vasoconstriction	Check ABG, avoid alkalosis, reduced FiO$_2$ if possible, consider increasing sedation to overcome intrinsic tachypnea. If hypertensive (or if systemic BP allows) consider short-acting systemic vasodilator. Optimize hemoglobin.
As (1) with additional markers of organ injury (e.g., elevation of creatinine, oliguria, liver dysfunction, irritability)	Excessive pulmonary blood flow with significant systemic "steal"	In addition to interventions in (1), provide supportive therapy for organ dysfunction, consider neuromuscular blockade. Discuss with cardiology and cardiac surgical team the need for additional interventions to limit pulmonary blood flow, including duct ligation if PDA still present, or potentially downsize the shunt.
Diastolic hypotension with or without signs of ischemia on ECG	Excessive pulmonary blood flow with significant coronary "steal"	This requires a careful balance between managing systemic perfusion without further compromising diastolic pressure. Interventions include optimizing ventilation, infusion of colloid, and addition of a low-dose vasopressin or norepinephrine infusion.
Differential flow apparent on CXR	Normal postoperative findings (plethoric shunted side) *or* obstructed flow to the non-shunted (oligemic) lung	Optimize ventilation. Discuss with cardiology and cardiac surgery. Requires further evaluation with echocardiogram / CTA / catheterization.
Desaturation and arterial hypoxemia without any focal lung pathology to explain it	Pulmonary cause or shunt malfunction (obstruction or occlusion)	Immediate CXR. In the absence of a respiratory etiology, this suggests *shunt malfunction* until proven otherwise. Oligemic lung fields or quiet or even absent shunt murmur will support this, but absence of these does not exclude shunt malfunction. After optimizing ventilation, there should be an immediate discussion with cardiac surgery and cardiology. Urgent echocardiography should be ordered and depending on the findings, further imaging including CTA or cardiac catheterization may be required. Depending upon the clinical condition of the patient, immediate surgical assistance at the bedside should be considered with readiness to provide urgent ECMO support.

285

PDA Stents

Percutaneous stent implantation can be performed to maintain ductal patency in patients with ductal-dependent pulmonary blood flow. Details of the ductal anatomy are vital to obtain prior to the procedure. Using TTE, the origin and insertion of the ductus, in addition to PA anatomy, should be ascertained. If not possible with TTE, further imaging with a cardiac CT scan may be necessary.

As these infants are maintained on PGE infusion, the size of the PDA is frequently too large to allow placement of an appropriately sized stent (i.e., a stent size that would not result in significant pulmonary overcirculation). PGE is usually stopped the day before the procedure (allowing for a constriction to occur with a safe level of desaturation) to provide an estimate of how long PGE will eventually need to be stopped before the cardiac catheterization procedure. The exceptions to this protocol are patients with ductal-origin of a PA who may not exhibit a change in oxygen saturation if PGE is stopped (the other PA is usually in continuity with the main PA). In this instance, ductal constriction can be gauged by TTE.

The cardiac catheterization procedure is performed under general anesthesia. Based on the origin of the ductus (i.e., from the descending aorta, underside of the aortic arch, innominate artery, subclavian artery, or ascending aorta), an access site is chosen that will result in the straightest trajectory. This may be from a percutaneous femoral artery, carotid artery, axillary artery, umbilical artery, or transvenous route. Patients are heparinized during the procedure to maintain activated clotting times of >250 seconds.

After the stenting procedure (Figure 38-1), patients are started on aspirin and in some instances, heparin therapy is administered until aspirin can be given. In addition to looking for signs of ductal stent patency on physical examination, it is important to interrogate the stented ductus in detail by TTE. Any patient with lower saturations than normal for a given physiology or signs of stent narrowing by echocardiography warrants prompt referral, and immediate catheter/surgical intervention may be indicated.

Imaging

A PDA usually courses from the undersurface of the aortic arch to the main PA. The best and more reliable echocardiographic view is a modified high-parasternal short-axis view with both branch PAs and the descending aorta in the same image ("3-finger view") (Figure 38-2). This view provides the best view of the entire length of the ductus arteriosus including its aortic and pulmonary sides, as well as the direction of blood flow. It is also a reliable view to use in order to "rule out" the presence of a PDA.

If the ideal ductal view cannot be obtained due to poor echocardiographic windows or to unsual anatomy (such as a right aortic arch), one can use a combination of an aortic arch view from the suprasternal notch (with the ascending aorta and the aortic isthmus present) and a high-parasternal short-axis view with both PA branches. It is important to keep in mind that the direction of blood flow might be reversed (right-to-left), in which case a large PDA could be easily be missed if one only focuses on a left-to-right shunt.

A PDA stent is expected to cover the entire length of the ductus without obstruction to blood flow in the proximal descending aorta and proximal left PA. Color and spectral

Doppler should be obtained not only within the PDA, but also in the descending aorta and proximal branch PAs (Figure 38-3).

An mBTTS in a patient with a left aortic arch will be located on the patient's right side, and course from the right subclavian artery to the proximal right PA. A suprasternal notch view of the aortic arch is the best place to start looking for the aortic origin of the shunt (Figure 38-4, A). The ultrasound probe should be angled superiorly towards the right shoulder, following the course of the innominate artery. Once the aortic side of the shunt is found, the course of the blood flow should be followed inferiorly, ideally to its entrance into the proximal right PA (Figure 38-4, B). The echocardiographic image should have the subclavian/innominate artery superiorly and the right PA inferiorly, with the entire length of the mBTTS coursing vertically.

Complete evaluation of an mBTTS includes evidence of any obvious narrowing or blood flow acceleration by color Doppler, as well as spectral Doppler evaluation. Pulse Doppler should be used before and after any level of obstruction. Continuous-wave Doppler should also be obtained, ideally along the entire length of the shunt, or proximally, medial, and distal, if proper alignment of the entire shunt is not possible.

After stenting of an mBTTS, it is important to evaluate for any evidence of obstruction in the innominate artery and proximal right PA. A final velocity inside the stent itself should also be reported.

Perioperative Care

An mBTTS or PDA stent placed during the neonatal period or early infancy should in general, be expected to provide appropriate pulmonary blood flow for adequate oxygenation, systemic oxygen delivery, and somatic growth for at least a period of a few months, if not longer. There is an acceptable mantra that a young infant may have to "grow into" the shunt, as the perfect shunt for a 3 kg newborn, may not remain perfect for very long. Thus, the "ideal shunt" may not appear physiologically ideal in the first instance, meaning that careful intensive care management and exquisite attention to detail are very important during the first days after surgery or PDA stent placement.

The mainstay of preoperative and postoperative management of infants undergoing shunt or PDA stent placement lies in the careful optimization of systemic oxygen delivery, while avoiding excessive pulmonary blood flow. Medical management includes attention to ventilatory management and gas exchange in order to avoid excessive pulmonary blood flow and simultaneously, careful fluid management, titration of vasoactive agents, and optimization of hematocrit to maximize systemic and myocardial oxygen delivery. Finally, avoidance of a hypercoagulable state and appropriate anticoagulation are essential to maintain shunt patency. Table 38-1 illustrates several clinical postoperative scenarios and recommended interventions.

Ventilation

In general, the basic principle that a shunt or stent provides a stable and controlled source of pulmonary blood flow means ventilation should be titrated only to avoid unwanted changes in PVR. The main drivers of PVR are pH and oxygen tension.

All newborns and the majority of young infants remain intubated and mechanically ventilated immediately after surgery. The duration of ventilation is variable and depends mainly on hemodynamics and systemic oxygen delivery, as well as other factors such as the status of the lungs or other comorbidities. In general, patients should progress to extubation within 48 hours of returning to the ICU.

We typically recommend maintaining a normal pH with the avoidance of alkalosis (respiratory or metabolic) with a normal $PaCO_2$. Inspired oxygen fraction should be titrated to provide a target PaO_2. This will in part depend on the underlying anatomy but would typically be <50 mmHg, though this number should not be overinterpreted in isolation. While ventilation can in theory be used to "control" pulmonary blood flow using hypoventilation or a respiratory acidosis to produce a deliberate elevation of PVR, this is not a recommended approach as acidosis can have unwanted effects on other organs including the brain and myocardium.

Hemodynamic Management

The first few hours after surgery represent a critical period in terms of establishing adequate systemic and myocardial perfusion. During this time, frequent reassessments of the patient should be performed focusing on the clinical assessment of systemic oxygen delivery and organ function. A physiologically generous shunt without careful and preemptive intensive care management, can produce systemic "steal" resulting in secondary organ dysfunction – most commonly acute kidney injury. Similarly, coronary "steal" can lead to myocardial ischemia. Meticulous attention to systemic BP (including diastolic pressure), acid-base balance including lactate, fluid balance, and other non-invasive markers of oxygen delivery including NIRS measurements are recommended at this early stage. It is also important to remember that hemoglobin is an important determinant of systemic oxygen delivery and is typically maintained at ~12-14 g/dL. IV vasoactive medications are often used early after surgery. Considerations include the use of milrinone to optimize systemic afterload, vasopressin, or norepinephrine to optimize diastolic BP and coronary perfusion, and low-dose epinephrine (<0.04 mcg/kg/min), particularly in the presence of any ventricular dysfunction.

Fluid Balance

There are no specific "goals" for early fluid management other than to avoid fluid overload (as this can delay postoperative recovery) and hypovolemia. Hypovolemia can be particularly undesirable early after a shunt – or even at any stage after surgery, as this may compromise shunt flow and can contribute to shunt occlusion. We recommend the careful use of diuretics in order to avoid fluid overload, but not necessarily as a routine.

Shunt Patency

The use of low-dose systemic unfractionated heparin infusion is recommended during the early postoperative period. We typically commence heparin once the coagulation studies are normal, or close to normal, and generally at around 4 hours after returning to the ICU. We typically infuse 10 Units/kg/hour and do not target any coagulation parameters. Indeed, at this low dose, we would not expect much change, if any, of the PTT. Enteral antiplatelet therapy with aspirin (~5 mg/kg/day) is commenced on postoperative day 1, aspirin responsiveness is tested after 3 doses, and if appropriate, heparin is discontinued (see Chapter 59).

39 Single-Ventricle Palliation

Elena C. Ocampo, Angela Gooden, Heather A. Dickerson, Nancy S. Ghanayem, Peter Ermis, Carlos M. Mery

Single-ventricle (SV) heart defects are a unique and heterogeneous group of complex congenital heart defects characterized by stenosis and/or atresia of the semilunar and/or AV valves, hypoplasia of the ventricles, and/or a segmental cardiac arrangement not conducive to a biventricular repair. The result is a "functional" SV that provides parallel support to the pulmonary and systemic circulations. Examples, to name a few, include hypoplastic left heart syndrome (HLHS), tricuspid atresia, double inlet left ventricle (DILV), and unbalanced atrioventricular septal defects (AVSD). Although initial presentation and management varies, most will require staged palliations to allow free flow of blood from the ventricle out to the body, protect the lungs from high pressure and extra blood flow, and create separate pathways for blood flow to the lungs and to the body.

Anatomical Considerations

There are several possible combinations of SV defects and clear anatomical descriptions are used to guide management. Initial and ongoing considerations in the evaluation of the anatomy of a patient with functional SV include:
- Ventricular morphology and function
- AV connections and function
- Ventriculoarterial connections
- Source of systemic and pulmonary blood flow
- Source of systemic and pulmonary venous return
- Atrial communication

Anatomically, most defects can be classified as follows:
- **Single-inlet AV defects** are characterized by atresia of one AV valve resulting in a functional SV with a single AV valve. Specific examples include HLHS, double-outlet RV (DORV) with mitral atresia and tricuspid atresia (See Chapter 27 for HLHS and Chapter 20 for tricuspid atresia).
- **Common-inlet SV defects** are characterized by a common AV valve connected to the ventricles in an unbalanced manner. Although there are commonly 2 complete ventricles, distribution of the common AV valve may be such that it is not possible to achieve a biventricular repair. The appropriate SV pathway will be determined by associated defects and blood flow obstruction. These defects often have associated systemic and pulmonary venous return abnormalities. Those with obstructed anomalous pulmonary venous return and unbalanced AVSD are a high-risk group and many were previously considered inoperable.
- **Double-inlet defects** are characterized by a SV that receives both AV valves. The ventricle may be of left (common), right, or indeterminate morphology (rare). Typically, there is a rudimentary or incomplete ventricle that is connected to the dominant chamber by a VSD (or bulboventricular foramen). A common example is

DILV. There are often associated lesions such as transposition of the great vessels, DORV, aortic coarctation, and varying degrees of subvalvar or valvar obstruction.
- **Other functional SV defects** may include situations in which a biventricular arrangement is not desirable such as patients with DORV and a remote VSD.

Pathophysiology and Clinical Presentation

The physiology associated with SV defects will depend on the relationship of pulmonary and systemic blood flow and the relative resistance of each pathway. Many infants with SV defects will have ductal-dependent systemic (SBF) or pulmonary blood flow (PBF) and require PGE infusion prior to initial palliation. They will often develop CHF symptoms secondary to excess PBF as the PVR falls. Infants with ductal-dependent SBF may also have signs of decreased systemic perfusion. Symptoms are worsened if there is a restrictive atrial-level shunt causing pulmonary venous congestion and limiting complete mixing of deoxygenated systemic and oxygenated pulmonary venous returns.

Infants with SV defects and ductal-dependent PBF are admitted to the NICU for preoperative evaluation and management while those with ductal-dependent SBF and/or heterotaxy with concern for pulmonary vein issues are admitted to the CICU. Preoperative feeding practices will vary based on type of SV defect and clinical status. However, most will remain NPO with TPN for nutrition. For those allowed to feed preoperatively, trophic PO feeds (20-40 mL/kg/day) with breast milk is preferred. The infant requires close monitoring of respiratory, GI, and circulatory status as the risk for necrotizing enterocolitis is increased in the setting of unbalanced PBF and SBF.

Diagnosis

- **Fetal echocardiogram.** Prenatal diagnosis of SV defects is common during routine fetal anatomy scans typically done at 18-20 weeks. Most families receive extensive prenatal counseling from multiple pediatric specialties based on perceived postnatal needs. The cardiologist will also determine if the infant requires postnatal PGE infusion for ductal-dependent lesions or urgent postnatal intervention such as septostomy to relieve atrial-level restriction. In high-risk patients who may require immediate intervention, the cardiologist attends the delivery and coordinates transfer to the cardiac catheterization laboratory for atrial septostomy and stenting.
- **CXR.** Useful to show cardiac position, size, and pulmonary vasculature markings (overcirculated or underperfused).
- **ECG.** Useful to evaluate for rhythm and measure axis and intervals. Ventricular hypertrophy, sometimes with a strain pattern, is a common finding.
- **Postnatal TTE.** Used to confirm the anatomy in addition to obtaining information about ventricular and valve function, and ductal- and atrial-level shunts. In some cases, additional imaging such as CTA is used to confirm systemic and pulmonary venous return, arch anatomy, or coronary artery origins.
- **Cardiac catheterization.** Typically not necessary unless atrial septostomy is needed or there is concern for coronary artery abnormalities and/or fistulae.
- **Renal ultrasound.** Routinely obtained to assess for renal anomalies. Renal

consultation is obtained in newborns undergoing surgery with CPB in anticipation of the need for peritoneal dialysis.
- **Preoperative brain MRI.** Obtained to evaluate for ischemic lesions or brain matter abnormalities sometimes seen in infants with CHD.
- **Genetics testing.** Tailored to syndromic features and known associations. For example, HLHS has a known association with Turner syndrome, Jacobsen syndrome, and trisomies 13 and 18. However, many SV defects are not associated with an identified genetic abnormality or there is unknown significance. Chromosomal microarray (CMA) is common as it allows detection of a wide array of chromosome gains and losses. Whole-exome sequencing may be obtained if the CMA is negative and there is a high suspicion for a genetic syndrome. More information about genetics testing can be found in Chapter 50.

Indications / Timing for Intervention

Symptoms vary based on defects, but most require close monitoring for cyanosis, CHF, or cardiogenic shock. Symptoms may worsen as the neonate transitions from fetal circulation.

The current paradigm of SV palliation includes generally 3 stages: an initial palliation at the newborn period that varies depending on the degree of pulmonary and systemic blood flow, a second-stage palliation consisting of a superior cavopulmonary shunt (bidirectional Glenn) at 4-6 months of age, and a third-stage palliation with a completion total cavopulmonary anastomosis (Fontan) at 3-5 years of age.

First-Stage Palliation

Most SV defects will fall into 1 of 4 categories: increased PBF, decreased PBF, decreased SBF, and balanced circulation. Patients within the first 3 categories will typically require a first-stage procedure with the goal of providing adequate systemic and pulmonary blood flow, and at the same time protect/prepare the lungs for the second stage of palliation. Those with a balanced circulation may be observed over time and later undergo a bidirectional Glenn as their initial palliation.

Increased PBF

Patients with increased PBF may require pulmonary artery banding (PAB) to limit flow and pressure to the lungs. Medically managing a SV patient with significant overcirculation is not desirable as the excess flow to the lungs may alter pulmonary vascular reactivity and make the patient a less suitable candidate for the second stage of palliation.

The PAB is typically placed using a median sternotomy. The upper pericardium is opened and the main PA (MPA) encircled. A small catheter is inserted into the distal MPA to measure pressure and help with adjusting of the PAB. Classically, the opening PA pressure will be equal to systemic pressure. A piece of umbilical tape is trimmed and marked at a distance corresponding to Trussler's rule (20 mm plus the weight in kg of the patient). The PAB is placed around the MPA with care not to impinge on the right PA or the pulmonary valve, and secured with a fine horizontal-mattress suture passed through both sides of the PAB. The PAB is then adjusted by placing additional sutures or clips while monitoring PA pressure, oxygen saturation, and PaO_2. The TEE is also used to monitor for PI, velocity across the PAB, and alterations in ventricular function. In general, the PAB is adjusted to achieve approximately 1/3 systemic PA pressure with oxygen saturation (SaO_2) levels in the 80s and PaO_2 in the 40s on an FiO_2 of 40-50%. When the PAB is applied to patients with a biventricular circulation (e.g., patients with multiple VSDs), the PAB is left slightly looser, with PA pressures approximately 35-50% systemic.

Postoperative management after PAB placement follows similar principles than postoperative Norwood palliation care (see Chapter 27) due to the need for precise partitioning of cardiac output but without the insult of CPB or, in some circumstances, reliance on an inferior systemic RV. Standardized monitoring for assessment of circulatory well-being, vasoactive support and ventilator management are similar to that used for Norwood palliation, though physiologic targets may vary depending on the underlying defect. For example, after Norwood palliation, the expectation is that SaO_2 that exceeds 90% places the patient at high risk for systemic hypoperfusion and persistent respiratory insufficiency. Whereas, a PAB placed to limit PBF in common-inlet SV defects might have persistent SaO_2 in the 90s with preserved lung function and good systemic output. Thus, therapeutic targets should include resolution of symptoms associated with CHF and pulmonary edema rather than targeting a specific SaO_2. Though intraoperative PAB adjustment targets the aforementioned SaO_2 and PaO_2, oxygenation often improves during the postoperative period due to resolution of the preoperative pulmonary edema-induced pulmonary venous desaturation. Oximetry targets ideally include narrowing of SaO_2 – cerebral rSO_2 (by NIRS) difference to <40% and SaO_2 – somatic rSO_2 difference to <20% (see Chapter 69). Widening of these oximetric gradients beyond the early postoperative period is an indication for systemic afterload reduction to optimize systemic oxygen delivery, and to further protect the lungs from excessive PBF and the subsequent development of irreversible pulmonary vascular disease.

Decreased PBF
Patients with decreased PBF will require an additional source of PBF in the form of a modified Blalock-Taussig-Thomas shunt (mBTTS) or a PDA stent. For details of these procedures and postoperative management, see Chapter 38.

Decreased SBF
Patients with impaired systemic outflow will usually require a Norwood-type operation that includes:
- **Creation of an unimpeded systemic outflow.** This usually entails creation of a Damus-Kaye-Stansel (DKS) anastomosis between the aortic and pulmonary trunks and an aortic arch reconstruction. For patients with a very small ascending aorta (such as those with HLHS and aortic atresia), the ascending aorta and aortic arch are opened longitudinally, an anastomosis is created between the transected PA and the side of the ascending aorta, and the entire ascending aorta/aortic arch is reconstructed with a homograft patch after removal of all ductal tissue (see Chapter 27). Patients with a sizable ascending aorta may undergo a modified Norwood

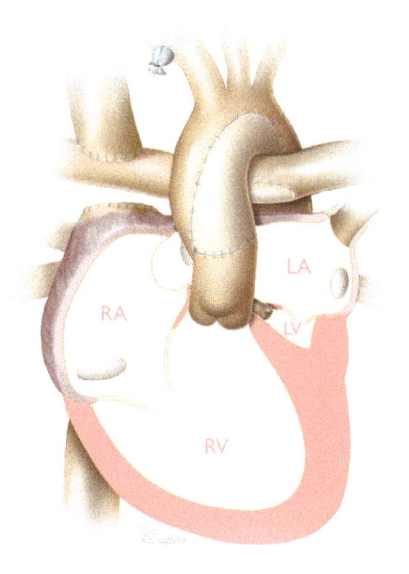

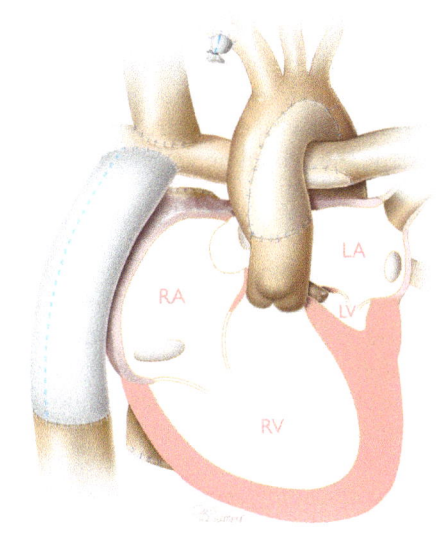

Figure 39-1. Bidirectional Glenn anastomosis in a patient after a Norwood procedure.

Figure 39-2. Extracardiac non-fenestrated Fontan procedure on a patient with a previous Norwood procedure and bidirectional Glenn anastomosis.

procedure (Lamberti modification). For these patients, both the ascending aorta and the PA are transected and anastomosed in a side-to-side fashion, therefore creating a double barrel. The aortic arch and ascending aorta are reconstructed using an aortic arch advancement technique (see Chapter 25) and a small patch. An end-to-end anastomosis is then created between the reconstructed ascending aorta and the double barrel. The advantage of this approach is that it decreases the time of antegrade cerebral perfusion since the DKS anastomosis and sometimes the ascending-aorta to double-barrel anastomosis is made under full-flow CPB.

- **Placement of a shunt or conduit to provide PBF.** This is usually achieved with either a mBTTS or an RV-PA (Sano) conduit. For patients with HLHS, an RV-PA conduit is favored unless there are prominent coronary arteries on the free wall of the RV. The conduit may be brought towards the left (traditional Sano) or towards the right (Brawn modification) of the aorta. Patients with other SV anatomy, such as those with DILV, usually undergo placement of a mBTTS.
- **Atrial septectomy** to provide unrestricted atrial-level shunting.

For details on the postoperative management of patients after a Norwood procedure, see Chapter 27.

Patients with DILV or tricuspid atresia with transposition of the great arteries may have a restrictive VSD leading to impaired SBF and aortic arch hypoplasia. Even though most centers will use a Norwood-type strategy to treat these patients, the anteroposterior arrangement of the vessels make a DKS anastomosis suboptimal and can lead to significant compression of the LPA by the dilated DKS with time. For these patients, if the coronary anatomy is conducive, a palliative arterial switch operation may be performed, usually with aortic arch reconstruction and sometimes requiring placement of a PAB on the neopulmonary trunk if the restriction at the VSD is not severe.

Interstage Period

The interstage is the period of time between the first and second palliation, which is associated with significant morbidity and mortality. Common issues include feeding difficulties, growth failure, residual defects, and difficulty achieving balanced circulation. Postoperative management will vary based on the specific SV defect, but generally the following clinical milestones should be achieved prior to transfer out of the CICU:
- Off continuous IV infusions
- All pacing wires and tubes removed (except PICC or peripheral IV access)
- Stable saturations on room air or minimal nasal cannula support
- Well-controlled arrhythmias with clear documentation of management plans
- Well-controlled BP with clear documentation of goals and medication plans
- All PO medications except IV antibiotic therapy as needed
- Tolerating narcotic weaning plan
- Tolerating at least 100 mL/kg/day of enteral feeds with no signs of feeding intolerance (emesis, bloody stools, etc.) and positive weight gain
- Recent postoperative echocardiogram with stable findings and no major residual lesions

Infants who have undergone a Norwood-type operation or have otherwise been identified for enrollment in SV home monitoring should be admitted to the Cardiology NP team. Generally, evening and weekend transfers should be avoided and face-to-face hand-off with members of the surgical, CICU, and cardiology teams should occur. A low threshold should be maintained for readmission to the CICU for red flag events, which include:
- Desaturation and/or cyanosis
- Tachypnea and increased work of breathing
- Feeding intolerance (emesis, hematochezia, loose stools)
- Increased irritability, fussiness, or fatigue
- Fever or other signs of illness

After discharge, surveillance should include biweekly echocardiograms to evaluate ventricular function, AV valve stenosis/regurgitation, shunt/conduit flow, atrial-level shunt, and systemic outflow tract/aortic arch. In addition, monthly ECGs are obtained and CXR imaging is performed as needed.

Discharge planning should start upon transfer out of the CICU with implementation of the standardized discharge checklist. Multidisciplinary collaboration is needed to achieve a successful discharge:
- Cardiology, CHS, and SV teams for treatment and surgical plan
- Dietician for growth goals and formula-mixing instruction

- Care management for home equipment (pulse oximetry, feeding supplies, Lovenox®, etc.)
- Social work for family support and resources
- Developmental pediatrics for neurodevelopmental evaluation and follow-up

Resources for difficult-to-obtain medications and formulas should be identified prior to discharge. Immunizations should be administered prior to discharge if >6 weeks postoperatively. Pavlizumab (Synagis®) should also be given during RSV season. Complete follow-up of genetic studies and newborn screens is needed for any abnormalities, and a plan should be documented.

The SV team and home monitoring program help families care for their infants at home with the support, resources, and clinical expertise needed to transition to stage 2 successfully. Before discharge, parents learn to measure daily weights, saturations, and heart rate. They enter information in a logbook along with feeding information. Once familiar with the red-flag action plan and comfortable with daily care, discharge occurs. Plans for pre-Glenn study (cardiac catheterization vs. CTA) and timing of stage-2 palliation should be tentatively decided/scheduled. Follow-up visits with Cardiology/SV team, pediatrician, and consulting services should be scheduled as well. Readmission during the interstage period is not uncommon.

Second-Stage Palliation

Preoperative Evaluation

Stage-2 palliation typically occurs at 4-6 months. The SV team is responsible for obtaining and reviewing pre-Glenn imaging and collaborating with the surgical team on the type of imaging and timing of stage-2 palliation. Imaging targets that should be assessed include the aortic arch (in particular if a Norwood-type procedure was performed), the morphology and dimensions of the branch PAs, and the anatomy of the systemic veins, in particular the SVC.

CTA is usually adequate and it can usually be completed on an outpatient basis without anesthesia. Cardiac catheterization is reserved for patients who have residual defects that may require intervention such as recurrent coarctation, shunt/conduit stenosis, pulmonary vein stenosis, or restrictive ASD, or those with concerns regarding PVR (e.g., patients that had repair of anomalous pulmonary veins or prematurity with chronic lung disease). MRI is an option as well, but requires anesthesia. A preoperative Holter should be done to evaluate for ectopy and arrhythmias. Studies should be reviewed prior to surgical consultation.

Surgical Approach

Stage-2 palliation usually involves the creation of a cavopulmonary connection (SVC to PA) with takedown of previous shunts or conduits (Figure 39-1). If a patient has bilateral SVCs, bilateral bidirectional Glenn anastomoses are created unless the patient has a bridging innominate vein that is at least the size of the contralateral SVC. The azygos and hemiazygos veins are routinely ligated and divided. Any branch PA stenosis or hypoplasia is liberally addressed with patching.

Sometimes, an additional source of PBF is left for patients with heterotaxy, systemic

PART III. SPECIAL CONSIDERATIONS

POD	CV Meds	Diuretics	Fluid	Nutrition	Respiratory	Chest Tubes	Mobilization	Pain Meds	Disposition
0	Inotropes	None	Crystalloid / blood product replacement	NPO then clears if stable	OR extubation vs <6 hrs in ICU		Head of bed 30 degrees	PCA IV acetaminophen	CICU
1	Wean inotropes	IV furosemide (1 mg/kg q12, max 20 mg/dose)	50% maintenance	Start enteral intake	Min: 0.5 L/min	Mediastinal out	Encourage highest degree of mobilization	PCA IV acetaminophen Consider ketorolac	CICU
2	Initiate ASA Consider resuming home meds	IV furosemide (1 mg/kg q8, max 20 mg/dose) PO chlorothiazide	75-80% maintenance	PO encouraged	Min: 0.5 L/min	Mediastinal out Pleural to bulb	Walk in ICU at least once per shift	PO opioid + acetaminophen Consider ketorolac	Transfer to acute care floor
3	ASA Consider resuming home meds	PO furosemide (1.5 mg/kg q8, max 20 mg/dose) PO chlorothiazide	75-80% maintenance	Full PO	Min: 0.5 L/min	Pleural to bulb	Walk x3	PO opioid + acetaminophen PO NSAID	Transfer to acute care floor
4	ASA	Optimize PO diuretics	75-80% maintenance	Full PO	Stop O_2 if sats >94%	Remove if <2 mL/kg/d each	Full mobilization as at home (min 3x)	PO NSAID PRN PO opioid	
5	ASA	Decrease or maintain	75-80% maintenance	Full PO	Stop O_2 if sats >94%	Remove if <2 mL/kg/d each	Full mobilization as at home (min 3x)	PO NSAID PRN PO opioid	D/c criteria met?
6	ASA	Decrease or maintain	75-80% maintenance	Full PO	Stop O_2 if sats >94%	Remove if <2 mL/kg/d each	Full mobilization as at home (min 3x)	PO NSAID PRN PO opioid	D/c criteria met?

Figure 39-3. Postoperative Fontan management protocol. Developed by the TCH Heart Center and the TCH Evidence-Based Outcomes Center. ASA: aspirin, CT: chest tube, NSAID: non-steroidal anti-inflammatory drug, PCA: patient-controlled analgesia, POD: postoperative day.

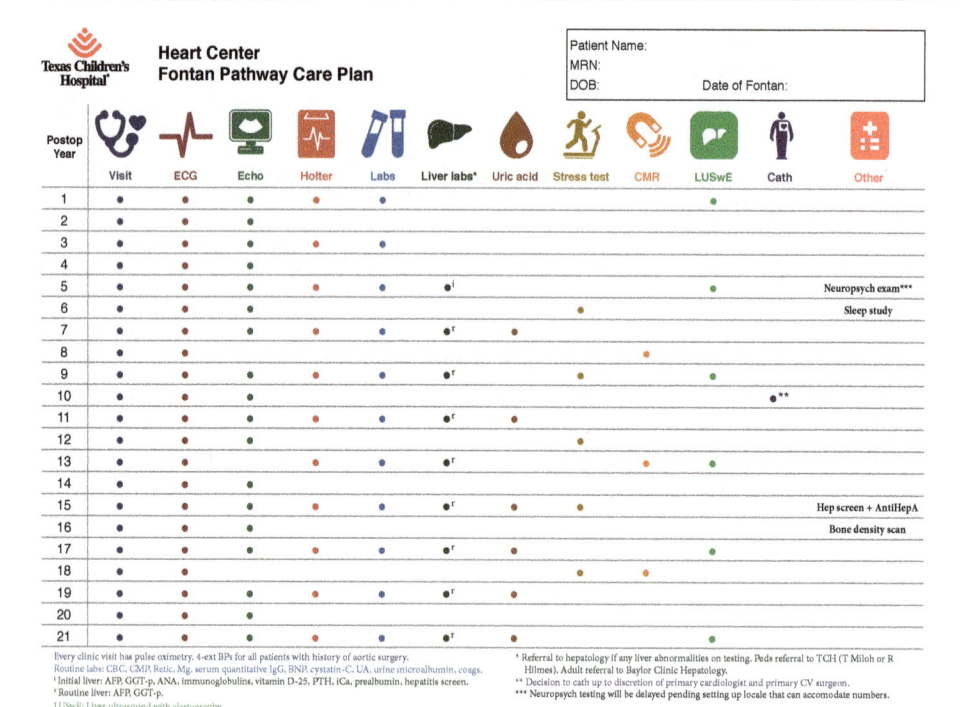

Figure 39-4. Heart Center Fontan Pathway Care Plan.

venous anomalies, genetic syndromes, or those in which it is unclear whether they will be adequate Fontan candidates in the future. This additional source of PBF is achieved by leaving some prograde flow across the RVOT; an existing PAB may be tightened or if there is not enough RVOT obstruction, a PAB may be placed. By providing additional PBF through the RVOT, these "pulsatile Glenns" may allow patients to be less desaturated as they grow, allow a delay in the next stage of palliation, and may decrease the creation of pulmonary arteriovenous malformations by allowing hepatic flow into the PAs.

The Glenn procedure is performed on CPB with the heart beating except in those patients that required intracardiac repairs, arch reconstruction, or pulmonary valve exclusion. If the RVOT is patent and a pulsatile Glenn is not planned, the heart is arrested, the main PA transected, the pulmonary valve oversewn, and the cardiac PA stump closed. Failure to oversew the pulmonary valve (or perform a valvectomy if the valve is very small) may lead to thrombus formation between the pulmonary valve and the MPA stump, which may then enter the ventricle and cause systemic embolization.

It is customary to place IJ and femoral venous catheters in patients undergoing Glenn procedures. This allows postoperative measurement of Glenn pressures and transpulmonary gradients. Adequate Glenn pressures at the end of the procedure are usually in the low-to-mid teens with a transpulmonary gradient between 3 and 8 mmHg. The IJ "Glenn" line is usually removed on the first postoperative day. Low-dose heparin may be started a few hours postoperatively and continued until the Glenn line is out if the SVC is small, especially in patients with bilateral SVCs.

Postoperative Management

Understanding cardiopulmonary interactions is implicit in postoperative management after the Glenn procedure. Because positive-pressure ventilation after cavopulmonary connection is associated with a decrease in PBF and thus cardiac output, early spontaneous breathing is desirable and extubation commonly occurs in the OR or shortly after arrival to the CICU. For those patients who are better served by positive-pressure ventilation in the early postoperative period (circumstances including ongoing bleeding, underlying airway disease, or depressed myocardial function), a ventilator strategy that allows for permissive hypercarbia at the lowest possible mean airway pressure (single digit) is optimal. Though acute hypocarbia and alkalosis have been shown to acutely reduce PVR, the benefit does not outweigh the negative impact of increased intrathoracic pressure on postoperative Glenn circulation. Alternatively, hypercarbia (pCO_2 45-55 mmHg) has been shown to increase PBF and oximetry measures likely through hypercarbia-induced increases in cerebral blood flow (cardio-pulmonary-cerebral interaction). In circumstances in which the transpulmonary gradient is wide and oxygenation concerning, iNO may be indicated.

The shift from dual-distribution circulation to superior cavopulmonary connection commonly results in postoperative hypertension. BP control through vasoactive infusions (milrinone + nipride or nicardipine) in the early postoperative period will assist in augmenting cardiac output through afterload reduction as well as lowering the end-diastolic pressures, allowing for optimal transpulmonary circulation. All patients will likely begin transitioning to angiotensing-converting enzyme (ACE) inhibitors on the first postoperative day. Diuretics are needed to maintain low Glenn pressures and to reduce the risk of pleural effusions. Even though the "Glenn" IJ line is typically removed on postoperative day 1, thorough physical exams including attention to the anterior fontanelle and facial edema assist in titration of diuretics.

It is common for patients after a Glenn procedure to have some degree of transient upper body edema that may lead to headaches. Alternating acetaminophen and non steroidal anti-inflammatory is effective to manage pain.

Third-Stage Palliation

Preoperative Evaluation

The Fontan operation is the third palliation and is usually done at 3-5 years of age. Timing varies based on individual degree of cyanosis. Evaluation includes:

- **ECG and Holter.** Patients with a Fontan circulation benefit from adequate AV synchrony. It is thus important to rule out arrhythmias or AV block that may require treatment.
- **CXR.** Assess cardiomegaly and pulmonary abnormalities.
- **Echocardiogram.** A complete echocardiogram is essential to assess abnormalities that may lead to failure of a Fontan circulation. These include lesions such as AV valve regurgitation, ventricular function, aortic arch or ventricular outflow tract obstruction, and other residual lesions.
- **Cardiac catheterization.** A successful Fontan circulation is dependent on low PVR. For this reason, all patients undergo a pre-Fontan cardiac catheterization for hemodynamics and to address residual lesions. Important hemodynamic values include Glenn pressures, PVR, Qp:Qs, end-diastolic pressure, transpulmonary gradient, and other intracardiac or aortic gradients. In addition, it is important to assess the IVC morphology and orientation (in particular in patients with heterotaxy), branch PA anatomy, patency of the Glenn anastomosis, the presence of collaterals (venovenous and arteriovenous) and arteriovenous malformations. Significant collaterals may be occluded in the lab.

Surgical Approach

The Fontan completion involves the creation of an extracardiac conduit (usually 18- or 20-mm Gore-Tex® graft) that connects the IVC to the PA (Figure 39-2). The procedure is performed using CPB via bicaval cannulation with the heart beating, unless intracardiac repairs are necessary. Any stenosis or hypoplasia of the branch PAs is managed with a patch plasty. If the RVOT is patent (pulsatile Glenn), the pulmonary valve is oversewn and the MPA sutured closed using a brief episode of cardiac arrest.

A fenestration (a communication between the Fontan conduit and the atrium) is created selectively in high-risk patients with hypoplastic PAs or high PVR in order to serve as a pop-off for elevated Fontan pressures. Currently, more than 75% of patients at TCH undergo a nonfenestrated Fontan.

Due to an expected higher venous pressure as part of the Fontan circuit, patients may have significant chest tube output postoperatively. It is therefore routine to open both pleural spaces and place bilateral pleural chest tubes in addition to the mediastinal chest tube. The mediastinal chest tube will usually be removed on postoperative day 2 while pleural chest tubes will remain in place until chest tube output decreases. Patients are routinely extubated in the OR since positive-pressure ventilation is unfavorable for the Fontan circuit.

Postoperative Management

Figure 39-3 depicts the TCH protocol for postoperative management of Fontan patients. The Fontan procedure "septates" the circulation in patients with SV physiology. PBF is a passive diastolic phenomenon (occurs during negative inspiration and is impeded with positive-pressure ventilation) and cardiac output is dependent on pulmonary venous return. This phenomenon dictates the postoperative management of patients with a Fontan circulation as pulmonary mechanics and volume status will determine cardiac output.

The transpulmonary gradient (CVP [which equals the PA pressure] minus LAP) is an important concept in Fontan management and must be low for good cardiac output. Strategies to decrease PVR will improve PBF and thus pulmonary venous return and cardiac output. Optimal Fontan physiology includes:
- CVP / PA pressure: 10-15 mmHg (most are >12 mmHg)
- LAP: 5-10 mmHg
- Transpulmonary gradient: 5-10 mmHg
- AV synchrony
- Lack of systemic hypertension

Some important tenants of postoperative Fontan management are:
- Negative-pressure ventilation improves hemodynamics; it is thus important to extubate early.
- Volume is needed in the early postoperative period (first 1-2 days) to maintain cardiac output. Avoid diuresis during this time. Low-dose vasopressin may help minimize excessive volume needs.
- Patients require eventual fluid restriction and diuresis to decrease chest-tube output toward discharge (days 2-3 until the time of discharge). Fluid restriction and diuresis is maintained at the time of discharge.
- AV synchrony is important to maintain cardiac output and avoid increases in atrial pressure that can impede pulmonary venous return.
- Avoid significant catecholamines as tachycardia decreases filling time and can lead to arrhythmias.
- A fenestration allows for maintenance of cardiac output in the face of less-than-optimal pulmonary hemodynamics. As such, it is used at TCH in high-risk patients with elevated PVR.
- Patients with SV physiology have high SVR and it is important to treat this to augment systemic perfusion.
- If there are persistent pleural effusions it is important to assure that they are not chylous (for management of chylothorax, see Chapter 77).

- If a patient has unexpected cyanosis after a Fontan procedure, evaluation should include:
  - Ventricular function/AV valve regurgitation (decreased mixed venous oxygenation)
  - Shunting through a fenestration or baffle leak
  - Systemic venous collateralization
  - Intrapulmonary arteriovenous malformations
  - Pulmonary pathology/diaphragm paresis
  - Hepatic venous connection to the atrium (not incorporated into the Fontan circuit)
  - Coronary sinus flow

Long-Term Follow-up

The unique nature of the Fontan physiology presents patients with a multitude of long-term issues. The Heart Center Fontan Pathway Care Plan (Figure 39-4), was developed so that longitudinal, standardized testing can be used to monitor specific long-term complications commonly encountered in Fontan patients. These include:
- **Cardiac**
  - *Structural* – There is universal diastolic dysfunction with any elevation in end-diastolic pressures leading to further elevation in Fontan pressures. Significant AV valve regurgitation independently predicts poor outcomes. Systolic dysfunction is less common, but still a noted concern.
  - *Electrical* – Bradycardia is common (mainly sinus node dysfunction). Tachycardia is common (atrial > ventricular), especially intra-atrial reentry tachycardia.
- **Liver.** Chronic congestive hepatopathy is the rule with most patients eventually developing some degree of cirrhosis. There are rare reports of hepatocellular carcinoma.
- **Fontan pathway obstruction.** Any obstruction in the Fontan pathway needs to be corrected since it will lead to elevation in Fontan pressures.
- **Pulmonary.** Any branch pulmonary stenosis needs to be corrected. Venovenous collateral vessels (from systemic to pulmonary veins) can lead to desaturations. Elevated PVR is rare but difficult to treat.
- **Vascular.** The diagnosis of protein-losing enteropathy (PLE) is made via clinical suspicion and can be confirmed with testing for fecal alpha-1-antitrypsin. Treatment is individualized (with medical treatment often unsuccessful) and ranges from medications (oral steroids, pulmonary vasodilators), to catheter interventions (fenestrating the Fontan circuit), to surgery (Fontan conversion, transplantation).
- **Hematologic.** Patients may present with coagulopathy. Thromboemboli are common with high risk of venous thromboemboli, pulmonary emboli, or stroke.
- **Renal.** Chronic kidney disease is likely underrecognized.

In a series of 610 patients undergoing Fontan procedures at TCH with a median follow-up of 7 years, freedom from any Fontan failure (defined as death, heart transplant, takedown or revision of the Fontan circuit, creation of fenestration, major reintervention, or development of plastic bronchitis or PLE), was 91% at 5 years and 89% at 10 years (Mery et al. 2019).

Suggested Readings

Castellanos DA, Ocampo EC, Gooden A, et al. Outcomes associated with unplanned interstage cardiac interventions after Norwood palliation. Ann Thorac Surg 2019;108:1423-1429.

Chacon-Portillo MA, Zea-Vera R, Zhu H, et al. Pulsatile Glenn as long-term palliation for single venticle physiology patients. Congenit Heart Dis 2018;13:927-934.

Heinle JS, Carberry KE, McKenzie ED, et al. Outcomes after the palliative arterial switch operation in neonates with single-ventricle anatomy. Ann Thorac Surg 2013;95:212-218.

Mery CM, De León LE, Trujillo-Diaz D, et al. Contemporary outcomes of the Fontan operation: a large single-institution cohort. Ann Thorac Surg 2019;108:1439-1446.

40 Pulmonary Valve Replacement

Varun Aggarwal, Henri Justino, Charles D. Fraser Jr.

Longstanding RVOT stenosis or regurgitation are common in patients with congenital anomalies involving the RVOT. There are 2 relatively distinct groups of patients requiring RVOT intervention. The first group consists of patients who underwent transcatheter or surgical intervention on the pulmonary valve (PV) or RVOT and now suffer from a *dysfunctional native RVOT* (i.e., without a preexisting conduit or artificial valve). The other group includes patients who received an RV-PA conduit or a bioprosthetic pulmonary valve and now suffer from a *dysfunctional conduit or bioprosthetic pulmonary valve*.

Chronic PR in the setting of repaired tetralogy of Fallot leads to RV dilation and dysfunction, which is linked to the development of exercise intolerance, arrhythmias and death. Current techniques for RVOT intervention include both transcatheter and surgical options.

Indications for Pulmonary Valve Replacement (PVR)

Criteria for PVR continue to be refined as information accrues concerning the late effects of compromised RV function. In the current era, surface echocardiography remains the primary screening tool and in most patients, it can provide semiquantitative information about RV size and function. Other important information includes level of RVOT obstruction, presence/degree of TR (and assessment of causation), and presence of intracardiac shunts. Anatomic and functional MRI has become the primary diagnostic modality for patient assessment for PVR and is possible in most patients. Pertinent information includes RV end-diastolic volume indexed for body surface area (RVEDVi), RV and LV ejection fraction, pulmonary regurgitant fraction, branch PA distortion, and assessment for intracardiac shunts. Less frequently, cardiac catheterization can be a useful adjunct to the decision-making process. Finally, in patients with pacing systems that are not MRI compatible, the decision to proceed with PVR may be facilitated by cardiac CTA.

The specific indications for PVR in patients with a dysfunctional conduit or bioprosthetic pulmonary valve are still debated. In general, PVR is indicated in the following circumstances (Tretter et al. 2016):

- Presence of symptoms from a dysfunctional RVOT
- For patients with predominant PI: an RVEDVi >150 ml/m2, ± pulmonary regurgitation fraction > 40%, or an indexed RV end-systolic volume (RVESVi) >80 ml/m2
- For patients with predominant PS: RVOT stenosis with mean Doppler gradient >35 mmHg

Additional criteria may include a dysfunctional RVOT with moderate-severe accompanying TR or the risk of long-term arrhythmia (QRS ≥180 msec) and progressive LV dysfunction.

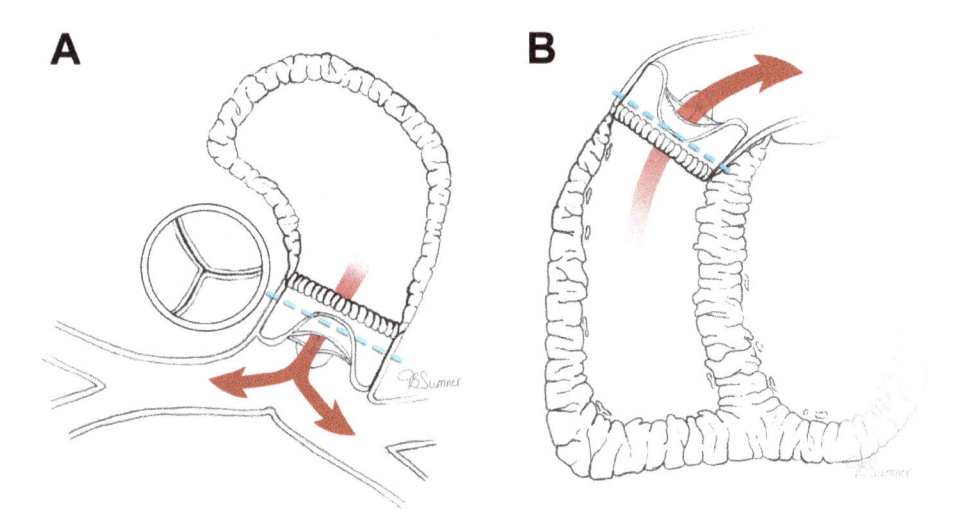

Figure 40-1. Axial and sagittal views illustrating the correct orientation of a surgically implanted PV in order to avoid branch PA obstruction.

Transcatheter Pulmonary Valve Replacement (TPVR)

Since the initial description of TPVR in 2000, TPVR has gained widespread acceptance as a nonsurgical alternative among patients who have dysfunctional RV-PA conduits or dysfunctional bioprosthetic valves. With the advent of larger transcatheter valves, the usage has also been extended to select patients with dysfunctional native RVOT without a preexisting conduit or bioprosthetic valve. The 2 FDA approved valves for pulmonic implantation are the Melody™ valve (Medtronic, Minneapolis, Minnesota, USA) and the Sapien™ XT valve (Edwards Lifesciences Inc., Irvine, CA).

Melody™ Valve

The first US implantation of the Melody™ valve was in 2007. The FDA approved the use of the Melody™ valve under humanitarian device exemption in January 2010 and subsequent premarket approval was given in February 2015. Currently available Melody™ transcatheter pulmonary valves in the US are composed of 16 mm or 18 mm bovine jugular veins sewn within a Cheatham-Platinum stent. These valves can be deployed using 18 mm, 20 mm, or 22 mm delivery systems. It is important to note that the diameter of the Melody™ valve therefore represents an *internal diameter* of 18, 20, or 22 mm.

In a recent meta-analysis (Virk et al. 2015), the overall periprocedural mortality was 1.4% and procedural complications included conduit rupture (2.6%), valve embolization (2.4%), coronary artery compression (1.2%), and PA obstruction (1.2%). Conversion to surgery was reported in 2.8% of patients. The incidence of stent fracture and infective endocarditis were 12.4% and 4.9%, respectively. The long-term outcome of the US Melody™ investigational device exemption trial (Cheatham et al. 2015) demonstrated 5-year freedom from reintervention and explantation of 76±4% and 92±3%, respectively. The main cause of valve dysfunction was stent fracture. It is noteworthy that the rate of

Melody™ stent fracture decreased by 65% when conduits were treated with placement of bare metal stents prior to implantation of a Melody™ valve, a practice known as "prestenting", which has become standard of care when Melody™ valves are placed within conduits.

Sapien™ Valve

Initially introduced for aortic valve replacement, the first use of the Sapien™ valve in the pulmonary position was reported in 2006. The COMPASSION trial (Kenny et al. 2011) demonstrated the successful deployment of the Sapien™ valve in 34 attempts in 33 patients. Valve migration was noted in 3 patients. Freedom from reintervention was 97%, with 1 patient undergoing elective placement of a second valve due to distortion of the initial implant.

Initially, the Sapien™ valve was available in the US in 23 mm and 26 mm sizes for use in RVOT ranges of 18-25 mm. In March 2016, the FDA approved the use of the Sapien™ XT valve (available in 23, 26, and 29 mm diameters) for the pulmonary position in patients with dysfunctional RV-PA conduits. The Sapien-3™ valve is available in 20, 23, 26, and 29 mm diameters, and represents a later iteration of the Sapien™ family. Although not FDA approved for pulmonic implantation, it is commonly being used off label in the pulmonary position. Of note, the Sapien™ valves are labeled by their *outer diameters* rather than by their internal diameters. Because they are available in larger diameters than the Melody™ valve, they are also commonly used off label in the native RVOT in patients who have received patch augmentation of the RVOT as part of tetralogy of Fallot repair.

Preprocedural Evaluation

TTE (2D, color, and spectral Doppler) is the first line imaging modality for all patients. Assessment of biventricular function, degree of RVOT/conduit stenosis and/or insufficiency, and evaluation of branch PAs is important. While Doppler-derived mean RVOT pressure gradients correlate reasonably well with catheter-derived gradients, echocardiography is often less accurate in estimating the severity of PR and RV size and function relative to cardiac MRI. Thus, in patients with predominant PR, cardiac MRI is generally an important component of the preprocedural evaluation.

Intraprocedural Evaluation

A complete right-heart catheterization is performed, carefully documenting the degree and levels of RVOT obstruction. A retrograde left-heart catheterization is generally also performed. Angiographic measurements of the conduit or bioprosthetic valve should be performed in several planes (ideally in a biplane catheterization laboratory). In general, degenerated conduits that are significantly shrunken down compared to their original (nominal) implanted diameters require successive balloon angioplasties to restore the conduits to an adequate diameter for TPVR. Balloon angioplasties are generally performed with noncompliant balloons, in 2 mm increments, with angiography after each angioplasty to look for signs of conduit disruption. Small pseudoaneurysms commonly develop as a consequence of conduit angioplasty. Ideally, conduits should be restored to a diameter suitable for the patient's body size and for TPVR; this implies generally a minimal diameter of 18 mm to implant a Melody™ valve. Of note, even relatively small conduits with nominal diameters <16 mm can frequently be overexpanded to enable TPVR.

Coronary angiography should be performed at baseline, and again after successive conduit angioplasty prior to TPVR. With the balloon inflated across the conduit using dilute contrast, coronary angiography is then performed to determine if there is coronary compression during balloon expansion of the conduit. Coronary compression is an absolute contraindication to conduit stenting and TPVR. Distally, aortic root angiography should be performed during test dilation of the conduit, to determine if there is significant distortion of the aortic root, as this would also preclude conduit stenting or TPVR. In the absence of coronary or aortic root compression, prestenting of the conduit is then performed with 1-3 heavy stainless steel stents to prevent conduit recoil, followed by TPVR. Prestenting is not necessary for the Sapien^{TM} valves because their stent is much less prone to fractures. Placement of a polytetrafluoroethylene (PTFE)-covered stent may be necessary to seal any substantial pseudoaneurysms or frank extravasations of contrast prior to prestenting and TPVR.

TPVR within bioprosthetic valves is similar to TPVR within conduits, with the exception that the frame of the bioprosthetic valve provides sufficient resistance from recoil, such that prestenting is often unnecessary, and pseudoaneurysms are much less common.

Off-label use of the current transcatheter valves has also been reported successful in native dysfunctional RVOT. In this case, a very compliant sizing balloon is used to determine if a suitable landing zone is present in the native RVOT. Generally, a suitable landing zone should be several millimeters smaller than the intended valve to be deployed. Similar precautions to look for signs of aortic root compression and coronary compression are necessary prior to TPVR in the native RVOT.

Postprocedural Care

Patients are observed overnight in the hospital for any arrhythmia and for hemodynamic monitoring. They undergo a 2-view CXR and echocardiogram on the following day to evaluate for valve position, any residual stenosis or insufficiency, perivalvar leaks, or pericardial effusion. The vascular access site is monitored for any bleeding or hematoma, given the large bore delivery sheaths needed for these procedures. Patients are started on aspirin 81 mg daily to be taken indefinitely, and maintenance of good oral hygiene and bacterial endocarditis prophylaxis cautions are required.

Surgical PVR

As per above, all patients with abnormal RV to PA connections face the ultimate need for surgical PVR. TPVR has become a very attractive and relatively safe option to *delay* the ultimate need for surgical PVR. Unfortunately, neither methodology confers lifelong security from need for reintervention, whether surgical or transcatheter. For a given patient, the goal should be to coordinate current technological alternatives in a careful strategic roadmap to optimize RV function and minimize morbity.

Preoperative Evaluation

Many patients undergoing surgical PVR have undergone previous cardiac surgery. They may have extra-anatomic RV-to-PA connections with calcified conduits, indwelling stent material, and other complex associations. The cardiac structures including aorta, PA, conduits, high-pressure cardiac chambers, and patches may be densely adherent to the sternum and/or other aspects of the chest wall. In the present era, even in the setting of multiple previous cardiac surgeries, safe sternal reentry should be expected and careful planning is paramount. CTA or MRI are very useful in determining the relationship of cardiac structures to the sternum. Options for peripheral cannulation for CPB should be carefully evaluated and the patient prepped accordingly. The OR team, including the perfusion team members, must be prepared to various contingency solutions for safe conduct of the operation. Some surgeons advocate for the routine use of femoral cannulation before sternal reentry in complex situations. We have found that with careful planning, this is not necessary in most cases.

Surgical Procedure

Sternal reentry is facilitated with the use of an oscillating saw that is used to divide the outer table and cortex, but *largely leave intact the inner table*. Using gentle upward traction and under direct vision, the adjacent cardiac structure are carefully dissected away from the undersurface of the sternum and the inner table progressively divided from a caudal to cranial direction. Once sternal reentry is gained, meticulous dissection facilitates the operation and optimizes hemostasis.

There are presently numerous options for surgical placement of a competent PV with or without a conduit. There are no data available to definitively demonstrate superiority of one over another. In our experience, in *small children and early adolescents* where significant somatic growth is still anticipated, human cadaveric cryopreserved valved conduits (pulmonary homograft valved conduits) or bovine jugular vein valved conduits (Contegra® conduits) offer attractive options. However, in our experience, bovine jugular vein conduits have a higher, and possibly prohibitive, risk of late endocarditis 7 years after implantation (Mery et al. 2016). Other options include the Hancock® composite porcine valved Dacron® conduits, which have the additional attractive feature of a supporting ring at the valve annulus. Some centers have utilized surgically constructed thin-walled Gore-Tex® valved conduits, although we do not have experience with that option. In extra-anatomic situations, where the distance from the RV to the PAs may be quite long, we have occasionally used aortic homograft valved conduits or have constructed composite extensions of homografts with Gore-Tex® tube grafts. Finally, in rare circumstances, surgeons do consider placing mechanical valves in the pulmonary position. We have uniformly avoided this alternative because of the need for significant anticoagulation.

For isolated PVR in *patients large enough to receive an adult-sized valve*, we have commonly used supported heterograft valves placed in an orthotopic position. We have favored porcine heterograft valves (such as the Epic™ and Epic™ Supra stented tissue valves) as their thin leaflets close better than bovine pericardial leaflets in the setting of the lower pressures that exist in the PA compared to the aorta. For implantation of these valves, the previous patch is longitudinally incised or removed, the valve is implanted by suturing the posterior two-thirds circumference to the RVOT at the level of the annulus, and a Dacron® patch is used to cover the anterior third of the RVOT. Attention is made to align the valve properly in order to avoid obstruction of the branch PAs (Figure 40-1). While these valves will eventually degenerate, they have the additional attractive feature of acting as a suitable "landing zone" for future transcatheter valves.

We frequently perform PVR on CPB support with a beating heart. It is therefore very important that no residual intracardiac shunts exist. A bubble-contrast TEE study is performed on all patients prior to initiating the operation. Any residual intracardiac shunts preclude beating-heart PVR. Where possible, all intracardiac shunts should be closed. The subject of tricuspid valve repair is frequently considered in the setting of RV dilation associated with PS or PI. A tricuspid repair is performed for any degree of TR greater than mild.

Suggested Readings

Cheatham JP, Hellenbrand WE, Zahn EM, et al. Clinical and hemodynamic outcomes up to 7 years after transcatheter pulmonary valve replacement in the US Melody valve investigational device exemption trial. Circulation 2015;131:1960-1970.

Kenny D, Hijazi ZM, Kar S, et al. Percutaneous implantation of the Edwards SAPIEN transcatheter heart valve for conduit failure in the pulmonary position: early phase 1 results from an international multicenter clinical trial. J Am Coll Cardiol. 2011;58:2248-2256.

McKenzie ED, Khan MS, Dietzman TW, et al. Surgical pulmonary valve replacement: a benchmark for outcomes comparisons. J Thorac Cardiovasc Surg 2014;148:1450-1453.

Mery CM, Guzmán-Pruneda FA, De León LE, et al. Risk factors for development of endocarditis and reintervention in patients undergoing right ventricle to pulmonary artery valve conduit placement. J Thorac Cardiovasc Surg 2016;151:432-439.

Tretter JT, Friedberg MK, Wald RM, et al. Defining and refining indications for transcatheter pulmonary valve replacement in patients with repaired tetralogy of Fallot: Contributions from anatomical and functional imaging. Int J Cardiol 2016;221:916-925.

Virk SA, Liou K, Chandrakumar D, et al. Percutaneous pulmonary valve implantation: A systematic review of clinical outcomes. Int J Cardiol 2015;201:487-489.

Warnes CA, Williams RG, Bashore TM, et al. ACC/AHA 2008 guidelines for the management of adults with congenital heart disease: a report of the American College of Cardiology/American Heart Association Task Force on Practice Guidelines (Writing Committee to Develop Guidelines on the Management of Adults With Congenital Heart Disease). J Am Coll Cardiol 2008;52:e143-e263.

41 Pacemakers and Defibrillators

Santiago O. Valdes, Iki Adachi, Christina Y. Miyake

Pacemakers and implantable cardioverter defibrillators (ICD) are made of 2 major components: the generator (battery) and the leads connecting the generator to the heart. The leads can be attached to the heart by screwing them into the myocardium from the inside (endocardium) via a transvenous approach or they can be sutured to the outside of the heart (epicardium) via an epicardial approach. The anatomy and size of the patients are the main considerations when deciding upon the approach for device placement. Patients with systemic shunts or lack of access to intracardiac chambers from subclavian access (Fontan or Glenn physiology) will require an epicardial approach. A transvenous approach can be considered in patients without shunting lesions who are generally at least 20 kg in weight for pacemakers and 30 kg for ICD.

After a transvenous implant, patients are admitted and kept on IV antibiotics until discharge. Arm movement on the side of device placement should be limited. Patients should not be allowed to lift the arm above 90° or put their arm behind them. The evening of the procedure, a portable CXR is performed to evaluate for the presence of a pneumo- or hemothorax and for lead placement (Figure 41-1). The morning of discharge, all patients must have a complete physical exam including evaluation of the device pocket, in addition to an anteroposterior (AP) and lateral CXR, device interrogation, and device teaching by the electrophysiology (EP) nurses. Patients are discharged home to complete a 3-7 day course of oral antibiotics.

ICDs are able to treat tachyarrhythmias either via electrical cardioversion or though antitachycardia pacing. Heart rate zones are set to tell the ICD when therapies should be delivered. ICDs will use several discriminators to differentiate supraventricular, ventricular, and sinus tachycardia.

The number and type of lead placed depends on the indication for pacing and size of the patient. Indications for pacing are based on published guidelines. Regardless of approach to implant, it is important that sensed P and R waves are of sufficient size for the lifetime of the lead. Epicardial bipolar leads should be placed at a distance <5 cm apart. The minimal P-wave amplitude is 1.5 mV with a goal of at least 2 mV. For R waves, the minimal amplitude is 6 mV with an optimal value of 10 mV. Capture thresholds should ideally be <1 V at 0.5 msec with a maximum value of 2.5 V at 0.5 msec. Battery life is dependent on the amount of pacing and capture threshold. The higher the threshold, the faster the battery will drain.

All medical teams caring for a patient with a pacemaker or ICD need to be aware of the device type and programming of the implanted device. Device programming should be located in the patient's chart. Device programming is indicated by a three-letter code with an additional fourth letter "R" for devices with rate response (Table 41-1). The first letter refers to the chamber paced. The second letter refers to the chamber sensed. The third letter refers to what the device does with the information. The fourth letter "R" is a pacing mode termed "rate response" which is typically used in patients with sinus node dysfunction. It allows the generator to sense activity or chest wall movement that

41. PACEMAKERS AND DEFIBRILLATORS

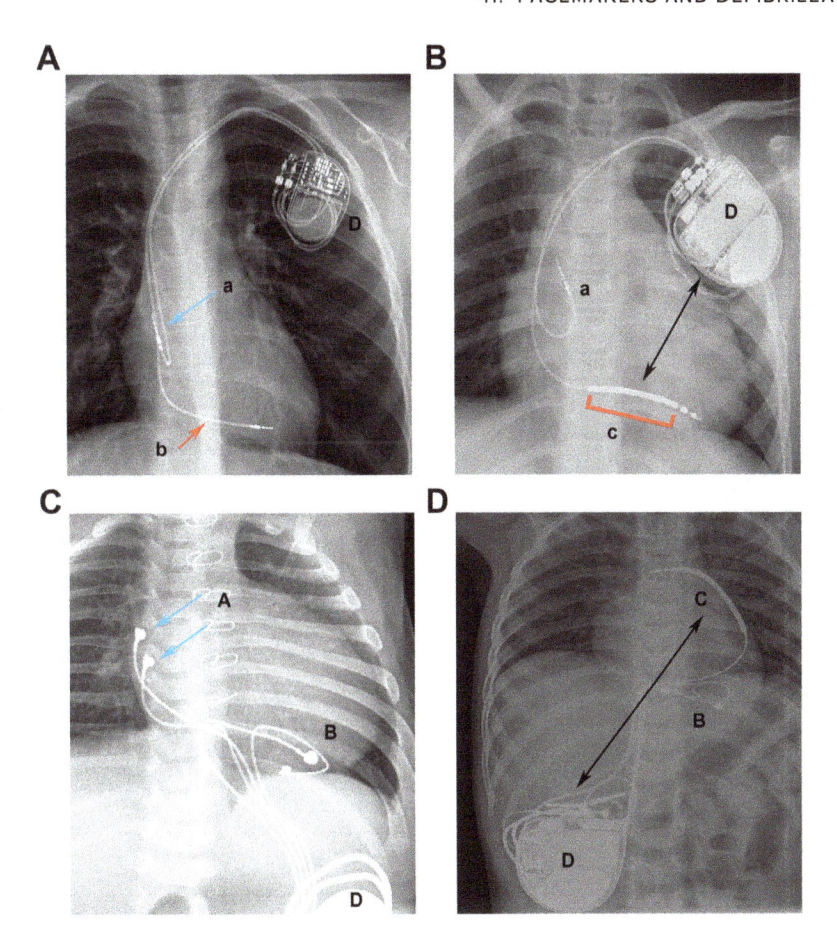

Figure 41-1. Images A-D are AP CXR views of transvenous (A-B) and epicardial (C-D) pacing and ICD systems. Lowercase letters refer to transvenous leads and uppercase letters refer to epicardial leads. A) Dual-chamber transvenous pacemaker. B) Dual-chamber transvenous ICD. C) Dual-chamber epicardial pacemaker. D) Single-chamber epicardial ICD. Transvenous and epicardial systems can be differentiated by imaging the lead and system. Transvenous systems utilize the subclavian veins to access the heart. The leads have a screw to attach the lead to the endocardial surface (a: atrial transvenous lead in the atrial appendage, b: ventricular transvenous lead in RV apex). Epicardial leads look like buttons which are sewn to the outside of the heart (A with blue arrows showing each of the buttons). If there is only one button, this means the systems is unipolar (not shown) and the other pole is the generator. Two buttons mean the lead is a bipolar lead. The generator (D) in transvenous systems is located in the prepectoral chest (most commonly left side, although the generator can also be placed in the right chest). For epicardial systems, the generator is typically in the abdomen. An ICD lead can be distinguished from a pacing lead by the presence of a thicker coil (see red bar labeled c and compare this to the pacing lead b). The ICD coil can be placed transvenously (c) or epicardially (C). The vector for the ICD system is important and one should imagine the coil as one shocking paddle and the generator as the second shocking paddle. Each "paddle" needs to surround the heart to defibrillate. The black arrows represent the shocking vector for the ICD system.

PART III. SPECIAL CONSIDERATIONS

Table 41-1. Pacemaker nomenclature.

	1st	2nd	3rd
	Chamber Paced	Chamber Sensed	Mode of Response
	A = Atrium V = Ventricle D = Both	A = Atrium V = Ventricle D = Both O = None	I = Inhibit (sensed event inhibits pacing) T = Trigger (sensed event triggers pacing) D = Both (inhibits and triggers pacing) O = None
AAI	This mode will sense the atrial activity and will pace the atrium at the lower rate limit (LRL) unless the sinus/atrial rate is above the LRL.		
VVI	This mode will sense the ventricular activity and will pace the ventricle at the LRL unless the ventricular rate is above the LRL.		
DDD	This mode can sense both the atrium and the ventricle. It can perform 4 different functions: AsVs = senses both the A and V AsVp = senses the atrium and paces the ventricle ApVs = paces the atrium and senses the ventricle ApVp = paces the atrium and ventricle		
AAI→ DDD	This mode (typically programmed in Medtronic devices) means the device will function in the AAI mode but if there are 2 out of 4 p waves without a QRS, the device will switch to the DDD mode to allow dual chamber pacing, if needed. This program is for patients with generally intact AV conduction with intermittent heart block. It encourages normal AV conduction as much as possible.		
AOO/ VOO DOO	This mode will pace the atrium (AOO) or ventricle (VOO) or both (DOO) at the set rate and will not look for any sensed beats. It is important that while pacing in this mode, one is well above the normal heart rate. Otherwise, inappropriate pacing can induce atrial or ventricular arrhythmias.		
VDI	This is an unusual mode to be programmed. The device will sense both the atrium and ventricle but will only pace the ventricle.		

occurs with physical activity. In response, the pacemaker will automatically increase the pacing rate of the chamber programmed.

Placing a magnet over the pacemaker will force the device to operate in an asynchronous mode: DOO in a dual-chamber device or VOO/AOO in a single-chamber device. Placing a magnet over an ICD will turn off therapies.

Pacemaker-mediated tachycardia (PMT) refers to tachycardia caused by interaction of the pacing system with the patient. Classically, this is an endless-loop tachycardia typically in a dual-chamber system when a premature ventricular contraction (PVC), loss of atrial capture, a prolonged PR, or atrial under- or oversensing result in retrograde atrial conduction that is sensed as an atrial event by the pacemaker, which then triggers DDD pacing.

Transesophageal Pacing

Transesophageal pacing (TEP) can be used for diagnostic and therapeutic intervention. The 5 Fr soft bipolar catheter is placed through the nares into the esophagus, similar to a feeding tube. It can be placed at the bedside. Once the lead is placed, the location is confirmed using a standard ECG. TEP is helpful to diagnose relationships between atrial and ventricular electrograms and can be used to pace the atrium to terminate reentrant supraventricular tachycardia (SVT). This method can be particularly helpful in the neonate with SVT or intra-atrial reentrant tachycardia (IART) in CHD.

Temporary Pacing

Temporary pacing wires are placed following certain cardiac operations. By convention, atrial wires usually exit to the right of the sternum and ventricular wires to the left. Temporary pacing wires are usually unipolar, have a single electrode, and require a second electrode to be able to pace. This can be achieved with a second temporary pacing lead or with a subcutaneous grounding wire. Pacing energy is delivered from the negative end of the temporary pacing box. The pacing wire is placed on the negative end and the grounding or second wire is placed on the positive end.

Programmable settings available in external temporary pulse generators include: pacing rate, atrial and/or ventricular output amplitude (milliamperes, mA), atrial and/or ventricular sensitivity (millivolts, mV) or asynchronous mode, A-V interval (milliseconds, msec), postventricular atrial refractory period (PVARP), and upper rate tracking. Programming of a temporary pacemaker should be guided by the clinical scenario and by testing of sensing and stimulation thresholds:

- **Rate.** Should be set at a physiological rate for age that provides adequate cardiac output for their postoperative hemodynamics. For overdrive suppression of an arrhythmia, the rate is set 10 to 20% higher than the arrhythmia rate.
- **AV delay.** This is the PR interval and is usually set automatically based on the rate, or between 100 and 150 msec.
- **Upper rate.** Represents the upper rate that the pacemaker will track the atrium in DDD mode. How high this is set is determined by the clinical scenario and by the total atrial refractory period (TARP) (AV delay + PVARP). The maximum the upper rate can be programmed will be 60,000/TARP.
- **Sensitivity.** The sensing threshold is the minimum electrical activity that the pacemaker is *able to sense*. The lower the sensitivity setting, the less electrical activity needed for the pacemaker to sense (i.e., greater sensitivity). In order to determine sensitivity, the patient must have an underlying rate in the chamber that is being tested. The pacemaker is set on a synchronous pacing mode (AAI, VVI, or DDD) and the rate is set lower than the underlying rate. The sensitivity setting is increased (i.e., decreasing sensitivity) until the pacemaker stops sensing and starts pacing. The sensitivity setting is then decreased (i.e., increasing sensitivity) until every cardiac depolarization is sensed. This represents the sensing threshold. The sensitivity should then be set at half of that sensing threshold. In patients with no underlying rhythm, sensitivity is typically set at 2 mV. If the sensitivity is set too high, the pacemaker can potentially not see electrical activity and overpace, which can lead to pacemaker-induced arrhythmias. If the sensitivity is set too low, the pacemaker might underpace due to inhibition by electrical noise.
- **Capture thresholds.** It is the minimum amount of energy required to stimulate the myocardium. To determine the threshold, the pacemaker rate is set above the underlying rate so the pacemaker is consistently pacing. The output is then decreased

until capture is lost. In order to provide a safety margin, the output should be set at twice the capture threshold.

For patients requiring temporary pacing, pacemaker settings should be interrogated daily. This should also include determining underlying rhythm and continued need for pacing. A second pulse generator and battery should be available at all times.

An atrial ECG obtained using temporary atrial pacing wires can provide diagnostic information in certain arrhythmias. To perform an atrial ECG, the temporary atrial wire can be hooked up to V1, or if two leads are available, hooked up to "right arm" and "left arm", which will display in lead I.

Suggested Readings

Valdes SO, Kim JJ, Miller-Hance WC. Arrhythmias: Diagnosis and management. In: Andropoulos DB, Stayer S, Mossad EB, Miller-Hance WC (eds). Anesthesia for Congenital Heart Disease. 3rd ed. John Wiley and Sons; 2015.

42 Ventricular Assist Devices

Sebastian C. Tume, Hari P. Tunuguntla, Jack F. Price, Barbara A. Elias, Robin Rae Schlosser, Iki Adachi

Treatment of children with end-stage heart failure has been revolutionized by the development of progressively smaller-in-size durable ventricular assist devices (VAD). The Texas Medical Center has played a crucial role in VAD development. In 1966, the first successful human VAD was implanted by Dr. DeBakey, and in 1969, Dr. Cooley attempted the first clinical application of the total artificial heart (TAH). Such historical background had a profound impact on the development of the VAD program at TCH, which is recognized as the largest program of its kind worldwide. VAD support has become the standard therapy for end-stage heart failure in adults, resulting in an exponential increase in the number of implants worldwide over the last decade. Likewise, VAD therapy is becoming a common practice in the pediatric field, although there still remains a substantial "lag" when compared with the adult field.

Patient Selection

A decision to offer VAD support involves careful clinical assessment and excellent interdisciplinary communication in an often limited timeframe. VAD therapy should be offered if its benefits are deemed to outweigh the expected risks. The risk-benefit profiles, however, vary across different age groups, cardiac diagnoses, and institutions. The timing of initiating VAD support is critical to ensure successful outcomes in all aspects of postoperative care. The decision for mechanical circulatory support in the setting of refractory cardiogenic shock should never be delayed. This assessment must be accompanied at times by rapid deployment of short-term VAD followed by careful assessment for durable VAD candidacy once shock is reversed and end-organ recovery emerges.

The common indications for durable VAD support in children include: bridge to recovery, bridge to transplantation, and at times, destination therapy. Undetermined transplant candidacy is not necessarily a contraindication for VAD support.

All inotropic-dependent patients with suboptimal circulation should be evaluated for VAD support. Patient's size (<5 kg) and anatomy may limit their long-term mechanical support options. It is important to identify those patients in need of long-term invasive support (invasive mechanical ventilation or circulatory support) before they develop significant secondary organ failure. End-organ dysfunction is the single most important predictor of patient mortality at the time of VAD implantation; careful monitoring of end-organ function cannot be overstated.

The commonly described conditions that preclude durable VAD therapy include extreme prematurity, low body weight (<2.5 kg), irreversible multiorgan failure, active systemic infection, coagulopathy not amenable to anticoagulation, intracranial hemorrhage or irreversible severe neurologic insult, major chromosomal aberrations, and irreversible pulmonary hypertension. Additionally, there are other complicating factors to be considered when providing VAD support in children. Anatomic variations pose technical challenges, and previous surgical procedures such as systemic-to-PA

PART III. SPECIAL CONSIDERATIONS

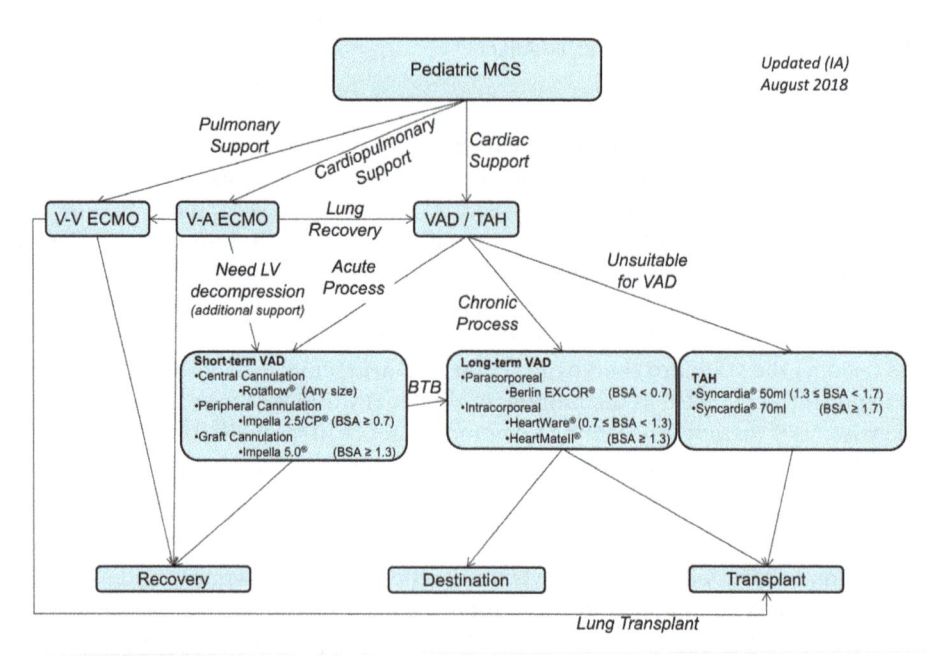

Figure 42-1. TCH mechanical circulatory support selection algorithm. BSA: body surface area, BTB: "bridge-to-bridge", ECMO: extracorporeal membrane oxygenation, LV: left ventricle, MCS: mechanical circulatory support, V-A: venoarterial, VAD: ventricular assist device, V-V: venovenous, TAH: total artificial heart.

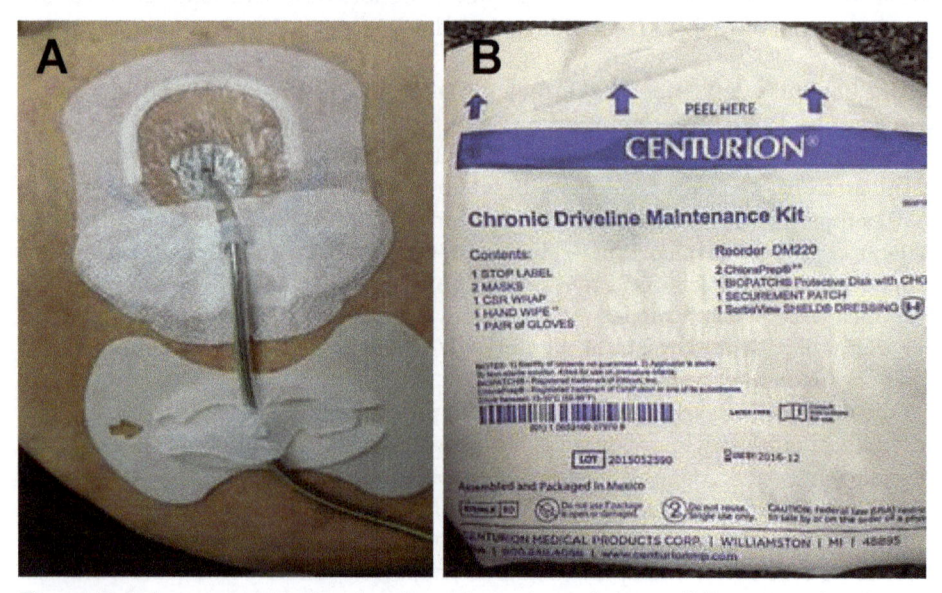

Figure 42-2. Appropriate driveline dressing and securing techniques. A) Dressing and anchoring device in place. B) Kit used for driveline maintenance and dressing.

Table 42-1. INTERMACS profiles. From Stevenson LW, Pagani FD, Young JB, et al. INTERMACS Profiles of Advanced Heart Failure: The Current Picture. J Heart Lung Transplant 2009;28:535-541.

INTERMACS profile	Profile description
1	Critical cardiogenic shock
2	Progressive decline
3	Stable but inotrope dependent
4	Resting symptoms
5	Exertion intolerant
6	Exertion limited
7	Advanced NYHA class III

shunts or disconnected caval veins after Glenn or Fontan operations may jeopardize the application of VAD therapy.

Timing of VAD implantation is crucial and to a large degree determines the trajectory of the patient's postoperative course and recovery. There continues to be a lack of accurate clinical pre-implantation assessment tools to aid with risk stratification. INTERMACS profiles (Table 42-1) are frequently used to recognize the severity of illness and make decisions. Databases such as PediMACS show that patients with low INTERMACS profiles are high-risk VAD candidates. At TCH, we have shifted away from offering durable VAD support to children with INTERMACS profiles 1 and 2, electing to first stabilize their circulation with short-term devices. The INTERMACS criteria also lacks assessment of end-organ function and fails to incorporate other comorbidities that are crucial for VAD candidacy and choice of optimal support technology. Figure 42-1 shows the TCH algorithm for selection of mechanical support.

Device Selection

Optimal device selection and avoidance of patient-to-device mismatch are critical to optimal outcome. VAD functions as a mechanical pump that augments the intrinsic function of the LV and RV to maintain cardiac output. In addition to generating cardiac output, the device must maintain function at appropriate preload and afterload pressures with minimal power consumption, have minimal activation of the inflammatory, hematologic, and immunologic systems, enable patient mobility and rehabilitation, and have a long-term endurance. Despite the variety of devices available for adults, the options for children remain limited.

The device armamentarium available at TCH is depicted in Table 42-2. Short-term devices include RotaFlow® (surgically implantable) and Impella® (percutaneous). Care must be taken when considering Impella® as it might have limited flow capability in patients with long-standing heart failure since they typically require substantially higher flows to facilitate end-organ recovery. The Berlin EXCOR® is a pulsatile-flow VAD (PF-VAD) and is the primary device for infants and small children with BSA <0.7 m^2. The HeartWare™ HVAD™ continuous-flow VAD (CF-VAD) remains our first choice

PART III. SPECIAL CONSIDERATIONS

Table 42-2. VAD selection available for circulatory support in children at TCH.

Device type	Device name	Characteristics	Patient selection	Considerations
Short-term	RotaFlow	Continuous centrifugal-flow LVAD or BiVAD	No size limitation	Used as bridge to decision
	Impella®	Continuous axial-flow Percutaneous RVAD: Impella® RP LVAD: Impella® 2.5, CP, 5.0* **Device flow, sheath size:** RP: 4 L/min, 11 Fr 2.5: 2.5 L/min, 13 Fr CP: 4 L/min, 14 Fr 5.0*: 5 L/min, 21 Fr Flows might be limited with RV failure or abnormal position *Impella® 5.0 requires surgical implant	**Patient selection:** based on size of the ventricle and access vessel, and the etiology of heart failure **Anatomic requirements:** LV long diameter >7 cm Aortic annulus >1.5 cm Severe hemolysis might restrict full flow/support	**Common uses:** High-risk cath procedures Acute circulatory support Examples: myocarditis, graft failure, refractory arrhythmias or as LA vent with VA-ECMO **Avoid with:** mechanical valves mod-severe AI/AS aortic disease LV thrombus intracardiac shunt
Long-term Pulsatile	Berlin EXCOR®	Paracorporeal LVAD or BiVAD	**Patient size:** >5 kg, BSA <0.7 m^2 **Available device sizes:** 10, 15, 25, 30, 50, and 60 mL pumps 5, 6, 9, 12 mm cannulas	**Use:** Bridge to transplant **Avoid:** severe AI severe MS CHD
	SynCardia (Total Artificial Heart)	Intracorporeal	**Patient size:** 50cc: BSA 1.2-1.7 m^2 70cc: T10 to sternum >10 cm, BSA >1.7 m^2	**Use:** Bridge to transplant Biventricular failure Examples: coronary vasculopathy **Avoid:** High PVR
Long-term Continuous Flow	HeartMate II	Intracorporeal Axial flow LVAD or BiVAD	**Patient size:** BSA ≥1.2 m^2 **Support parameters:** 6000-15000 RPM, up to 10 L/min	**Use:** Bridge to transplant or destination
	HeartWare	Intracorporeal Centrifugal flow LVAD or BiVAD	**Patient size:** BSA ≥0.7 m^2 **Support Parameters:** 1800-3200 RPM, up to 10 L/min	**Use:** Bridge to transplant or destination

BiVAD: biventricular assist device, LVAD: left ventricular assist device, RVAD: right ventricular assist device, VA: Venoarterial

Table 42-3. Structural and physiologic differences between pulsatile and continuous flow VADs

Pulsatile-flow devices	Continuous-flow devices
Positive displacement pumps undergoing filling and ejection period Pneumatic mechanism drives filling and ejection Flow (output) = HR x SV (chamber volume) Arterial pressure tracings reflect systole and diastole with palpable pulses	Continuous flow dependent on the rotational speed of the impeller and the pressure differential (aorta to ventricle) across the pump Sensitive to inflow (preload) and outflow (afterload) environments Presence of pulsatility is dependent on the intrinsic ejection of the native ventricle

HR: heart rate, SV: stroke volume

for children with BSA >0.7 m^2. Biventricular support can be achieved using any of the devices as biventricular support (BiVAD) or SynCardia TAH (where size permits).

Surgical Implantation
The key principle of surgical implantation of a VAD, irrespective of the type of device, is to complete the implant procedure while preserving end-organ function and RV function. If the end organs are severely compromised, the patient may not tolerate the invasive operation, even in the setting of optimal cardiac output. This is why timing of VAD implantation is so critical. In adults, there has been a dramatic change over the last decade shifting away from implant for impending death or progressive decline on inotropes (i.e., INTERMACS profiles 1 or 2) to elective surgery in more stable outpatients with chronic heart failure (i.e., INTERMACS profiles 3 or 4). As the pediatric field still lags behind the adult field, pediatric patients typically undergo surgery at a more advanced stage, requiring more careful management and end-organ preservation.

Intraoperative monitoring is crucial to determine appropriate device setting and optimize its function. LA lines and central venous catheters (CVC) are inserted in all patients, and pressures are monitored to assess the degree of ventricular unloading and evidence of right heart failure (RHF). The LAP is used to establish intraoperative degree of LV unloading at the time of device support titration. Intra- and postoperative TEE imaging allows assessment of the aortic valve for evidence of AI, position of the outflow cannula, and presence of ASDs. TEE is also used to measure the effects of VAD function such as degree of MR, ventricular septal position, and severity of RV dysfunction, which will help guide postoperative CICU management.

Postoperative Management
Familiarity with the basic function and structure of VADs is essential for optimal postoperative patient management and troubleshooting of VAD-related issues. Table 42-3 describes the major physiologic and structural differences between pulsatile- and continuous-flow VADs. In general, a VAD has 5 basic elements: the pump, the inflow and outflow cannulas, a controller/driver, and connection to the power source (battery or power adapter).

The postoperative course can be accompanied by numerous complications related to the preoperative clinical state of the patient, as well as physiologic/hemodynamic changes associated with VAD support. Table 42-4 lists some of the most common postoperative scenarios and their effect on VAD function. The use of hemodynamic monitoring is essential to provide optimal care and prevent some of the common complications. Each patient should have left- and right-heart pressure monitoring to provide accurate information in case of acute hemodynamic changes. Arterial BP should be monitored in all patients. In patients with CF-VADs that have minimal pulsatility, cuff pressure and pulse oximetry are unreliable, and BP should be measured manually using a Doppler and a cuff. We also encourage monitoring of oxygen delivery using NIRS technology.

Appropriate ventilator management and optimization of lung volume to reduce PVR cannot be overstated. PVR can be elevated due to atelectasis, pleural effusions, or pulmonary edema, which should be immediately treated. Typically, patients are extubated within 48 hours after surgery unless chronically ventilated prior to VAD placement.

Postoperative bleeding may be a problem after VAD placement. In addition to surgical bleeding, VAD therapy predisposes patients to additional bleeding risks through the use of anticoagulation for the device or coagulopathies such as acquired von Willebrand disease or liver dysfunction. Chest tube output should be monitored carefully, especially when titrating anticoagulation. Ongoing significant bleeding (>2 mL/kg/hr) must be urgently addressed as it can result in tamponade physiology, leading to suboptimal VAD preload and compromised flows.

RHF after VAD implantation is associated with significant morbidity and mortality. Commonly, right heart dysfunction may be observed in the OR, where initial therapies such as iNO and inotropic medications are instituted and the chest may be left open. In an attempt to prevent worsening of RHF, caution should be taken to control heart rate and rhythm, optimize RV afterload, avoid volume overload, and institute inotropic therapies when appropriate. CVP monitoring is very helpful. A rising CVP in the face of low LAP is suggestive of RHF and should be treated urgently. If elevated PVR is suspected, iNO and/or nebulized prostacyclin should be utilized. Some high-risk patients or those with significant RHF may require transition to sildenafil to enable early extubation and prevention of potential exacerbation of the disease. Right VAD support is rarely necessary but may be entertained in cases of severe refractory RHF.

Cerebrovascular events are a significant cause of morbidity and mortality in VAD patients. Neurologic injury is more common in PF-VAD compared with CF-VAD, and should be kept in mind as the patient transitions to full anticoagulation. Patients with poor device output and suction events are at a higher risk of thrombus formation due to stasis and turbulence. Close neurologic monitoring is essential and any behavioral or neurologic changes should be immediately addressed. Head CT is the primary imaging modality as current VAD technologies are not MRI compatible. CT may lack the diagnostic sensitivity to identify ischemic events, especially early in the course of the event, but should be able to identify hemorrhagic events.

Infections remain frequent in pediatric VAD patients. Nondevice infections are most common and can be easily treated with medical therapy. Device-related infections might require device replacement. Fever should be evaluated immediately with blood

42. VENTRICULAR ASSIST DEVICES

Table 42-4. Common continuous-flow VAD scenarios

Pump flow change	Clinical condition	Hemodynamic changes					Pump parameters			
		CVP	LA/PCWP	MAP	SvO$_2$/NIRS	Power	Pulsatility/Filling	Flow
Decreased flow index	Right heart failure	←	→	<->	→	<->	→	→
	Tamponade	←	↑ or no change	→	→	→	→	→
	Hypovolemia	→	→	→	<->	<->	→	→
	Hypertension	<->	← or no change	←	<->	<->	←	→
	Inlet obstruction or inlet clot	←	←	→	→	→ less than expected	→	<->
Increased flow index	Fluid overload	←	←	←	←	←	←	←
	Vasodilation	→	→	→	<->	<->	→	←
	Aortic insufficiency	<->	←	→	→	←	→	←
	Motor clot	←	←	→	→	←	→	← falsely high

CVP: Central venous pressure, LA: left atrial pressure, MAP: Mean arterial pressure, PCWP: Pulmonary capillary wedge pressure, SVO$_2$: Mixed venous saturation

319

cultures and appropriate antibiotic therapy. The driveline entry site requires frequent dressing changes as minimizing entry-site irritation helps facilitate wound healing.

Acute renal failure is commonly related to preoperative renal injury. CPB, use of diuretics, or elevated CVP due to RHF can further exacerbate renal injury. Optimizing systemic perfusion pressures and maintaining a low CVP helps optimize renal perfusion pressures and facilitate renal recovery. If present, hemolysis should be urgently addressed, as elevated levels of plasma-free hemoglobin can exaggerate renal injury.

Driveline Care and Transition to Home Environment

Driveline care is managed initially by the VAD coordinator and then by family members. Sterile driveline dressing changes occur daily until the wound sutures are removed and then transition to changes every Monday, Wednesday, and Friday, plus as needed after showering. Dressing kits that utilize BIOPATCH® and Tegaderm™ are the most convenient. Figure 42-2 shows appropriate driveline dressings and anchoring. Aquacel® Ag is used for those patients with signs of driveline infection or fat necrosis. Minimizing driveline mobility and irritation of the skin is crucial for optimal healing. We routinely document driveline sites and photo images in order to track healing.

Physical and occupational therapy are an integral part of the multidisciplinary team. Patients begin mobilizing as soon as medically tolerated, focusing on activities of daily living, strengthening, and mobility. The 6-minute walk test and functional mobility are monitored to track progress. Patient and family education is reinforced in all therapy sessions and local field trips are encouraged between hospital floors and play areas.

VAD education begins prior to implantation and escalates after. Education manuals including videos help reinforce new concepts and terminology. Advanced education should concentrate around driveline care, understanding controller and battery/power connection, common alarm simulations, and controller-exchange sessions with all caregivers taking part. The discharge binder contains emergency contacts, a letter to emergency medical services (EMS), a copy of the medication sheet, clinic appointments, device log, patient manual, EMS-controller exchange card, and a VAD luggage tag. In addition, patients are given an equipment bag to house batteries, charger, AC- and DC-power adaptors, and dressing supplies. Competency checklists are helpful to document progress and adherence to protocols, and to ensure a successful discharge and success in the community.

Full community involvement is encouraged. VAD teaching to the local fire department/EMS, place of worship, and schools is arranged by the VAD coordinator. A phone landline must be in place for secure emergency contact. Emergency phone contacts must be established and include a VAD-emergency line. Out-of-town patients are required to reside close to TCH for at least 3 months, with regular clinic visits. When cleared by the medical team, patients are allowed to return to their local home area with monthly clinic visits. The ultimate goal is to return the VAD-supported patient to a "new mode of normalcy and lifestyle" in which quality and safety are a priority.

Suggested Readings

Adachi I. Continuous-flow ventricular assist device support in children: A paradigm change. J Thorac Cardiovasc Surg 2017;154:1358-1361.

Adachi I, Khan MS, Guzmán-Pruneda FA, et al. Evolution and impact of ventricular assist device program on children awaiting heart transplantation. Ann Thorac Surg 2015;99:635-40.

Rich JD, Burkhoff D. HVAD flow waveform morphologies: Theoretical foundation and implications for clinical practice. ASAIO J 2017;63:526-535.

Rosenthal DN, Almond CS, Jaquiss RD, et al. Adverse events in children implanted with ventricular assist devices in the United States: Data from the Pediatric Interagency Registry for Mechanical Circulatory Support (PediMACS). J Heart Lung Transplant 2016;35:569-577.

43 Extracorporeal Membrane Oxygenation

Patricia Bastero, James A. Thomas, Cole Burgman, Aimee Liou, Iki Adachi

Extracorporeal membrane oxygenation (ECMO) refers to several interdependent technologies that operate in concert to support cellular respiration in patients with respiratory failure, cardiac failure, or both. It consists on removing deoxygenated blood through a cannula inserted into a vein (or venous reservoir such as the RA), driving the blood through an oxygenator that removes CO_2 and oxygenates the blood, and pumping it back into the body through a cannula placed into an artery (venoarterial [VA] ECMO) or a vein or venous reservoir (venovenous [VV] ECMO).

Cardiac ECMO (VA ECMO)

Indications
VA ECMO substitutes the gas exchange function of the lungs and the systemic distribution of blood performed by the heart. It is used for either isolated cardiovascular disease (e.g., ventricular stunning, arrhythmias, cardiomyopathy), or combined respiratory and cardiovascular disease (e.g., sepsis) poorly responsive to medical support alone.

Cardiac output (CO) on VA ECMO is defined by the following formula:

$$CO = \text{flow in circuit} + \text{residual intrinsic CO}$$

Flow on ECMO depends on:
- Cannula size (the larger the cannula, the better the flow)
- Cannula location
- Intravascular volume
- SVR

Cannulation Strategies
The patient's flow requirements and vessel size drive the cannulation strategy discussion. Patients with normal metabolic requirements need normal or mildly increased flow (typically 75-110% of their estimated CO), whereas patients with dramatically increased metabolic needs (e.g., high-output septic shock) may need flows that exceed 200-300% of normal CO. The cannula size (both diameter and length) determines flow rates through the ECMO circuit, but vessel diameter dictates cannula size.

VA cannulation can be accomplished in 2 ways:

Flow Calculations and Dilutional Calculations

CICU/PICU:
Patients weighing <10 kg
  Flow = Wt (kg) x 150 mL/min

Patients weighing >10 kg
  Flow = BSA x Cardiac Index

NICU:
All patients
  Flow = Wt (kg) x 100 mL/min

$$BSA = \sqrt{\frac{Ht\ (cm) \times Wt\ (kg)}{3600}}$$

Note: If no height can be found to calculate BSA, then mL/kg/min can be used until a height can be determined. See mL/kg/min chart.

Cardiac Index		mL/kg/min	
0-2 yrs:	3.0	0-10 kg:	150
2-4 yrs:	2.8	10-15 kg:	125
4-6 yrs:	2.6	15-30 kg:	100
6-10 yrs:	2.5	30-50 kg:	75
>10 yrs:	2.4	>50 kg:	65

Figure 43-1. Chart used to calculate appropriate ECMO flows depending on age and size.

43. EXTRACORPOREAL MEMBRANE OXYGENATION

- **Peripheral cannulation.** Venous cannulation is performed most commonly through the right IJ vein or a femoral vein, and arterial cannulation is performed through the right carotid artery or a femoral artery. Femoral access is more commonly used in larger children (>30 kg), adolescents, and adults.
- **Central cannulation.** Used when the patient's flow requirements exceed the flow limits of cannulas placed peripherally or when direct cannulation and venting of the LA is required. Short, wide-bore cannulas are placed directly into the RA and the ascending aorta through a median sternotomy.

Avoidance of left-heart distention is important, especially when trying to optimize myocardial recovery. Inadequate left-heart decompression can also lead to pulmonary edema. As such, active cardiac decompression is particularly important when the cardiac function is so depressed that the heart is unable to pump against the pressure generated by the ECMO circuit. Options for active cardiac decompression include: creation of an ASD in the cath lab (for patients on peripheral VA ECMO), placement of a vent into the LA (for patients on central ECMO), or insertion of an Impella® device in the cath lab through either the femoral or axillary arteries (for patients >30 kg).

TCH General Guideline to VA ECMO Canulation

Patient Weight	Neck (Medtronic Biomedicus) Venous	Neck Arterial	Groin (Maquet HLS) Venous	Groin Arterial	Central (Medtronic DLP) Rt Atrial	Central Lt Atrial	Central Arterial	Tubing
< 2kg	8/10	8			14	12	8	1/4
2-2.9 kg	10	8			16	12	8	1/4
3-3.9 kg	12	10			16	12	10	1/4
4-4.9 kg	12	10			18	14	10	1/4
5-5.9 kg	12	10			20	14	12	1/4
6-6.9 kg	14	10			20	14	12	1/4
7-7.9 kg	14	10			20	16	12	1/4
8-8.9 kg	14	12			20	16	12	1/4
9-9.9 kg	14	12			20	16	12	1/4
10-12 kg	14	12			20	16	14	3/8
13-14 kg	14	14			22	18	14	3/8
15-16 kg	14	14			22	18	14	3/8
17-18 kg	May need neck cannula due to size		19	15	22	18	14	3/8
19-20 kg	May need neck cannula due to size		19	15	24	18	14	3/8
21-25 kg	May need neck cannula due to size		19	15	24	18	16	3/8
26-30 kg			21	15	24	18	16	3/8
31-35 kg			21	15	24	18	16	3/8
36-40 kg			23	17	26	18	16	3/8
41-45 kg			25	17	26	20	16	3/8
46-50 kg			25	17	26	20	16	3/8
51-60 kg			29	19	28	20	18	3/8
61-65 kg			29	21	28	20	20	3/8
66-70 kg			29	21	28	20	20	3/8
>70 kg			29	21	30	20	22	3/8

Figure 43-2. Cannulation and circuit selection chart for VA ECMO.

PART III. SPECIAL CONSIDERATIONS

Prime Constituents

CV/PICU Neonate/Infant - 200 mL (1/4-1/4) <10 kg

1. Fresh RBC	2 units
2. FFP	1 unit
25% albumin	100 mL (if FFP not available)
3. Heparin	200 units
4. NaH$_2$CO$_3$	25 mEq*
5. CaCl$_2$	500 mg*

NICU Neonate - 200 mL (1/4-1/4) <10 kg

1. Fresh RBC	2 units
2. Heparin	200 units
3. NaH$_2$CO$_3$	15 mEq*
4. Ca gluconate	200 mg*

CV/PICU Pediatric/Adult - 500 mL (3/8-3/8) >10 kg

Without Blood:	With Blood Only:	With Blood & FFP:
1. Plasmalyte 400 mL	1. RBC 2 units	1. RBC 2 units
2. 25% albumin 200 mL	2. Heparin 1000 units	2. FFP 1 unit
3. Heparin 1000 units	3. NaH$_2$CO$_3$ 15 mEq	3. Heparin 1000 units
4. NaH$_2$CO$_3$ 10 mEq	4. CaCl$_2$ 200 mg	4. NaH$_2$CO$_3$ 25 mEq
5. CaCl$_2$ 200 mg		5. CaCl$_2$ 500 mg

*These amounts are what you should start with. After prime gas, you may need more.

Figure 43-3. Prime constituents for different patient populations.

Management

VA ECMO for Cardiac Support

VA ECMO for cardiac support aims to optimize tissue oxygen delivery (DO$_2$) to meet local metabolic demands and decrease myocardial work. VA ECMO helps with myocardial recovery by "unloading" the heart. This is accomplished by: 1) decreasing ventricular end-diastolic pressure, which optimizes coronary perfusion pressure and decreases wall stress, 2) improving BP, and 3) decreasing myocardial work by assuming much of the "pumping" function of the heart. Coronary perfusion occurs in a retrograde manner from blood returning into the ascending aorta from the arterial cannula, and in a prograde manner if there is aortic valve opening. Proper oxygenation of that blood is important to prevent coronary ischemia.

The CO provided by VA ECMO usually approximates 80% of the total CO, as there is always some blood return to the pulmonary veins from bronchial and collateral vessels that is then ejected through the aortic valve (provided there is enough cardiac function to do so). This residual endogenous CO helps prevent blood stasis and inappropriate cardiac unloading. Sometimes, to achieve aortic valve opening, inotropic agents and/or vasodilators to decrease SVR may be required. If this is inadequate, active cardiac decompression will be necessary.

CO on VA ECMO depends on preload (circulating volume), flows (dependent on cannula size and location), and afterload (dependent on SVR and return cannula size and position). DO_2 depends on all of these factors in addition to oxygen carrying capacity, which is determined by hemoglobin (Hb) concentration. As such, DO_2 on ECMO can be enhanced by optimizing intravascular volume, increasing ECMO flows, controlling SVR, and increasing the Hb concentration >10 g/dL.

ECMO-CPR
ECMO-CPR refers to VA-ECMO cannulation while providing CPR due to the lack of return of spontaneous circulation. The best results are obtained when ECMO is instituted within 25-30 minutes of the start of a witnessed arrest. The most common cannulation strategy is peripheral VA ECMO as the procedure is faster than central cannulation (unless there is a fresh sternotomy). For details about ECMO-CPR, see Chapter 72.

Circulatory Support for Sepsis
VA ECMO is used as a rescue therapy in selected cases of refractory septic shock. Patients with severe vasoplegia and sepsis-induced myocardial dysfunction may be cannulated centrally and placed on high-flow VA ECMO. These patients have experienced better-than-expected survival rates, given prior dismal experiences with peripheral VA ECMO for this condition. These ECMO runs are usually short, with circulatory recovery occurring 2-4 days following cannulation.

Respiratory Support While on VA ECMO
ECMO takes over the ventilation and oxygenation function of the lungs. Mechanical ventilation support is therefore only needed to prevent lung collapse. The strategy used at TCH is to minimize ventilator-associated lung injury by limiting the rate to 8-10 breaths per minute, optimizing the PEEP to prevent lung collapse (8-10 cmH_2O), and minimizing the PIP (maximum of 20-25 cmH_2O). The use of the ventilator to optimize CO_2 removal and oxygenation is limited to those circumstances where there is still significant RV preload and output, as the gas exchange for that blood will depend on lung parenchymal conditions and thus affected by the mechanical ventilation strategies.

In general, at full VA-ECMO flows and with minimal RV preload and output (indicated by a low end-tidal CO_2), a lung-protective strategy would be set using the following parameters: PIP 20-25 cmH_2O, inspiratory time 1 sec, PEEP 8-12 cmH_2O, FiO_2 30-40%. Lung recruitment is followed with daily CXRs, and the ventilatory support is titrated to optimize PVR and achieve functional residual capacity (FRC) (see Chapter 56).

In situations where there is significant cardiogenic pulmonary edema (e.g., severe MR) and/or pulmonary hemorrhage, PEEP levels may need to be increased to provide a "tamponade" effect. PEEP helps by opening airways, recruiting alveoli and, possibly, redistributing excess lung water to sites where it interferes less with gas exchange.

Weaning
Weaning patients from VA ECMO for cardiac support requires evidence of improving cardiovascular function. Return of heart rate variability, control of dysrhythmias,

decreased vasoactive medication requirements, and improving pulse pressure indicate a recovering myocardium. A preliminary assessment of weaning readiness may involve decreasing ECMO flows to 30-50% predicted CO. This increases cardiac preload, and permits evaluation of the myocardial contractile response to that increased load. If a patient becomes tachycardic, hypotensive, and/or develops lactic acidosis, the patient may not be ready to wean or may need additional inotropic support for a successful separation from ECMO. Contractile function should also be assessed by echocardiogram on decreased ECMO flows to help predict how the heart will perform off mechanical support.

It is important to prepare the patient for a successful wean. To that end, it is essential to optimize ventilator support, institute appropriate inotropic therapy before weaning (to give the vasoactive medication time to work), optimize hematocrit level (>30%), and minimize excess oxygen consumption with adequate sedation and analgesia.

Respiratory ECMO (VV ECMO)

Most ECMO in CICU patients is VA. It provides both cardiovascular and respiratory support. Rarely, cardiac patients develop isolated severe gas exchange problems (oxygenation or ventilation). In these instances, they may be placed on VV ECMO until their respiratory disease improves enough to continue treatment with mechanical ventilation and adjunctive medical therapies.

CICU patients needing VV ECMO arrive by one of two routes. First, they may have been initially treated for multisystem disease, including heart and lung disease, with VA ECMO. As the cardiac dysfunction resolves but severe respiratory illness persists, the patient is converted from VA to VV ECMO until lung function recovers. Alternatively, patients in the CICU recovering from surgery or acquired heart disease, develop new or worsening respiratory failure, necessitating primary VV cannulation.

Indications

The indications for respiratory ECMO are severe, progressive respiratory failure unresponsive to conventional or unconventional mechanical ventilation. Several criteria can be used to determine the severity of respiratory failure:
- Oxygenation Index (OI) >30-40. OI is calculated by the following formula:
$$OI = (FiO_2 \times \text{mean airway pressure} \times 100) / PaO_2$$
- Oxygen Saturation Index (OSI) >12.3. OSI substitutes PaO_2 in the OI formula for SaO_2:
$$OSI = (FiO_2 \times \text{mean airway pressure} \times 100) / SaO_2$$
- P/F Ratio <70. This is calculated as: PaO_2 / FiO_2.
- Hypercapnic respiratory failure as manifested by pH <7.2 or $PaCO_2$ >90 mmHg on 2 or more blood gases
- Milder defects in oxygenation or ventilation combined with severe air leak syndrome

In general, the OI is the preferred method to score oxygenation defects in invasively ventilated patients (OSI would be alternative, though no ECMO thresholds have been accepted), as it accounts for the mean airway pressure and not just the ventilator FiO_2 and patient PaO_2.

Cannulation Strategies

When possible, patients who are candidates for respiratory ECMO should be cannulated at a single site. The preferred cannulation site is the right IJ vein with a double lumen VV-ECMO cannula, with or without a second cephalad venous drain in the same vessel. In this setup, deoxygenated blood is drained from the IVC and either the RA or intrahepatic IVC (as well as the jugular bulb with a cephalad drain), and oxygenated blood is returned to the RA directed towards the tricuspid valve to enter the RV and then be ejected to the lungs.

Alternatively, 2-site VV-ECMO cannulation is an option. The IJ and femoral veins are the most commonly cannulated vessels, with catheter tips in the RA and intrahepatic IVC. The ECMO circuit is usually configured so that deoxygenated blood is drained from the RA and returned to the IVC, though there may be circumstances when this is reversed.

Management

Ensuring Adequate Tissue Oxygen Delivery (DO_2)

VV-ECMO runs tend to be much longer than VA-ECMO runs since the lungs take more time to recover. As such, it is important to maximize conditions that ensure adequate DO_2, favor pulmonary recovery, and avoid sedation toxicity.

The major determinants of DO_2 are arterial blood oxygen content (CaO_2) and CO. CaO_2 is calculated according to the following formula:

$$CaO_2 \text{ (mL/100 mL of blood)} = 1.34 \times [Hb] \times SaO_2 + 0.003 \times PaO_2$$

DO_2 is the product of CaO_2 and CO, as expressed in the following formula:

$$DO_2 \text{ (mL/min)} = 10 \times CO \times CaO_2$$

In VV ECMO, SaO_2 will be – and *should be* – lower than in VA-ECMO patients, usually in the 70-80% range. The most common way to increase DO_2 in patients on VV ECMO is to increase their Hb concentration with transfusion of RBCs. It is not uncommon to maintain patients with a Hb of 13-15 g/dL and SaO_2 of 70-75%, as long as their SvO_2 is >60%, their lactate remains low, and their cerebral NIRS are stable. More infrequently, DO_2 can be increased by either adding inotropic support (to increase CO), or, even more rarely, reducing oxygen consumption (using sedation, neuromuscular blockade, or mild cooling).

Managing Recirculation

Recirculation occurs when oxygenated blood from the circuit is captured by the venous limb of the circuit and passed again through the ECMO circuit. Signs of recirculation include dropping patient arterial saturations and rising saturations of the venous drainage. The blood on the venous side of the circuit will have almost the same bright-red color as the blood postoxygenator. Recirculation is quantified using the following equation:

$$\text{Recirculation (\%)} = (S_{pre}O_2 - SvO_2) / (S_{post}O_2 - SvO_2) \times 100$$

$S_{pre}O_2$ and $S_{post}O_2$ refer to the blood oxygen saturations pre- and postoxygenator, respectively.

Managing recirculation may require multiple maneuvers to ensure adequate DO_2

including decreasing pump flow rates, adding inotropic support, infusing volume, correcting anemia, repositioning cannulas, reducing intrathoracic or intra-abdominal pressures, and adding venous drains at different sites.

Fostering Pulmonary Recovery

Optimizing the conditions to allow for pulmonary recovery is an important goal when managing patients on VV ECMO. Some important strategies to foster this include:

- **Reduce ventilator settings.** In the CICU, lung disease requiring VV ECMO is usually the result of infection or inflammation and some degree of ventilator-induced injury. How much the ventilator contributes to overall lung injury is unknown. However, it seems reasonable to assume that higher pressures, higher rates, and more days on the ventilator cause more damage than lower pressures and fewer cycles of distention and release. The therapeutic goal should be to minimize or eliminate the iatrogenic contribution to lung injury. In general, if a patient remains intubated or ventilated during VV ECMO, PEEP is reduced to 8-10 cmH$_2$O, PIP is limited to 20-25 cmH$_2$O, respiratory rate is set at 8-12 breaths per minute, and FiO$_2$ is reduced to 21-30% until the lungs begin to show spontaneous recovery.

- **Maintain airway clearance.** It is important to maximize efforts to clear the airway including discontinuation of neuromuscular blockade, mechanical clearance treatments, and frequent direct bronchoscopy, in order to prevent large-airway obstruction and promote distal-airway secretion removal.

- **Low threshold for diagnostic curiosity.** Many patients on VV ECMO will experience complete lung "whiteout" during their course. Lack of alveolar air renders intrathoracic structures indistinguishable on CXR and may hide processes preventing spontaneous reaeration of the lungs, such as a pleural effusion or intraparenchymal hematoma. When a patient's lungs remain consolidated longer than expected for the disease process, this should trigger a search for plausible causes including intrapleural processes (revealed by ultrasound or CT) or large-airway obstruction (identified by bronchoscopy).

Weaning

Weaning patients from VV ECMO is different from tapering them off VA ECMO. The question to be answered is straightforward: "Have the patient's lungs recovered sufficiently to support adequate oxygenation and ventilation?". Ideally, the patient should remain on VV ECMO until pulmonary recovery permits return to "nontoxic" ventilator settings. A patient who is starting to improve will experience reaeration of consolidated lungs, increasing SaO$_2$ without changes in ECMO FiO$_2$, and improving tidal volumes on stable pressure settings.

To determine the patient's readiness to wean off ECMO, ventilator settings must be increased to full-support levels and the oxygenator taken offline. To do this, both the inlet and exhaust gas ports must be capped off. If the patient tolerates this "capping trial" for 1-2 hours, the patient is decannulated.

ECMO Circuit and Monitoring

Prior to initiation of ECMO, it is important to determine: 1) the optimal blood flow range to optimize DO_2 for the patient, 2) the optimal cannula and circuit size, and 3) the blood products and solutions required for priming of the pump. Appropriate blood flows are calculated based on either mL/kg/min for patients <10 kg or based on BSA and cardiac index (CI) for patients >10 kg (Figure 43-1). Once the necessary blood flow is calculated, the optimal cannula and circuit size are selected based on the chart on Figure 43-2. The blood products and medications needed for priming of the ECMO circuit are detailed on Figure 43-3. All of these charts and flowsheets are attached to each of the ECMO pumps.

Renal-support devices are routinely used during ECMO. The most common type of renal assistance is ultrafiltration. This is the process of small-protein fluid passing through a semipermeable membrane by the use of a hydrostatic pressure difference. The byproduct is the passive movement of solutes through convection. The removal of fluid in the ultrafiltrator is controlled by the transmembrane pressure and blood flow. Fluid removal can be increased by increasing transmembrane pressure, increasing blood flow into the ultrafiltrator, restricting blood outflow, or changing the waste-side pressure. The use of the ultrafiltrator must be monitored closely. If too much fluid is removed, the patient can develop acute renal failure.

If the patient has renal failure, ultrafiltration may need to be transitioned to dialysis. Dialysis can be performed with the current ultrafiltrator if the patient is <20 kg by running the dialysate countercurrent to the blood. Larger patients require placement of a separate dialysis pump, which can be placed inline with the ECMO circuit or by using a separate dialysis catheter inserted into the patient.

Cannulation Strategies and Technique

The decision as to which cannulation technique (i.e., central vs. peripheral) is offered should be made on an individual basis considering the goal of ECMO support and overall picture of the patient (e.g., coagulopathy). The usual cannulation approach on peripheral VA ECMO is the neck (common carotid artery and IJ vein) in small children (<30 kg) and femoral cannulation in larger children. There is still some debate about the appropriateness of carotid cannulation in older patients, because of the risk of stroke on the ipsilateral side, though large retrospective studies have failed to find significant evidence to support the claim.

VA cannulation can be accomplished via ultrasound-guided percutaneous approach, the "open percutaneous" technique (surgical vascular exposure followed by needle puncture under direct visualization and Seldinger-guided serial vessel dilation and cannulation), or surgical cutdown with venotomy/arteriotomy and direct cannula insertion. No technique has demonstrated superiority and different operators are more comfortable with different techniques. The two latter techniques allow for the surgeons to secure the cannula directly to the vessels. This decreases the risk of cannula dislodgement, but may complicate decannulation, sometimes requiring the incision to be reopened.

In case of VV cannulation, placement of a double-lumen cannula in the right IJ vein is our method of choice. Similar to VA cannulation, this can be achieved percutaneously or surgically. It is critical to optimize the depth and direction of the cannula so the outlet port of the cannula (i.e., where the oxygenated blood exits) points toward the tricuspid valve. This optimization can be done with echocardiographic guidance (at the bedside) or fluoroscopy (at the bedside, in the OR, or in the cath lab).

Anticoagulation

At this time, our anticoagulation strategy of choice is IV heparin. At the time of cannulation, an IV heparin bolus is given (50-100 Units/kg), which will cause a transitory elevation of activated clotting time (ACT). A continuous heparin drip is typically started when ACT is <200 sec. The anticoagulation plan should be made when the patient is stabilized on ECMO support at the end of cannulation. The range parameters for ACT, heparin level, PTT, and fibrinogen are set for every patient and left documented by the patient's bedside. In general, desired parameters are 180-220 sec for ACT, 0.2-0.4 U/mL for heparin levels, 60-80 sec for PTT, and >250 mg/dL for fibrinogen. In addition, we aim for an antithrombin (AT) ≥80%, a platelet count >100,000 /mcL, and normal INR. The ECMO panel includes all the previously labs as well as D-Dimer and PT levels. The ECMO panel is checked every 6 hours, with the exception of ACT, which is measured every 1-2 hours. A ROTEM® is run daily for a better understanding of each ECMO patient's homeostasis. Plasma-free Hb levels, a marker of hemolysis, are checked daily and the goal is to keep them <150 mg/dL, as higher levels may cause kidney injury. If the plasma-free Hb levels are >150 mg/dL, the ECMO circuit, or parts of it, may need to be changed. These are obviously reference goal parameters and may vary based on the patient's specific needs.

Bivalirudin is an alternative anticoagulant that is gaining widespread acceptance for VAD management at TCH, as well as other pediatric heart centers in North America. Bivalirudin has also been used in select ECMO patients at TCH. The strength of bivalirudin over heparin is the fact that the former is much less dependent on the inflammatory status of the patient, which can result in less fluctuation in the anticoagulation effects.

The transfusion medicine team at TCH rounds with the CICU team daily on every ECMO patient to help optimize their anticoagulation management.

Sedation on ECMO

Within minutes of ECMO initiation, or after a circuit change, the patient will require additional sedation and analgesia boluses, as sedative concentrations in the fresh-blood prime are much lower than they were in the blood prior to cannulation (or in the old circuit). Preferred starting agents include continuous infusions of a benzodiazepine (e.g., midazolam) and morphine or hydromorphone as opioids (less adherence to ECMO circuit as per a TCH pharmacy study).

On VA ECMO, an acute rise on SVR is commonly seen right after ECMO flows start. Appropriate sedation is fundamental to manage that SVR and be able to run at desired flows to adequately support the patient and optimize DO_2.

Since many respiratory ECMO runs are longer than cardiac ones, intubated ECMO patients develop sedation complications, including habituation, tolerance, delirium, and need for multiple medications with different mechanisms of action. Removing major irritants like the endotracheal tube (by extubating or placing a tracheostomy) may be more effective in preventing sedation complications than treating those complications with polypharmacy.

Sedation is monitored hourly using an objective sedation scale, the State Behavioral Scale (SBS) (see Chapter 55). The goals of sedation are discussed on daily rounds and vary depending on the patient's condition. Daily holidays, brief cessations of continuous infusions, should be part of the respiratory ECMO sedation regimen.

Catheter-Based Procedures in Patients Requiring Mechanical Support

Impella®
The Impella® device is a catheter that bears an impeller pump. It can be placed percutaneously or surgically, and drives blood forward coaxially through the vessel in which it is situated. It supports the patient by augmenting forward CO and promoting ventricular unloading, allowing for improved end-organ perfusion and decreased myocardial workload.

Versions of the Impella® device can be used for support of the systemic or pulmonary circulation. Impella® catheters designed for systemic circulatory support (2.5, CP, 5.0, LD) are positioned across the aortic valve such that they draw blood through an inlet port in the LV and impel it through the catheter and out of an outlet port in the ascending aorta. The Impella® RP is designed for pulmonary circulatory support and is placed such that it draws blood from the inferior vena cava and impels it through an outlet port in the PA.

The function of the Impella® catheter is monitored and controlled via a controller console that remains by the patient's side. The console allows for titration of output and displays information on catheter position and hemodynamics in real time. Additional information on catheter position can be obtained as needed by bedside echocardiography.

Currently, the Impella® is used primarily for short-term support of CO, although successful medium-term use has been reported. Impella® devices can also be used as temporary support during cath procedures. Rapid percutaneous Impella® catheter placement can be performed in clinical scenarios demanding emergent support of cardiac output. It can also be used as an adjuvant for left-heart decompression while on VA ECMO.

The Impella® device can be placed in the femoral artery, axillary artery, ascending aorta, or femoral vein (for RP).

ASD Creation
In various clinical scenarios, patients with an intact atrial septum who are supported with VA ECMO may develop LA hypertension and pulmonary edema secondary to incomplete left-heart unloading. In these cases, catheter-based atrial septal interventions are performed to decompress the left heart. Infrequently, a conventional balloon atrial septostomy performed in the style of Rashkind procedure can be employed. In many patients, however, the atrial septum is too thick for this technique. An ASD is

therefore created by one of various other means, including transseptal puncture followed by static balloon dilation, blade septostomy, or atrial-septal stent placement.

Suggested Readings

Coleman RD, Goldman J, Moffett B, et al. Extracorporeal membrane oxygenation mortality in high-risk populations: an analysis of the Pediatric Health Information System Database. ASAIO J 2019; doi: 10.1097/MAT.0000000000001002.

Philip J, Burgman C, Bavare A, et al. Nature of the underlying heart disease affects survival in pediatric patients undergoing extracorporeal cardiopulmonary resuscitation. J Thorac Cardiovasc Surg 2014;148:2367-2372.

44 Heart Transplantation

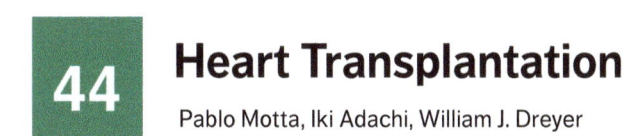

Pablo Motta, Iki Adachi, William J. Dreyer

TCH performed its first successful heart transplant in an 8-month-old child with dilated cardiomyopathy in November, 1984. Since that time, the heart transplant program has grown to be one of the largest and most successful programs of its kind in the world. In 2018, the program surpassed 400 transplants performed.

Indications and Contraindications

Heart transplantation becomes an option in any patient with end-stage heart disease (ESHD) that cannot be managed by other medical or surgical intervention. This includes any of the cardiomyopathies (dilated, hypertrophic, restrictive, or LV non-compaction) or CHD. Most patients with CHD have had prior surgical palliation, which has failed. Other patients are born with such complex CHD that there is no good surgical palliation available to them. Cardiac retransplantation may be indicated in patients whose primary grafts fail. The most common cause of graft failure is transplant-associated coronary vasculopathy.

At TCH, there are a few conditions that are considered absolute contraindications to cardiac transplant (Table 44-1).

Recipient Evaluation

Patients being considered for cardiac transplantation undergo a comprehensive evaluation process. That process begins with a detailed conversation with family members discussing evaluation, listing, the surgery itself, and postoperative follow-up. That discussion also includes the indications, risk and benefits of transplant as well as an expected lifestyle and prognosis for the patient. There is also a review of our institutional volumes and outcomes relative to other centers across the country.

The evaluation process includes an extensive panel of bloodwork designed to assess end-organ function in the patient, provide a roadmap of prior infection, and assess the patient's current immune status and human leukocyte antigen (HLA) sensitization. Imaging beyond standard CXR and echocardiograms may be required. Imaging is tailored to the individual needs of the patient but might include chest CT or MRI, as well as cardiac catheterization. A baseline ECG and Holter are required. In addition to transplant cardiology and CV surgery evaluations, the patient is seen by the transplant immunology and transplant infectious disease services. The patient is also seen by pharmacy, occupational and physical therapy, and nutrition. Consultation is required with our medical social worker, child life, and financial counselor. If possible, neuropsychological and developmental testing is also obtained. If this initial screening evaluation determines any additional concerns, additional consults may be obtained. Patients are commonly seen by the renal, neurology, and pulmonary services in order to complete their evaluation. Following acquisition of all of this information, a multidisciplinary medical review board meeting is held. Each consultant is asked

PART III. SPECIAL CONSIDERATIONS

Table 44-1. Contraindications to cardiac transplantation.

Absolute contraindications	Comments
• Untreatable malignancy	
• Progressive and untreatable liver disease	
• Severe fixed elevated PVR	PVR >6 Woods units per m² measured in the cath lab, despite intervention with pulmonary vasodilator therapy
• Severe chronic obstructive pulmonary disease	
• Psychiatric disorder	Prevents a patient from adhering to or being able to comprehend their posttransplant care
• Hemodynamic compromise	MSOF such that the patient is unlikely to recover despite transplantation

Relative contraindications	Comments
• Active infection	
• Recent pulmonary infarction	
• HIV infection	
• Peripheral vascular disease	
• Chronic systemic illness with multiorgan involvement	
• History of noncompliance	
• Absence of a responsible caretaker	
• Current drug and/or alcohol addiction	Patient or parent caretaker
• Absence of resources to support transplantation and posttransplant follow-up	Including medications, living expenses and/or proper maintenance of a transplant environment, transportation, and medical care
• BMI >35 kg/m²	
• Severe neurologic impairment	
• Pregnancy	

BMI: body mass index, MSOF: multi-systemic organ failure

to present their findings to the group at large and, finally, a vote for the candidacy of transplantation is obtained.

Listing Status
The United Network of Organ Sharing (UNOS) maintains the listing status for all patients (pediatric and adult) awaiting all solid organ transplantation. Their protected website is accessed through the internet. Potential pediatric donor heart recipients are actively listed into 1 of 3 separate categories:
- **Status 1A.** The highest priority category is status 1A. Patients meet criteria for status 1A listing if 1) they require continuous mechanical ventilation; 2) they require assistance with an intra-aortic balloon pump; 3) they have a ductal-dependent systemic or pulmonary circulation with ductal patency maintained by stent or prostaglandin infusion; or 4) they have hemodynamically significant CHD and require infusion of multiple IV inotropes or high doses of a single IV inotrope. Any patient that requires the assistance of mechanical circulatory support, either temporary or durable, meets 1A listing status.
- **Status 1B.** Patients qualify for 1B status if they require infusion of one or more inotropic agents but do not qualify for pediatric 1A status, or if a patient is <1 year of age at the time of initial registration and has the diagnosis of hypertrophic or restrictive cardiomyopathy.
- **Status 2.** All patients that are actively listed but do not meet status 1A or status 1B criteria are then listed status 2.

Patients are eligible for ABO incompatible heart offers if they are <2 years of age and their isohemagglutinin titers are ≤1:16. When a patient is eligible to receive a potential donor offer, our center is contacted to review the donor offer and determine if the donor offer is medically and surgically acceptable. Our center remains open 24/7 to receive donor offers.

Donor Evaluation
The donor evaluation process begins with a thorough review of the donor medical history. In particular, the cause of death and the presence or absence of downtime/CPR are important. Infectious history, malignancy, social history, and high-risk behaviors are important too. However, this crucial information is often unclear. Objective data (e.g., echocardiography, inotrope use, serum sodium, troponins) are also critical. The final decision regarding organ suitability is made by the procuring surgeon under direct vision. Typically, the recipient surgery starts only after the final decision has been made.

Surgical Technique
At TCH, we prefer to utilize the "bicaval" technique, in which the systemic venous return is reconstructed at the level of the caval veins (i.e., SVC and IVC). This is superior to the classic "biatrial" technique where the donor and native right atria are sewn together, as it preserves tricuspid valvar competency as well as electrical conduction. The downside includes the possibility of anastomotic stenosis, particularly at the SVC in small recipients. In patients with complex CHD, significant technical challenges exist, which may require modifications to the standard technique. One example is the

Table 44-2. Anesthetic and perioperative considerations following heart transplantation.

	Mechanism	Consideration	Treatment
Early considerations			
Sinoatrial dysfunction	Disruption of sinoatrial node	Severe bradyarrthmias	Temporary pacing, alpha 1-agonist (e.g., isoproterenol or epinephrine)
Ventricular dysfunction	Ischemia-reperfusion injury Recipient pulmonary hypertension Suboptimal organ preservation	Diastolic dysfunction RV dysfunction	Inodilators (milrinone) Epinephrine Optimize ventilation with 100% FiO_2 iNO Temporary VAD or ECMO
Late considerations			
Denervation of the donor heart	Disruption of baroreceptor reflex	Minimal HR response to: - Hypovolemia - Orthostatic changes - Anticholinergics	Use of direct agonist pheniléphrine to increase SVR Epinephrine to increase CO and HR
Graft dysfunction	Chronic rejection	Ventricular dysfunction	Inotropic need Temporary VAD
Coronary artery vasculopathy		Coronary perfusion-pressure dependent	Maintain CPP Phenylephrine Correct anemia if present Temporary VAD

CO: cardiac output, CPP: coronary perfusion pressure, HR: heart rate.

presence of bilateral Glenn anastomoses; in select situations, the left Glenn is left in place, while the right Glenn is taken down for reconstruction with the donor right SVC.

Anesthetic and CPB Management

The conduct of anesthesia varies depending on the etiology of heart failure (CHD vs. no CHD) and/or the need for pretransplant VAD support. Patients on VAD support are usually physiologically more stable and tolerate better the induction of anesthesia. All repeat-sternotomy patients (e.g., palliated CHD and VADs) have a longer intraoperative course due to increased surgical complexity and a higher risk of postoperative bleeding.

Since ESHD is exquisitely sensitive to changes in loading conditions and contractility, the goals of induction of anesthesia are to maintain preload, afterload, heart rate, and contractility. The majority of ESHD patients have long-term IV access (e.g., PICC line) due to the need for chronic inotropic support. IV induction with etomidate (0.3 mg/kg), ketamine (1-2 mg/kg), or a combination of fentanyl (5-10 mcg/kg) and midazolam (0.05-0.1 mg/kg) is the usual approach to achieve the established hemodynamic goals. Preoperative inotropic therapy, usually milrinone, is continued during the induction and pre-CPB period. Escalation of inotropic needs, such as adding epinephrine, is indicated in patients with evidence of poor systemic perfusion (e.g., low SvO_2, poor cerebral oximetry, or lactic acidosis). Maintenance of anesthesia is achieved with a balance technique of synthetic opioids, low-dose inhalation anesthetics, and non-depolarizing muscle relaxants.

In addition to standard ASA monitors, heart transplant patients need invasive hemodynamic monitoring (arterial and central line), cerebral oximetry, hourly diuresis monitoring, and TEE. Ultrasound-guided vascular access is needed in continuous-flow VAD patients due to a lack of pulsatility. In addition, ultrasound is invaluable to diagnose the patency of vessels.

CPB is accomplished by bicaval and aortic cannulation, mild hypothermia, and aortic cross-clamping for the left atrial and aortic anastomoses. The left heart is deaired under TEE guidance and the aortic cross-clamp is usually removed after completion of these anastomoses. After unclamping of the aorta and while rewarming, the IVC, pulmonary artery, and SVC are anastomosed. Exchange transfusion is used in infants with ABO incompatibility. Patients with CHD who have aortic arch hypoplasia or a prior Norwood procedure require deep hypothermia and aortic reconstruction with the donor arch under circulatory arrest or antegrade cerebral perfusion. Donor heart ischemic times are minimized with the goal of staying under 4 hours.

Once all anastomoses are completed and inotropes are started (milrinone and low-dose epinephrine), the patient is weaned off CPB. TEE is useful to assess ventricular function (especially RV function), visualize the venous anastomoses (exclude IVC/SVC stenosis), and rule out major valvar anomalies. iNO is used in patients with evidence of RV failure and at risk for pulmonary hypertension. Rarely, temporary VAD and/or ECMO are needed in case of primary graft dysfunction. The majority of the patients are kept intubated postoperatively until the transplanted heart function is stable and coagulation abnormalities are corrected. Dexmedetomidine is often used for postoperative sedation. Although previously a standard medication, the use of isoproterenol has been in decline because of supply shortages, but may constitute an adjuvant for chronotropy and even inotropy when pacing and standard inotropes are insufficient.

Table 44-2 describes some anesthetic and postoperative considerations on patients after heart transplantation.

Posttransplant Surveillance

Following heart transplantation, patients recover postoperatively as any other surgical patient. Patients are immunosuppressed, which increases the risk of infection and changes the use of other drugs which may interact with their immunosuppression drugs. Unless the donor and recipient are both cytomegalovirus (CMV) negative, CMV prophylaxis is required. This includes administration of CMV immunoglobulin (Cytogam®) early posttransplant and every 2 weeks posttransplant for the first 3 months. Patients also receive daily IV ganciclovir and are then transitioned to PO valganciclovir when appropriate, and continue for the first 3 months.

Patients must undergo surveillance for rejection. Routine surveillance biopsies are performed at 2, 4, 8 and 12 weeks after transplant. An additional biopsy is performed

Table 44-3. TCH cardiac transplant steroid protocol.

Intraoperatively	Methylprednisolone[a] 10 mg/kg/dose	Every 12 hours while in OR
POD # 1	Methylprednisolone[a] 5 mg/kg/day	Divided in 3 doses
POD # 2	Methylprednisolone[a] 2.5 mg/kg/day	Divided in 3 doses
POD # 3-6	Methylprednisolone[a] or oral prednisone[b] 1 mg/kg/day	Divided in 2 doses
POD # 7-13	Methylprednisolone[a] or prednisone[b] 0.8 mg/kg/day	Divided in 2 doses
POD # 14	Prednisone 0.5 mg/kg/day	One dose
	NO REJECTION	**REJECTION (only one)**
1 month	Prednisone[b] 0.4 mg/kg daily	0.5 mg/kg daily
2 months	Prednisone[b] 0.3 mg/kg daily	0.4 mg/kg daily
3 months	Prednisone[b] 0.2 mg/kg/daily	0.3 mg/kg daily
4 months	Prednisone[b] 0.2 mg/kg/daily	0.2 mg/kg daily
6 months	Prednisone[b] 0.1 mg/kg daily	0.1 mg/kg daily
8 months	Prednisone[b] 0.05 mg/kg daily	
9 months	Prednisone[b] 0.05 mg/kg every other day	
10 months	STOP	

Dosing guidelines for steroids: Use 50 kg as max weight – initial postoperative dose should not exceed 250 mg. Chronic/recurrent rejection within the first year will require individualized wean.
[a] Intravenous administration. [b] Oral administration.
POD: postoperative day.

at 6 months posttransplant and then annually, beginning one year after transplant. Patients <7 kg are monitored noninvasively without biopsy.

Surveillance biopsies for younger patients are usually done under general anesthesia. Patients older than 8-12 years old are catheterized under sedation with spontaneous ventilation. This is commonly achieved with a combination of propofol, ketamine, and/or dexmedetomidine.

Acute cellular rejection is determined by the pathologist using light microscopy and is scored according to the revised International Society for Heart and Lung Transplantation (ISHLT) biopsy grading system as 0R (no rejection), 1R (mild rejection), 2R (moderate rejection), or 3R (severe rejection). Rejection scores 2R or 3R require treatment with enhanced immunosuppression. Antibody-mediated or humoral rejection (AMR) is determined by immunostaining for C4d deposition in a vascular pattern within the biopsy and by corroboration of donor specific antibodies (DSA) when C4D positive.

Patients are also seen between their biopsies for the first year posttransplant at varying intervals. Following the first year posttransplant, patients are routinely seen every four months, twice during the year for clinic visits, and once for cardiac catheterization and biopsy.

Table 44-4. TCH posttransplant medication protocol.

Tacrolimus	
Start 48 hours posttransplant. Dose start at: 0.08/mg/kg/day BID PO/NG. Therapeutic levels: • 0-12 months: 10-12 ng/mL • 1-2 years: 8-10 ng/mL • >3 years: 6-8 ng/mL	
Cyclosporine (CYA)	
Start 48 hours posttransplant if not able to take Tacrolimus PO/NG or previously on CYA. Dose start 1 mg/kg/24hrs continuous IV (levels usually ~200 ng/mL). When used as chronic oral immunosuppressive, therapeutic levels: • 1st 3 months: 300-350 ng/mL • 3-12 months: 250-300 ng/mL • 1-2 years: 200-250 ng/mL • >3 years: 150-200 ng/mL	
Mycophenolate	
Start immediately pretransplant and continue posttransplant. Dose start at: 20 mg/kg/dose IV/PO every 12 hours. Max dose: 1500 mg. If WBC 4,000-5,000 /mcL, reduce therapy by 50%.	
Steroids	
Start intraoperatively and then continue posttransplant per protocol.	
CMV therapies	
Only for donor- and recipient-positive and when there is donor and recipient mismatch. • **Cytogam**®. Give within 24-48 hours post-transplant. Dose: 150 mg/kg/dose every 2 weeks for the 1st three months. • **Ganciclovir.** Give 48-72 hours posttransplant (1 day after Cytogam). Dose: 5 mg/kg/dose IV Q12 hours. Need to adjust dose for abnormal kidney function.	
Sirolimus	
Not immediately after transplant. Usually added when there is posttransplant coronary artery vasculopathy or for renal sparing. Usual level: 2-5 ng/mL If used in conjunction with CYA or tacrolimus: • CYA: run CYA level 80-120 ng/mL. • Tacrolimus: run Tacrolimus + Sirolimus (combo) at 10-12 ng/mL	

BID: bis in die (twice a day), CMV: cytomegalovirus, CYA: cyclosporine, NG: nasogastric, PO: per os (by mouth).

Immunosuppression and Management of Rejection

Routine immunosuppression at TCH includes mycophenolate mofetil (Cellcept®) 20 mg/kg IV given pretransplant and every 12 hours thereafter, as well as methylprednisolone 10 mg/kg/dose given intraoperatively and every 12 hours. Postoperatively, steroids are weaned according to protocol (Table 44-3). When the patient can tolerate enteral administration, tacrolimus (Prograf®) is started. Dosing is highly variable dependent upon absorption and metabolism. The starting dose is 0.08 to 0.1 mg/kg/day divided every 12 hours and levels are required to establish a therapeutic dose. Tacrolimus dosing is highly affected by other medications, particularly antibiotics. Therapeutic target tacrolimus levels are based on time out from transplant (Table 44-4). Initially, we attempt to achieve serum levels of 10 to 12 ng/mL. Given its WBC-count suppression properties, Cellcept® dosing is determined using WBC (target >4,000 cells/μL) rather than serum level.

Empirically, rejection treatment is started with IV methylprednisolone 10 mg/kg/dose for a total of 4 doses (every 8 hours). Additional treatment of rejection is determined by endomyocardial biopsy results. In grade 2R acute cellular rejection with normal cardiac function, no additional therapy is required. If a patient has grade 2R cellular rejection with hemodynamic compromise or grade 3R acute cellular rejection, a course of antithymocyte globulin is typically required for 3 to 7 days. If a biopsy suggests the presence of AMR, additional therapy is required and is directed at both the reduction of circulating anti-HLA antibody (plasmapheresis) and prevention of additional production of anti-HLA antibody (IV immunoglobulin G). To prevent further production, patients typically receive rituximab, which is a monoclonal antibody directed at CD20-positive B lymphocytes. Circulating B-cell elimination is accomplished with 1 to 4 doses provided on a weekly basis. A repeat biopsy following treatment of both acute cellular rejection or AMR is typically performed to determine therapeutic effect. In cases of unrelenting AMR, eculizumab (C5 complement protein blocker) or bortezomib (proteasome inhibitor to target plasma cells) may be used.

Outcomes and Complications

Transplant outcomes include waitlist mortality and posttransplant outcomes. In general, the higher the pretransplant complexity, the higher the risk of waitlist mortality. At TCH, there has been a substantial improvement in waitlist survival with the introduction of VAD support as a bridge to transplant. There are 2 groups of patients in whom waitlist mortality remains suboptimal; one subset is neonates/infants with complex single ventricle on which VAD support options are limited, and the other is small infants with cardiomyopathy on which VAD support has been offered less frequently over time.

In terms of posttransplant outcomes, there has been a substantial improvement in early mortality. Such improvement is likely multifactorial and includes better donor selection, organ preservation, and perioperative management. Late outcomes saw dramatic improvement following the introduction of cyclosporine in the 1980s, but nothing as significant since. Chronic rejection and/or transplant coronary vasculopathy are the primary reasons for late attrition. TCH-specific outcome data are publically available online (https://www.srtr.org/transplant-centers/texas-childrens-hospital-txtc/?organ=heart&recipientType=adult&donorType=).

45 Heterotaxy Syndrome

Heather A. Dickerson

Heterotaxy syndrome (HS) constitutes a constellation of defects based on issues with laterality in the body's organs. Several gene loci have been identified and initial genetic screening should be offered in every child diagnosed with HS. HS affects many organs but the most clinically relevant in infancy are cardiac defects, which can be severe.

In general, HS can be classified into right-atrial isomerism (RAI; asplenia) or left-atrial isomerism (LAI; polysplenia), depending on whether there's predominance of right-sided or left-sided structures, respectively. Patients with RAI have 2 morphologic RAs and lungs, and usually no spleen. On the contrary, patients with LAI have 2 morphologic LAs and lungs, in addition to polysplenia. This classification, although not 100% specific, can help categorize cardiac defects as the rhythm and venous anomalies follow the "duplicated" and "missing" atria. Patients with RAI have a higher likelihood of pulmonary venous issues and tachyarrhythmias. Those with LAI are more likely to lack sinus and AV nodes and are at a higher risk for bradyarrhythmias. They are also more likely to have an interrupted IVC with separate hepatic vein insertion.

Cardiac Involvement

Initial management of patients with HS focuses on palliating their cardiac defects. Very frequently, these patients have single ventricle cardiac lesions – most commonly, unbalanced atrioventricular septal defects (AVSD) with double-outlet right ventricle and malposed great vessels. Initial surgical/interventional management is based on whether the pulmonary valve is normal, stenotic, or atretic, and whether the patient needs a PA band or an additional source of pulmonary blood flow. Care must be taken to evaluate the pulmonary veins, as anomalous veins are frequently present and can require urgent repair if obstructed. It is important in the face of obstructed pulmonary veins not to over- or underestimate the amount of obstruction across the pulmonary valve. Patients will be more cyanotic due to elevated PVR and thus it is more helpful to evaluate the pulmonary valve anatomically than by the gradient obtained by echocardiography. Due to many of these patients having a single RV and AVSD-type atrioventricular valve, they are less able to handle pulmonary overcirculation, leading to ventricular dilation and increased AV valve regurgitation. For this same reason, care should be taken to assure adequate afterload reduction and diuresis.

Repair of total anomalous pulmonary venous return (TAPVR) on patients with HS can pose significant challenges for future single-ventricle palliation. In particular, the site of anastomosis of the pulmonary veins to the atria may be on the way of future Fontan completion. Patients with dextrocardia and a right-sided IVC (or hepatic veins) may require creation of an extracardiac Fontan conduit behind the mass of the heart (usually with a reinforced ringed Gore-Tex® graft).

Patients with HS are particularly prone to having arrhythmias (Niu et al. 2018). Those with RAI often have dual sinus and AV nodes that can set them up for reentrant supraventricular tachycardia and atrial tachycardia. Many patients will also have atrial suturelines (after TAPVR repair) that can also put them at risk for atrial tachycardia. Those with LAI may present with complete heart block that will need to be paced early due to their associated anatomic cardiac abnormalities.

Extracardiac Involvement

Patients with HS tend to have extracardiac organ-system involvement. All patients with HS should be assumed to be functionally, if not anatomically, asplenic. Even those with polysplenia should be treated with prophylactic antibiotics as the splenules are generally hypofunctional. Patients are especially susceptible to infections with encapsulated organisms. The literature supports prophylactic treatment at least through 5 years of age. Patients should also receive the pneumococcal vaccine. At TCH, the standard of care is to treat with amoxicillin during this period. The absence of Howell-Jolly bodies (especially in infancy) can be misleading and nuclear medicine scanning can be helpful to assess splenic function beyond infancy, but it is not reliable before this time.

Inversion of abdominal organs should be evaluated and can affect appropriate placement of a nasogastric/orogastric tube. Care should be taken to look for location of the hepatic mass and stomach bubble on initial radiography. Malrotation is frequently diagnosed and all patients should have an upper GI series to confirm this diagnosis. Initially at TCH, all patients with malrotation underwent an elective Ladd's procedure after they had stabilized from their Glenn palliation or any surgeries required in infancy. The approach has recently changed after reviewing all patients and concluding that postoperative complications after Ladd's procedure (mainly bowel obstruction) exceeded the risk of developing a volvulus (Abbas et al. 2016). Patients are now not offered surgical intervention prophylactically. All parents are now instructed that children with HS should be evaluated with any abdominal pain, obstructive symptomatology, and/or vomiting to rule out volvulus as the cause. It is also important in these children to remember that their appendix is infrequently in the "normal" position and appendicitis can present without the classic right-lower-quadrant pain. Any abdominal pain associated with fever should be thoroughly worked up. If patients have any intra-abdominal surgery, they should have an incidental appendectomy at that time for this same reason.

Bronchial anatomy follows whether patients have RAI or LAI. Patients with RAI have bilateral trilobed lungs and eparterial bronchi, while patients with LAI have bilateral bilobed lungs and hyparterial bronchi. Generally, these anatomic changes in the lungs are of no clinical consequence though should be kept in mind in those with RAI as they can have bilateral upper lobe collapse. Patients with HS can also have problems with ciliary dyskinesia and should be evaluated for this, especially if they are having recurrent pulmonary infections or obstruction.

Long-Term Follow-Up

Long-term follow-up of patients with HS needs to take into account the systemic nature of the syndrome and that multiple organ systems may be involved. In patients with pulmonary vein repairs, special attention should focus on evaluating for reobstruction and if present, proceeding with early intervention. Afterload reduction is important as the AV valves are more likely to become regurgitant than normal mitral or tricuspid valves.

It is important to control rhythm disturbances in these patients. Frequent Holter monitoring should be performed to evaluate for occult arrhythmias, as they are more frequent than in other cardiac lesions. Timing of the bidirectional Glenn procedure should be based on oxygen saturation and whether or not the patients have ventricular dysfunction and/or AV valve regurgitation, as these can improve with ventricular offloading. Some of these patients may undergo creation of a "pulsatile" Glenn (leaving some degree of prograde flow across the RVOT) due to the higher likelihood that systemic venous anatomy or PVR may preclude them from further single-ventricle palliation.

Evaluation prior to a Fontan procedure is focused at assessing hemodynamics, but also at evaluating anatomic variations that may make Fontan completion challenging, in particular systemic and pulmonary venous abnormalities. It is our preference to delay Fontan completion in these patients until symptomatically required rather than at a certain age, as baffling of anomalous venous structures is usually required and can be less challenging in larger patients. Preoperative assessment should also include evaluation for arteriovenous malformations and portosystemic shunts that can lead to cyanosis after the Fontan procedure. Portosystemic shunts should be occluded.

Transplantation is not automatically precluded in these patients as some patients can have reasonable outcomes. However, anomalies in systemic and pulmonary venous anatomy may preclude heart transplantation from a technical standpoint.

In general, the management of patients with HS involves early anatomic delineation and staged surgical palliations. Appropriate surveillance for the development of rhythm disturbances, ventricular dysfunction, significant AV valve regurgitation, or pulmonary venous obstruction is imperative. In addition, the clinician should be aware of the associated organ system abnormalities that can impact the lives of these children.

Suggested Readings

Abbas PI, Dickerson HA, Wesson DE. Evaluating a management strategy for malrotation in heterotaxy patients. J Pediatr Surg 2016;51:859-862.

Broda CR, Salciccioli KB, Lopez KN, et al. Outcomes in adults wiht congenital heart disease and heterotaxy syndrome: a single-center experience. Congenit Heart Dis 2019;doi: 10.1111/chd.12856.

Niu MC, Dickerson HA, Moore JA, et al. Heterotaxy syndrome and associated arrhythmias in pediatric patients. Heart Rhythm 2018;15:548-554.

46 Connective-Tissue Disorders

Taylor Beecroft, Lisa C. A. D'Alessandro, Justin Zachariah, Shaine A. Morris

TCH conducts a comprehensive Cardiovascular Genetics Clinic to evaluate, diagnose, and manage children with connective tissue disorders that affect the heart as well as other conditions associated with significant aortic or arterial disease. Initial evaluation of a patient in this clinic includes:
- A thorough medical history, including a detailed family history and creation of a 3-generation genetic pedigree
- Review of any prior imaging, interventions, and genetic testing
- A complete physical examination, including:
    - A standard cardiovascular and pulmonary assessment
    - An evaluation for dysmorphic features
    - A Marfan syndrome systemic score (see below)
    - A Beighton score for joint hypermobility

If appropriate genetic testing has not been performed, it will be ordered as indicated. Due to the phenotypic similarity and genetic heterogeneity observed in many of these syndromes, the most often ordered test is an aortopathy panel, which typically includes sequencing and deletion/duplication analysis for genes causing Marfan syndrome, the Loeys-Dietz syndromes, classical and vascular Ehlers-Danlos syndromes, *ACTA2* and *FLNA* smooth muscle diseases, and arterial tortuosity syndrome, among others. For ease for the family, a saliva sample is obtained in the office for this testing. Knowing that children may not meet clinical criteria for genetic testing and that some connective tissues disorders are not well-characterized in children, the threshold for testing is often low. Testing is performed if one of the conditions below is suspected, or if there is significant aortic dilation in the presence of at least one of the following: skeletal features consistent with connective tissue disorder, a Beighton score >4, a family history of a similar condition, or significant mitral valve prolapse. Results are discussed with the family by the genetic counselor and/or the cardiologist once resulted. If genetic testing identifies a pathogenic variant, genetic counseling and cascade testing are recommended for all appropriate first-degree relatives to evaluate the need for cardiovascular screening and surveillance.

Marfan Syndrome

Marfan syndrome is the most prevalent connective tissue disorder. It is a multisystem genetic disorder caused most commonly by autosomal dominant missense, premature termination, or splice-variant pathogenic mutations in the *FBN1* gene, although *FBN1* exon deletions may also cause the condition. Individuals with Marfan syndrome exhibit significant variability in features and severity, even among relatives who share the same pathogenic variant, and there is minimal genotype-phenotype correlation. The hallmark features include tall stature with disproportionately long limbs, long fingers and toes, pectus excavatum or carinatum, progressive scoliosis, myopia, ectopia lentis, aortic root dilation, and mitral valve prolapse. The cardiovascular manifestations

Table 46-1. Calculation of systemic score for Marfan syndrome by Revised 2010 Ghent Nosology. A score ≥7 is a positive systemic score (Loeys et al. 2010).

Feature	Point Value
Wrist AND thumb sign	3
Wrist OR thumb sign	1
Pectus carinatum deformity	2
Pectus excavatum or chest asymmetry	1
Hindfoot deformity	2
Pes planus	1
Spontaneous pneumothorax	2
Dural ectasia	2
Protucio acetabulae	2
Scoliosis or thoracolumbar kyphosis	1
Reduced elbow extension	1
3 of 5 facial features: malar hypoplasia, downward slanting palpebral fissures, retrognathia, enophthalmos, and dolichocephaly	1
Skin striae	1
Severe myopia	1
Mitral valve prolapse	1
Reduced upper segment/lower segment ration and increased arm span/height ratio	1

are the leading driver of early mortality in Marfan syndrome, but recent advances in management are mitigating the excess risk to approach that of the general population.

When evaluating for Marfan syndrome in the pediatric population, it is important to remember that the features of this syndrome are often more subtle in children, and additional clinical findings may evolve over time. A diagnosis of Marfan syndrome can be established in a proband with 1) a confirmed pathogenic variant in *FBN1* in addition to aortic root dilation (z-score ≥2.0) or ectopia lentis; or 2) aortic root dilation in addition to ectopia lentis or a systemic score ≥7 (Table 46-1). It is also crucial to assess the family history for signs of additional affected relatives, as Marfan syndrome is inherited in approximately 75% of cases.

Management of patients with Marfan syndrome at TCH includes:
- Cardiology follow-up and imaging.
    - Lifelong cardiology follow-up with at least annual cardiovascular evaluation and echocardiography.
    - For patients with severe dilation or an absolute root measurement ≥4 cm, we will often perform a cardiac MRI with angiography (MRA) to best assess the aorta. We will also assess the vertebral-artery tortuosity index to assist in risk stratification.
- Initiation of medical management with beta-blocker and/or angiotensin-receptor

blocker (ARB, typically losartan) in the setting of aortic root dilation; consideration should be given to initiation of prophylactic medical management at the time of diagnosis even with a normal root dimension.
    - For beta-blockers, propranolol will be prescribed to infants and toddlers, atenolol will be prescribed to grade-school children and adolescents, and metoprolol XL will be prescribed to adolescents and adults.
    - For most patients with severe dilation, or more rapid growth than is expected, dual therapy with both a beta-blocker and ARB will be recommended, if tolerated.
    - During follow-up, medication doses will gradually be increased to achieve adequate beta-blockade (heart rate drop of at least 20% from baseline or 70s bpm in younger children, 60s bpm in older children/adolescents), and maximum-dose ARB (goal 1-1.5 mg/kg losartan in most patients), as tolerated, until minimum aortic growth is noted. We define optimum treatment in growing children as an unchanging aortic dimension and a declining z-score.
- First-degree relatives should undergo known familial mutation testing whenever possible as they have a 50% chance to be affected. If genetic testing cannot be performed, we will order an echocardiogram in potentially affected relatives, although those affected can be missed by echocardiography alone.
- Encourage routine aerobic exercise with strong counseling about avoidance of competitive and contact sports and high-strain activities depending upon severity of cardiovascular manifestations.
- The indication for surgical intervention in aortic root dilation is an absolute aortic dimension >5.0 cm. In the pediatric population, this may not be applicable and the rate of change of aortic root dimension is an important consideration. Counseling is given to families regarding valve-sparing aortic root replacement versus valve-replacing root replacement (Bentall procedure). Most families of young patients will opt for valve-sparing surgery to avoid bleeding complications and lifetime anticoagulation. Intervention may be indicated at >4.0 cm in any of the following situations:
    - A woman planning a pregnancy
    - Another cardiac surgery is planned
    - A family history of dissection at an aortic root dimension <5.0 cm is noted
    - Severe vertebral-artery tortuosity is present, defined as vertebral artery tortuosity index ≥50).
    - The patient reaches 4.0 cm at a very young age (i.e., <5 years old)

Ehlers-Danlos Syndromes

The Ehlers-Danlos syndromes (EDS) are a group of genetically and phenotypically heterogeneous connective tissue disorders primarily characterized by joint hypermobility and skin hyperextensibility. There are now more than 10 recognized subtypes of EDS, which are distinguished by genotype and the presence of specific additional phenotypic features. There are 3 subtypes of EDS that most commonly present to the cardiology clinic: classical, vascular, and hypermobile EDS.

Classical EDS (cEDS)

cEDS is an autosomal dominant condition caused by pathogenic variants in *COL5A1* (and less commonly in *COL5A2* and *COL1A1*). The clinical features of cEDS include hyperelastic, fragile skin that is soft and doughy to the touch, poor wound healing with atrophic scarring, significant joint hypermobility (and complication of joint hypermobility including sprains, subluxations, etc.), easy bruising, hernias, and fatigue. While cardiovascular manifestations are uncommon, aortic root dilation and mitral valve prolapse have been reported. These patients are only typically followed in the Cardiovascular Genetics Clinic if cardiovascular manifestations are present.

Management of patients with cEDS includes:
- Cardiology follow-up and imaging.
  - If no cardiovascular features noted on initial echocardiography, either no follow-up or intermittent echocardiographic follow-up (every 5 years with echocardiography) is performed.
  - If aortic dilation or significant mitral valve prolapse is present, annual evaluation with echocardiography is performed.
  - With severe dilation or an absolute root measurement ≥4 cm, we may perform cardiac MRA to best assess the aorta.
- Medical therapy
  - Patients are not typically treated with medical therapy unless aortic dilation is moderate, as aortic dissection is exquisitely rare in cEDS.
  - If moderate-to-severe dilation is present, monotherapy with a beta-blocker or ARB may be started, with same goals as in treatment for Marfan syndrome.
- First-degree relatives should undergo known familial mutation testing whenever possible as they have a 50% chance to be affected.
- Activity limitations are usually not prescribed from a cardiac perspective, although contact sports and weightlifting are sometime advised against to protect again subluxations, hernias, and skin injury in more severely affected patients.
- Aortic surgery is rarely indicated in cEDS. If aortic dilation is present nearing surgical consideration, additional/alternative diagnoses should be considered.

Vascular-type EDS (vEDS)

vEDS encompasses a more severe spectrum of cardiovascular features, including a substantial risk for arterial aneurysm, dissection, and rupture. It is a rare, autosomal dominant disorder caused by pathogenic variants in the *COL3A1* gene. The significant fragility of the vasculature in vEDS can lead to rupture even in the absence of dilation/aneurysm or trauma. Other common features include thin, translucent skin with a propensity for easy bruising, joint hypermobility, chronic joint subluxation and dislocation, congenital hip dislocation, and pneumothorax, as well as fragility and rupture of the GI tract, uterus, and other organs. The average lifespan for individuals with vEDS is 48 years.

Management of patients with vEDS includes:
- Cardiology follow-up and imaging.
  - Lifelong cardiology follow-up is necessary. In our clinic, we perform at least annual cardiovascular evaluation. Most years include either MRA from head

to pelvis or echocardiography, although for some very stable patients with no apparent cardiovascular events or aneurysm, intermittent evaluations may only include a physical examination and BP monitoring.
    - For patients with known dilation/aneurysms, or who have had a vascular event, at least annual MRA or CTA from head to pelvis is performed.
    - BP should be monitored regularly, and hypertension should be treated promptly.
- Initiation of medical management with beta-blocker is recommended for all patients with vEDS, given a European trial that showed reduced events after celiprolol, a beta-blocker, was given. Celiprolol, a third-generation beta-blocker, is not available in the US. Therefore, we recommend similar beta-blockers, including labetalol and carvedilol, even in the absence of aortic/arterial dilation or hypertension.
- First-degree relatives should undergo known familial mutation testing whenever possible as they have a 50% chance to be affected.
- All patients are counseled extensively about risks in vEDS, and to have emergency medical provider contact information and emergency plans. Patients are provided with written material to carry with them to inform emergency personnel about vEDS.
- Encourage routine aerobic exercise with strong counseling about avoidance of competitive and contact sports and high strain activities.
- Vascular interventions and surgery are avoided as much as possible, as many reported deaths in vEDS are a result of diagnostic and prophylactic interventions, including cardiac catheterization. Surgery and arterial intervention should only be considered in collaboration/communication with a team familiar with complications of vEDS or in an absolute life-threatening emergency. Colonoscopy should also be avoided for risk of colonic rupture.
- Affected women should be counseled extensively regarding pregnancy, as pregnancy confers at least a 5.3% risk for death as a result of uterine or arterial rupture.

Hypermobile EDS (hEDS)

In contrast to vEDS, the features of hEDS occur on the milder end of the phenotypic spectrum in terms of cardiovascular features. The genetic etiology of hEDS is unknown and genetic testing is therefore *not indicated* for this condition, except in circumstances where vEDS or cEDS need to be ruled out. In hEDS, the joints are hypermobile and while the skin may still be soft and doughy, it is often less hyperextensible than other EDS subtypes. Affected individuals may also exhibit spontaneous subluxations and dislocations, easy bruising, and bowel disorders, as well as cardiovascular autonomic dysfunction with frequent episodes of syncope or near syncope. Postural orthostatic tachycardia syndrome is common and may need to be treated. Chronic pain secondary to degenerative joint disease is also a common manifestation and can be debilitating. Approximately 11-33% of individuals have mild aortic root dilation, but the risk for dissection is very low and the size typically remains stable. Therefore, mild root dilation is rarely treated with medical therapy in patients with hEDS.

Loeys-Dietz Syndromes

The Loeys-Dietz syndromes (LDS) are another group of multisystem connective tissue disorders with demonstrating similar skeletal, craniofacial, cutaneous, and cardiovascular features. All known LDS subtypes are autosomal dominant and inherited from an affected parent approximately 25% of the time. Several genes have been implicated, but pathogenic variants in *TGFBR2* (causing LDS2) and *TGFBR1* (LDS1) have been observed in 55% and 20% of cases, respectively. Less frequently, pathogenic variants in *SMAD3* (LDS3), *SMAD2* (LDS5), *TGFB2* (LDS4), and *TGFB3* (LDS5) have also been reported, but the cardiac phenotype in these patients appears milder than in LDS1 and LDS2. Given this genetic heterogeneity, panel testing is most appropriate when a diagnosis of LDS is suspected.

Similar to other disorders, LDS occurs on a phenotypic spectrum from mild to severe, and variable expressivity is observed even among relatives with the same pathogenic variant. The physical findings of LDS include pectus excavatum or carinatum, joint hypermobility, scoliosis, widely spaced and prominent eyes, bifid uvula, cleft palate, craniosynostosis, easy bruising, and translucent, velvety skin with occasional dystrophic scarring. Severe cardiovascular manifestations may be observed, including widespread abdominal, thoracic, and cerebral arterial aneurysms with significant risk for dissection and rupture. More than 95% of affected individuals have some degree of aortic root dilation. There is also frequent tortuosity of the head and neck vessels. Inflammatory disease is another common symptom, including manifestations such as eczema, asthma, inflammatory bowel disease, and increased allergic reactions to dietary and environmental allergens. Spontaneous pneumothorax, recurrent hernias, and myopia can also occur.

Arterial aneurysms in LDS may be more aggressive than those observed in Marfan syndrome. In particular, the aorta has a higher risk to dissect at smaller diameters, and dissections typically have a younger age of onset, at least in the LDS1 and LDS2 subtypes.

- Cardiology follow-up and imaging.
    - Lifelong cardiology follow-up with at least annual cardiovascular evaluation.
    - Head to pelvis MRA (or occasional CTA) is recommended every 1-3 years. In years without MRA/CTA, echocardiography is performed. We will also assess the vertebral artery tortuosity index on MRA/CTA to assist in risk stratification.
- Patients should be treated with beta-blockers and/or ARBs to decrease stress to the arterial walls and reduce the risk for dissection. Commonly, patients in our clinic are placed on dual therapy.
- First-degree relatives should undergo known familial mutation testing whenever possible.
- Encourage routine aerobic exercise. Competitive and contact sports as well as isometric exercise, including lifting weights above 30 pounds, should be strictly avoided.
- Aortic root surgery is indicated when the aortic dimensions reach 4.0-4.4 cm in patients with LDS1/2. Less is known about other LDS syndromes; we assess case by case, and recommend surgery between 4.0 and 5.0 cm.
- Pregnancy may be dangerous in women with LDS, as there is risk for aortic dissection or rupture as well as uterine rupture and death, although many women tolerate

pregnancy without a problem. Comprehensive counseling should be performed prior to pregnancy planning, and should depend on each patient's individual risks. Affected individuals who become pregnant should follow closely with a high-risk obstetrician and receive frequent aortic imaging both during and after the pregnancy.

Arterial Tortuosity Syndrome

Arterial tortuosity syndrome (ATS) is a rare connective tissue disorder. Unlike most connective tissue disorders, ATS exhibits an autosomal recessive inheritance pattern, and requires a pathogenic change to both copies of the *SLC2A10* gene. As such, both parents of the affected patient are likely to be unaffected carriers, and each of their offspring has a 25% chance of having ATS, a 50% chance of being an unaffected carrier, and a 25% chance of being an unaffected noncarrier.

As its name suggests, it causes severe vascular arterial tortuosity. In addition to significant cardiovascular findings, ATS is also characterized by skeletal, craniofacial, and generalized connective tissue features. The cardiovascular features include severe elongation and tortuosity of the aorta and other mid-sized arteries, significant risk for aneurysm and dissection, and stenosis of the aorta and pulmonary arteries. There is also an increased risk for mitral valve prolapse, valvar regurgitation, dilation of the large veins, and ischemic events affecting cerebrovascular and abdominal circulation. As with most connective tissue disorders, the cardiovascular features are the primary cause of morbidity and mortality in ATS. The extracardiac manifestations of ATS include scoliosis, joint laxity and/or contractures, arachnodactyly, camptodactyly, pectus carinatum or excavatum, high-arched palate, dental crowding, myopia, hypotonia, as well as abdominal, inguinal, and/or diaphragmatic hernia.

Patients with confirmed ATS should be monitored closely by a cardiologist. Treatment depends on specific cardiovascular findings. For those with aortic dilation, medical therapy is typically limited to a beta-blocker, as the risk of renal artery stenosis may limit the use of ARBs. They should have regular echocardiograms as well as head-to-pelvis MRAs or CTAs with 3D reconstruction to evaluate aortic dimensions and stenoses.

Heritable Thoracic Aortic Disease (HTAD) caused by *ACTA2*

HTAD is a group of disorders characterized by genetically-mediated predisposition to thoracic aortic aneurysms and dissections. While there are several genes implicated in HTAD, this section will discuss features specific to HTAD caused by autosomal dominant pathogenic variants in *ACTA2*, the most frequent cause of nonsyndromic familial HTAD. Individuals with this type of HTAD typically have fusiform aortic aneurysms that involve the aortic root, ascending aorta, and aortic arch. Arch hypoplasia and coarctation are common, as is PDA. While descending and abdominal aortic aneurysms are also possible with *ACTA2* pathogenic variants, these are less common. Syndromic forms of HTAD have also been observed in association with *ACTA2*, with some pathogenic variants conferring increased risk for early-onset stroke, coronary artery disease, and/or cerebrovascular disease. A recurrent pathogenic variant disrupting the arginine 179 (R179) residue in *ACTA2* has syndromic anomalies that include aortic coarctation, pulmonary hypertension, large PDA, gut malrotation, hypotonic bladder, congenital mydriasis, and Moyamoya-like cerebrovascular disease.

Treatment is challenging for aneurysms caused by *ACTA2*. Treatment efficacy has not yet been studied to data, but we traditionally will use ARBs or beta-blockers. However, patients are prone to baseline low diastolic pressure and high risk of stroke, especially if they have the R179 pathogenic variant. For them, hypotension can be quite risky, and often antihypertensive medications are strictly avoided. Anesthesia that is necessary for cardiac surgery may also introduce significant risk. Therefore, treatment is individualized and based on coexisting risks and morbidities.

FLNA-Related Periventricular Nodular Heterotopia (PVNH)

While *FLNA*-related PVNH is characterized as a seizure disorder caused by abnormal neuronal migration, there are associated connective tissue and cardiovascular manifestations. As its name suggests, *FLNA*-related PVNH is caused by pathogenic variants in the *FLNA* gene. In addition to seizures which are not typically observed in other connective tissue disorders, another distinguishing feature of *FLNA*-related PNVH is its inheritance pattern. This is an X-linked condition that most often exhibits prenatal or neonatal lethality in males. As such, a majority of affected individuals are female. A family history of cardiac anomalies and/or seizures primarily affecting females in an X-linked manner should indicate the need for *FNLA* or panel testing.

The cardiovascular manifestations of this condition include thoracic aortic aneurysm and dissection, coarctation of the aorta, PDA, ventricular and atrial septal defects, as well as mitral and aortic valve insufficiency. Pulmonary hypertension is also common. The unique combination of pulmonary hypertension and ascending aortic dilation should trigger suspicion for *FLNA* disease. The extracardiac features in this disorder include seizures, congenital strabismus, joint laxity, short digits, and dyslexia. The phenotype may range from mild to severe. While seizures have historically been considered the presenting feature of *FLNA*-related PVNH, recent data suggests that these patients may present to a cardiologist well before receiving a diagnosis from neurology. This indicates a need for earlier recognition and diagnosis of this disorder, which can be aided by recognizing key features in the family history in conjunction with the above cardiac manifestations.

Treatments for *FLNA*-associated aortopathy and arteriopathy have not been studied, and guidelines have not been established. For most patients, given the often severe dilation, we use a combination of ARBs and beta-blockers in affected girls. As many patients may have undergone lung transplant for the sometimes severe pulmonary manifestations, renal function must be monitored when on posttransplant medications and ARBs. There are no surgical guidelines for *FLNA* aneurysms at this time.

Suggested Readings

Loeys BL, Dietz HC, Braverman AC, et al. The revised Ghent nosology for the Marfan syndrome. J Med Genet 2010;47:476–485.

47 The Adult Fontan

Peter Ermis, Wilson Lam, David F. Vener, Charles D. Fraser Jr.

Coordinated management of patients suffering from single-ventricle anatomy and physiology has improved outcomes dramatically over the past several decades. As such, survival to adulthood following the final stage of palliation, the Fontan operation, is expected for the great majority of single-ventricle patients. The unusual nature of Fontan physiology as well as the changing modes of Fontan palliation present a multitude of challenges in caring for the adult Fontan patient. Most patients who have undergone Fontan palliation within the past 20 years have received a "modern-style" Fontan operation in the form of a total cavopulmonary connection (TCPC). This has been accomplished most commonly through the construction of a lateral atrial tunnel or more recently, through the use of extracardiac conduits. This is in distinct contrast to those Fontan connections constructed more than 25-30 years ago, which were predominantly atriopulmonary (A-P) Fontan connections. Given the long-term necessities of care and the frequent transitory nature of many patients, it is incumbent on the healthcare team to obtain surgeons' records of previous Fontan operations (or if unavailable through the use of advanced imaging) to determine the exact type of Fontan connection in a given patient. In general, patients with A-P Fontan connections tend to present with more frequent atrial arrhythmias, particularly reentrant tachycardias, than patients with TCPC Fontans, although this may be a feature of length of follow-up. Even in the absence of arrhythmias, most A-P Fontan patients should be considered for Fontan conversion surgery (see below).

Fontan Complications

Fontan palliation presents many challenges related to chronic cardiac and noncardiac complications. At approximately 20-25 years following Fontan palliation, many patients start to display some signs of these issues. As discussed in Chapter 39, close follow-up and longitudinal testing should be used to monitor Fontan patients. TCH has developed a long-term pathway care plan for these patients (Figure 39-4).

Cardiac Complications

Cardiac complications can be divided into several categories including structural, functional, and electrical. In the complex constellation of anatomic variants undergoing Fontan operations, there are many opportunities for residual or new structure abnormalities. These may include semilunar valve insufficiency, systemic outlet obstruction, pulmonary venous drainage obstruction, coronary sinus obstruction, AV valve regurgitation or stenosis, anastomotic strictures, or other pathway distortions. Any of these problems can result in compromised Fontan physiology and may be sufficient indication for a revision operation. AV valve regurgitation is an independent predictor of poor prognosis.

Fontan patients frequently develop diastolic dysfunction often leading to elevated end-diastolic pressures (EDP). This exacerbates a multitude of issues leading to elevated Fontan pressures. Systolic dysfunction tends to be less frequent, but if present, should be treated with optimizing heart failure medications and considering mechanical/surgical support in extreme cases.

From an electrical perspective, bradycardia occurs eventually in many adult Fontan patients due to sinus node dysfunction. This can lead to a marked decline in functional status due to chronotropic incompetence and should be addressed, in many cases, with pacemaker implantation. Tachycardia is common, especially intra-atrial reentry tachycardia (IART). This is often difficult to diagnose as telemetry appears similar to a sinus tachycardia with a heart rate of 120-130s. However, anytime a Fontan patient is noted to have a relatively fixed heart rate above 110s, IART should be considered.

Noncardiac Complications

A multitude of noncardiac complications in adult Fontan patients can occur stemming from elevated systemic venous pressures. Any obstruction in the Fontan pathway or branch PAs should be aggressively managed. Congestive hepatopathy is the rule, often leading to signs of cirrhosis. Routine liver surveillance is required and a hepatology team, with particular understanding and experience of Fontan physiology, should probably follow most adult Fontan patients. While liver fibrosis is commonly seen, it is relatively rare to see any classic findings of portal hypertension, and hepatic synthetic dysfunction is not typically present, particularly in early stages.

Fontan patients are also at an elevated risk for thromboembolic events on both the systemic and pulmonary sides of the circulation. Most practitioners believe that Fontan patients should be treated, at the very least, with daily aspirin and many of the more complex patients may require full oral anticoagulation. Other complications that should be monitored, and treated if present, include protein-losing enteropathy (PLE), chronic kidney disease, pulmonary venovenous collaterals, and coagulopathy.

The Failing Fontan

The term "failing Fontan" encompasses a broad spectrum of conditions from various hemodynamic and conduction abnormalities to extracardiac end-organ issues, including most frequently, the GI tract. A useful acronym – **FACET** – helps to address issues related to **F**unction, **A**rrhythmia, **C**yanosis, **E**nteropathy, and **T**hrombosis:

- **Function.** Systolic and diastolic dysfunction develop in many patients and initial anticongestive medical management is reasonable with limited data showing benefit.
- **Arrhythmia.** Brady- and tachyarrhythmias are common in adult Fontan patients. Antiarrhythmic medications can delay the need for ablation or Maze procedures. Most defibrillators are placed epicardially, but there may be a role for subcutaneous technology.
- **Cyanosis.** Cyanosis may develop from increasing Fontan pressures leading to systemic-to-pulmonary venous collaterals or due to prior surgical fenestration, both of which are amenable to catheter occlusion. However, cyanosis may recur with Fontan pressure elevation. Liver disease or misdirection of hepatic venous flow may contribute to the development of intrapulmonary arteriovenous malformations and intrapulmonary shunting, also leading to cyanosis. These may require redirection of the IVC baffle or liver transplantation.

- **Enteropathy.** Should PLE occur, reversible hemodynamic causes such as Fontan circuit obstruction or valvulopathy causing atrial hypertension should be addressed. However, this may be insufficient in advance stages. Multiple medical therapies and fenestration creation have been reported to be useful in some patients, but heart transplantation remains the mainstay in treatment of PLE.
- **Thrombosis.** As mentioned above, Fontan patients are at a higher risk for thromboembolic events. Antiplatelet therapy and anticoagulation are commonly used.

Certain patients with failing Fontan circulation may benefit from surgical interventions:
- The Fontan conversion (revision from older A-P to newer extracardiac or lateral tunnel versions combined with atrial Maze and epicardial pacemaker implantation) is an antiarrhythmic surgery for medication-refractory atrial arrhythmias best performed when ventricular function is preserved and in the absence of cyanosis.
- With newer reactive antitachycardia pacing devices, a dual-chamber epicardial pacemaker without Maze or Fontan conversion can benefit patients with chronotropic incompetence, poor hemodynamics from lack of AV synchrony, and/or medication-refractory atrial dysrhythmias.
- For medication-refractory systolic heart failure, a systemic ventricular assist device can be considered as a bridge to transplant or destination therapy after weighing the risks of thrombosis, anticoagulation, and infection.
- Heart transplantation is beneficial for pump failure, diastolic heart failure, PLE, or significant liver fibrosis prior to cirrhosis.

Anesthesia Considerations for the Fontan Patient

Anesthesia for the adult Fontan patient is aimed at assuring cardiopulmonary stability throughout the intraoperative period into the ICU transition. Because these patients have had multiple previous cardiac operations, they are at a much higher risk of bleeding during redo-sternotomy and from scar tissue during dissection. At least 1, preferably 2, large bore IVs (>18 gauge) are appropriate along with central venous access. Blood volume replacement should be geared to maintaining and/or restoring normal colloid osmotic pressure by the use of albumin 5% or FFP and PRBC as appropriate. Many of these patients have had chronic hepatic congestion and may have impaired liver synthetic function, thus impairing clotting factor production.

Some older Fontans may have had "classic" BT shunts with loss of the ipsilateral subclavian artery at some point in their care. It is necessary to know this ahead of time in order to guide noninvasive BP measurement and arterial-line location. Because of the high incidence of arrhythmias in these patients, it is appropriate to continue antiarrhythmic therapy through the day of surgery and to place external pacing/defibrillator pads on the patient once in the OR. Many of these patients also have pacemaker systems and it is strongly suggested that pacing devices be placed in a mode to avoid interference from the use of electrocautery. Ventilation should be adjusted to minimize intrathoracic pressure by utilizing as little PIP and PEEP as necessary to maintain alveolar patency and appropriate blood gases. If plastic bronchitis is present, the ETT should be irrigated and suctioned regularly to minimize airway obstruction.

Post-CPB care is directed towards normalizing intravascular status, assuring minimal surgical bleeding by the use of blood products (including factor supplements and prothrombotic agents such as Kcentra® and activated Factor 7 as appropriate). Ideally, these patients should have a postoperative hemoglobin >13 g/dL in order to maximize oxygen carrying capacity. Many of these patients will benefit from the use of low-dose vasopressin infusions, especially if they have been on angiotensin-converting enzyme (ACE) inhibitors preoperatively. Epinephrine and milrinone should be titrated based upon cardiac function as determined by intraoperative TEE.

Many of these patients will have been on aspirin therapy and will require platelet transfusion; transfusion goals may be directed by the use of advanced clotting studies such as ROTEM®. Attempts should be made to promote perioperative extubation as soon as possible, ideally in the OR, to take advantage of the supplementary effects of negative inspiration on pulmonary blood flow in the Fontan circuit. This is facilitated by the limited use of narcotics and benzodiazepines, and the use of dexmedetomidine and acetaminophen IV. Appropriate perioperative pain control with judicious use of a narcotics and nonnarcotic analgesia to minimize splinting and postoperative atelectasis is very important. As soon as the use of intraoperative electrocautery has been completed, the pacing system, if in place, should be adjusted to the most appropriate mode (typically DDD). Transfer of care to the CICU should include a complete handover including such factors as cardiac rhythm (and pacing mode), function postrepair, blood product usage, intraoperative pressures in the Fontan circuit, antibiotic and analgesia plans, and goals for airway management if not extubated.

Fontan Revision

In properly selected patients, a Fontan revision operation can confirm considerable benefit in allowing patients to have improved Fontan physiology, mitigation of secondary hemodynamic and symptomatic consequences of the failing Fontan, and the avoidance (or at least delay) of cardiac transplantation. As noted above, indications for a Fontan revision are centered on improving a correctable anatomic, functional, or electrical problem with the existing Fontan circuit. Historically, Fontan revision operations were predominantly utilized in patients with failing A-P Fontan connections. More recently, it has become clear that other forms of Fontan connection may also develop correctable problems that merit intervention.

In selecting patients for a Fontan revision, it is critical to conduct an exhaustive preoperative functional and physiologic assessment. As noted above, it is enormously useful to obtain and carefully study old operative records, including all previous palliations. Cardiac assessment should include detailed echocardiography (transthoracic or transesophageal), diagnostic (and where indicated interventional) cardiac catheterization, cardiac MRI and/or chest CTA, pulmonary function testing, and 24-hour Holter monitoring. Detailed blood work should include serum chemistries, complete blood count/indices, liver function testing, coagulation profile, and thyroid function testing (many patients are chronically treated with amiodarone and are at risk of hypothyroidism). In some patients, liver biopsy may be considered, particularly in the setting of borderline synthetic function, although interpretation of biopsy results in these patients may be very challenging. It is also critical to perform an extensive survey of vascular access as all of these patients have undergone multiple previous interventions and there may be chronic occlusions of important access vessels including the femoral arteries and/or veins, issues that need to be understood for operative planning. In patients with any history of neurologic dysfunction, a detailed evaluation by a neurologist and in most cases, brain imaging, is mandatory prior to proceeding with a surgical procedure.

In counseling patients for the revision operation, the proposed operation is discussed usually during several lengthy preoperative sessions. Patients must be informed of the very complex nature of the operation. These are typically very long procedures; operations extending for as long as 10-12 hours are not infrequent. It is very important to inform patients that revision operations were formerly associated with a very high perioperative risk of morbidity and mortality. Fortunately, in the current era, in properly selected patients, several centers have reported outstanding outcomes (our overall perioperative survivorship for all Fontan revision operations from 1995-2018 was >99%). Nonetheless, patients should know that there are alternatives. The historical mainstay of the failed Fontan has been cardiac transplantation. While a complete review of this topic is beyond the scope of this chapter, cardiac transplantation in a Fontan patient can be a very challenging and risk-laden proposition with variable results being reported. Previous anatomic distortions, situs abnormalities, chronic multiorgan dysfunction (particularly hepatic insufficiency), patient sensitization with preformed circulating antibodies, and other challenges all combine to make transplantation in Fontan patients a potentially challenging intervention. Finally, bailout strategies are always discussed, including support with ECMO and temporary and durable VAD support.

The revision operations require detailed preparation by the anesthesia team as noted above. For the surgeon, carefully planned sternal reentry is paramount. Patients with failing A-P Fontan connections may have massively dilated systemic atria, often immediately underneath the sternum. In others, the aorta or PAs may be intimately associated with the sternum. Our approach has been to proceed with careful, deliberate sternal reentry without the routine use of preemptive femoral cannulation. In most cases, with meticulous direct vision dissection, reentry can be safely accomplished. The critical, immutable key features are meticulous dissection, under direction vision and without need of hurry. Breaching these principles can be catastrophic.

Once sternal reentry has been achieved, the anatomy is carefully dissected, again with careful attention to hemostasis. CPB is then instituted with the use of separate, direct vena caval cannulation. Our routine has been to use mild hypothermia (nasopharyngeal temperature of 32 °C) for most cases. The operative plan should include complete takedown of the previous Fontan connection, often with considerable debulking of the massively dilated RA. Previous ASD patches are often calcified and should be removed, if possible. All structural deficiencies that are amenable to correction should then be addressed. These include AV valve repair or replacement, semilunar valve replacement, subaortic (systemic outlet) resection, pulmonary venous pathway obstruction relief, and repair of PA stenosis. A modified cryo-Maze procedure is performed to include isolation of potential reentrant pathways on both right and left atrial aspects. After reconstruction of the debulked common atrium, the new Fontan channel is constructed with an extracardiac tube graft (typically 24 mm Gore-Tex®) anastomosed between the divided IVC and the branch PAs. If the patient did not have superior cavopulmonary connections previously, bidirectional (bilateral in appropriate situations) Glenn shunts are constructed. Finally, it is critically important to place a dual-chamber epicardial pacing system at the end of the operation. We have favored bilateral, epicardial steroid eluting "button" electrodes. Finding an acceptable lead site can be a challenging proposition in patients who have undergone multiple previous surgeries, but with diligence, the surgeon will be able to find appropriate locations. The pulse generator is selected in coordination with the collaborating cardiac electrophysiologist (a critical relationship in the management of these patients) and should be a sophisticated device with overdrive pacing capabilities. Despite the length of these operations, we favor early extubation (typically in the OR) and rapid progress through the CICU. The typical hospital length of stay is around one week. Despite the use of Maze operations and epicardial pacing, most patients are at risk of recurrent atrial reentrant tachycardias, particularly during the first 6 months after the revision operation. As such, many centers prefer to maintain patients on oral amiodarone therapy, but this remains a somewhat controversial subject.

Cardiac Replacement Therapy

In patients with refractory heart failure in the setting of systemic ventricular dysfunction, treatment with a VAD and/or cardiac transplantation may be the only options. While each subject could merit its own separate chapter, several points are worth mentioning. We first "discovered" the utility of placing continuous flow devices in patients with failing Fontans when we placed a HeartMate II™ continuous flow device in an adult Fontan patient with profound ventricular dysfunction. We were uncertain how the Fontan circulation would perform in this setting and were pleased to observe excellent hemodynamics with improvement in Fontan pressures. This reemphasizes the critical nature of ventricular dysfunction in overall Fontan circuit performance. The patient was quickly progressed through the hospital and this experience led us to become more liberal with the use of VADs as either a bridge to transplantation or chronic "destination" therapy in appropriate patients.

Cardiac transplantation in failing Fontan patients is variously reported by different centers as prohibitively risky or of acceptable risk profile. This fact, of course, has to do with patient selection and technique. By way of patient selection, it is important to emphasize the general rule that in a failing Fontan with preserved ventricular function, something else is wrong (distorted PAs, obstructed pulmonary veins, elevated PVR to name a few) and great caution should be exercised in proceeding with cardiac transplantation. The transplant operation itself can be very challenging. Patients with multiple reoperations have increased bleeding risk, exacerbated by hepatic dysfunction, arteriovenous and venovenous collateral burden, anatomic distortion, and other features. Patients with complex venous connections, distorted branch PAs, situs abnormalities (e.g., left-sided venae cavae) require creative technical solutions, but these patients are candidates for transplantation. We believe that an experienced congenital heart surgeon should be involved in complex transplantation operations in patients with complex structural congenital heart anomalies, particularly in failing Fontan patients, to optimize outcomes.

Long-Term Follow-Up

Patients with a Fontan circulation require diligent, frequent, lifelong surveillance by an adult congenital cardiologist who works in close association with a congenital heart surgeon well versed in adult remedial operations. While the question of how long one can live with a Fontan circulation is, as of yet, unanswered, we have several patients who are now in their early 60s with very satisfactory cardiorespiratory physiology in the setting of a Fontan connection. It is incumbent on the medical community to properly shepherd these patients through the stages of life in an expectant, vigilant manner.

48 Simulation in the Heart Center

Patricia Bastero, Premal M. Trivedi, Kerry Sembera

Simulation is a tool for educational, quality, safety, advocacy, research, and competency assessment endeavors that has proven not only to improve learning and retention, but also to improve patient outcomes. Simulation replaces real-patient experiences with "guided experiences that evoke or replicate substantial aspects of the real world in a fully interactive manner" (Gaba 2004). Simulation allows us to learn, practice, and test our knowledge as well as experiment and evaluate new systems, processes, and spaces safely. An error made in simulation is a potential error prevented in real life.

Simulation has applications in:

- **Education.** Simulation applies adult learning theories, making it an excellent tool for team training. As andragogy describes, adults learn by doing. According to Kolb's experiential learning circle, there are 4 key elements to adult learning: 1) *experience* (simulation participants are exposed to a simulated scenario close to a real-life situation and they perform based on previous learning), 2) *reflection* (during the debriefing phase, learners are guided through an exploration of their thought processes by the debriefer to analyze why they did what they did), 3) *conceptualization* (after analyzing their paradigms, adult learners adopt new perspectives, define optimal performance, and "take home" specific points), and 4) *experimentation* (participants apply new or modified behaviors and/or skills to future simulations and real-life situations).
- **Quality and safety.** There is evidence that various simulation activities can improve patient outcomes (e.g., cardiac arrest). In addition, by system testing, it is possible to identify possible latent threats and intervene before they reach patients, potentially also improving their outcomes.
- **Advocacy.** Mainly focused on the training of family members of children that are technology dependent (e.g., tracheostomies, gastrostomy tubes).
- **Research.** All simulation-based research is performed in liaison with the TCH Simulation Center. The vast majority of studies are related to education, advocacy, or quality and safety research projects.
- **Competency assessment.** This area has not been formally introduced yet.

The goal of the simulation group at TCH is to improve patient safety outcomes by implementing evidence-based simulation activities following best practice. Simulation activities are performed either in situ or at the TCH Simulation Center. For the purpose of this chapter, we will focus on the in situ simulation activities that take place in the Heart Center. The main focus and type of in situ simulation activities at the Heart Center are:

- **Multidisciplinary team training.** These sessions are in situ / point of care (POC) sessions that include all different disciplines involved in the care of cardiac patients (e.g., physicians, nurses, respiratory therapists, ECMO specialists, physical and occupational therapists). These sessions may have different objectives: 1) *cognitive* (wide range of different cardiac emergencies and related complications), 2) *technical* (spanning from code cart and defibrillator use to invasive procedures, such as intubation or vascular access), and 3) *behavioral* (crisis resource management and leadership skills directed to improve effective communication, situational awareness, mental modeling, resource

utilization, and role assignment to optimize team performance). These sessions take place 3-4 times weekly.
- **Just-in-time simulation.** POC simulation is performed with the treating team of an acute-care or intensive-care patient to practice any possible event that the patient may encounter. The objective is to improve patient care and team performance at the time, should that complication happen in real life. These sessions are embedded in the multidisciplinary team training activities.
- **Simulation-based system testing.** In situ simulation activities to train and/or evaluate new processes and new spaces, such as a new ECMO-CPR algorithm, or the opening of a new unit. These sessions take place as needed. Failure Modes and Effect Analysis (FMEA) scoring-based reports are created after each session and then submitted to leadership so processes can be improved before a possible failure reaches one of the patients. These sessions include the whole Heart Center.
- **Advocacy.** Sessions for the training of health care providers and families in the care of patients who are technology dependent (e.g., tracheostomies, VADs).
- **Technical skills stations.** These sessions are usually single discipline and the skills taught vary based on the discipline involved. For example, using task trainers, the anesthesia fellows are taught techniques for obtaining vascular access, securing difficult airways, performing a focused cardiac assessment using transthoracic echocardiography (FATE), and achieving one-lung ventilation.

Two basic rules are followed in simulation: 1) the basic assumption is that all participants are intelligent, are doing their best, and are willing to learn; and 2) confidentiality (actions that take place in the simulation environment are not shared, and those actions will not impact performance evaluations for the participants). The main objective is to provide a safe learning environment.

Following a simulation activity, there is always a debriefing. Debriefing is where the real learning happens. Different debriefing techniques (e.g., advocacy and inquiry, plus/delta, direct feedback, rapid-cycle deliberate practice) are used, based on the level of expertise of the participants, the allocated time for the simulation activity, and type of activity performed.

Senior simulation instructors also apply their simulation debriefing techniques for the debriefing of real-life events. All codes in the CICU are debriefed in two modalities:
- **Warm debriefings.** Debriefings within an hour of the event with focus on team and clinical performance.
- **Cold debriefings.** Debriefings within a week of the event with focus on crisis resource management, facility issues, clinical performance issues, process or system issues, and resource issues. The data obtained from the cold debriefings are used to develop FMEA scoring-based reports that are taken back to the safety and Heart Center leadership. Any patient safety event or potential safety threat is studied, and action plans to address them are made.

Suggested Readings

Gaba DM. The future of simulation in health care. Qual Saf Health Care 2004;13(Suppl 1):i2-i10.

Stocker M, Burmester M, Allen M. Optimization of simulated team training through the application of learning theories: a debate for a conceptual framework. BMC Med Educ 2014. April 3;14:69

Kolb DA. Experiential learning: Experience as the source of learning and development (Vol. 1). Prentice-Hall; 1984.

49 Cardiac Developmental Outcomes

Estrella Mazarico de Thomas, Lara S. Shekerdemian

Thanks to medical and surgical advances, children with CHD now receive treatment early in life and most of them survive into adulthood and thrive. However, children with CHD are at greater risk for and have higher rates of developmental delays and behavior and learning disorders than the general population. The prevalence and severity of developmental disorders and disability (DD) and developmental delays increases with the complexity of CHD.

The TCH Heart Center Cardiac Developmental Outcomes Program (CDOP) serves children with CHD by providing neurodevelopmental monitoring, screening, and assessments to diagnose and treat neurodevelopmental disorders. The program aims to enhance children's opportunities in life by focusing on medical, developmental, and social health to help them reach their maximum individual potentials. The program provides family-centered care, where the child's parents and caregivers are directly involved in the child's assessment and interventions to enhance her/his developmental progress. The program also helps families find resources that support their child's developmental needs in their local communities. The CDOP follows the guidelines established by the AHA and provides patients with CHD with the neurodevelopmental care they need. Patients that are at particular risk for impaired development include:

- Children with CHD that require open heart surgery during infancy
- Children with cyanotic heart lesions not requiring open heart surgery during infancy
- Children with CHD and other comorbidities including prematurity, genetic syndromes, chromosomal abnormalities, history of mechanical support (ECMO or VAD), heart transplantation and/or prolonged hospitalization

CDOP Clinic

The CDOP Clinic provides children referred to program with neurodevelopmental and neuropsychological assessments, monitoring, referral to subspecialties, and therapeutic and ancillary services in a family-centered environment.

The CDOP Clinic team is composed of developmental pediatricians, psychologists, medical social work, and a program coordinator. Infants and children are evaluated and monitored starting at 6 months of age and continuing at 12, 18, and 24 months. Follow-up thereafter occurs yearly or as clinically indicated.

Outpatient referral patients receive a full baseline neurodevelopmental assessment and may be referred for further evaluation to psychology, medical social work, and/or other ancillary services. Follow-up after initial evaluation would be as medically indicated.

The clinic team helps families find resources in their communities that help to support their child's developmental needs. Written reports are provided to parents and referring physicians.

CDOP Referral Criteria
- CHD requiring cardiac surgery at less than 6 months of age

- Heart transplant recipients
- History of mechanical support / ECMO
- Catheterization procedure
- Any child with CHD and developmental, behavioral and/or school concerns
- Children with CHD from birth to 18 years of age

The following are exclusions to CDOP referral:
- Down Syndrome (Developmental Pediatrics has a specialty clinic for these children)
- PDA ligation only

Referral Process

Inpatient Referral

Inpatient infants with CHD who have undergone cardiac surgery at <6 months of age should be referred to CDOP after transfer out of the CICU to an acute care floor. The program coordinator identifies those patients that meet criteria for inclusion in the program.

The process is as follows:
1. The resident or advance practice provider enters a consult order to Developmental Pediatrics (Epic).
2. The program coordinator introduces CDOP to parents, gives educational material, and offers to schedule the 6-month evaluation appointment at the CDOP outpatient clinic.
3. A developmental pediatrician/neurologist evaluates patient before discharge.
4. Outpatient evaluations at 6, 12, 18, and 24 months of age will take place at the CDOP clinic after discharge. Follow-up thereafter will be yearly or as clinically indicated.

Outpatient Referral

Patients with CHD and developmental, behavioral, and/or school concerns can also be referred as outpatients. The process is as follows:
1. TCH requesting providers enter an outpatient referral to the CDOP (Epic). Non-TCH providers send a referral to the CDOP via fax. For parent self-referral, the family calls the program coordinator requesting an evaluation.
2. The program coordinator calls the family and confirms criteria for CDOP, introduces program, and offers first available appointment for an evaluation.

50 Genetic Testing

Lisa C. A. D'Alessandro, Christina Y. Miyake, Shaine A. Morris

Individuals cared for in the Heart Center from fetal life through adulthood may have heart disease arising secondary to an underlying genetic disorder. Identification of genotype has the potential to transform how we care for cardiac patients by defining optimal surveillance and therapeutic strategies, and improved accuracy in prognostication and evaluation of recurrence risk. Currently, there are clear guidelines outlining the role of genetic testing in cardiomyopathy, inherited arrhythmias, and aortopathy. Genetic testing is also indicated in those with multiple congenital anomalies and intellectual disability, and is increasingly being offered to patients with apparently isolated structural heart disease. Broadly speaking, approximately 20-30% of individuals with CHD have a syndromic phenotype, although additional features and extracardiac manifestations may not initially be apparent in the neonatal period. Accurate clinical assessment and meaningful interpretation of genetic testing results is dependent upon accurate cardiac phenotyping, identification of extracardiac manifestations and dysmorphic features, and family history.

Genetic Test Overview

Chromosomal Microarray (CMA)

CMA is a technology that compares patient DNA to reference DNA to detect copy number variations, i.e., deletions and duplications. There are different types of CMA studies, each with specific advantages and limitations. For most indications, a "Comprehensive CMA" is ordered, which includes a combination of aCGH (array comparative genomic hybridization) and SNP (single nucleotide polymorphism) techniques to assess the whole genome.

Turnaround time: 2 weeks
Best for:
- When a microdeletion or microduplication disorder is clinically suspected
- Multiple congenital anomalies
- Intellectual disability
- Autism spectrum disorders

CMA is now routinely offered for syndromic and apparently nonsyndromic CHD (although yield in the latter is lower and has not been fully delineated). Comprehensive CMA will detect aneuploidy, unbalanced translocations, regions of absence of heterozygosity indicating consanguinity or uniparental disomy, and triploidy. Mosaicism can be detected depending on the fraction of abnormal cells in the blood. Very low level mosaicism can be missed by this study.

If the comprehensive CMA is *negative*, microdeletion and microduplication syndromes are excluded. Consideration should be given to single-gene disorders, imprinting disorders, and trinucleotide-repeat conditions (e.g., Fragile X, congenital myotonic dystrophy).

PART III. SPECIAL CONSIDERATIONS

Fluoresecent In-Situ Hybridization (FISH) and Multiplex Ligation Probe-Dependent Analysis (MLPA)
FISH and MLPA are targeted tests to detect copy-number variations at specific regions. These tests have been largely replaced by CMA as the first-line test. The exception to this is the use of rapid FISH for trisomy 13, 18, 21, and sex chromosomes in a newborn/unstable patient in whom identification of one of these diagnoses may affect urgent management.
Turnaround time: Rapid FISH 2-3 days

Chromosomal Karyotype
Chromosomal Karyotype is visual inspection of the chromosomes to assess number, large structural abnormalities, and banding patterns.
Turnaround time: 3 weeks
Best for:
- Aneuploidy
- Large translocations, balanced translocations
- Complex chromosomal rearrangements
- Mosaicism

Karyotype is no longer recommended as the first-line test for multiple congenital anomalies. If the karyotype is *negative*, aneuploidy and large translocations are excluded. Consider submicroscopic copy-number variations and single-gene disorders.

Single-Gene Sequencing
Single-gene sequencing determines the nucleotide sequence of individual genes to assess for mutations causing single-gene disorders.
Turnaround time: 3-4 weeks
Best for:
- When a single-gene disorder with a single underlying gene is suspected
- Laboratory confirmation of mutations identified through alternate sequencing modalities (whole-exome sequencing, panel testing)

If single-gene sequencing is *negative*, a mutation in that gene is excluded, however small deletions or duplications within the gene may not be detected. If gene sequencing with deletion/duplication testing is negative, then consider other genes, copy-number variations and chromosomal rearrangements.

Whole-Exome Sequencing (WES)
WES is a large-scale (next-generation) sequencing technology to simultaneously determine the nucleotide sequences of all the exons (protein-coding regions) of all the genes (the whole exome). Analysis of WES data relies heavily on the clinical information provided in order to focus the report to relevant findings. Detection of incidental findings and variants of uncertain significance require significant pretest and posttest counseling with the family.
Turnaround time: 3-4 months
Best for:
- Assessment of multiple single-gene disorders simultaneously in the setting of complex phenotypes or numerous discordant phenotypes

Table 50-1. Recommended genetic testing by lesion.

Left-sided lesions	
HLHS	Male: CMA Female: CMA and rapid FISH for sex chromosomes to screen for Turner syndrome (if outside the newborn period or non-urgent, do only CMA) If CMA negative, with any of the following: renal anomalies, hypotonia, ear anomalies: consider Kabuki panel (may also do WES)
Coarctation of the aorta, moderate-to-severe aortic stenosis	CMA If CMA negative, with any of the following: renal anomalies, hypotonia, ear anomalies: consider Kabuki panel (may also do WES)
BAV in female with any of the following: coarctation, PAPVR, LSVC, absent ductus arteriosus, cystic hygroma, lymphedema, shield chest, short stature, webbed neck	Karyotype
Supravalvar aortic stenosis	CMA If CMA negative, elastin gene (*ELN*) sequencing with deletion/duplication testing

Right-sided lesions	
Pulmonary stenosis with any of the following: hypertrophic cardiomyopathy, conduction abnormalities, fetal chylous effusions, short stature, webbed neck, shield chest, developmental delay, cryptorchidism, dysmorphic features	Noonan panel

Conotruncal defects	
TOF (PS or PA-VSD)	CMA If seen with bile duct paucity, cholestasis, butterfly vertebrae, ocular anomalies, growth delay, hearing loss, horseshoe kidney: also do *JAG1* and *NOTCH2* gene sequencing (or CHD panel that includes these)
Truncus arteriosus, DORV, IAA with VSD	CMA
Right aortic arch (even if isolated)	CMA

PART III. SPECIAL CONSIDERATIONS

Aortic disease	
Aortic root dilation without CHD and features concerning for Marfan-like disorder	Aortopathy panel
Ascending aortic dilation with lung disease and /or pulmonary hypertension	Aortopathy panel

Others	
AVSD	Features suggestive of T21: karyotype (unless diagnosis critical, then rapid FISH for chromosome 21) No concerning facial features, or features not consistent with T21: CMA (will also detect T21) With short stature, conduction abnormalities, hypertrophic cardiomyopathy, webbed neck, shield chest, developmental delay, cryptorchidism, abnormal facies: consider Noonan panel
Heterotaxy	CMA and heterotaxy panel
All other CHD with the exception of isolated muscular VSDs, nonsyndromic isolated ASDs, isolated BAV, isolated LSVC	CMA

ASD: atrial septal defect, AVSD: atrioventricular septal defect, BAV: bicuspid aortic valve, CHD: congenital heart disease, CMA: chromosomal microarray, DORV: double-outlet right ventricle, FISH: fluorescent in-situ hybridization, HLHS: hypoplastic left heart syndrome, IAA: interrupted aortic arch, LSVC: left superior vena cava, PA: pulmonary atresia, PAPVR: partial anomalous pulmonary venous return, PS: pulmonary stenosis, T21: trisomy 21, TOF: tetralogy of Fallot, VSD: ventricular septal defect, WES: whole-exome sequencing.

- Identification of new genes causing inherited disorders

If WES is *negative*, then pathogenic mutations in protein-coding regions of genes related to the specific phenotype reported on the test requisition are not detected. However, single-gene disorders cannot be completely excluded as there are numerous technological limitations and as of yet undiscovered genes. Copy number variations and aneuploidy are also not completely excluded. Data from WES can be periodically reinterpreted as the patient's phenotype evolves and knowledge surrounding genetic disorders continues to expand.

Next-Generation Sequencing Panels
These studies are an adaptation of WES technology to simultaneously determine the nucleotide sequence of a specific set of genes.
Turnaround time: 2 weeks to 2 months (lab dependent)
Best for:
- Suspected Mendelian disorder known to be caused by multiple genes (e.g., Noonan syndrome, Loeys-Dietz syndrome)

If a panel is **negative**, the disorder tested for may not be completely excluded (technological limitations, other genes implicated that are not on the panel). Consider also other single-gene disorders, copy-number variants, large chromosomal rearrangements.

Test Selection Considerations

1. **What diagnosis is suspected?**
   - Consider the cardiac phenotype, extracardiac phenotype, dysmorphic features and family history. Genetic-test interpretation relies heavily on accurate phenotyping.
   - Select the best test for the suspected diagnosis. The exception is use of rapid-FISH for trisomy 13,18, 21, and sex chromosomes in order to rapidly determine an aneuploidy diagnosis in a critically ill/newborn patient when the diagnosis may affect prognosis and/or management.
   - If a specific diagnosis is not clinically suspected, CMA is the first-line test for multiple congenital anomalies/dysmorphic features, intellectual disability, autism spectrum disorder, and increasingly for syndromic and nonsyndromic heart disease.
2. **What is the test yield?**
   - What percentage of patients with the phenotype will have a positive test?
   - Consider pretest probability. There is a higher yield with extreme phenotypes. If multiple family members are affected, the individual with the most severe phenotype should be tested as the proband.
3. **Test interpretation**
   - What does a positive, negative, or uncertain test result mean?
   - What are the technical limitations of the test?
4. **What are the implications of a positive or negative test for the family?**
   - Can the disorder be diagnosed or excluded with certainty?
   - Cascade screening in family members, inheritance, recurrence risk, and surveillance
   - Risk of detecting variants of uncertain significance and incidental findings
5. **Follow-up and counseling**
   - Pretest counseling and consent for genetic testing must be performed
   - All genetic tests require insurance preapproval in the outpatient setting but this may not be required in the inpatient setting. Not all tests are covered by all insurance plans. This can result in a large out-of-pocket cost to families.
   - Testing results may be returned weeks or months after the testing is performed and frequently after the patient has been discharged from the hospital. It is essential that results are obtained, reviewed, and communicated to the family.

Genetic Testing Algorithms

Positive Fetal Genetic Testing

Biomarker screening (i.e., maternal serum screening, integrated prenatal screening) is performed routinely for most pregnancies. A "screen positive" result is given when

PART III. SPECIAL CONSIDERATIONS

Table 50-2. Recommended genetic testing by suspected diagnosis.

Suspected diagnosis	Testing
Down syndrome	Karyotype If the diagnosis is critical in the newborn period, rapid FISH for chromosome 21 Will also be detected by CMA, but won't identify rearrangement, low-level mosaicism
Trisomy 13, 18	Newborn rapid FISH for chromosome 13, 18 and karyotype Will also be detected by CMA, but won't identify rearrangement, low-level mosaicism
Turner syndrome	With HLHS: rapid FISH for sex chromosomes If strongly suspect or to confirm diagnosis: karyotype with FISH for Y centromere Will also be detected by CMA, but won't identify rearrangement, low-level mosaicism
Williams syndrome	Best: CMA Will also be detected with FISH for Williams region If CMA negative or if family history of SVAS, strongly consider elastin gene (*ELN*) sequencing with deletion/duplication testing
22q11.2 deletion syndrome (DiGeorge syndrome, velocardiofacial syndrome)	Best: CMA Will also be detected with FISH for DiGeorge (usually includes chromosomes 22 and 10)
Noonan syndrome	Best: Noonan syndrome panel (adding deletion/duplication will diagnose an additional 5%) Will also be detected on WES
Marfan syndrome	Best: Aortopathy panel Will also be detected on WES
Loeys-Dietz syndrome	Best: Aortopathy panel Will also be detected on WES
Holt-Oram syndrome	TBX5 gene sequencing Will also be detected on WES and most CHD gene panels
Ehlers-Danlos syndrome	
- Hypermobile type (type 5)	There is no current diagnostic test (but there are clinical diagnostic criteria). If personal history of easy bruising/bleeding, or abnormal skin (atrophic scars, poor wound healing, highly elastic), or family history of vascular/organ rupture, must exclude other types of EDS with EDS or aortopathy panel
- Vascular EDS (type 4)	Best: EDS panel (unless there is root dilation, then do aortopathy panel) Will also be detected on aortopathy panel or WES
- Classical EDS/Classical-like EDS/Cardiac-valvular EDS (types 1-3)	Best: EDS panel (unless there is root dilation, then do aortopathy panel) Will also be detected on aortopathy panel or WES
CHARGE syndrome	Best: CHD7 sequencing with deletion/duplication Will also be detected on WES

CHD: congenital heart disease, CMA: chromosomal microarray, EDS: Ehlers-Danlos syndrome, FISH: fluorescent in-situ hybridization, HLHS: hypoplastic left heart syndrome, SVAS: supravalvar aortic stenosis, WES: whole-exome sequencing.

the risk of aneuploidy based on biomarker testing is higher than maternal age-related risk. This is not a specific genetic test and does not yield a specific diagnosis. Biomarker screen results should not influence the decision to evaluate and perform genetic testing postnatally.

Non-Invasive Prenatal Testing (NIPT) is analysis of cell-free fetal DNA in the maternal blood stream to assess for aneuploidy (most commonly 13, 18, 21, and sex chromosomes). Some companies also offer testing for select microdeletion/duplications; however this technology has yet to be validated in population studies. NIPT is a screening test for specific aneuploidy conditions and requires confirmation with a diagnostic test (i.e., via amniocentesis or postnatal testing):

- **Positive NIPT without prenatal confirmatory testing:** complete evaluation and postnatal confirmatory testing of the NIPT screen-positive result
- **Negative NIPT:** Should not influence a postnatal decision to perform genetic testing when clinically indicated

If amniocentesis or chorionic villus sampling (CVS) was performed to obtain a sample for genetic testing, then genetic counseling, karyotyping, CMA and/or FISH may have been performed. The reports detailing the type of testing performed and the results should be obtained and scanned to the patient's medical record.

- **Positive genetic test result (karyotype, CMA, FISH) on sample obtained by amniocentesis/CVS:** Consult genetics to determine if the patient's phenotype is consistent with the prenatal diagnosis and if confirmatory/additional testing is required
- **Negative genetic test result on sample obtained by amniocentesis/CVS and genetic disorder is suspected:** Confirm what type of testing was performed (e.g., CMA by amniocentesis will not rule out Noonan syndrome). Consult genetics for additional evaluation and testing.

CHD and Aortopathy
Table 50-1 lists the recommended genetic testing by CHD lesion. Table 50-2 lists the recommended genetic testing by suspected diagnosis.

Cardiomyopathy
Genetic testing in cardiomyopathy is recommended for patients who have undergone a comprehensive evaluation (including clinical history, detailed 3-generation family history, examination, ECG, echocardiography) and have been given a clinical diagnosis of cardiomyopathy. Testing is not recommended for individuals with non-diagnostic clinical features (e.g., athlete's heart). Accurate genetic test interpretation relies upon accurate clinical phenotyping, therefore evaluation of a patient with cardiomyopathy must include consideration of:

- Syndromic features (dysmorphic features, multisystem organ involvement, developmental delay, developmental regression)
- Arrhythmia and conduction system involvement
- Skeletal myopathy
- Family history and inheritance pattern

PART III. SPECIAL CONSIDERATIONS

Table 50-3. Considerations and genetic testing in patients with cardiomyopathies.

Cardiomyopathy	Considerations	Testing
Hypertrophic cardiomyopathy (HCM)	Highest yield of all cardiomyopathies; highest in familial HCM	Comprehensive or HCM-targeted panel testing Also consider Rasopathy panel if features of Noonan-spectrum disorders are present
Dilated cardiomyopathy (DCM)	Highest yield in those with DCM and conduction system disease, family history of sudden death and familial DCM	Comprehensive or dilated-targeted panel Also consider muscular dystrophy, metabolic cardiomyopathy, mitochondrial disorders
Restrictive cardiomyopathy	Numerous modes of inheritance, rare diagnosis	Comprehensive panel testing Also consider skeletal myopathy, storage disorders, Noonan-spectrum disorders
Arrhythmogenic cardiomyopathy (ARC)	Numerous modes of inheritance and complex genetics (e.g., compound heterozygosity) make test interpretation challenging High incidence of false positives is suspected	Comprehensive or ARC-targeted panel testing may be recommended but should be undertaken by Cardiomyopathy Team/Electrophysiology Team
LV non-compaction cardiomyopathy	Numerous modes of inheritance, numerous implicated genes, broad phenotypic spectrum, and considerable overlap with other forms of cardiomyopathy Lower yield than for other forms of cardiomyopathy	Comprehensive or LVNC-targeted panel testing may be recommended but should be undertaken by Cardiomyopathy Team/Electrophysiology team Also consider Barth syndrome, muscular dystrophy, mitochondrial disease, ARC

ARC: arrhythmogenic cardiomyopathy, DCM: dilated cardiomtyopathy, HCM: hypertrophic cardiomyopathy, LVNC: left-ventricular non-compaction.

Evaluation and genetic testing should be guided by the Cardiomyopathy Team. The role of genetic testing in cardiomyopathy includes:
- Identification of a specific disorder with altered management:
  - Hypertrophic cardiomyopathy in Fabry disease, Danon disease
  - Dilated cardiomyopathy in muscular dystrophy
  - Metabolic cardiomyopathy for which enzyme-replacement is available
- Permits mutation-specific testing of family members who might otherwise require long-term clinical surveillance

Next Generation Comprehensive Cardiomyopathy Panel Testing ("Pancardiomyopathy Panel") is a panel that encompasses genes known to cause hypertrophic, dilated, restrictive, non-compaction, and arrhythmogenic cardiomyopathy. It is often used due to the overlap in clinical cardiomyopathy phenotypes within families and evolution of cardiac phenotype over the lifespan. This approach also helps identify specific genetic disorders with altered management (e.g., identification of Fabry disease in hypertrophic cardiomyopathy or muscular dystrophy in dilated cardiomyopathy). However, some data suggest that pancardiomyopathy testing is not more effective than phenotype-targeted testing and may increase the risk of detecting a variant of uncertain significance. Additionally, this approach will not necessarily identify the cause of cardiomyopathy associated with syndromic disorders (e.g., Noonan syndrome), skeletal myopathies, or metabolic and mitochondrial disorders. Therefore, a thorough and thoughtful approach to test selection must be employed.

Table 50-3 lists the recommended genetic testing and important considerations for patients with cardiomyopathies. For details on diagnosis and management of the different cardiomyopathies, see Chapter 32.

Inherited Arrhythmias
Details on genetic testing for inherited arrhythmia syndromes and workup of cardiac arrest can be found in Chapter 35.

51 Transition Medicine in Pediatric Cardiology

Keila N. Lopez

CHD encompasses multiple different diseases, ranging from mild to severe. Many children born with complex CHD who previously would have died at an early age are now surviving into adulthood. Advances in medical and surgical care for CHD children have resulted in ~85% survival into adulthood and there are now roughly 1.4 million survivors of CHD reaching adulthood. However, despite improved treatments, CHD survivors are often palliated rather than cured. As such, lifelong surveillance and disease management are critical to maintain healthy and productive lives.

Poor transition and transfer of care significantly and adversely affect health outcomes for CHD adolescents, particularly minorities. CHD adolescents have unique medical, social, emotional, and functional needs throughout their lives. As such, a successful transition from pediatric to adult care is critical to reduce lapses in care.

Transition is a multifaceted process for adolescents with CHD, and needs to be understood from five different perspectives: the patient, the parents, the pediatrician, the pediatric cardiologist, and the adult cardiologist. In addition, the aspects of developmental progression and the impact of their chronic illness on adolescent and family development have to be fully incorporated. Major developmental milestones (e.g. self-care, social interaction) typically achieved during adolescence are often disrupted and underdeveloped in children with a chronic illness such as CHD. Furthermore, information transfer from pediatric to adult cardiologist is often lacking or incomplete. Transition- and transfer-related intervention efforts have largely failed to address this multifaceted process for chronic-disease adolescents. Studies show that <30% of adults with CHD are seen by appropriate specialized congenital heart physician providers, and that many have lapses in care. These lapses of care translate into a higher likelihood of needing an urgent surgical or catheter-based intervention. Transition outcomes are particularly suboptimal among ethnic minorities

At TCH, we have created a transition program for adolescents and young adults with CHD between the ages of 15 and 21 years. This program was created by using transition medicine guidelines, best practices for pediatric cardiology transition, and understanding the needs of stakeholders, including the patient, their parents, and the medical providers (pediatric cardiologists, adult CHD specialists, and the pediatric and adult primary care physicians). The program incorporates our transition education and skill training into the pediatric cardiology clinic, with the transition team introducing the program to CHD families at 14 years of age. Starting at 15 years, the transition team meets independently with the adolescent with CHD and administers a CHD knowledge and transition skills assessment. A thorough formal needs assessment is then conducted, including collecting information about their understanding of navigating the medical system, their mental health and coping skills, their understanding of health insurance, and their understanding of living with CHD (including risky behaviors, recognizing medical emergencies, an the need for long-term follow-up). Based on this data, the transition team creates an individualized learning plan (ILP) for each patient, tailoring their education to suit their knowledge and skill deficits. This information is

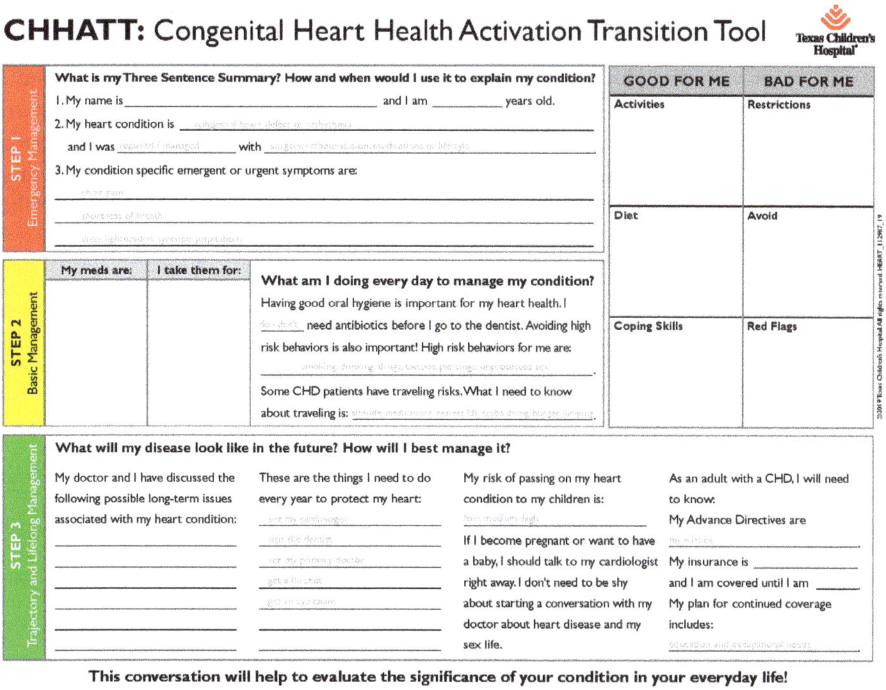

CHHATT: Congenital Heart Health Activation Transition Tool — Texas Children's Hospital

STEP 1 — Emergency Management

What is my Three Sentence Summary? How and when would I use it to explain my condition?

1. My name is ________ and I am _____ years old.
2. My heart condition is congenital heart defect or arrhythmia
   and I was repaired / managed with surgery, catheterization, medications or lifestyle
3. My condition specific emergent or urgent symptoms are:
   chest pain
   shortness of breath
   dizzy, lightheaded, syncope, palpitations

STEP 2 — Basic Management

My meds are:	I take them for:

What am I doing every day to manage my condition?

Having good oral hygiene is important for my heart health. I do / don't need antibiotics before I go to the dentist. Avoiding high risk behaviors is also important! High risk behaviors for me are: smoking, drinking, drugs, tattoos, piercings, unprotected sex.

Some CHD patients have traveling risks. What I need to know about traveling is: altitude, medications, nearest ER, scuba diving, bungee jumping.

GOOD FOR ME	BAD FOR ME
Activities	Restrictions
Diet	Avoid
Coping Skills	Red Flags

STEP 3 — Trajectory and Lifelong Management

What will my disease look like in the future? How will I best manage it?

My doctor and I have discussed the following possible long-term issues associated with my heart condition:

These are the things I need to do every year to protect my heart:
see my cardiologist
visit the dentist
see my primary doctor
get a flu shot
get an eye exam

My risk of passing on my heart condition to my children is: low, medium, high

If I become pregnant or want to have a baby, I should talk to my cardiologist right away. I don't need to be shy about starting a conversation with my doctor about heart disease and my sex life.

As an adult with a CHD, I will need to know:
My Advance Directives are my wishes.
My insurance is ________
and I am covered until I am ____.
My plan for continued coverage includes: education and occupational needs

This conversation will help to evaluate the significance of your condition in your everyday life!

Figure 51-1. Transition team "chalk talk".

then entered into an adolescent database and a special section of the electronic medical record that we created for the purposes of a) tracking potential improvements in CHD knowledge and transition skill acquisition with each transition team encounter, and b) providing that information to the pediatric cardiologist caring for the patient.

The transition team uses a 3-sentence summary format to help our patients better understand their condition (primary diagnosis or disease), their treatments (procedures, surgical repairs, medications, and the importance of compliance), and their disease trajectory (symptoms that may require emergent care and how to self-monitor) (Figure 51-1).

Confidence in communicating their condition is important to all patients; however, it can really help young adults establish independence. Thus, beyond educating on their disease process, the transition team teaches adolescents with CHD transition skills (making their own appointments, asking the physician questions directly, etc.), provides important medical system navigation resources ("MyChart"), and helps with coping strategies (to deal with stress, anxiety, etc.).

The team also covers challenging topics including birth control, high-risk behaviors, and activity restrictions. The team provides referral information for adult cardiologists specializing in CHD, subspecialty providers trained to work with CHD patients (e.g., obstetricians and gynecologists, gastroenterologists), and additionally teaches about insurance, future career, and family planning.

An adult planning visit happens at the 18-year-old pediatric cardiology visit, and includes discussion with the transition team, parent, patient, and pediatric cardiologist. This visit includes a formal recommendation for following to an adult congenital heart physician, discussion of an advanced directive, a formal transfer summary, and discussions of other ways to empower the young adult with CHD. As individual needs are met and transition skills are gained, the adolescent continues at each visit to meet with the transition team until they are ready for transfer to adult care. Official policy at TCH includes transfer to adult CHD care at 21 years of age.

Suggested Readings

American Academy of Pediatrics, American Academy of Family Physicians, American College of Physicians, Transitions Clinical Report Authoring Group, Cooley WC, Sagerman PJ. Supporting the health care transition from adolescence to adulthood in the medical home. Pediatrics 2011;128:182-200.

Hudsmith LE, Thorne SA. Transition of care from paediatric to adult services in cardiology. Arch Dis Child 2007;92:927-930.

Lotstein DS, Kuo AA, Strickland B, et al. The transition to adult health care for youth with special health care needs: do racial and ethnic disparities exist? Pediatrics 2010;126 Suppl 3:S129-S136.

Marelli AJ, Mackie AS, Ionescu-Ittu R, et al. Congenital heart disease in the general population: changing prevalence and age distribution. Circulation 2007;115:163-172.

Pless IB, Cripps HA, Davies JM, et al. Chronic physical illness in childhood: psychological and social effects in adolescence and adult life. Dev Med Child Neurol 1989;31:746-755.

Sable C, Foster E, Uzark K, et al. Best practices in managing transition to adulthood for adolescents with congenital heart disease: the transition process and medical and psychosocial issues: a scientific statement from the American Heart Association. Circulation 2011;123:1454-1485.

ant
IV. Perioperative Care

52 Preoperative Evaluation

Jennifer Yborra, Kimberly Krauklis

General Considerations

Patients undergoing cardiac surgery should have a thorough preoperative evaluation within 7 days of surgery. This evaluation is done by the congenital heart surgery team, cardiac anesthesia team, child-life specialist, and social worker. In addition to meeting with the team, the patient also undergoes a series of laboratory tests.

The history should be detailed and include specific questioning, including:
- Previous complications with anesthesia
- Easy bruising or known bleeding disorders
- Neurological complications
- Developmental delay or previous seizures
- Previous methicillin-resistant Staphylococcus aureus (MRSA) or methicillin-sensitive Staphylococcus aureus (MSSA) infections
- Symptoms of infection (cough, runny nose, fever, vomiting, diarrhea, sore throat, etc.) in the last 4 weeks
- Immunization status

The family history questioning should include whether there are family members with congenital heart defects, congenital deafness, pacemakers, heart muscle problems, reactions to anesthesia, bleeding or clotting disorders, as well as sickle-cell disease or trait.

As part of the preoperative evaluation, all patients undergo the following routine tests:
- Complete blood count with differential
- Chemistry
- Coagulation studies
- Urinalysis
- Blood type and crossmatch
- CXR (both posteroanterior and lateral views); this is particularly important for patients undergoing repeat sternotomy to evaluate the location of the heart behind the sternum
- ECG within the last 30 days

For patients with repeat sternotomy, a CT may also be indicated if there are increased concerns for complications during reentry. All recent echocardiograms, cardiac catheterization images, CT scans, and MRI images should be available. Operative reports from all previous cardiac operations should be obtained.

Special Considerations

If the patient has symptoms of an upper respiratory infection, viral studies should be sent. If positive and the procedure is elective, surgery should be rescheduled 4-6 weeks later.

In addition, neonates undergoing cardiac procedures with CPB require preoperatively:
- Brain MRI (see Table 52-1)
- Renal ultrasound
- Clearance from all consulting services

Table 52-1. Genetic and neuromonitoring schedule for infants undergoing cardiac surgery during the first month of life.

	Preoperative	
Genetic testing	Genetic testing recommended prior to surgery: **CMA**	
Imaging	**Preoperative MRI**	
	To be requested by CICU or NICU medical team. Ideally within 72 hours prior to surgery, and before the day of surgery.	
	Where possible, to be scheduled on an existing MRI list and not out of hours or at weekends unless a significant clinical concern.	
	The patients will be scanned during a routine list, without sedation or anesthesia if feasible, and will be monitored throughout by a CV anesthesiologist. Consent will be obtained as routine. The MRI will be performed only if the patient is deemed stable by the cardiac ICU, surgical, and CV anesthesiology teams. Patients should be fasted prior to transfer to MRI. MRI sequences will include Sagittal T1-w 3D imaging, axial 15-30 direction DRI, axial GRE, axial T1-2, and coronal T2 FLAIR imaging, taking a total of 25-30 minutes.	
	Head Ultrasound	
	Routine head ultrasound is not recommended in nonsyndromic, asymptomatic term newborns with a normal clinical neurological examination.	

	Postoperative	
Brain Monitoring	NIRS – Single site (brain)	
	NIRS will be monitored with a probe on the right side of the forehead for 48-72 hours postoperatively. Longer periods may be utilized at the discretion of the clinical team. Target rSO2 should be >50%. An rSO2 <50% will be cause to notify the physician team. Persistent low rSO2 or clinical signs such as seizures, new focal neurological deficit, or coma are indications for urgent neuroimaging.	
Brain Imaging	**Postoperative MRI**	
	7-10 days postoperatively when the infant is stable for transport to MRI. To be requested by CICU or inpatient cardiology team.	
	The patients will be scanned during a routine list, and will be monitored throughout by a CV anesthesiologist. Consent will be obtained as routine. The default will be for a nonsedated scan. IV sedation, or if the infant is still intubated, inhaled or intravenous general anesthesia, *may* be used at the discretion of the attending anesthesiologist. Patients should be fasted prior to transfer to MRI.	
Developmental	**Cardiac Developmental Outcomes Clinic**	
	To be referred to the Cardiac Developmental Outcomes Program (CDOP) team after transfer from CICU to the cardiac inpatient unit. The initial assessment by the CDOP team will ideally occur as an inpatient on the cardiology floor. Outpatient assessment will take place in the CDOP at 6, 12, 18, and 24 months of age. Follow-up thereafter will be yearly or as clinically indicated.	

CICU: Cardiac Intensive Care Unit, CMA: chromosomal microarray, MRI: magnetic resonance imaging, NICU: Neonatal Intensive Care Unit, NIRS: near-infrared spectroscopy, rSO2: regional oxygen saturation

Table 52-2. Additional testing and special considerations for particular patient populations.

Patient population	Additional testing
DiGeorge syndrome	Calcium, magnesium, and phosphorus levels. CMV negative, irradiated, and leukoreduced blood necessary.
Down syndrome	Thyroid-function studies. A TSH level >6 mU/L warrants discussion with Endocrinology and a TSH >10 mU/L may warrant a delay in surgery. Cervical X-rays for patients >2 years of age to rule out atlantoaxial instability.
Girls >10 years of age	Serum HCG levels to rule out pregnancy.
Patients with tattoos, body piercings, or high-risk behavior	Hepatitis and HIV screening.
Sickle-cell disease and sickle-cell trait	Hemoglobin electrophoresis. If HbS >30%, exchange transfusion will be considered at the time of CPB.
Patients with known arrhythmias, left-hand topology (L-looping), or those undergoing a Fontan procedure	Holter within the 6 months prior to OR.

CMV: cytomegalovirus, HbS: hemoglobin S, HCG: human chorionic gonadotropin, HIV: human immunodeficiency virus, TSH: Thyroid-stimulating hormone.

- Renal consultation of patients undergoing complex neonatal repairs for postoperative peritoneal dialysis

Table 52-2 lists some special considerations for other patient populations.

Other Preoperative Preparations

All medications should be reviewed and consideration to holding certain medications should be made. Aspirin should be held for 1 week, unless the patient has shunt-dependent pulmonary blood flow. Lovenox® should be held for 2 doses prior to surgery. Coumadin® needs to be converted to heparin or Lovenox® prior to surgery and then held. Angiotensin-converting enzyme (ACE) inhibitors and beta-blockers may be held for 3-5 days, as deemed appropriated by the surgeon and primary cardiologist. Vaccines (except influenza and Synagis®) should not be administered in the 2 weeks leading up to surgery. MRSA screening and universal decolonization are completed per the protocol in Table 52-3.

Child-life specialists meet with the children and their families the day before surgery to discuss age-appropriate expectations, engage in therapeutic play, and take a tour of the Heart Center.

Table 52-3. Staphylococcus aureus infection prevention protocol for pediatric patients undergoing cardiac surgery.

Recommendation	Description
Universal MRSA screening	• **Population:** All patients undergoing cardiac surgery • **Action:** Using a single swab, swab the nares, axilla, and groin of the patient for MRSA PCR testing. (If positive these swabs will automatically be saved for culture) • **Timing:** Perform at least 3-4 hours prior to surgical procedure
Universal decolonization	• **Population:** All patients undergoing cardiac surgery • **Action A:** Apply a small amount of topical mupirocin to both anterior nares BID for 5 days • **Timing:** When possible, start 5 days prior to surgical procedure date (complete a 5-day course even postoperatively) • **Action B:** Use chlorhexidine bath clothes (2% chlorhexidine gluconate antiseptic wipes) as directed according to patient weight daily for 5 days • **Timing:** When possible, start 5 days prior to surgical procedure date (Continue as long as central lines remain in place) *At preop visit, patients will be given packets containing: a patient instruction sheet, chlorhexidine wipes, and a prescription for mupirocin*
Preoperative bath	• **Population:** All patients undergoing cardiac surgery • **Action:** A preoperative bath with soap and water or chlorhexidine containing solution or wipe • **Timing:** The night before and/or morning of surgery
Screening-directed preoperative antibiotic[a]	• **Population:** All patients undergoing cardiac surgery • **Action:** Administer cefazolin[b] • **Timing:** 0-60 minutes prior to incision; re-dose every 4 hours • **Population:** MRSA-positive patients undergoing cardiac surgery should receive cefazolin in addition to the following: • **Action:** Administer vancomycin • **Timing:** 0-120 minutes prior to incision; no re-dosing

[a] Per ASHP national guidelines, the data regarding efficacy of antimicrobial prophylaxis is extrapolated from adult studies.
[b] In patients with a documented β-lactam allergy, may refer to A&I for penicillin allergy testing. If β-lactam allergy confirmed, administer clindamycin and re dose every 6 hours or a one-time dose of vancomycin for Gram-positive coverage.
A&I: Allergy and Immunology, ASHP: American Society of Health-System Pharmacists, BID: twice a day, MRSA: methicillin-resistant Staphylococcus aureus, PCR: polymerase chain reaction.

Clearances

Adult patients require clearance from their primary care provider. All patients over 2 years of age need dental clearance and dental caries addressed at least 2 weeks prior to surgery. All subspecialists who follow the patient should see the patient and provide clearance and recommendations for perioperative care.

PART IV. PERIOPERATIVE CARE

Table 52-4. TCH CVOR preoperative blood ordering guidelines.[a,b,c]

Pump cases[d,e]		
Weight	**Standard**	**Redo**
<3 kg Norwood, TAPVR, Truncus, IAA, Arterial Switch, Arch Advancement, Palliative Switch	2 U PRBC, ≤5 days old 1 U PRBC 2 U FFP ½ (0.5) U apheresis platelet 1 U cryoprecipitate	2 U PRBC, ≤5 days old 1 U PRBC, 2 U FFP ½ (0.5) U apheresis platelet 1 U cryoprecipitate Stay ahead 2 U PRBC and ½ (0.5) U apheresis platelet
<8 kg	1 U PRBC, ≤5days old 2 U PRBC 2 U FFP ½ (0.5) U apheresis platelet 1 U cryoprecipitate	1 U PRBC, ≤5 days old 2 U PRBC, 2 U FFP ½ (0.5) U apheresis platelet 1 U cryoprecipitate Stay ahead 2 U PRBC and ½ (0.5) U apheresis platelet
8-18 kg	1 U PRBC, ≤5days old 2 U PRBC 2 U FFP ½ (0.5) U apheresis platelet 1 U cryoprecipitate	1 U PRBC, ≤5 days old 2 U PRBC, 2 U FFP 1 U apheresis platelet 1 U cryoprecipitate Stay ahead 2 U PRBC and ½ (0.5) U apheresis platelet
>18 kg	3 U PRBC, 2 U FFP ½ (0.5) U apheresis platelet 2 U cryoprecipitate Stay ahead 2 U PRBC and ½ (0.5) U apheresis platelet	4 U PRBC, 2 U FFP 1 U apheresis platelet 2 U cryoprecipitate Stay ahead 6 U PRBC and 2 U apheresis platelet

Non-pump cases (thoracic cases, PDA ligation, CoA repair, pacemaker generator change)	
Weight	**Order**
<8 kg	1 U PRBC/low K+, split into halves for CVOR
8-18 kg	1 U PRBC, ≤5 days old (stay ahead 2 U PRBC, ½ (0.5) U apheresis platelet for aortic procedures)
>18 kg	2 U PRBC (stay ahead 4 U PRBC, ½ (0.5) U apheresis platelet for aortic procedures)

[a] IRR/LR for <4 months old and transplant patients. Please note that we no longer irradiate blood for single ventricles (unless they are active transplant candidates).
[b] CMV-/IRR/LR for DiGeorge patients, neonates with pending CMA, and SCID patients.
[c] If no blood transfusion or pregnancy in the last 3 months, can extend specimen expiration to 14 days. Check box on initial order. New blood order to be sent with new surgery date for cancelled CVOR cases.
[d] Add comment "CBP protocol 7-25" to PRBC orders for patients weighing 7 kg to 25 kg. CPB protocol 7-25 triggers the blood bank to purposefully send the largest PRBC unit available.
[e] Transplants follow guidelines as outlined above. Additional blood product orders per transplant team on individual basis (e.g., exchange transfusion).
CMA: chromosomal microarray, CMV: cytomegalovirus, CoA: aortic coarctation, IRR: irradiated, FFP: fresh frozen plasma, IAA: interrupted aortic arch, LR: leukoreduced, PRBC: packed red blood cells, SCID: severe combined immunodeficiency.

The Night Before Surgery

All patients undergoing surgery are made NPO at midnight but allowed to have clear fluids until 2 hours prior to the scheduled OR start time. If the patient is hospitalized, maintenance IV fluids are started at midnight.

A preoperative bath must be administered after 5 pm the night prior to surgery in accordance with the Surgical Site Infection Prevention guidelines.

Blood is ordered based on TCH CVOR Preoperative Blood Ordering Guidelines (Table Table 52-4). Directed blood donation can be arranged if donors are the same blood type, older than 17 years, and have not traveled outside of the US for the last year. Donations must be done 3-5 days prior to surgery. Paperwork must be completed in advance to ensure proper handling.

53 Anesthesia for Congenital Heart Disease

Stuart R. Hall

Congenital heart surgery is unique in that it is perhaps the only area of medicine in which a patient can enter the OR with one abnormal physiology and leave with a different abnormal physiology. It is important to be aware of the various physiologic states seen in these patients and to understand how their physiology affects and is affected by anesthesia.

General Considerations

Intraoperative monitoring is according to ASA standard, with the addition of bilateral cerebral NIRS probes, which can be placed before or after induction.

In patients with IV access, induction is commonly achieved with a combination of midazolam and fentanyl in slowly titrated doses. This can be augmented with inhaled sevoflurane, if desired.

The patient's physiology will dictate the FiO_2 used in induction: small, overcirculated neonates may tolerate supplemental oxygen, but those with already low BP might benefit from an FiO_2 approaching room air. Patients without IV access are often induced with sevoflurane, with IV access established as soon as possible. Nearly all patients will be muscle-relaxed for intubation.

Access

In the CVOR, nearly all patients will need arterial and central venous access. Arterial access should take into account the patient's anatomy. The anesthesiologist will review the anatomy to determine the optimal sites for access and monitoring. For example, if there is an aberrant subclavian artery, an ipsilateral arterial line fed by that subclavian artery may dampen with TEE probe placement. Does the patient have a coarctation, and if so, where is it? Will antegrade cerebral perfusion be used, in which case, is a right-upper-extremity arterial line desired? If the patient will end the operation with a Blalock-Taussig-Thomas shunt, should the arterial line be placed on the contralateral side?

Usually, the radial artery is accessed, but after discussion, sometimes an ulnar artery (verified by ultrasound) is used. Long cases, such as lung transplants and redo heart transplants, will often require femoral arterial access if possible because the upper-extremity arteries can be unreliable after long CPB runs. As a rule, the brachial artery is not cannulated.

Central venous access is typically femoral in patients <5 kg. Most patients ≥5 kg will receive an IJ central venous catheter. In most cases, a double- or triple-lumen line is used. For Glenn procedures, the CVP catheter is placed femorally, while the IJ is cannulated with a single-lumen 3F line to allow transduction of PA pressures after CPB.

All neck lines are placed using ultrasound visualization; some staff use ultrasound for femoral lines as well while others prefer to use a Doppler. Once the patient has central venous access, an epsilon-aminocaproate infusion is started.

Pre-CPB Period

During the pre-CPB period, the goal is to maintain acceptable hemodynamics and patient-physiologic oxygen saturation. Anesthesia is maintained with a volatile agent, usually isoflurane, and intermittent boluses of fentanyl and muscle relaxant. Pressors may be needed; their use is usually discussed between the anesthesiologist and surgeon. In patients for whom the bypass pump will be primed with blood (patients less than aproximately 15 kg), there are often fresh PRBCs available for pre-CPB transfusion.

When the procedure involves arch reconstruction and antegrade cerebral perfusion will be used, the surgeon will generally ask for "shunt-dose heparin". At this point, 100 units/kg of heparin are given to prevent thrombosis as vessels are clamped to facilitate placement of a Gore-Tex® graft for arterial cannulation. When the surgeon is ready for full cannulation, he or she will ask for "full-dose heparin"; this means a dose of 400 units/kg to ensure adequate anticoagulation for CPB: the target initial ACT is >350 seconds.

It is important to make sure that the perfusionist has an appropriate bolus dose of epsilon-aminocaproate and antibiotic for the prime, as per institutional guidelines.

CPB

As CPB is initiated, ventilation of the lungs is stopped. The first minutes of CPB are a good time to ensure adequate hypnosis, analgesia, and muscle relaxation with boluses of whichever drugs are being used for the case. In some cases, the perfusionist will need to bolus phenylephrine to reach an adequate perfusion pressure. Conversely, especially in small children, phentolamine may be given for adequate vasodilation. Goal perfusion pressure depends on age:
- Neonates: ~35-40 mmHg
- Toddlers and small children: ~45 mmHg
- Younger teenagers: ~50 mmHg
- Larger teenagers and adults: 55-60 mmHg

For a complete discussion on CPB, see Chapter 6. The attending anesthesiologist should be present for initiation and weaning from CPB, initiation of antegrade cerebral perfusion, and unclamping of the aorta, at a minimum.

Once the cross-clamp has been removed and after sinus rhythm has returned, or pacing has been started, it is time to start whichever vasoactive medications might be necessary to facilitate weaning from CPB. This can range from nothing for a straightforward, healthy ASD, to vasopressin, epinephrine, and calcium for a small, sick neonate. It is also time to begin thinking about what blood products, in the way of platelets, cryoprecipitate, and FFP, will be needed after CPB. This is also a good time to send any studies such as a ROTEM®, which might help with those decisions (see Chapter 59).

Post-CPB Period

After weaning from CPB, hemostasis becomes a priority. In first-time operations in healthy patients, reversal of the heparin (10-13 mg protamine / 1000 units heparin) may be all that is needed. In others, platelets/cryoprecipitate/FFP may also be needed. After giving what is termed "a couple of rounds," of these products, which is admittedly vague, it should be discussed with the surgeon whether more procoagulants (such as recombinant Factor VIIa) might be helpful. For details on postoperative hemostasis, see Chapter 60). The chest may be left open, with the edges of the sternum strutted apart and the chest cavity covered with a Gore-Tex® membrane in cases of extreme hemodynamic instability or persistent bleeding.

While many patients will go to the CICU intubated after surgery, many patients may be suitable for extubation in the OR. In these patients, it is helpful to limit the dose of narcotic to <30 mcg/kg for the duration of the case. Preoperative discussion with the surgeon regarding the intent to extubate in the OR is therefore paramount. Some staff advocate the use of a dexmedetomidine infusion to supplement the anesthetic after CPB and to provide some postoperative sedation. Per institutional protocol, most patients aimed at extubation should also be given a dose of ondansetron in the OR.

Transport to the CICU is perhaps one of the most critical points in the case for the anesthesia team. Ensure that all drips are running and have sufficient quantities left in their syringes or bags to allow for several hours of infusion. Bring along emergency airway equipment and appropriate resuscitation drugs and volume. Air-oxygen blenders are available for transport when 100% oxygen is inappropriate for transport. Patients on iNO can be ventilated using the side port on the iNO delivery system. Once in the CICU, monitors will be switched to the CICU system, and the CICU, surgery, and anesthesia teams will meet at the bedside for detailed handoff of care.

54 Admission to the Intensive Care Unit

Sebastian C. Tume, Guill Reyes

Admission of a patient after cardiac surgery involves extensive preparation to ensure safe patient arrival, handoff, rapid clinical assessment, and flawless transition and initiation of hemodynamic monitoring. The admission process at TCH is typically carried out in 3 phases. First, the team prepares for admission to ensure transition with minimal distractions. Second, the patient arrives, and monitoring and supportive therapies are transitioned. Handoff of clinical information takes place at that time. Last, laboratory and radiological assessment is accompanied by device securement and a comprehensive discussion of the care plan between the critical care team members. Appropriate adherence to these steps will ensure safe transition and preparation for any unexpected clinical events during the postoperative recovery period.

Phase 1: Preparation in Advance of Patient Arrival

The nurse and the patient-care assistants will set up the room. Consistency in this process can be ensured by formulating a standard equipment setup checklist (Figure 54-1). The respiratory therapist (RT) will set-up appropriate respiratory support therapies. It is also encouraged that the team reviews and understands the cardiac lesion and postoperative physiology.

After the patient transitions off CPB, the OR nurse calls the CICU with a patient status report that includes demographics, summary of surgical procedure, vascular access, drains, infusions, and planned respiratory support. The admitting nurse will share the report with the admitting team verbally and using a signout template. The postoperative orders should be placed at this time to ensure timely arrival of medications, laboratory tests, and radiological services. The RT should be updated to ensure that the appropriate equipment is available.

Phase 2: Patient Arrival

This phase consists of actual patient arrival and transfer of critical information between the surgical, anesthesia, and CICU teams. As the patient approaches the assigned room, the unit staff should ensure the hallway is clear, the door is fully open, and the equipment is out of the way for easy movement into the room. A supporting nurse should be available for charting and help with admission. As the patient is rolled into the room, the IV pole and other equipment should be positioned so it does not obstruct the view of the monitor or restrict access to supportive devices. The bed or infant warmer is plugged in and locked in position. Transition to the bedside monitor from the transport monitor should be seamless and with uninterrupted monitoring. Once all invasive pressures are displayed, calibration (zeroing) should be performed to ensure accuracy. To ensure consistency and avoid missed steps in the transition process, a checklist designed for this phase of admission should be followed (Figure 54-2).

An uninterrupted communication and clear exchange of information is crucial for safe transfer of vital clinical information. Members of the surgical, anesthesia, and CICU

PART IV. PERIOPERATIVE CARE

Room Setup Checklist

- Ventilator, ETCO2 cable, Bag and mask
- Supplemental O2 (Nasal cannula and Face Mask)
- Blood pressure cuff and cable
- Chest Tube tubing and wall suction
- Temperature cables (rectal and skin)
- Suction canisters and catheters
- Mucus trap for NG tube
- Tape to secure chest tubes and atrium
- Hemostats and clamps to secure chest tubes
- Medical Restraints
- Admission labs collection tubes
- Lab request stickers
- Saline Flushes and syringes for blood draws
- 1 Unit/ml Heparin for pressure lines
- Filtered and non-filtered medication tubing
- IV fluid pumps (3 syringe pumps)
- Code sheet with verified weight
- Emergency medications if patient is unstable

Figure 54-1. Setup checklist

Admission Checklist

- Open doors and clear equipment
- Release Orders and call for X-ray and EKG
- Plug in the bed/warmer and lock in place
- Connect chest tubes to suction and tape and strip
- Transfer monitor box (PDM) to the bedside monitor and allow to load data
- Display of two ECG leads (II, V), ST segment trends.
- Set alarm parameters at 20% from baseline. Adjust alarms again if needed following handover
- Transfer patient onto ventilator and connect ETCO2
- Calibrate (zero) all invasive PA, LA, CVP and arterial lines.
- Check all pressure tubing for air
- Draw labs (check ID band with specimens)
- Noninvasive monitoring setup: NIRS both cerebral and somatic, temperature probes rectal and toe, and cuff blood pressure.
- Confirm drip concentrations and dosing with pharmacy before anesthesia leaves bedside
- Flush and check existing PIV and central line ports for patency
- Finalize the post-operative care plan with critical care team (parameters, goals etc.)
- Check available blood products in cooler
- Remove pressure bags from pressure tubing and transition to syringe carriers
- Call family to bedside

Figure 54-2. Admission checklist

medical and surgical teams, as well as RT and pharmacy must be present for handoff. Our institutional practice is to have all attending-level providers at handoff to ensure that crucial information is elicited and relayed. All team members should devote full attention to the handoff process and refrain from performing any procedures during the handoff. Extra nursing personnel are required to attend to the patient during the handoff process so that the receiving nurse can devote full attention to the discussion.

The handoff consists of a brief patient history and surgical interventions by the cardiac surgeon followed by the CV anesthesiology report, which includes airway details, vascular access, anesthetic course, imaging findings, timing of perioperative medications, optimal filling and systemic pressures on separation from CPB, current inotropic/vasoactive infusions, blood product administration, sedative management, and any other pertinent information. The team discusses a postoperative care plan, hemodynamic and ventilator goals, as well as alarm parameters. At the conclusion of the handoff, the CICU staff "reads back" the plan to insure that communication has been effective.

Phase 3: Assessment and Studies

The last phase of admission includes baseline clinical and hemodynamic-state assessment followed by collection of laboratory and radiologic studies. A full clinical assessment should be performed by the bedside nurse and the medical team with special attention to skin assessment, perfusion, drain and catheter insertion sites, surgical site, and neurologic function. The nurse will also examine for air in the pressure lines. If present, atrial and ventricular temporary pacing wires should be labeled and secured. If paced, settings and thresholds should be confirmed. Chest tubes are reinforced at the connection site and secured to the bed. The chest-tube container should be taped to the floor and checked for water seal and appropriate suction. The urinary catheter bag is set to below the level of the patient with the catheter secured to the thigh. Nasogastric tubes should be at gravity in patients <5 years old and low-intermittent suction in older children.

The bedside monitor is set up to enable rapid hemodynamic assessment in case of complications. Alarm parameters are set to previously discussed parameters (usually 20% from baseline). Two ECG leads (preferably leads II and V6) are displayed with ST-segment monitoring enabled. A baseline 12-lead ECG is performed within 1 hour of admission. Invasive pressures should be color labeled. Cerebral and somatic NIRS should be used if invasive venous oximetry is not available. Temperature is monitored using rectal and peripheral probes with the goal of normothermia unless otherwise indicated. Rewarming should be gradual to prevent excessive vasodilatation.

Laboratory studies such as arterial blood gas, complete blood count, chemistry, and coagulation panel should be collected after handoff and CXR, within 30-60 minutes of admission. An adequate CXR can be achieved by ensuring that the precordium is free of cables and tubing, and the head is positioned at midline, in a neutral position.

Additional considerations include a four-extremity BP assessment after aortic arch repair. Drip concentration and dosing verification should occur with a pharmacist, ensuring that there is sufficient volume available to avoid having to switch vasoactive medication drips in the immediate postoperative period. A cooler with blood products should be present at the bedside for every admission and kept overnight for patients with intracardiac lines, open chest, VADs, or ECMO. Those on significant amounts of vasoactive support will remain supine and head elevation should be gradual.

The postoperative recovery can be associated with some expected hemodynamic lability. Adherence to protocols and checklists will limit variation in care. Each patient should be treated according to their postoperative physiology but ensuring strict adherence to all the phases of postoperative admission to ensure a safe and flawless transition.

55 Sedation and Analgesia in the Cardiac Intensive Care Unit

Barbara-Jo Achuff, Ashraf Resheidat, Zoel A. Quinonez, Lara S. Shekerdemian

The majority of patients in the CICU require and receive analgesia and/or sedation in order to provide comfort, manage pain, and minimize their stress response to pain or noxious stimuli. Analgesia is most often required to preempt and treat postoperative pain, but can also help in managing overall comfort while in the ICU environment. Sedation is used to maximize comfort, reduce the stress response, and avoid excessive oxygen consumption at a time of actual or potential hemodynamic instability. The depth of sedation ranges from minimal (anxiolysis) to decrease stress and maintain a natural airway, to deep sedation with depression of consciousness requiring intubation and mechanical ventilation. The desired depth of sedation requires there to be a balance between undersedation, which can lead to hemodynamic instability, poor healing, and other untoward events such as self-extubation; and oversedation, which can lead to hemodynamic instability, delirium, and long-term habituation. In addition, a growing awareness of the long-term effects of some agents on neurodevelopment, coupled with the 2016 FDA Drug and Safety Communication regarding this concerns, has added further emphasis on the need for careful consideration of analgesic and sedating agents in the ICU as well as in the OR.

Analgesia and sedation requirements are variable and no ideal medication or regime fits every patient, but optimizing sedation and analgesia through protocols provides safe and adequate titratable pain/sedation control and allows communication among providers. Thus, at TCH, our multi-disciplinary *S.T.A.R. (Sedation Targeted Assessment and Review)* team of *physicians, nurses, pharmacists, and administrators* has undertaken a comprehensive review of sedation and analgesia practice in the CICU, and has used this data coupled with the existing literature to formulate a systematic approach to sedation and analgesia in the unit. This requires a consensus-based approach to assessing pain and sedation, deciding on the target for "wakefulness" of an individual patient, and then following a logical algorithm of how to achieve this, with frequent reassessment.

Assessment of Pain and Sedation

Our bedside CICU providers utilize validated objective scoring systems for pain and sedation. The pain score mainly used at TCH is the FLACC scale (Face, Legs, Activity, Cry, Consolability) (Table 55-1). The State Behavioral Scale (SBS) (Table 55-2) is used to describe the *desired* level of sedation (from -3 meaning unresponsive to +2 meaning agitated) for the *intubated* patient who is not receiving neuromuscular blockade. The SBS target is decided by the team on bedside rounds and the observed score is documented regularly by the bedside nurse.

Postoperative Pain Management

With an emphasis on minimizing side effects while avoiding excessive "catch-up" dosing, we use a multimodal approach to analgesia for patients that have been *extubated* in the CVOR or shortly after. Opioid patient- (or nurse-) controlled analgesia (PCA) helps

55. SEDATION AND ANALGESIA IN THE CARDIAC INTENSIVE CARE UNIT

Table 55-1. FLACC scale - Face, Legs, Activity, Cry, Consolability Observational Tool as a Measure. The specific scores for each of the areas are added to create the overall score. From: Merkel SI, Voepel-Lewis T, Shayevitz JR, et al. The FLACC: a behavioral scale for scoring postoperative pain in young children. Pediatr Nurs 1997;23:293-297. © 1997 The Regents of the University of Michigan (reprinted with permission).

	0	1	2
Face	No particular expression or smile	Occasional grimace or frown, withdrawn, disinterested	Frequent to constant frown, clenched jaw, quivering chin
Legs	Normal position or relaxed	Uneasy, restless, tense	Kicking, or legs drawn up
Activity	Lying quietly, normal position, moves easily	Squirming, shifting back and forth, tense	Arched, rigid, or jerking
Cry	No cry (awake or asleep)	Moans or whimpers, occasional	Crying steadily, screams or sobs, frequent complaints
Consolability	Content, relaxed	Reassured by occasional touching, hugging, or talking to; distractible	Difficult to console or comfort

match the patient's requirement in a timely and safe manner. In addition to opioids, IV acetaminophen as well as antinociceptive nonsteroidal anti-inflamatory drugs (ketorolac), local anesthetics, adjunctive alpha-2 agonists (clonidine and dexmedetomidine), and antihyperalgesic N-methyl-D-aspartate (NMDA)-receptor antagonists (ketamine) can be used alone or in in combination. Conversion to oral analgesics occurs once the patient is able to tolerate oral intake. We also integrate complementary and alternative medicine (CAM) techniques with environmental controls, behavioral modification, and physical therapy for longer-term patients.

Clinical Pathways

Standardized clinical pathways improve provider, nursing, and patient satisfaction while providing less variation in analgesia and sedation practice. In our unit, we utilize color-coded age and weight-based clinical pathways for *intubated* patients who are not on neuromuscular blockade. These pathways offer initial medication choices according to age group and desired SBS level, as well as a roadmap to guide bolus dosing for the bedside nurse.

Neonatal (*Blue*) Sedation Pathway

The neonatal sedation pathway (Figure 55-1) applies for intubated patients <30 days old. It includes:

1. Fentanyl infusion as single agent with dexmedetomidine as secondary if required.
2. If the SBS score is greater than desired, consider non-pharmacologic interventions to decrease environmental stress including bundling (if possible), noise reduction, distraction, and soothing techniques.
3. If the SBS score remains elevated, then bolus doses are given with dosing matching

Table 55-2. State Behavioral Scale (SBS) to describe the desired level of sedation for the intubated patient not receiving neuromuscular blockade. Score as patient's response to voice, then touch, then noxious stimuli (planned endotracheal tube suctioning or nailbed pressure for <5 seconds). From: Curley MA, Harris SK, Fraser KA, et al. State Behavioral Scale: a sedation assessment instrument for infants and young children supported on mechanical ventilation. Pediatr Crit Care Med 2006;7:107-114. © 2006 Wolters Kluwer Health, Inc. (reprinted with permission).

Score	Description	Definition
-3	Unresponsive	No spontaneous respiratory effort No cough or coughs only with suctioning No response to noxious stimuli Unable to pay attention to care provider Does not distress with any procedure (including noxious) Does not move
-2	Responsive to noxious stimuli	Spontaneous yet supported breathing Coughs with suctioning/repositioning Responds to noxious stimuli Unable to pay attention to care provider Will distress with a noxious procedure Does not move/occasional movement of extremities or shifting of position
-1	Responsive to gentle touch or voice	Spontaneous but ineffective non-supported breaths Coughs with suctioning/repositioning Responds to touch/voice Able to pay attention but drifts off after stimulation Distresses with procedures Able to calm with comforting touch or voice when stimulus removed Occasional movement of extremities or shifting of position
0	Awake and able to calm	Spontaneous and effective breathing Coughs when repositioned/Occasional spontaneous cough Responds to voice/No external stimulus is required to elicit response Spontaneously pays attention to care provider Distresses with procedures Able to calm with comforting touch or voice when stimulus removed Occasional movement of extremities or shifting of position/increased movement (restless, squirming)
+1	Restless and difficult to calm	Spontaneous effective breathing/Having difficulty breathing with ventilator Occasional spontaneous cough Responds to voice/ No external stimulus is required to elicit response Drifts off/Spontaneously pays attention to care provider Intermittently unsafe Does not consistently calm despite 5 minute attempt/unable to console Increased movement (restless, squirming)
+2	Agitated	May have difficulty breathing with ventilator Coughing spontaneously No external stimulus required to elicit response Spontaneously pays attention to care provider Unsafe (biting ETT, pulling at lines, cannot be left alone) Unable to console Increased movement (restless, squirming or thrashing side-to-side, kicking legs)

ETT: Endotracheal tube.

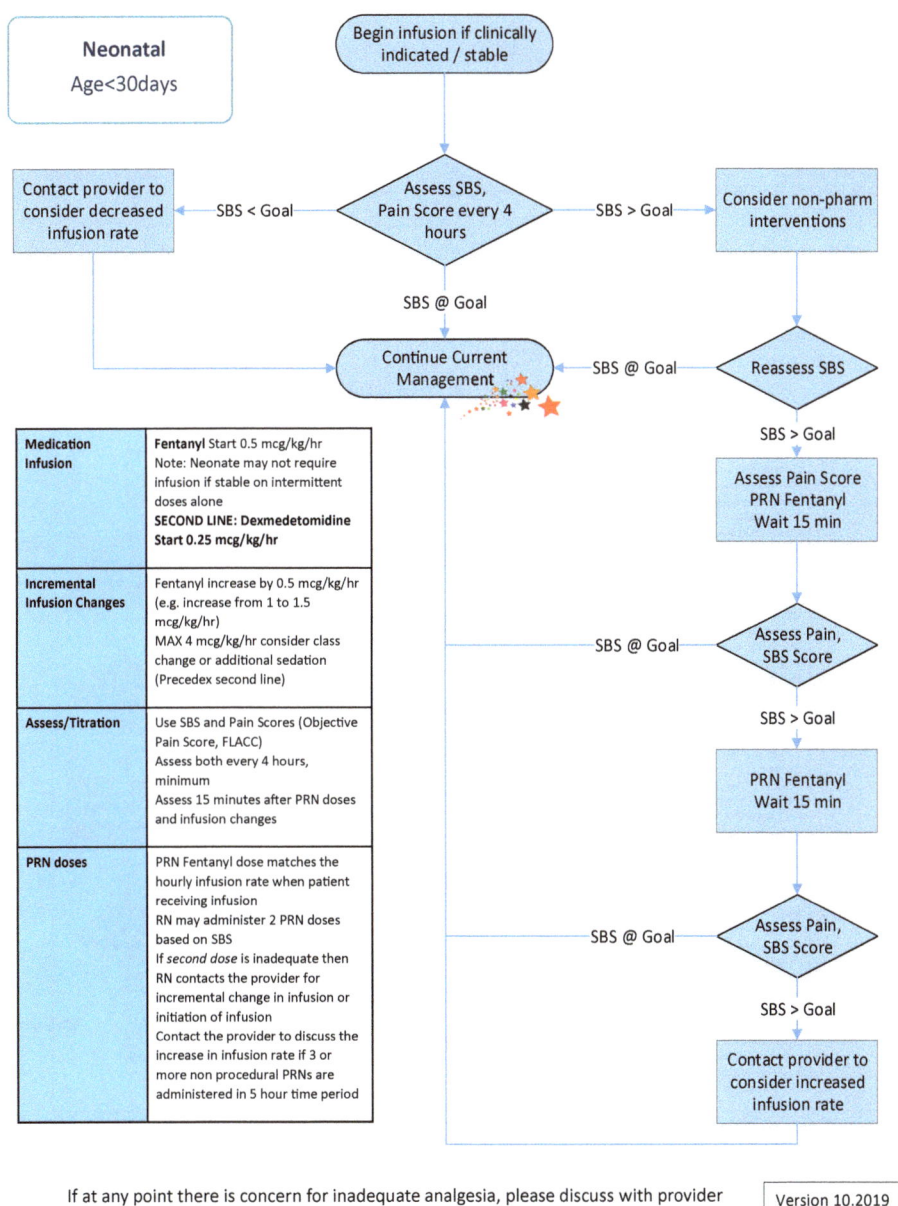

55. SEDATION AND ANALGESIA IN THE CARDIAC INTENSIVE CARE UNIT

Figure 55-1. Neonatal (blue) sedation pathway.

PART IV. PERIOPERATIVE CARE

Figure 55-2. Infant/child (orange) sedation pathway.

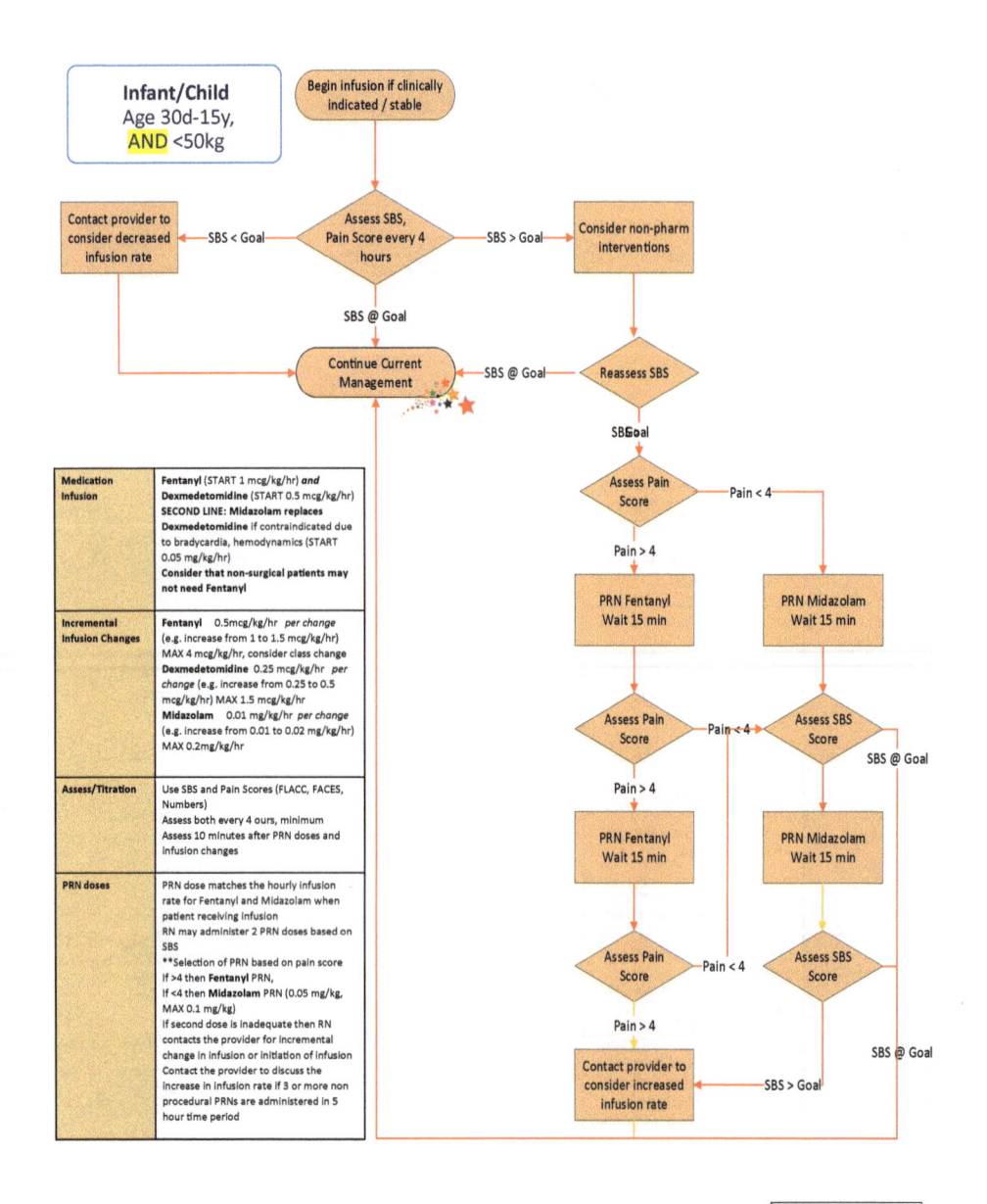

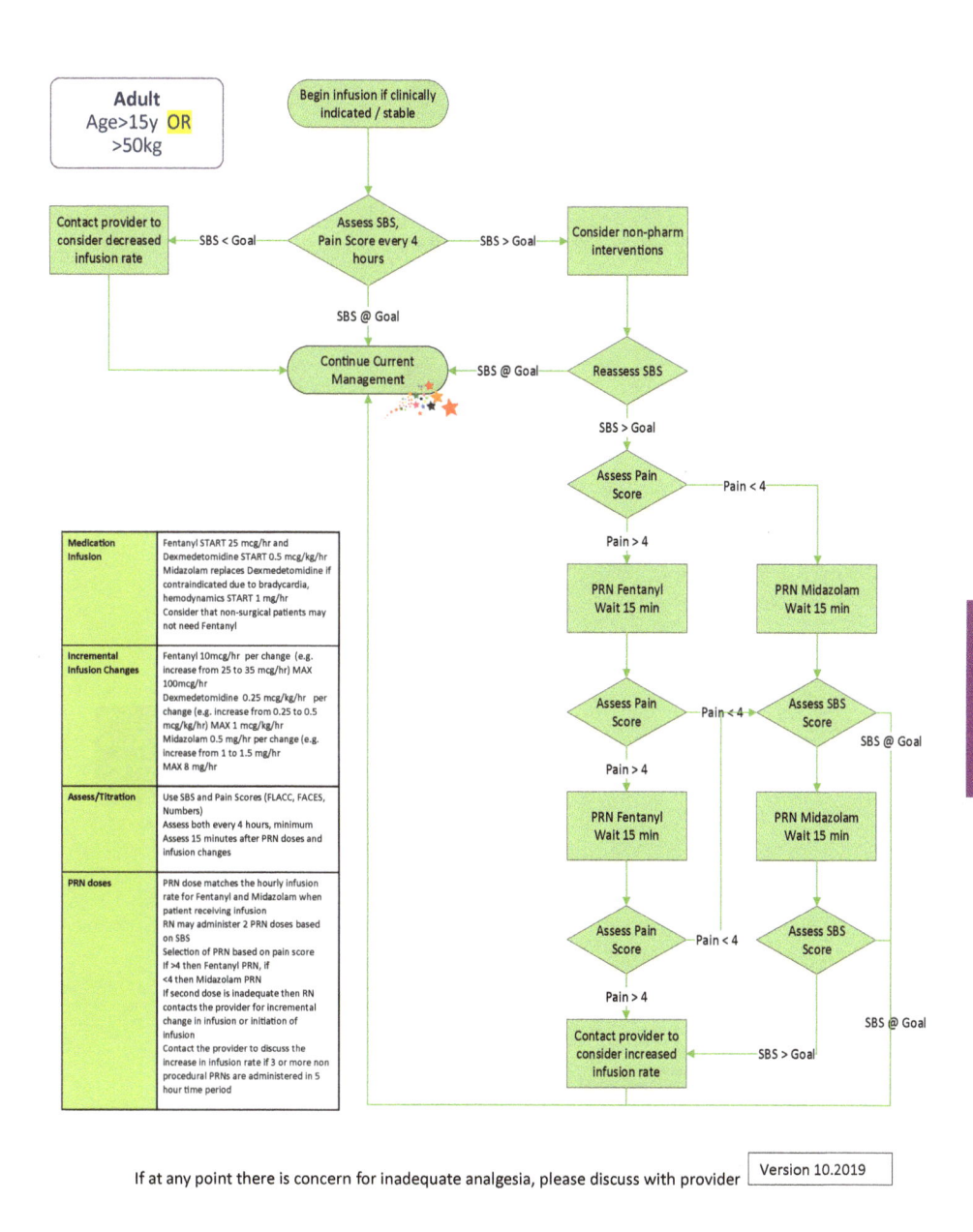

55. SEDATION AND ANALGESIA IN THE CARDIAC INTENSIVE CARE UNIT

Figure 55-3. Adult (green) sedation pathway.

PART IV. PERIOPERATIVE CARE

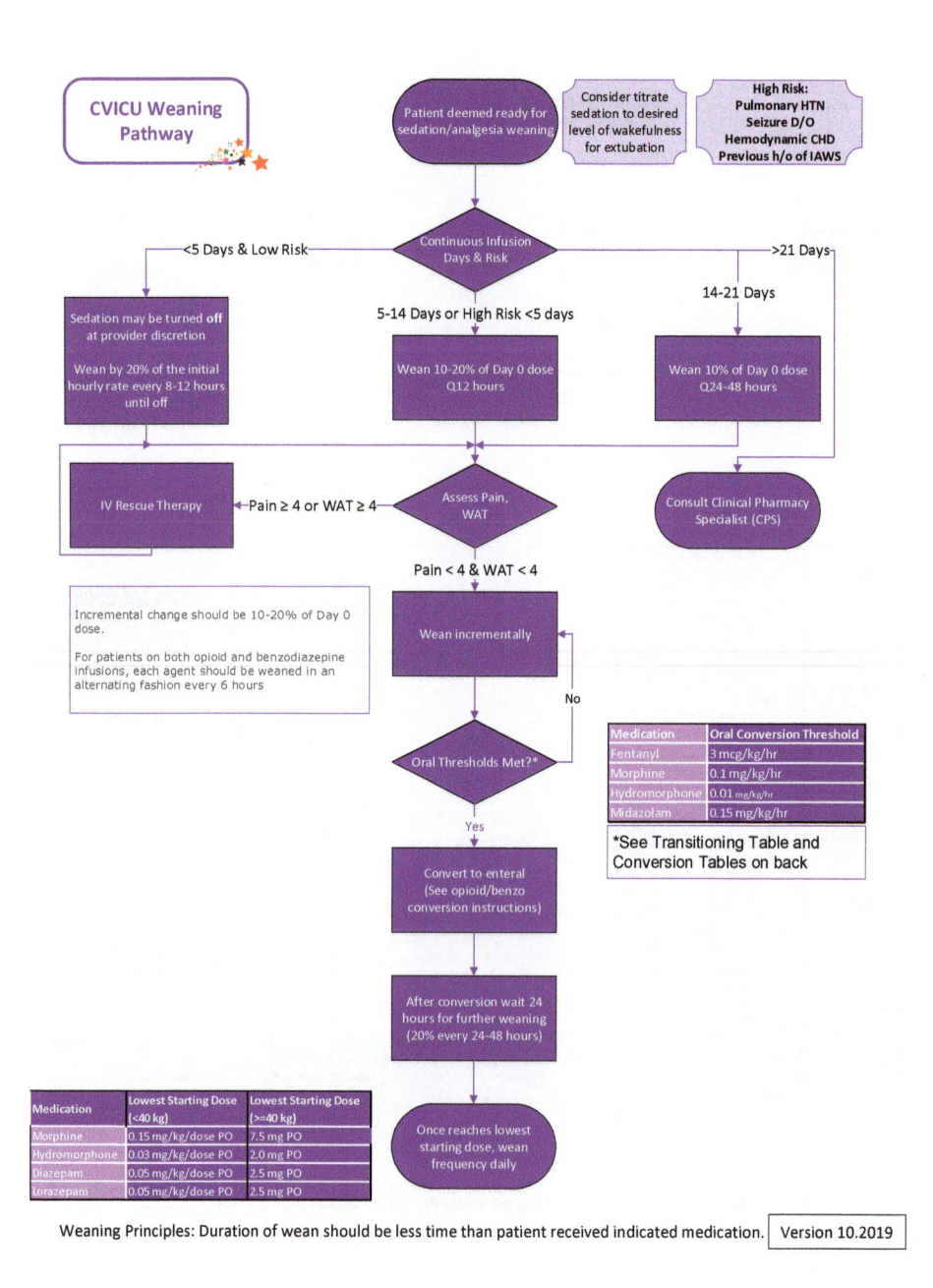

Figure 55-4. CICU weaning (purple) pathway.

55. SEDATION AND ANALGESIA IN THE CARDIAC INTENSIVE CARE UNIT

Transitioning from Continuous IV Sedation to Intermittent PO regimen (IV to PO Opioid)	
Step 1	Start ENTERAL opioid agent at dose calculated
Step 2	Wean opioid infusion by 50% 30 minutes after the 2nd ENTERAL opioid dose
Step 3	Turn off the opioid infusion 30 minutes after the 3rd ENTERAL opioid dose

Transitioning from Continuous IV Sedation to Intermittent PO regimen (IV to PO Benzo)	
Step 1	Start ENTERAL benzo agent at the dose calculated
Step 2	Wean benzo infusion by 50 % 30 minutes after the 1st ENTERAL benzo dose
Step 3	Turn off the benzo infusion 30 minutes after the 2nd ENTERAL benzo dose

Continuous Infusion	Enteral Agent (PO/GT/JT/NG/NJ/ND) Max Dose 6mg per dose
Midazolam 0.15 mg/kg/hr	Lorazepam 0.15 mg/kg/dose q 4h
Midazolam < 0.15 mg/kg/hr	Midazolam ___ mg/kg/hr x ___kg x 1.0 = ___ mg enteral Lorazepam/dose q4h
Midazolam 2 mg/hr	Lorazepam *** mg enteral q4hr
Midazolam <2 mg/hr	___ mcg/hr x *** = ___mg enteral Lorazepam /dose q4h

Continuous Infusion	Enteral Agent (PO/GT/JT/NG/NJ/ND) Max Dose 30mg per dose
Fentanyl 3 mcg/kg/hr	Morphine 0.55 mg/kg/dose q 4h
Fentanyl < 3 mcg/kg/hr	Fentanyl ___ mcg/kg/hr x ___ kg x 0.18 = ___mg enteral Morphine/dose q4h
Fentanyl 100 mcg/hr	Morphine 18 mg enteral q4h
Fentanyl < 100 mcg/hr	Fentanyl ___ mcg/hr x 0.18 = ___mg enteral Morphine/dose q4h
Morphine 0.1 mg/kg/hr	Morphine 0.6 mg/kg/dose q 4h
Morphine < 0.1 mg/kg/hr	Morphine ___ mg/kg/hr x ___ kg x 6 = ___ mg enteral morphine/dose q4h
Morphine 4 mg/hr	Morphine 24 mg enteral q4h
Morphine < 4 mg/hr	Morphine ___ mg/hr x 6 = ___ mg enteral morphine/dose q4h
Hydromorphone 10 mcg/kg/hr	Morphine 0.4 mg/kg/dose enteral q4h
Hydromorphone < 10 mcg/kg/hr	Hydromorphone ___ mcg/kg/hr x ___ kg x 0.04 = ___ mg enteral Morphine/dose q4h
Hydromorphone 500 mcg/hr	Morphine 20 mg dose enteral q4h
Hydromorphone < 500 mcg/hr	Hydromorphone ___ mcg/kg/hr x ___ kg x 0.04 = ___ mg enteral Morphine/dose q4h

Figure 55-4. CICU weaning (purple) pathway (Continuation).

1 hours' worth of infusion as a "rescue". SBS should be reevaluated after each PRN dose and each dose can be given at 10-minute intervals to achieve desired sedation.
4. Incremental increases in infusion dosages are suggested if 2-3 bolus doses are inadequate. The bedside nurse is instructed to notify the provider for infusion changes.
5. If SBS less than ordered level, decrease the infusion to maintain the SBS at desired level and titrate to effect of sedation level.

Infant/Child (*Orange*) Sedation Pathway

The infant/child sedation pathway (Figure 55-2) is used for patients aged 31 days old to 15 years old, or <50 kg. Fentanyl and dexmedetomidine infusions are initiated with a substitute of midazolam infusion for those patients for whom dexmedetomidine is contraindicated, or not tolerated for hemodynamic reasons. If SBS is greater than desired, consider nonpharmacologic interventions as above. The pathway continues as points 3-5 above.

Adolescent/Adult (*Green*) Sedation Pathway

The adolescent/adult sedation pathway (Figure 55-3) is used for patients aged >15 years old or those that weigh ≥50 kg. This pathway differs from the orange pathway because it is no longer weight based (per kg) for opioids and benzodiazepines and is dosed appropriately at an hourly rate for infusion.

Tolerance and Withdrawal

Patients with prolonged narcotic or benzodiazepine exposure can develop tolerance (decreased response to the same doses of medications), dependence and withdrawal, hyperalgesia (heightened sensitization to pain), allodynia (pain elicited by nonpainful stimuli), or delirium. Sedation holidays and opioid rotation may not be effective or feasible. Continuous infusions may need to be weaned carefully in these patients.

Weaning (*Purple*) Pathway

For patients at high risk for iatrogenic withdrawal syndrome (IAWS) including those receiving infusion >5 days and particularly those in which hemodynamics would not tolerate withdrawal symptoms (pulmonary hypertension, history of seizure disorder, significant hemodynamic instability, history of previous withdrawal syndrome), a weaning pathway is desired. Figure 55-4 illustrates the weaning pathway. Nonopioid drugs may also be considered (ketamine, chloral hydrate, gabapentin) while weaning narcotics.

The Withdrawal Assessment Tool (WAT-1) score (Figure 55-5) should be documented twice daily starting on the *first day of weaning* in at risk patients, and should be continued until 72 hours after the last dose.
1. If a patient received an infusion ≤5 days, then it can be stopped at the provider's discretion or weaned by 20% of the initial hourly rate every 8-12 hours. WAT-1 scores can be followed and PRN bolus doses given as required to keep WAT-1 score <4.
2. Patients receiving infusions for >5 days or at high risk for IAWS should wean the infusions incrementally until oral thresholds are met

WITHDRAWAL ASSESSMENT TOOL VERSION 1 (WAT – 1)

© 2007 L.S. Franck and M.A.Q. Curley. All Rights reserved. Reproduced only by permission of Authors.

Patient Identifier										
	Date:									
	Time:									
Information from patient record, previous 12 hours										
Any loose /watery stools	No = 0 / Yes = 1									
Any vomiting/wretching/gagging	No = 0 / Yes = 1									
Temperature > 37.8°C	No = 0 / Yes = 1									
2 minute pre-stimulus observation										
State	SBS[1] ≤ 0 or asleep/awake/calm = 0 / SBS[1] ≥ +1 or awake/distressed = 1									
Tremor	None/mild = 0 / Moderate/severe = 1									
Any sweating	No = 0 / Yes = 1									
Uncoordinated/repetitive movement	None/mild = 0 / Moderate/severe = 1									
Yawning or sneezing	None or 1 = 0 / ≥2 = 1									
1 minute stimulus observation										
Startle to touch	None/mild = 0 / Moderate/severe = 1									
Muscle tone	Normal = 0 / Increased = 1									
Post-stimulus recovery										
Time to gain calm state (SBS[1] ≤ 0)	< 2min = 0 / 2 - 5min = 1 / > 5 min = 2									
Total Score (0-12)										

WITHDRAWAL ASSESSMENT TOOL (WAT – 1) INSTRUCTIONS

- Start WAT-1 scoring from the **first day of weaning** in patients who have received opioids +/or benzodiazepines by infusion or regular dosing for prolonged periods (e.g., > 5 days). Continue twice daily scoring until 72 hours after the last dose.
- The Withdrawal Assessment Tool (WAT-1) should be completed along with the SBS[1] at least once per 12 hour shift (e.g., at 08:00 and 20:00 ± 2 hours). The progressive stimulus used in the SBS[1] assessment provides a standard stimulus for observing signs of withdrawal.

Obtain information from patient record (this can be done before or after the stimulus):
- ✓ **Loose/watery stools**: Score 1 if any loose or watery stools were documented in the past 12 hours; score 0 if none were noted.
- ✓ **Vomiting/wretching/gagging**: Score 1 if any vomiting or spontaneous wretching or gagging were documented in the past 12 hours; score 0 if none were noted.
- ✓ **Temperature > 37.8°C**: Score 1 if the modal (most frequently occurring) temperature documented was greater than 37.8 °C in the past 12 hours; score 0 if this was not the case.

2 minute pre-stimulus observation:
- ✓ **State**: Score 1 if awake and distress (SBS[1]: ≥ +1) observed during the 2 minutes prior to the stimulus; score 0 if asleep or awake and calm/cooperative (SBS[1] ≤ 0).
- ✓ **Tremor**: Score 1 if moderate to severe tremor observed during the 2 minutes prior to the stimulus; score 0 if no tremor (or only minor, intermittent tremor).
- ✓ **Sweating**: Score 1 if any sweating during the 2 minutes prior to the stimulus; score 0 if no sweating noted.
- ✓ **Uncoordinated/repetitive movements**: Score 1 if moderate to severe uncoordinated or repetitive movements such as head turning, leg or arm flailing or torso arching observed during the 2 minutes prior to the stimulus; score 0 if no (or only mild) uncoordinated or repetitive movements.
- ✓ **Yawning or sneezing** > 1: Score 1 if more than 1 yawn or sneeze observed during the 2 minutes prior to the stimulus; score 0 if 0 to 1 yawn or sneeze.

1 minute stimulus observation:
- ✓ **Startle to touch**: Score 1 if moderate to severe startle occurs when touched during the stimulus; score 0 if none (or mild).
- ✓ **Muscle tone**: Score 1 if tone increased during the stimulus; score 0 if normal.

Post-stimulus recovery:
- ✓ **Time to gain calm state** (SBS[1] ≤ 0): Score 2 if it takes greater than 5 minutes following stimulus; score 1 if achieved within 2 to 5 minutes; score 0 if achieved in less than 2 minutes.

Sum the 11 numbers in the column for the total WAT-1 score (0-12).

[1]Curley et al. State behavioral scale: A sedation assessment instrument for infants and young children supported on mechanical ventilation. Pediatr Crit Care Med 2006;7(2):107-114.

Figure 55-5. Withdrawal Assessment Tool Version 1 (WAT-1). © 2007 L.S. Franck and M.A.Q. Curley (reprinted with permission). For more information on the WAT-1, see https://familynursing.ucsf.edu/withdrawal-assessment-tool-1-wat-1.

3. For patients with intermediate exposure (8-14 days), wean medications 10-20% every 12 hours.
4. For patients with long-term exposure (>14 days), wean medications 10-20% every 24 hours. For those with very long-term exposure (>21 days), please consult the clinical pharmacy specialist for a wean plan.
5. After oral conversion, wait 24 hours for further weaning.
6. If FLACC >4 or WAT-1 >4 then IV rescue therapy is utilized. If multiple rescue doses required per shift or there are hemodynamic status changes, hold further weaning.
7. Once the "basement dose" is reached, wean the frequency daily until off.

NOTE: For patients on both opioid and benzodiazepine infusions, each agent should be weaned in an alternating fashion every 4 hours.

For patients with indwelling nerve block catheters, the pain service should be called to provide recommendations and to assess the patient before initiating pain alleviating interventions, when possible. Additionally, in *challenging* patients with prolonged sedation complications from opioids and hypnotics, the pain service and pharmacy can be consulted for help with weaning.

Delirium

Delirium is a disturbance of both consciousness and cognition with the cardinal features of acute change or fluctuation in mental status and inattention. The phenotypes of delirium include hyperactive, hypoactive, and mixed types, with the hypoactive type being the most common in the pediatric population although patients may alternate between types. *Hyperactive delirium* is characterized by agitation, restlessness, hypervigilance, and combative behavior. In contrast, *hypoactive delirium* is notable for lethargy, inattention, and decreased responsiveness. Other symptoms can include profound sleep disturbances, auditory and/or visual hallucinations, and waxing and waning behaviors. Delirium can be associated with increased severity of illness, time to extubation, hospital length of stay, healthcare costs, and mortality. It has been linked in children to delusional memories, perceptual-motor and behavioral problems, and posttraumatic stress disorder.

According to the literature, factors associated with increased risk of delirium include CPB surgery, use of specific medications including benzodiazepines and opiates, physical restraints, and the intensive care environment. Given the risks present in the cardiac population, there is a need for heightened and targeted delirium screening in the CICU to potentially improve outcomes in this vulnerable patient population.

Treatment for ICU delirium is largely preventive and focuses on appropriate screening and decreasing iatrogenic factors through nonpharmacological methods. While pharmacologic therapies are available, the medications utilized can have significant side effects and there is limited data on efficacy. Implementation of a delirium screening tool has been associated with decreased delirium prevalence, and early recognition and treatment may decrease long-term cognitive impairment and improve the neurodevelopmental trajectory.

55. SEDATION AND ANALGESIA IN THE CARDIAC INTENSIVE CARE UNIT

Please answer the following questions based on your interactions with the patient over the course of your shift:						
	Never	Rarely	Sometimes	Often	Always	Score
	4	3	2	1	0	
1. Does the child make eye contact with the caregiver?						
2. Are the child's actions purposeful?						
3. Is the child aware of his/her surroundings?						
4. Does the child communicate needs and wants?						
	Never	Rarely	Sometimes	Often	Always	
	0	1	2	3	4	
5. Is the child restless?						
6. Is the child inconsolable?						
7. Is the child underactive—very little movement while awake?						
8. Does it take the child a long time to respond to interactions?						
					TOTAL	

Figure 55-6. Cornell Assessment of Pediatric Delirium (CAPD) revised. From: Traube C, Silver G, Kearney J, et al. Cornell Assessment of Pediatric Delirium: a valid, rapid, observational tool for screening delirium in the PICU. Crit Care Med 2014;42:656-663 (reprinted with permission).

Assessment of Delirium

The Cornell Assessment of Pediatric Delirium (CAPD) tool (Figure 55-6) was validated in 2014 for patients 0-21 years of age, including those with developmental delay (Traube et al. 2014). This tool specifically allows discrimination between delirium and other causes of altered mental status in critically ill children. The CAPD is designed to take into account a period of extended observation (rather than being used as a point-in-time), and a score of 9 or higher is considered diagnostic for delirium in developmentally typical patients. In those with developmental delay, a diagnosis of delirium requires both a CAPD score >9 and confirmation of a change from neurologic baseline. Developmental anchor points are available to be used in conjunction with the CAPD to provide reference for the screener (https://www.icudelirium.org/medical-professionals/pediatric-care).

Delirium (*Teal*) Pathway

The delirium (teal) pathway is shown in Figure 55-7. Twice a day (once a shift), the nurse completes the SBS assessment (Table 55-2) and if the SBS is -2 or higher, delirium is assessed using the CAPD tool (Figure 55-6). Patients with an SBS score of -3 or patients that are paralyzed are excluded from this pathway.

PART IV. PERIOPERATIVE CARE

Delirium Screening

Definition: Delirium is a disturbance of both consciousness and cognition with the cardinal features of acute change or fluctuation in mental status and inattention.

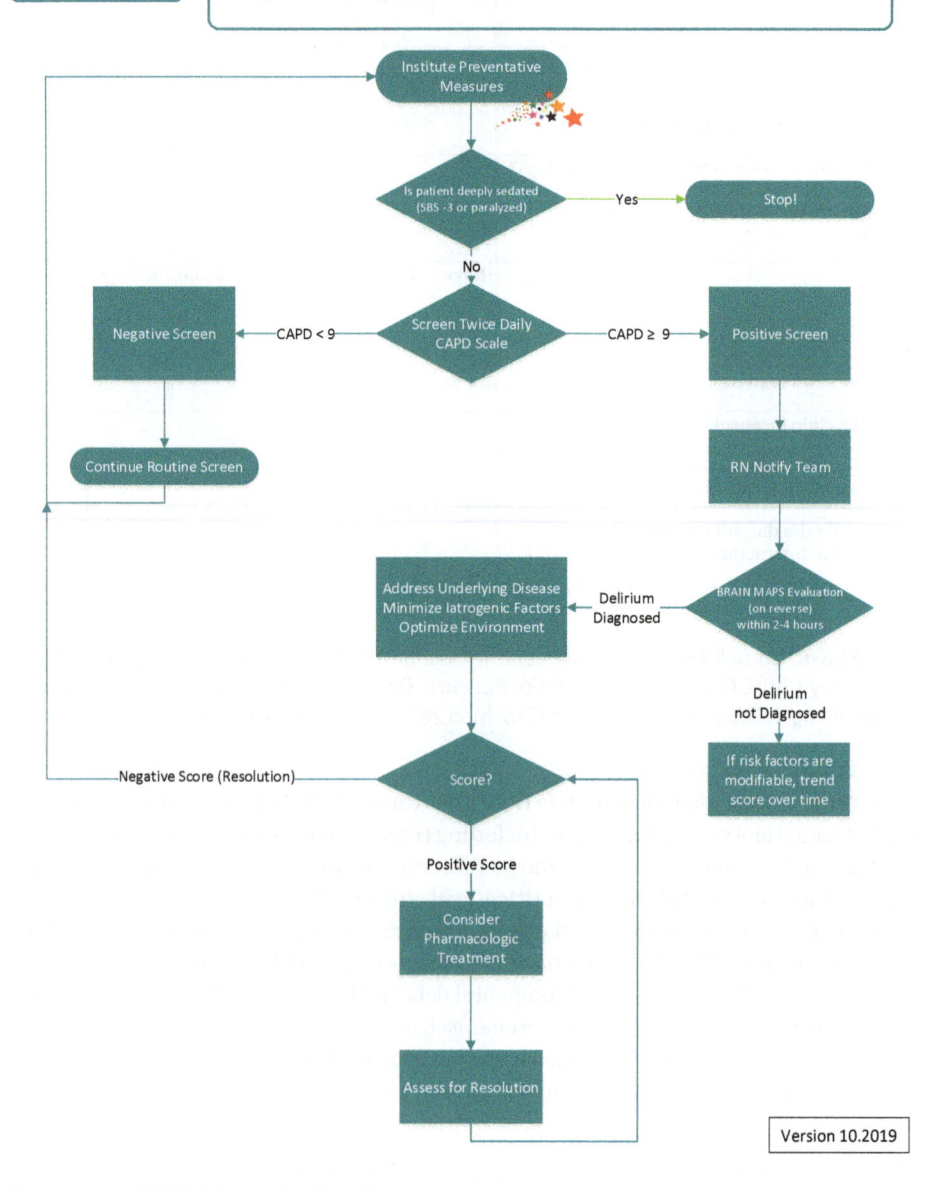

```
                    Institute Preventative
                          Measures
                              │
                              ▼
                    Is patient deeply sedated ──Yes──▶ Stop!
                      (SBS -3 or paralyzed)
                              │
                              No
                              ▼
   Negative Screen ◀──CAPD < 9── Screen Twice Daily ──CAPD ≥ 9──▶ Positive Screen
                                    CAPD Scale                          │
          │                                                             ▼
          ▼                                                      RN Notify Team
   Continue Routine Screen                                              │
                                                                        ▼
                                                              BRAIN MAPS Evaluation
   Address Underlying Disease     ◀──Delirium                   (on reverse)
   Minimize Iatrogenic Factors       Diagnosed                 within 2-4 hours
   Optimize Environment                                                 │
          │                                                     Delirium not Diagnosed
          ▼                                                             │
  ──Negative Score (Resolution)──  Score?  ◀─────────────         If risk factors are
                                     │                            modifiable, trend
                                  Positive Score                  score over time
                                     ▼
                                 Consider
                              Pharmacologic
                                Treatment
                                     │
                                     ▼
                            Assess for Resolution
```

Version 10.2019

Figure 55-7. CICU delirium (teal) pathway.

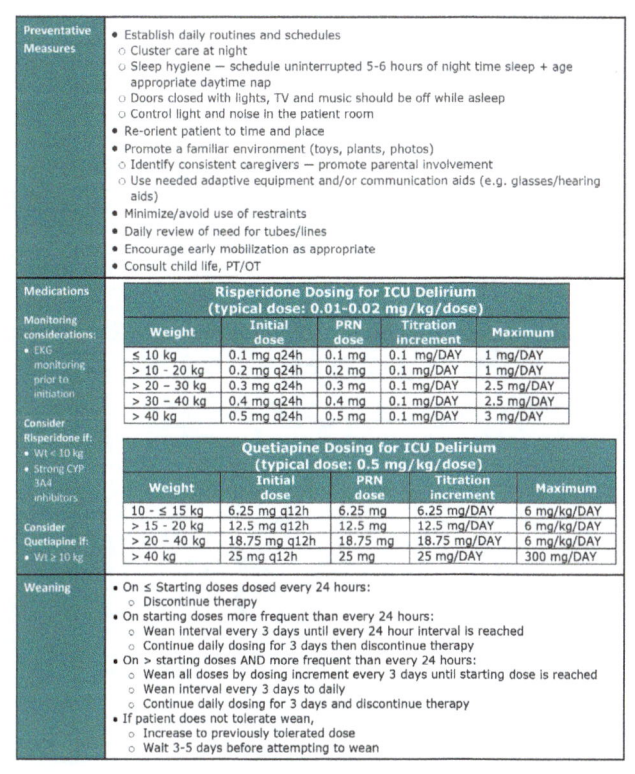

55. SEDATION AND ANALGESIA IN THE CARDIAC INTENSIVE CARE UNIT

Preventative Measures	• Establish daily routines and schedules ○ Cluster care at night ○ Sleep hygiene — schedule uninterrupted 5-6 hours of night time sleep + age appropriate daytime nap ○ Doors closed with lights, TV and music should be off while asleep ○ Control light and noise in the patient room • Re-orient patient to time and place • Promote a familiar environment (toys, plants, photos) ○ Identify consistent caregivers — promote parental involvement ○ Use needed adaptive equipment and/or communication aids (e.g. glasses/hearing aids) • Minimize/avoid use of restraints • Daily review of need for tubes/lines • Encourage early mobilization as appropriate • Consult child life, PT/OT
Medications **Monitoring considerations:** • EKG monitoring prior to initiation **Consider Risperidone if:** • Wt < 10 kg • Strong CYP 3A4 inhibitors **Consider Quetiapine if:** • Wt ≥ 10 kg	**Risperidone Dosing for ICU Delirium** **(typical dose: 0.01-0.02 mg/kg/dose)** 	Weight	Initial dose	PRN dose	Titration increment	Maximum
---	---	---	---	---
≤ 10 kg	0.1 mg q24h	0.1 mg	0.1 mg/DAY	1 mg/DAY
> 10 - 20 kg	0.2 mg q24h	0.2 mg	0.1 mg/DAY	1 mg/DAY
> 20 - 30 kg	0.3 mg q24h	0.3 mg	0.1 mg/DAY	2.5 mg/DAY
> 30 - 40 kg	0.4 mg q24h	0.4 mg	0.1 mg/DAY	2.5 mg/DAY
> 40 kg	0.5 mg q24h	0.5 mg	0.1 mg/DAY	3 mg/DAY | **Quetiapine Dosing for ICU Delirium** **(typical dose: 0.5 mg/kg/dose)** | Weight	Initial dose	PRN dose	Titration increment	Maximum
---	---	---	---	---
10 - ≤ 15 kg	6.25 mg q12h	6.25 mg	6.25 mg/DAY	6 mg/kg/DAY
> 15 - 20 kg	12.5 mg q12h	12.5 mg	12.5 mg/DAY	6 mg/kg/DAY
> 20 - 40 kg	18.75 mg q12h	18.75 mg	18.75 mg/DAY	6 mg/kg/DAY
> 40 kg	25 mg q12h	25 mg	25 mg/DAY	300 mg/DAY	
Weaning	• On ≤ Starting doses dosed every 24 hours: ○ Discontinue therapy • On starting doses more frequent than every 24 hours: ○ Wean interval every 3 days until every 24 hour interval is reached ○ Continue daily dosing for 3 days then discontinue therapy • On > starting doses AND more frequent than every 24 hours: ○ Wean all doses by dosing increment every 3 days until starting dose is reached ○ Wean interval every 3 days to daily ○ Continue daily dosing for 3 days and discontinue therapy • If patient does not tolerate wean, ○ Increase to previously tolerated dose ○ Wait 3-5 days before attempting to wean

Figure 55-7. CICU delirium (teal) pathway (Continuation).

1. Start with emphasizing environmental factors including day and night activities in the ICU and limitation of stimulation at night. Understand the child's usual routine and mimic home activities.
2. If the CAPD score ≥9 and the patient is not at neurologic baseline, the patient screens positive for delirium. The ICU advance practice provider or the fellow should be notified. After completing the history and medical assessment, the clinical team should consider the causes of delirium and recommendations using the BRAIN MAPS acronym (Figure 55-8) to minimize iatrogenic factors and optimize environment.
3. Is the pain adequately treated? Is the patient adequately sedated? Is the patient withdrawing from opioids or benzodiazepines?
4. If delirium persists >48 hours or is particularly hyperactive, then consider medication. If there is sleep/wake cycle dysregulation, consider starting melatonin every night. Otherwise, consider the use of antipsychotics such as risperdone or quetiapine (Figure 55-7).
5. If the patient is exposed to medications known to increase the odds of developing delirium (benzodiazepines or anticholinergic agents), consider safely weaning them off.
6. Consider consulting child psychiatry.
7. Assess for resolution and consider stopping medication (if prescribed).

PART IV. PERIOPERATIVE CARE

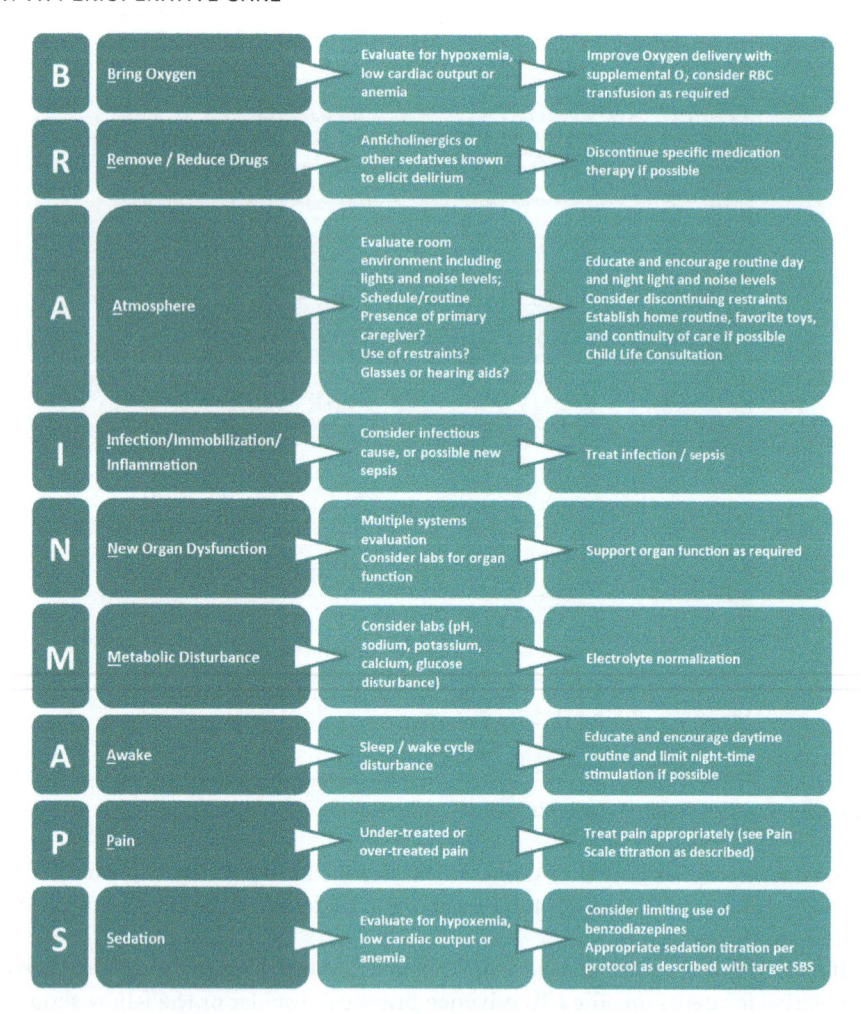

B	Bring Oxygen	Evaluate for hypoxemia, low cardiac output or anemia	Improve Oxygen delivery with supplemental O₂, consider RBC transfusion as required
R	Remove / Reduce Drugs	Anticholinergics or other sedatives known to elicit delirium	Discontinue specific medication therapy if possible
A	Atmosphere	Evaluate room environment including lights and noise levels; Schedule/routine Presence of primary caregiver? Use of restraints? Glasses or hearing aids?	Educate and encourage routine day and night light and noise levels Consider discontinuing restraints Establish home routine, favorite toys, and continuity of care if possible Child Life Consultation
I	Infection/Immobilization/ Inflammation	Consider infectious cause, or possible new sepsis	Treat infection / sepsis
N	New Organ Dysfunction	Multiple systems evaluation Consider labs for organ function	Support organ function as required
M	Metabolic Disturbance	Consider labs (pH, sodium, potassium, calcium, glucose disturbance)	Electrolyte normalization
A	Awake	Sleep / wake cycle disturbance	Educate and encourage daytime routine and limit night-time stimulation if possible
P	Pain	Under-treated or over-treated pain	Treat pain appropriately (see Pain Scale titration as described)
S	Sedation	Evaluate for hypoxemia, low cardiac output or anemia	Consider limiting use of benzodiazepines Appropriate sedation titration per protocol as described with target SBS

Figure 55-8. BRAIN MAPS acronym with causes of delirium and recommendations. Adapted with permission from: Wolfe H, Mack A, Warrington S, et al. CICU/PCU/PICU Clinical Pathway for Delirium, Clinical Team to Bedside to Assess Patient: BRAIN MAPS. The Children's Hospital of Philadelphia - The Center for Healthcare Quality and Analytics - The Clinical Pathways Program (https://www.chop.edu/clinical-pathway/picu-pcu-delirium-brain-maps). Based on: Smith HA, Brink E, Fuchs DC, et al. Pediatric Delirium - Monitoring and Management in the Pediatric Intensive Care Unit. Pediatr Clin North Am. 2013; 60:741-760.

Suggested Readings

Patel AK, Biagas KV, Clarke EC, et al. Delirium in children after cardiac bypass surgery. Pediatr Crit Care Med 2017;18:165-171.

Simone S, Edwards S, Lardieri A, et al. Implementation of an ICU bundle: an interprofessional quality improvement project to enhance delirium management and monitor delirium prevalence in a single PICU. Pediatr Crit Care Med 2017;18:531-540.

Traube C, Silver G, Kearney J, et al. Cornell Assessment of Pediatric Delirium: a valid, rapid, observational tool for screening delirium in the PICU. Crit Care Med 2014;42:656-663.

56 Mechanical Ventilation

Patricia Bastero

Cardiorespiratory Interactions in Mechanically Ventilated Patients

The ultimate goal of mechanical ventilation is to optimize the balance between oxygen delivery (DO_2) and oxygen consumption (VO_2). Positive pressure ventilation (PPV) can impact cardiovascular status. However, in health, the body is able to compensate for intrathoracic pressure changes without significant hemodynamic impact. The main parameter that affects cardiorespiratory interactions is the mean airway pressure (Paw), as it directly affects the intrathoracic pressure.

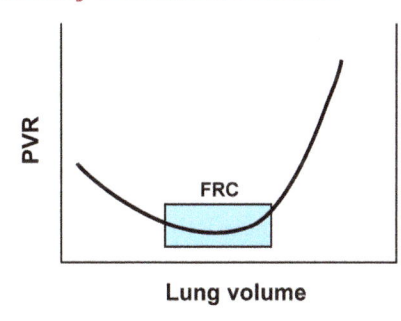

Figure 56-1. PVR-lung volume relationship.

PPV has the following effects:
- **On the RV:** reduces preload and affects RV output based on its effects on RV filling, and to a variable extent, on PVR (Figure 56-1). In health, these effects can be minimal, but in the abnormal circulation or in the presence of ventricular dysfunction or pulmonary hypertension, they can be more marked. Optimal PVR is achieved at functional residual capacity (FRC). PPV increases intrathoracic pressure and can both elevate or decrease PVR based on whether it overdistends the lungs, therefore increasing PVR, or on the contrary, helps achieve FRC by recruiting atelectatic lungs.
- **On the LV:** reduces afterload, thus may be beneficial when there is systolic dysfunction such as cardiomyopathy or myocarditis.

In general, it is desirable to aim for an optimal Paw (to achieve FRC) to help with RV and LV performance, and interventricular dynamics.

The ventilator management will focus on the use of protective mechanical ventilation strategies while supporting and optimizing ventilation and oxygenation in the cardiac patient. The ventilation modality and settings will vary based on each patient's respiratory dynamics, the type and severity of lung injury, and the need to modify intrathoracic pressure, among others.

It is important to follow appropriate parameters to ensure safe and adequate ventilation and oxygenation. Ventilator alarms should be appropriately set up, depending on the patient's age and size, status of the lungs, wakefulness, and timing of weaning.

Postoperative Ventilation

The standard invasive mechanical ventilator settings for a fresh postoperative patient are most commonly as follows:
- **Mode:** SIMV-VC+PS
- **Vt:** 8 ml/kg
- **Respiratory rate (RR):** Neonates: 25-30, infants: 25, 1-5 years: 20, >5 years: 12-16

- **PEEP:** 5 cmH$_2$O
- **Pressure support (PS):** 8-10 cmH$_2$O
- **Trigger:** 0.5 L
- **Inspiratory time (Ti):** 0.5-1 sec
- **FiO$_2$:** 21% (most single-ventricle patients) - 50% (other); higher if needed
- **Alarms:** PIP 30-35 cmH$_2$O

Parameters are modified depending on the particular patient's needs:
- Optimizing SaO$_2$/PaO$_2$: higher FiO$_2$, higher PEEP, longer Ti, consider adding iNO. Consider optimizing PEEP and/or adding iNO before increasing FiO$_2$ >60%.
- Decreasing high CO$_2$ levels: higher RR, larger Vt (in general not greater than 10 ml/kg to prevent volutrauma), optimize inspiratory:expiratory (I:E) ratio (assess for need for longer E time).
- Optimize respiratory rate and I:E ratio: in most conventional ventilators the respiratory rate is set directly. In order not to invert the I:E ratio and give patients a longer inspiratory than expiratory time with high risk of air trapping, pneumothorax, etc., monitor I:E ratio and watch for complete exhalation (auscultation, graphs, and loops).

Severe Lung Injury/ARDS

The following lung protective strategies are followed:
- PEEP levels to prevent alveolar collapse (in general higher than usual: 8-12 cmH$_2$O)
- Low Vt (6 mL/ideal weight kg)
- Maximum inspiratory plateau pressure, in general, 35 cmH$_2$O
- Recruitment maneuvers
- Neuromuscular blockade <48 hours (continuous)
- Prone positioning should be avoided on fresh postoperative cardiac patients

High-Frequency Oscillatory Ventilation (HFOV)

HFOV is a mode that uses a constant Paw with high-frequency pressure oscillations around the Paw, therefore creating very small tidal volumes. It helps with oxygenation by maintaining lung recruitment without causing overdistention.

Consider giving volume (5-10 mL/kg) prior to converting a patient from conventional ventilation to HFOV, as higher maintained Paw can decrease preload to the RV and affect cardiac output. Reasonable initial settings are:
- **Paw:** Equal or 2 cmH$_2$O higher than Paw measured while on conventional ventilator (may start higher and then decrease while monitoring the patient)
- **FiO$_2$:** 100%, then titrate for desired SaO$_2$
- **Ti:** 33%
- **Delta P:** Adjusted for proper "body shaking" down to the lower part of the abdomen
- **Hz:** 12 (neonates) – 6 (adults)

We recommend a CXR at 30-60 minutes after commencing HFOV to ensure that the lungs are not overdistended, and to rule out any associated barotrauma.

If using cuffed ETTs, the cuff should be deflated to allow for a minimal leak to ensure CO_2 clearance. Adjustements are made using the following principles:
- Optimizing SaO_2/PaO_2: higher FiO_2, higher Paw, consider adding iNO. Consider optimizing Paw and/or adding iNO before increasing FiO_2 >60%.
- Decreasing high CO_2 levels: higher delta P, lower Hz.

Prevention of Ventilator-Associated Pneumonia (VAP)
- Hand hygiene
- Oral nystatin
- Mouth care with antiseptic solution
- Patient's head of bed at 30-45 degrees
- Remove ventilator's condensate away from the patient
- Cuffed ETT pressure maintenance
- Aseptic in-line suction when needed to provide pulmonary toilet (bag and suction)
- Minimal ventilator circuit change
- Gastric residue checks to prevent aspiration

Mechanical Ventilation and ECMO
The goal of mechanical ventilation while on ECMO is to prevent atelectasis, VAP, and pulmonary edema. While the patient is on full venoarterial ECMO support, standard initial "rest" settings are:
- **PEEP:** 8-10 cmH_2O with a maximum PIP of 25 cmH_2O to prevent lung injury
- **Ti:** 0.8-1 sec
- **RR:** 10

Provide frequent pulmonary toilet but prevent trauma, especially in an anticoagulated patient. Ventilation settings will vary as soon as ECMO support is decreased, adapting for optimal ventilation and oxygenation while continuing lung-protective strategies. Full ventilator support, deep sedation and/or neuromuscular blockade, and/or iNO is instituted at least 12-24 hours prior to attempting an ECMO wean.

Extubation
Assessing the readiness for extubation is important. The following system-based evaluation for extubation and planning ahead for possible noninvasive mechanical ventilatory (NIMV)-support needs can be helpful:
- **Cardiovascular**
  - Run PS trials (or minimal RR back-up: 5-10 in neonates) and assess signs/symptoms of LCOS (e.g., diaphoresis, tachycardia, lower cerebral NIRS).
  - Consider extubation to NIMV support for patients with known systolic cardiac dysfunction and/or significant AV valve regurgitation, particularly if they previously failed an attempted extubation.

PART IV. PERIOPERATIVE CARE

- **Respiratory**
  - Assess compliance, pulmonary edema, effusions, recurrence of atelectasis, obstructive-airway patterns, suctioning requirements, and secretion characteristics.
  - Consider extubation to noninvasive mechanical ventilation support for patients with history of recurrent atelectasis, chronic lung disease, previous extubation failure, difficulty managing secretions, known airway malacia, residual lung edema.
  - Difficult airway: *always* make sure the patient is "baggable". If not, consider muscular blockade. These extubations should happen in the OR with Anesthesia and ENT present.
- **Neurological**
  - Assess level of consciousness, ability to clear airway, myopathy and/or general weakness or deconditioning, asymetric chest rise (phrenic nerve injury?).
  - Consider NIMV support in patients with significant general deconditioning such as those that have been intubated for long periods of time (7 days), especially if they have required muscular blockade, or those patients with known neurological disorders affecting respiratory dynamics (scoliosis, spasticity, hypotonia).
- **Other**
  - Severe abdominal distension compromising lung volumes: if ready to extubate, consider NIMV support.
  - Known difficult airway: address with CV Anesthesia and ENT for possible need of an OR extubation.

Noninvasive Mechanical Ventilation (NIMV)

High-Flow Nasal Cannula (HFNC)

HFNC requires a specific type of nasal cannula. The maximum support (flow) that can be achieved with HFNC will depend on the patient's size and therefore nasal cannula size. The maximum flow is associated to cannula size, and it is color-coded as described below:
- Yellow / red: 6 L/min
- Violet / blue: 7 L/min
- Green: 8 L/min
- Clear pediatric: 10 L/min
- Adult: 20-40 L/min

In general, maximum flow is 7 L/min for neonates and 25-30 L/min for adults.

Continuous Positive Airway Pressure (CPAP)

CPAP is usually started at 5-10 cmH$_2$O. Pressure is increased according to the patient's work of breathing, atelectasis, SaO$_2$, and CO$_2$ levels.

Bilevel Positive Airway Pressure (BiPAP)

On BiPAP, the inspiratory pressure (IPAP) and expiratory pressure (EPAP) are set. It can be supported with a baseline RR (ST mode).

Start at low pressures (8 / 4) and increase up to the desired level slowly for better patient adaptation (maximum 16 / 8-10). Adjustments are made as follows:
- Optimizing SaO_2/PaO_2: higher FiO_2, higher EPAP.
- Decreasing high CO_2 levels: increase delta P or the pressure difference between EPAP and IPAP by optimizing EPAP and increasing IPAP, adjust RR (ST mode).

57 Fluids and Electrolytes

Patricia Bastero, Antonio G. Cabrera

Careful fluid management in the postoperative period is important to prevent fluid overload and edema after surgery. During CPB, blood flow to the renal cortex may be diminished and may contribute to postoperative acute kidney injury. In addition, capillary leak may be present for at least 48 hours after surgery, requiring volume replacement with blood products or colloids. Periods of LCOS will result in increased antidiuretic hormone (ADH) secretion, resulting in diminished water clearance and exacerbating fluid retention.

Fluids

Daily maintenance IV fluids (IVFs) are calculated based on Holliday and Segar's equation as follows:
- First 10 kg of body weight: 100 mL/kg
- 10-20 kg of body weight: 50 mL/kg
- Each kg over 20 kg of body weight: 20 mL/kg

Divide the total volume by 24 hours for a full (100%) maintenance (mL/h). When we refer to full, half, or quarter maintenance in this handbook, we refer to the total mL/h calculated by Holliday and Segar's equation.

Example, for a 23 kg patient:
- First 10 kg: 10 x 10 = 1000 mL +
- Between 10 and 20 kg: 10 x 50 = 500 mL +
- Above 20 kg of body weight: 3 x 20 = 60 mL
- Total IVF = 1560 mL/24 hours
  - Full maintenance: 65 mL/h
  - Half maintenance: 32 mL/h (32.5 mL/h)
  - Quarter maintenance: 16 mL/h (16.25 mL/h)

Standard IVF maintenance is composed of D10% for neonates (include sodium and potassium after the first 24-48 hours of life; neonates may need calcium and magnesium supplements early on) and D5% + 0.45% NaCl for the rest of the patients. Adolescents and adults can receive Ringer's Lactate or Plasmalyte as maintenance IVF.

The fluid management goal of the first 24 hours should be carefully considered to attain an optimal hemodynamic state. Balancing the capillary leak syndrome with changes in cardiac output imposes a significant challenge, as high CVP may promote additional fluid retention due to decreased perfusion gradient across the renal vascular bed. The following are general recommendations for fluid management:
- **CPB cases.** Start at 25% (quarter) maintenance IVFs and advance 15-25% per day to 100%. Exceptions:
  - Postoperative Fontan patients. Advance 10-25% daily to a maximum of 50-75% maintenance IVFs.
  - Postoperative adult patients and postoperative heart transplant patients. Begin at 35-40% maintenance IVFs and advance accordingly.

- **Non-CPB cases.** Start at 50% (half) maintenance IVFs and advance 25% each day to 100%.

NOTE: Initial IVF should not include potassium until renal function and urine output have been adequately assessed.

Potassium
Potassium levels may affect arrhythmia threshold and myocardial function. In the cardiac population with active arrhythmias or history of recent arrhythmias, the goal is to keep potassium levels >4 mEq/L.

Hypokalemia
Potassium serum levels <3.5 mEq/L.

Etiology
Hypokalemia can be secondary to drugs such as furosemide; inadequate potassium supplementation; excessive GI (emesis, diarrhea), cutaneous (diaphoresis), CNS (central diabetes insipidus), or renal (dialysis, nephritic diabetes insipidus) losses; hyperaldosteronism; or hypomagnesemia.

Signs and Symptoms
Mild hypokalemia may be asymptomatic. Potassium levels <2.5 to 3 mEq/L may present with constipation, muscle weakness, and arrhythmias.

Treatment
Hypokalemia should always be treated if symptomatic. In the cardiac population, in order to prevent arrhythmias, potassium levels should be kept >3.5 mEq/L, and >4 mEq/L in patients with active arrhythmias that need treatment.

Potassium supplements can be given:
- Enterally: usually used for chronic replacements in patients already tolerating feeds and with potassium levels >3 mEq/L.
- IV: 0.5-1 mEq/kg over 60 minutes. Maximum dose at a time: 20 mEq. Infusion rate should not exceed 1 mEq/kg/h.

Potassium levels must be checked within an hour of any IV potassium bolus administered, or within 3 hours after an enteral bolus administered.

Hyperkalemia
Potassium serum levels >5.5 mEq/L.

Etiology
Most cases of hyperkalemia will be secondary to renal injury and inability to excrete potassium properly (acute kidney injury, renal tubular disease, hypoaldosteronism). Hyperkalemia could also be secondary to excessive administration of potassium in IVF, parenteral nutrition, or blood transfusions. Additionally, it can be caused by, or exacerbated by the use of potassium-sparing diuretics or angiotensin-converting-enzyme inhibitors. Potassium's distribution can also be altered, increasing its serum levels, during acidosis or insulin deficits.

PART IV. PERIOPERATIVE CARE

Signs and Symptoms
Clinical manifestations of hyperkalemia include muscle weakness, dizziness, nausea and tachyarrhythmia (including ventricular tachycardia and fibrillation).

The ECG can show peaked T waves, followed by flat P waves, an increasing PR time, and finally, a wider QRS with ST-segment changes leading to tachycardia and ventricular fibrillation.

Treatment
Hyperkalemia should be treated when serum potassium reaches 6.5 mEq/L, or even lower if the increase is fast. The goal is to stabilize the myocyte's membrane (arrhythmia threshold) with calcium; drive the potassium into the myocytes with sodium bicarbonate, insulin with glucose, and albuterol; and increase potassium elimination with furosemide, dialysis, and/or kayexalate (exchange resin):
- Calcium chloride: 20 mg/kg IV over 5-10 minutes
- Dextrose 25% (D25W) + regular insulin 0.05 Units/mL: 2 mL/kg IV over 30-60 minutes (monitor glucose to prevent hypoglycemia)
- Sodium Bicarbonate: 1-2 mEq/kg IV over 10-20 minutes
- Furosemide: 1 mg/kg IV over 20 minutes
- Kayexalate: 1 g/kg enteral or rectal
- Salbutamol neb (0.15 mg/kg) or IV (5 mg/kg over 15 minutes)

Sodium
Sodium levels may affect arrhythmia thresholds and their management can have a significant neurological impact. Chronic sodium dysregulation is much better tolerated than acute changes in sodium levels.

Hyponatremia
Serum sodium levels <135 mEq/L.

Etiology
Hyponatremia is most commonly secondary to the use of diuretics or hypotonic intravenous fluids, but it can also be secondary to diarrhea, heart failure (pseudohyponatremia), liver disease, renal disease, inappropriate ADH secretion (SIADH), and cerebral salt-wasting disease.

Signs and Symptoms
Clinical manifestations include nausea, vomiting, confusion, decreased level of consciousness, and seizures.

Treatment
When correcting sodium levels, one must ensure an adequate intravascular volume state, eliminate water excess, and secure a continuous source of sodium while increased losses persist.

Acute severe symptomatic hyponatremia is an emergency. Administer NaCl 3% at 5 mL/kg IV over 15 minutes until sodium levels are over 120 mEq/L. In case of SIADH, add furosemide 1 mg/kg IV.

For hyponatremia with hypovolemia, restore intravascular volume with 20 mL/kg IV of NS 0.9% over 20 minutes. Repeat as needed, monitoring pulmonary status.

While correcting hyponatremia, it is important not to allow sodium levels to rise beyond 0.5 mEq/L/hour, to prevent central pontine myelinolysis.

Hypernatremia
Sodium serum levels >145 mEq/L.

Etiology
Hypernatremia is most commonly due to excessive water losses due to fever, hyperventilation, diabetes insipidus, burns, osmotic diuresis, etc.

Signs and Symptoms
Arrhythmias and CNS symptoms (irritability, seizures, coma) are the most common clinical signs of hypernatremia.

Treatment
It is important to avoid rapid correction of hypernatremia (aim for a decrease in sodium levels <0.5 mEq/L/hour), to prevent the development of cerebral edema.

It is also important to determine hydration level and correct fluid losses accordingly. Hypernatremic dehydration should be corrected over 48-72 hours. If diabetes insipidus is the cause, desmopressin (DDAVP) should be administered.

Calcium
The neonatal myocardium is especially sensitive to calcium levels. There are 3 forms of calcium: ionized (more active form), nonionized, and protein-bound. For patients with active arrhythmias or a recent history of arrhythmias, the goal is to keep ionized calcium (iCa^{++}) levels >1.2 mmol/L.

Hypocalcemia
Hypocalcemia is defined as an iCa^{++} <1.1 mmol/L or a total calcium <8.9 mg/dL. It is preferable to check levels of the active or ionized calcium form (iCa^{++}). Given the relationship between total calcium levels and serum albumin, we would recommend basing any interventions for hypocalcemia upon the iCa^{++} levels.

Etiology
Causes of hypocalcemia include renal failure, liver failure, blood transfusions, burns, sepsis, polytrauma, hypomagnesemia (check Mg^{++} levels when facing refractory hypokalemia), hypoalbuminemia, renal-replacement therapies, or drugs such as furosemide, heparin, steroids, bicarbonate, gentamycin, excessive use of calcium-channel blockers, and others. In the CHD population, it is also always important to remember the possibility of DiGeorge syndrome and associated hypoparathyroidism as a possible cause of hypocalcemia.

Signs and Symptoms
Clinical manifestations include impaired myocardial contractility, tetany, seizures, and laryngospasm. Myocardial dysfunction is worse in the setting of concomitant hyperkalemia. A prolonged QT may be found on ECG.

Treatment
Hypocalcemia can be treated in 2 ways:
- Calcium chloride: 10-20 mg/kg IV over 15-30 minutes. Calcium chloride should be administered via a central line.
- Calcium gluconate: 50-100 mg/kg IV over 15-30 minutes. Calcium gluconate may be administered via a peripheral line.

Hypercalcemia
iCa^{++} >1.4 mmol/L or total calcium >10.7 mg/dL.

Etiology
Hypercalcemia may be due to excessive supplements of calcium or Vitamin D, thiazide diuretics, renal failure, immobilization, hyperparathyroidism, or malignancy.

Signs and Symptoms
Hypercalcemia is characterized by abdominal pain, nausea and vomiting, and constipation. One may also see calcium deposits in soft tissues, corneas, or kidneys (nephrocalcinosis) if associated with an elevated phosphorus.

Treatment
Treatment of severe hypercalcemia (total calcium >15 mg/dL) is mandatory. Administer NS 0.9% IV and furosemide to induce diuresis, increase calcium wasting, and control potassium levels. Prednisone (decreases intestinal absorption of calcium), calcitonin, and bisphosphonates may also be used. Patients may need hemodialysis.

Magnesium
Magnesium levels are important to keep adequate potassium and calcium balances. The goal magnesium level in cardiac patients with active arrhythmias or recent history of arrhythmias is >2 mg/dL.

Hypomagnesemia
Magnesium levels <1.5 mg/dL.

Etiology
Hypomagnesemia is commonly secondary to renal losses due to drugs such as diuretics, amphotericin B, or aminoglycosides.

Signs and Symptoms
Clinical manifestations include arrhythmias, seizures, muscle weakness, fatigue, tremors, irritability, and confusion.

Treatment
Correct magnesium levels using magnesium sulfate 25-50 mg/kg IV over 60-120 minutes. Magnesium infusion can cause hypotension.

Hypermagnesemia
Magnesium levels >2.3 mg/dL.

Etiology
Hypermagnesemia is usually iatrogenic due to excessive magnesium supplementation.

Signs and Symptoms
Signs and symptoms of hypermagnesemia usually occur when the levels are >5 mg/dL. They include arrhythmias, muscle weakness, loss of reflexes, and neurological depression. Muscular paralysis may occur with levels >7.5 mg/dL.

Treatment
There is no specific treatment for hypermagnesemia. Calcium chloride or gluconate may be used to stabilize the myocardial membrane. Dialysis may be necessary if there are significant neurological or cardiac symptoms.

58 Nutrition

D. Jeramy Roddy, Natalie Cannon, Lauren Hannigan, David E. Wesson

Infants with CHD requiring surgical intervention shortly after birth, are at increased risk for growth failure. This can be attributed to higher energy expenditure required to support postoperative healing, genetic syndromes, hemodynamic derangements, or GI issues such as malrotation, decreased absorption, delayed gastric emptying, gastroesophageal reflux, villous atrophy, gut dysbiosis, necrotizing enterocolitis (NEC), medication effect, or neurologic sequela. Additionally, imposed fluid restrictions in the postoperative period can further potentiate a negative nutritional balance. Moreover, literature links increased hospital length of stay and worse neurodevelopmental outcomes to malnutrition. It is imperative that infants with CHD receive adequate nutrition to maintain normal growth and support neurological development.

Patients with lesions that have a physiology with a potential imbalance in Qp:Qs are considered *high-risk lesions* (i.e., hypoplastic left heart syndrome, other single-ventricle lesions [e.g., unbalanced atrioventricular septal defects, double-inlet LV, double-outlet RV with unrestricted pulmonary blood flow], truncus arteriosus, aortopulmonary window, aortic coarctation, interrupted aortic arch) and are at an increased risk of GI morbidity, including feeding intolerance, ischemia, and NEC. Even though the GI risk is lower in patients with other lesions, frequent assessment of these patients is also necessary.

Nutritional Assessment

Table 58-1 and Table 58-2 can be used to calculate the nutritional needs of cardiac infants <4 months of age and 4 months to 1 year of age, respectively.

Table 58-1. Nutritional needs of cardiac infants <4 months of corrected gestational age (from the Texas Children's Hospital Pediatric Nutrition Reference Guide).

	Preterm	Term
Energy Needs (Parenteral)	90-110 kcal/kg/day	90-110 kcal/kg/day
Energy Needs (Enteral)	100-130 kcal/kg/day	100-130 kcal/kg/day
Protein Needs	3.5-4.5 g/kg/day	2-4 g/kg/day

Table 58-2. Nutritional needs of cardiac infants >4 months of corrected gestational age (from the Texas Children's Hospital Pediatric Nutrition Reference Guide).

	4 months – 1 year
Energy Needs (Parenteral)	BMR (Schofield) x 1.1-1.3
Energy Needs (Enteral)	BMR (Schofield) x 1.3-1.5
Protein Needs	2-4 g/kg/day

Estimated needs can be adjusted based on medical status (level of cardiopulmonary support, sedation, or paralytics), or degree of malnutrition and growth history.
BMR: Body metabolic rate.

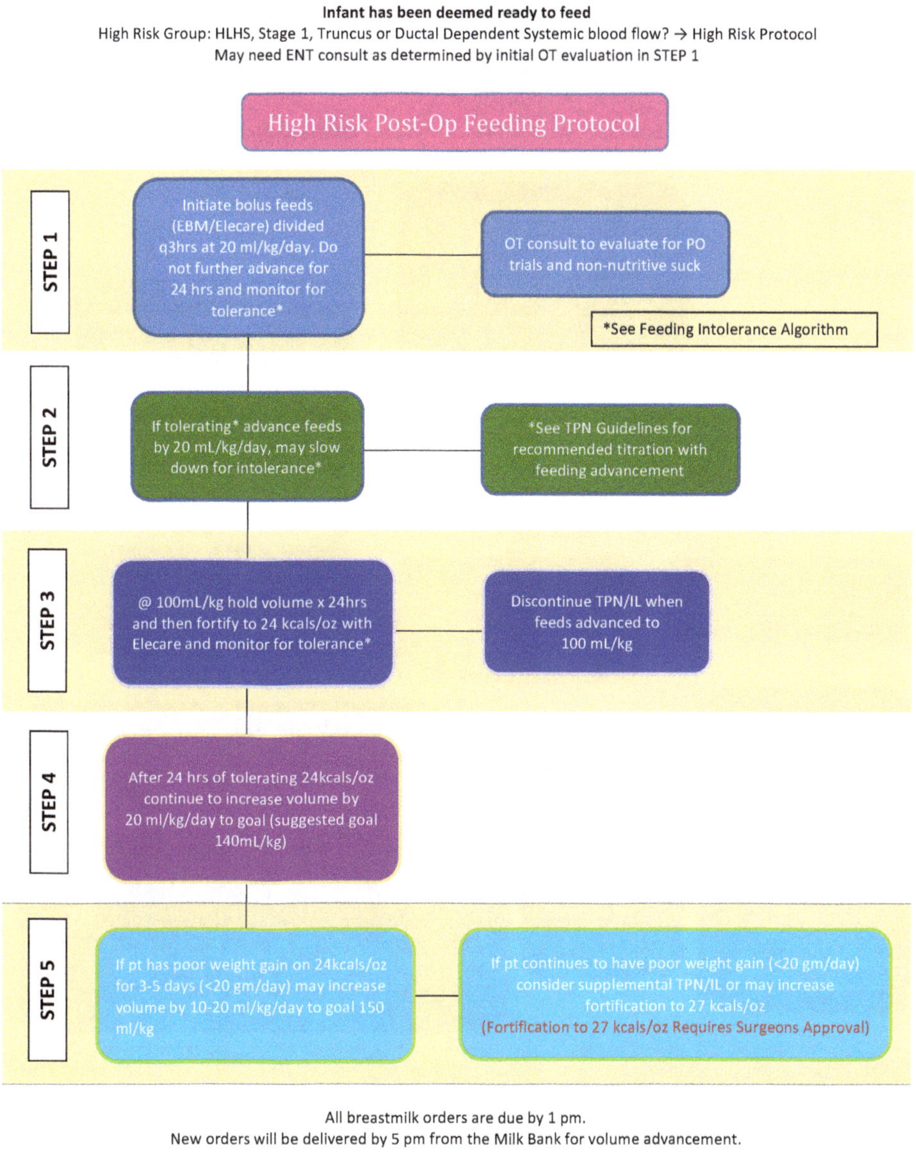

58. NUTRITION

Infant has been deemed ready to feed
High Risk Group: HLHS, Stage 1, Truncus or Ductal Dependent Systemic blood flow? → High Risk Protocol
May need ENT consult as determined by initial OT evaluation in STEP 1

High Risk Post-Op Feeding Protocol

STEP 1
- Initiate bolus feeds (EBM/Elecare) divided q3hrs at 20 ml/kg/day. Do not further advance for 24 hrs and monitor for tolerance*
- OT consult to evaluate for PO trials and non-nutritive suck

*See Feeding Intolerance Algorithm

STEP 2
- If tolerating* advance feeds by 20 mL/kg/day, may slow down for intolerance*
- *See TPN Guidelines for recommended titration with feeding advancement

STEP 3
- @ 100mL/kg hold volume x 24hrs and then fortify to 24 kcals/oz with Elecare and monitor for tolerance*
- Discontinue TPN/IL when feeds advanced to 100 mL/kg

STEP 4
- After 24 hrs of tolerating 24kcals/oz continue to increase volume by 20 ml/kg/day to goal (suggested goal 140mL/kg)

STEP 5
- If pt has poor weight gain on 24kcals/oz for 3-5 days (<20 gm/day) may increase volume by 10-20 ml/kg/day to goal 150 ml/kg
- If pt continues to have poor weight gain (<20 gm/day) consider supplemental TPN/IL or may increase fortification to 27 kcals/oz
(Fortification to 27 kcals/oz Requires Surgeons Approval)

All breastmilk orders are due by 1 pm.
New orders will be delivered by 5 pm from the Milk Bank for volume advancement.

Figure 58-1. Postoperative feeding protocol for high-risk patients (i.e., hypoplastic left heart syndrome, other stage-1 single-ventricle palliation patients, truncus arteriosus, or ductal-dependent systemic circulation).

PART IV. PERIOPERATIVE CARE

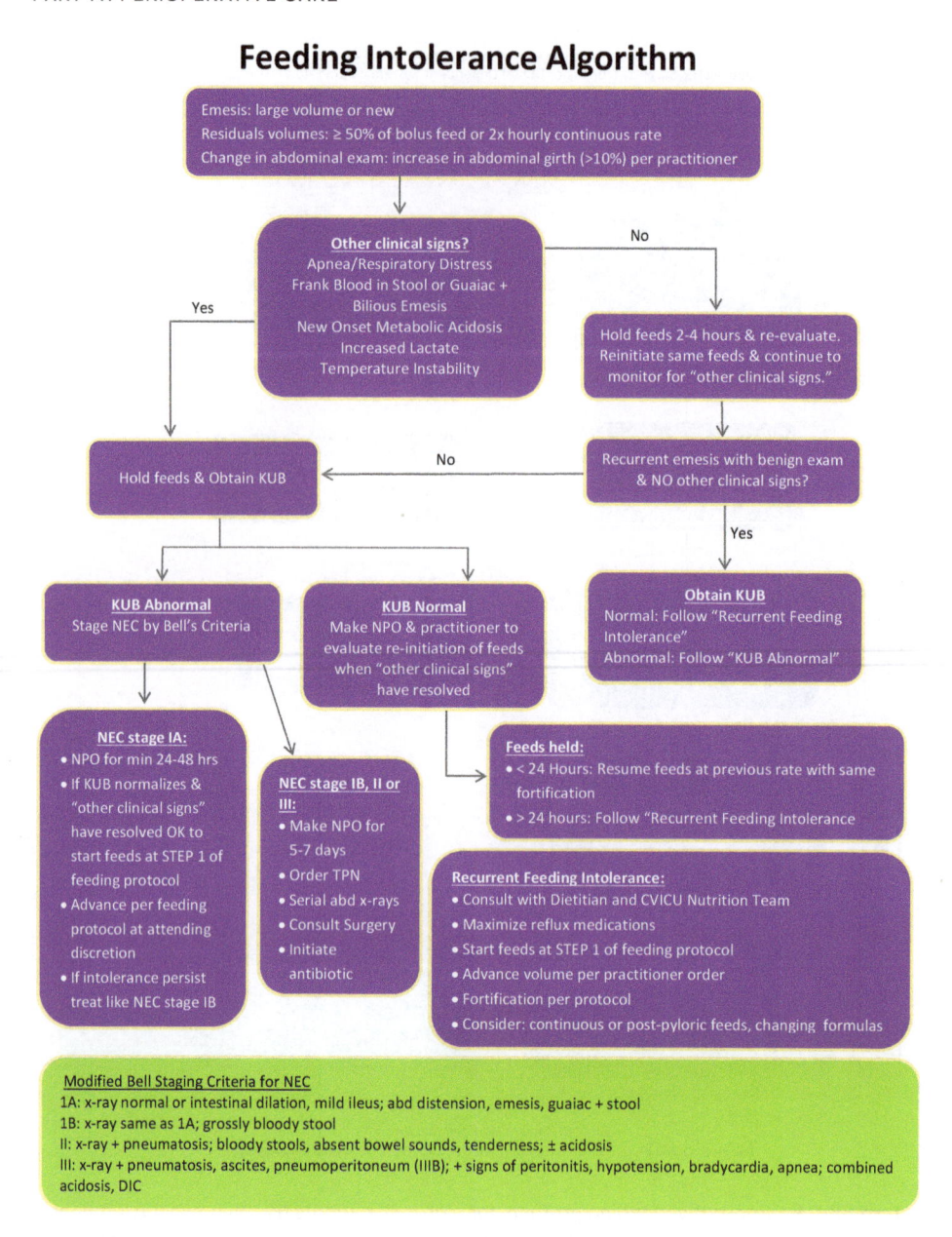

Feeding Intolerance Algorithm

Emesis: large volume or new
Residuals volumes: ≥ 50% of bolus feed or 2x hourly continuous rate
Change in abdominal exam: increase in abdominal girth (>10%) per practitioner

↓

Other clinical signs?
Apnea/Respiratory Distress
Frank Blood in Stool or Guaiac +
Bilious Emesis
New Onset Metabolic Acidosis
Increased Lactate
Temperature Instability

— No → Hold feeds 2-4 hours & re-evaluate. Reinitiate same feeds & continue to monitor for "other clinical signs."

↓ Yes

Hold feeds & Obtain KUB ← No — Recurrent emesis with benign exam & NO other clinical signs?

↓ Yes

Obtain KUB
Normal: Follow "Recurrent Feeding Intolerance"
Abnormal: Follow "KUB Abnormal"

KUB Abnormal
Stage NEC by Bell's Criteria

KUB Normal
Make NPO & practitioner to evaluate re-initiation of feeds when "other clinical signs" have resolved

NEC stage IA:
- NPO for min 24-48 hrs
- If KUB normalizes & "other clinical signs" have resolved OK to start feeds at STEP 1 of feeding protocol
- Advance per feeding protocol at attending discretion
- If intolerance persist treat like NEC stage IB

NEC stage IB, II or III:
- Make NPO for 5-7 days
- Order TPN
- Serial abd x-rays
- Consult Surgery
- Initiate antibiotic

Feeds held:
- < 24 Hours: Resume feeds at previous rate with same fortification
- > 24 hours: Follow "Recurrent Feeding Intolerance"

Recurrent Feeding Intolerance:
- Consult with Dietitian and CVICU Nutrition Team
- Maximize reflux medications
- Start feeds at STEP 1 of feeding protocol
- Advance volume per practitioner order
- Fortification per protocol
- Consider: continuous or post-pyloric feeds, changing formulas

Modified Bell Staging Criteria for NEC
1A: x-ray normal or intestinal dilation, mild ileus; abd distension, emesis, guaiac + stool
1B: x-ray same as 1A; grossly bloody stool
II: x-ray + pneumatosis; bloody stools, absent bowel sounds, tenderness; ± acidosis
III: x-ray + pneumatosis, ascites, pneumoperitoneum (IIIB); + signs of peritonitis, hypotension, bradycardia, apnea; combined acidosis, DIC

Figure 58-2. Feeding intolerance algorithm.

Table 58-3. Parenteral nutrition guidelines for postoperative CPB infants (from the Texas Children's Hospital Pediatric Nutrition Reference Guide).

Infants 0-4 months Corrected Gestational Age			
Postoperative	Day 1	Day 2	Day 3
TPN volume	45 mL/kg/day	65 mL/kg/day	85 mL/kg/day
IL volume	5 mL/kg/day	10 mL/kg/day	15 mL/kg/day
Total volume	50 mL/kg/day (50% maintenance)	75 mL/kg/day (75% maintenance)	100 mL/kg/day (100% maintenance)
GIR goal	6-8 mg/kg/min	8-10 mg/kg/min	12 mg/kg/min
Aminoacid goal	2-2.5 g/kg/day	3-4 g/kg/day	3-4 g/kg/day

Goal to achieve estimated body metabolic rate (BMR) within 48 hours post cardiac surgery.
GIR: glucose infusion rate, IL: intralipids, TPN: total parenteral nutrition.

Human Milk Diet and Qualifications for Donor Human Milk

TCH promotes the use of breast milk or expressed breast milk (EBM) in all cardiac infants due to its numerous benefits. If maternal EBM is not available, then donor human milk is recommended, with parental consent, for qualifying infants:
- Current gestational age <34 weeks
- Used as a bridge while establishing mother's milk supply (≤2 weeks)
- High-risk CHD lesions (as per above)

Transitioning from donor human milk to formula may be done as follows:
- Day 1: Add 1 formula feeding
- Day 2: Add 2 formula feedings
- Day 3: Add 4 formula feedings
- Day 4: All formula feedings

Preoperative Feeding

Infants benefit from early initiation of oral motor therapy with nonnutritive and/or nutritive intervention. The goal of preoperative intervention is to establish oral motor skills that are essential for progression to full oral feeds postoperatively. Infants who do not orally feed or establish nonnutritive skills prior to surgery typically require greater length of time to reach full oral feeds postoperatively.

High-risk infants receive the majority of their nutrition via central parenteral nutrition prior to surgery. Intubated infants receive fresh colostrum/breast milk oral care every 6-12 hours while NPO. Patients with a duct-dependent systemic circulation preoperatively are allowed up to 20 mL/kg/day of oral EBM or donor EBM divided every 3 hours as trophic feeds prior to surgery.

Postoperative Feeding

Our standard practice is to fluid-restrict patients after surgery with CPB to 25% maintenance on postoperative day 0. Total fluid volume is advanced on subsequent days per the parenteral nutrition guidelines in Table 58-3.

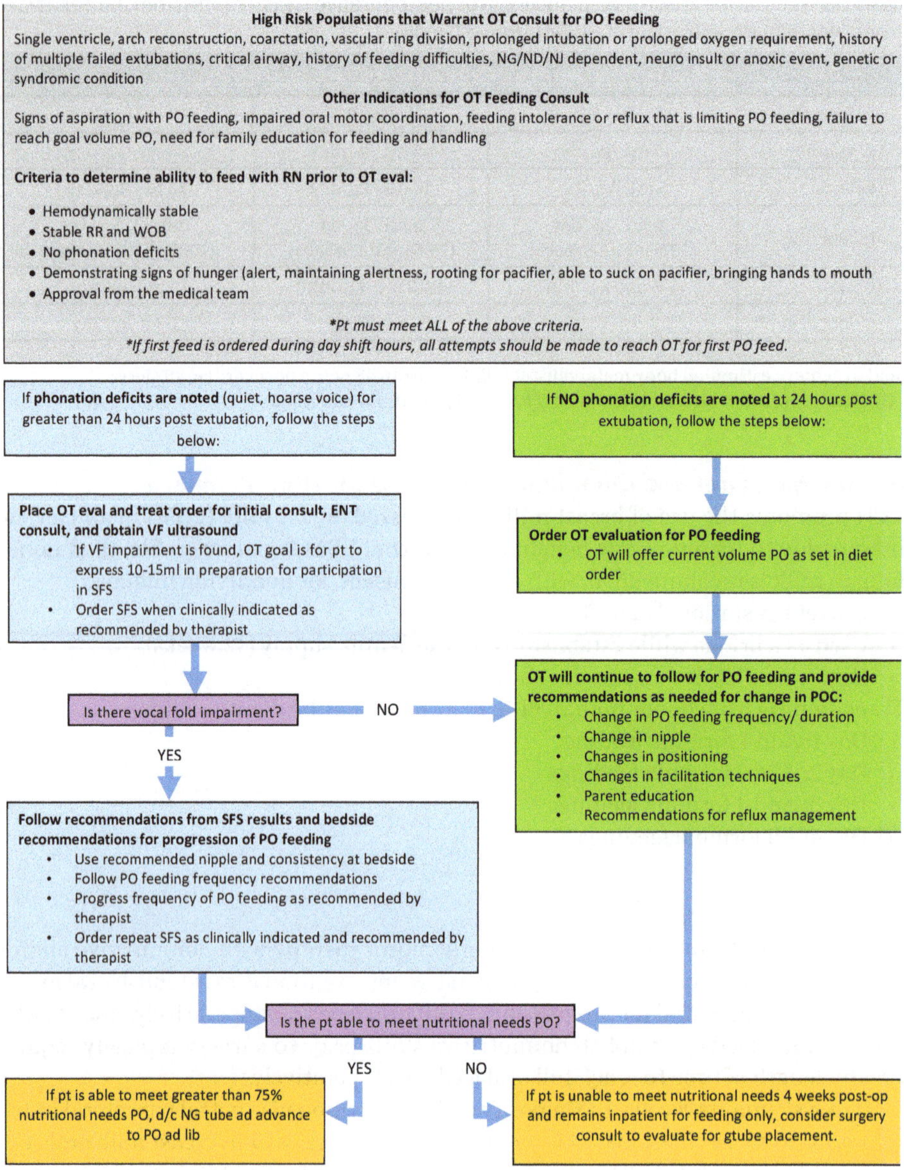

PART IV. PERIOPERATIVE CARE

High Risk Populations that Warrant OT Consult for PO Feeding
Single ventricle, arch reconstruction, coarctation, vascular ring division, prolonged intubation or prolonged oxygen requirement, history of multiple failed extubations, critical airway, history of feeding difficulties, NG/ND/NJ dependent, neuro insult or anoxic event, genetic or syndromic condition

Other Indications for OT Feeding Consult
Signs of aspiration with PO feeding, impaired oral motor coordination, feeding intolerance or reflux that is limiting PO feeding, failure to reach goal volume PO, need for family education for feeding and handling

Criteria to determine ability to feed with RN prior to OT eval:
- Hemodynamically stable
- Stable RR and WOB
- No phonation deficits
- Demonstrating signs of hunger (alert, maintaining alertness, rooting for pacifier, able to suck on pacifier, bringing hands to mouth)
- Approval from the medical team

Pt must meet ALL of the above criteria.
If first feed is ordered during day shift hours, all attempts should be made to reach OT for first PO feed.

If **phonation deficits are noted** (quiet, hoarse voice) for greater than 24 hours post extubation, follow the steps below:

↓

Place OT eval and treat order for initial consult, ENT consult, and obtain VF ultrasound
- If VF impairment is found, OT goal is for pt to express 10-15ml in preparation for participation in SFS
- Order SFS when clinically indicated as recommended by therapist

↓

Is there vocal fold impairment? —— NO ——→

YES ↓

Follow recommendations from SFS results and bedside recommendations for progression of PO feeding
- Use recommended nipple and consistency at bedside
- Follow PO feeding frequency recommendations
- Progress frequency of PO feeding as recommended by therapist
- Order repeat SFS as clinically indicated and recommended by therapist

↓

Is the pt able to meet nutritional needs PO?

YES ↓   NO ↓

If pt is able to meet greater than 75% nutritional needs PO, d/c NG tube ad advance to PO ad lib

If pt is unable to meet nutritional needs 4 weeks post-op and remains inpatient for feeding only, consider surgery consult to evaluate for gtube placement.

If **NO phonation deficits are noted** at 24 hours post extubation, follow the steps below:

↓

Order OT evaluation for PO feeding
- OT will offer current volume PO as set in diet order

↓

OT will continue to follow for PO feeding and provide recommendations as needed for change in POC:
- Change in PO feeding frequency/ duration
- Change in nipple
- Changes in positioning
- Changes in facilitation techniques
- Parent education
- Recommendations for reflux management

Figure 58-3. Occupational therapy algorithm.

TCH has a variety of postoperative feeding protocols. Figure 58-1 illustrates the feeding protocol for high-risk patients. Figure 58-2 shows the algorithm for feeding intolerance. Figure 58-3 shows the algorithm for OT and ENT consult on patients after CHD.

Nutrition-Related Postoperative Complications

Chylothorax
Infants with chylous effusions are changed to a formula with low long-chain fatty acids and high medium-chain fatty acids, such as Enfaport™ or Portagen®. Children >1 year of age with chylothorax are restricted to a minimal-fat diet (<5 g/day of fat) for 6 weeks after diet initiation. For details on management of chylothorax, see Chapter 77.

Oral-Motor Issues
Infants with CHD frequently have impaired oral-motor coordination and skills. Impaired oral-motor coordination of the suck, swallow, breathe triad is highly prevalent due to tachypnea, increased work of breathing, level of sedation, and disuse of the swallow mechanism while being NPO. Furthermore, delay in skill development is common in infants who are not able to feed orally at birth and become dependent on parental nutrition or supplemental tube feeding. Finally, infants with CHD may have associated syndromes or neurological or anatomic comorbidities that may impact their ability to feed by mouth.

It is very important that the OT team works with patients to build oral motor skills and improve coordination with the ultimate goal of meeting nutritional needs orally. Some supplemental techniques include alternative positioning, paced oral feeding, and working with different types of nipples.

Gastrostomy Tubes
Some patients with CHD will be unable to reach full oral feeds prior to discharge. The etiology is often multifactorial and often includes a combination of factors such as feeding intolerance, reflux/GERD, poor endurance, limited motivation and hunger cues, genetic conditions, developmental delay, oral aversion or avoidance, aspiration, and impaired oral-motor skills. If oral feeding is not possible after 4 weeks, a feeding gastrostomy may be warranted. This will allow for removal of the indwelling nasogastric or orogastric tube, which may make oral feeding easier for the baby, reducing the amount of GERD and improving the baby's comfort.

The gastrostomy can be placed by an open or laparoscopic approach at the surgeon's discretion, as there is limited evidence to support the superiority of one versus the other. Many neonates and infants with cardiac disease have symptoms of GERD, just as other normal children. In most cases, the reflux will resolve spontaneously. Transesophageal feeding tubes may cause or exacerbate the reflux. Since the reflux will improve or resolve in the vast majority of cases, a fundoplication is seldom indicated. Furthermore, adding a fundoplication to a gastrostomy placement increases morbidity and mortality in cardiac patients (Short et al. 2017).

Monitoring and Evaluation

At TCH, bedside nutrition rounds including a multidisciplinary team of dietitians, nurses, neonatologists, and cardiac intensivists, are conducted weekly on high-risk infants. Interventions include optimization of current nutrition support, changes in route of nutrition delivery (enteral vs. parenteral), rate of enteral nutrition (bolus vs. continuous), and type of enteral nutrition (breast milk vs. formula).

Continuous anthropometric monitoring is assessed on a daily to weekly basis to assure achievement of growth goals. Monitoring includes consistent daily weights on an infant scale, weekly lengths via length boards, and weekly occipital-frontal head circumferences.

Suggested Readings

Beaver BB, Carvalho-Salemi J, Hastings E, Ling H, Spoede E, Wrobel M (eds). Texas Children's Hospital Pediatric Nutrition Reference Guide. 12th edition. Texas Children's Hospital; 2019.

Short HL, Travers C, McCracken C, et al. Increased morbidity and mortality in cardiac patients undergoing fundoplication. Pediatr Surg Int 2017;33:559-567.

59 Anticoagulation

Mubbasheer Ahmed, Iki Adachi, Jun Teruya

Thrombotic complications are a common morbidity in the CHD population. A myriad of factors lead to higher rates of thrombosis including baseline coagulopathies, genetic disorders, postsurgical inflammation, low-flow states, factor loss in chylous effusions, exposure to prosthetic material, extracorporeal support (including CPB) leading to platelet activation, and turbulent flow patterns due to anatomical defects. The unique underlying profile of the CHD patient necessitates a careful anticoagulation strategy in both the pre- and postoperative periods, while incorporating the risk of bleeding during this phase.

Anticoagulation management requires an individualized approach for each patient. The information provided in this chapter should be considered as a general guidance that would likely necessitate modification individually.

Single-Ventricle Prophylaxis

Children with single-ventricle physiology require 3 stages of palliation with differing thrombotic risk following each stage. Interstage patients (between first and second stage) commonly have systemic-to-pulmonary shunts or PDA stents, which are associated with a risk of thrombotic occlusion. Later, the Glenn and the Fontan circulations create passive blood flow through the pulmonary vessels. Acute thrombotic complications risk creating severe hypoxemia and hypercarbia in the Glenn patient, while they can cause obstructive shock in Fontan patients.

The anticoagulation protocol for patients with systemic-to-pulmonary shunts (i.e., modified Blalock-Taussig-Thomas shunts, central shunts, Mee shunts) or PDA stents is:
1. Start Heparin 10 U/kg/hr, 4 hours after arriving to the CICU if no bleeding concerns. There are no therapeutic endpoints.
2. On postoperative day 1, start aspirin and continue heparin. After 3 doses, test for aspirin responsiveness via VerifyNow®. Discontinue heparin if responsive to ASA.
3. Patients should remain on aspirin even if they are on therapeutic heparin or enoxaparin for thrombosis.

For patients with Glenn and Fontan circulation, start aspirin on postoperative day 2. Consider warfarin (in addition to aspirin) if there is a genetic predisposition to thrombophilia, protein-losing enteropathy, *chronic* pleural or chylous effusions, or a history of previous thrombosis.

Aspirin dosage is 5 mg/kg PO every day rounded to the nearest ¼ tablet (i.e., 20.25 mg, 40.5 mg, or 81 mg)

Prosthetic valves

Table 59-1 lists the recommended anticoagulation for bioprosthetic and mechanical valves.

Table 59-1. Anticoagulation for bioprosthetic and mechanical valves. From: Nishimura RA, Otto CM, Bonow RO, et al. 2017 AHA/ACC Focused update on the 2014 AHA/ACC Guideline for management of patients with valvular heart disease. J Am Coll Cardiol 2017;70:252-289.

	Prophylaxis			
	Aortic Valve	**Mitral Valve**	**Class recommendation**[1]	**Level of evidence**[2]
Mechanical	Warfarin INR 2.5 (2-3) INR 3 (2.5-3.5) if (+) risk factors (AF, hypercoagulability, LV dysfunction, previous thromboembolism) + ASA (5 mg/kg), 81 mg max	Warfarin INR 3 (2.5-3.5) + ASA (5 mg/kg), 81 mg max	I	A & B
Bioprosthetic	ASA (5 mg/kg), 81 mg max vs. Warfarin, INR 2.5 (2-3) for 3-6 months if low bleeding risk		IIa IIa	B B-NR

	Thrombosed valve		
	Therapy	**Class recommendation**[1]	**Level of evidence**[2]
Mechanical	Left-sided valve + clinical symptoms: Urgent low-dose fibrinolytic infusion or surgery	I	B-NR
Bioprosthetic	Vitamin-K antagonist if suspected or confirmed thrombosis (if hemodynamically stable)	IIa	C-LD

[1] Class recommendation: I - strong recommendation, IIa – moderate recommendation (reasonable).
[2] Level of evidence: A – high-quality, B – moderate-quality, B-NR – moderate-quality from nonrandomized trials, C-LD – limited data.

Management of VAD and ECMO patients

Overall, the Division of Transfusion Medicine and Coagulation provides guidance on how to monitor and interpret coagulation tests, and suggests therapeutic options in VAD and ECMO patients. The following are general protocols.

ECMO

- Preanticoagulation: rotational thromboelastometry (ROTEM®) and ECMO coagulation panel (prothrombin time [PT], partial thromboplastin time [PTT], PTT hepzyme, fibrinogen, antithrombin (AT), D-dimer, heparin level [anti-Xa assay], platelet count)
- Begin heparin when no concerns for active bleeding AND activated clotting time (ACT) <200 seconds
- Initiate heparin at 20 U/kg/h (max 1000 U/h), per team discussion after cannulation
- Monitor for bleeding at all times

59. ANTICOAGULATION

Table 59-2. Antithrombotic and fibrinolytic medications.

	Properties	Indications	Dose	Monitoring
Unfractionated heparin (UFH)	Potentiates inhibition of clotting factors by AT. t½ dose dependent ~ 1h. Hepatic/Renal clearance.	Thrombosis or risk of thrombosis when bleeding risk is high (e.g., perioperative period).	Prophylaxis: 6 U/kg/h. <12 mo: 28 U/kg/h. ≥12 mo: 20 U/kg/h. Max: 1000 U/h. Bolus: 75 U/kg (max 5000 U).	Anti–factor Xa: 0.35–0.7 U/mL. PTT: 1.5-3x normal. Levels 4h after change, then q12-24h.
Low-molecular weight heparin (enoxaparin)	Greater inhibition of factor Xa. t½=3-6h. Low dependence on AT. Renal clearance.	Thrombosis or thromboprophylaxis, bridge on or off warfarin.	<2 mo: 1.7 mg/kg/dose q12h SQ ≥2mo: 1 mg/kg/dose q12h SQ.	Lovenox level 4h after 2nd dose from initiation and 4h after each change. Therapy: 0.5-1 U/mL Prophylaxis: 0.2–0.4 U/mL.
Bivalirudin	Direct thrombin (IIa) inhibitor. Enzymatic 80%, renal 20% clearance. t½=25 min.	HIT in VADs, ECMO. Poor anticoagulation control with heparin.	Infusion: 0.03–0.3 mg/kg/h. Bolus: 0.1–0.2 mg/kg. Increment by 25–50%.	PTT hepzyme. PTT: 1.5-2.5x normal, check q2h with changes, then q12h.
Alteplase (tPA)	Converts plasminogen to plasmin. Plasmin degrades fibrin & fibrinogen. t½=4 min.	Venous or arterial thrombosis with threaten loss of limb, massive PE, MI.	Per Hematology or Transfusion Medicine. Continue heparin during alteplase treatment.	Close neurologic monitoring, muco cutaneous bleeding.
Aspirin	Inhibits platelet aggregation. t½ dose dependent, irreversible binding. Discontinue 7d prior to surgery (unless shunted circulation).	Thromboprophylaxis of stents, shunts, Glenn, Fontan, prosthetic valves.	5 mg/kg (max 81 mg).	
Clopidogrel	Inhibition of platelet aggregation. t½=7 h. Renal clearance, hepatic metabolism	Additional need for antiplatelet therapy.	≤24 mo: 0.2 mg/kg qd. >24 mo: 0.2–0.3 mg/kg qd (max 75 mg).	
Warfarin (Coumadin®)	Inhibits formation of vitamin K-dependent factors. t½= ~25–60h, duration of action ~2–5 days.	Long-term anticoagulation, VADs, Fontan.	Initial Dose: 0.1 - 0.2 mg/kg/dose (initial max 5 mg/dose). See text for initiation.	Obtain INR qd until 2 therapeutic levels, then q1-4wks.

AT: antithrombin, ECMO: extracorporeal membrane oxygenation, HIT: heparin-moulded thromboplastinia INR: international normalized ratio, PE: pulmonary embolus, MI: myocardial infarction, PTT: partial thromboplastin time, SQ: subcutaneous, t½: half life, VAD: ventricular assist device.

- Goals for anticoagulation: Anti-Xa 0.2-0.5 U/mL, PTT 60-80 seconds
- Titrate by 10-20% every 2 hours until therapeutic
- Obtain anti-Xa levels and PTT 2 hours after a change and then every 6-8 hours
- ECMO coagulation panel every 6-8 hours, daily ROTEM® and plasma hemoglobin level

Implantable Continuous-Flow VAD (HeartWare and HeartMate)
Acute Phase:
- Preanticoagulation: ROTEM® and ECMO coagulation panel (PT, PTT, PTT hepzyme, fibrinogen, AT, D-dimer, heparin level, platelet count)
- Correct underlying coagulopathy or thrombocytopenia as clinically indicated by transfusion of plasma, cryoprecipitate, or platelets
- Begin heparin after 24-48 hours postimplantation
- Initiate heparin at 10 U/kg/h (max 1000 U/hr), per team discussion
- Monitor for bleeding at all times
- Goals for anticoagulation: Anti-Xa 0.2-0.4 U/mL, PTT 60-80 seconds
- Titrate up by 10-20% every 4 hours until therapeutic
- Obtain anti-Xa levels and PTT 4 hours after a change and then every 12-24 hours
- ECMO coagulation panel every 6-8 hours, daily ROTEM® and plasma hemoglobin level

Chronic Phase:
- Initiate warfarin when the patient resumes stable enteral feeding
- Once INR reaches a therapeutic range (usually 2-3), consider stopping heparin and adding aspirin.

Management of Catheter-Related Arterial and Venous Thrombosis

Arterial Thrombosis
TCH has a clinical algorithm for management of arterial thrombosis. In brief, if suspected catheter-related arterial thrombosis:
- Remove catheter
- Order stat Doppler ultrasound (US)
- Consult Hemostasis and Thrombosis (HAT) team
- If limb ischemia and/or compartment syndrome are suspected, consult interventional radiology, plastic surgery, orthopedic surgery, and/or vascular surgery without delay (this is an emergency)
- Thrombolytic (i.e., alteplase) therapy or surgical intervention may be indicated (recent major surgery is a contraindication to thrombolytic therapy)
- Start anticoagulation with heparin or enoxaparin
- Therapy is a minimum of 7 days; then repeat a Doppler US

Deep Venous Thrombosis (DVT)
TCH also has a clinical algorithm for deep vein thrombosis. Briefly, if DVT is suspected:
- Order stat Doppler US
- Consult HAT team
- Start anticoagulation with heparin or enoxaparin

Table 59-3. Monitoring of hemostasis and thrombosis.

Lab	Property	Abnormal values	Use
PTT	Assess the intrinsic and common pathways of clotting, including fibrinogen	von Willebrand disease, lupus anticoagulants, factor deficiencies	Heparin, bivalirudin, ECMO, perioperative
PT / INR	Assess the extrinsic & common pathways of clotting, including fibrinogen; INR standardizes for different PT testing mechanisms	DIC, warfarin, liver disease, vitamin-K deficiency	Warfarin, ECMO, perioperative
D-dimer	Product of fibrin degradation. Elevated levels indicate recent intravascular blood coagulation and then fibrinolysis.	Procoagulant and fibrinolytic mechanisms: DIC, surgery, trauma, hematomas, thromboembolism, hypercoagulable state	
Thrombin time	Measures the final step of the clotting pathway, conversion of fibrinogen to fibrin	Heparin, direct-thrombin inhibitors (bivalirudin), fibrin products, hypofibrinogenemia	
ACT	Contact-activated whole blood to measure clotting time in secs; poor marker for heparin effect	Factor deficiency, severe hypofibrinogenemia, low AT levels, low temperature, thrombocytopenia, anemia, heparin	CPB, ECMO, VAD
Thromboelastogram: ROTEM®	Dynamic POCT providing data on kinetics of hemostasis in whole blood from clot formation through lysis, includes platelet function and coagulation profile		CPB, ECMO, VAD, perioperative bleeding

ACT: activated clotting time, AT: antithrombin, CPB: cardiopulmonary bypass, DIC: disseminated intravascular coagulation, ECMO: extracorporeal membrane oxygenation, INR: international normalized ratio, POCT: point-of-care testing, PT: prothrombin time, PTT: partial thromboplastin time, VAD: ventricular assist device.

- Therapy should be continued for a minimum of 6 weeks for neonates and 3 months for children and adolescents; then repeat a Doppler US

Medications

Table 59-2 lists the properties, indications, and doses for antithrombotic and fibrinolytic medications.

PART IV. PERIOPERATIVE CARE

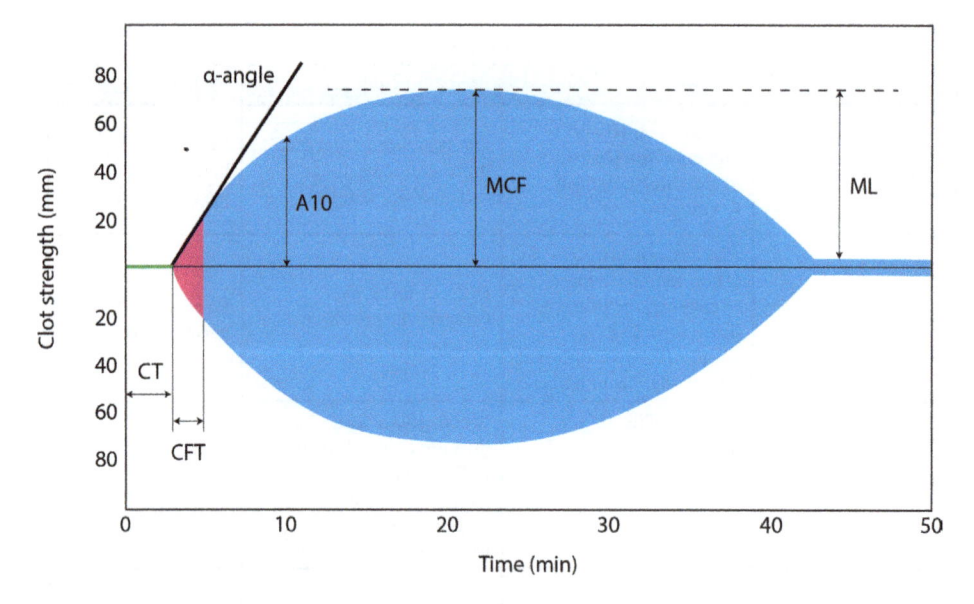

Figure 59-1. Depiction of ROTEM® results. The X-axis measures time elapsed and the Y-axis depicts clot strength in mm. Clot time (CT) is the time required for a 2 mm clot to form. Clot-formation time (CFT) is the time elapsed between formation of a 2 and a 20 mm clot. Maximal clot firmness (MCF) is the maximum amplitude prior to clot breakdown. Maximum lysis (ML) is the percentage reduction of clot amplitude by lysis at the end of the test. A10 is the amplitude of the clot at 10 min. See Table 59-5 for details.

Initiation of Warfarin (Coumadin®)

Warfarin has a half life of 25-60 hours and a duration of action of 2-5 days. Most patients require 3-5 days before achieving a sable phase. Please see Appendix A for dosing guidelines. Once the INR is therapeutic, stop therapy with unfractionated heparin or low-molecular weight heparin. After achieving a stable phase, routine monitoring includes INR checks every 1-4 weeks based on patient's age, compliance, and risk of thrombosis.

Table 59-4. Tests included as part of the ROTEM®.

Test	Description
EXTEM	Activation by tissue factor. Assesses the extrinsic pathway, like PT. Measures effects of warfarin and factor 7 deficiency.
FIBTEM	EXTEM with platelets blocked with cytochalasin D. Assesses fibrinogen effect.
APTEM	EXTEM with fibrinolysis blocked with tranexamic acid. Assesses clot formation without fibrinolysis.
INTEM	Assesses the intrinsic pathway, like PTT. Measures the effects of heparin and factor 8 deficiency.
HEPTEM	INTEM with heparin neutralized. Assesses heparin effect or uncovers underlying coagulopathy.

Antithrombotic Medication Changes with Major Surgery
- **Aspirin:** hold 7 days prior to surgery (except for shunted patients).
- **Enoxaparin:** Hold 2 doses (minimum 24 hours between last dose and procedure).
- **Heparin:** Hold 4 hours prior to procedure. Hold for LA line removal.
- **Warfarin**
  - *Urgent procedures:* FFP or factor concentrates (KCentra®) can be administered for rapid reversal.
  - *Elective procedures:* Stop warfarin 72 hours prior to the procedure **AND** either 1) start enoxaparin 72 hours prior to procedure (stop enoxaparin 24 hours prior to surgery) **OR** 2) admit 24 hours prior to surgery and start unfractionated heparin with no bolus (stop heparin 6 hours prior to surgery).
  - *Postoperatively*, discuss with the surgical team and resume heparin without bolus. Warfarin may be resumed when condition permits and adjust as necessary.
- **Bivalirudin:** Half-life is 25 min for older infants/adults and 15 min for newborns. Stop accordingly, based on the particular circumstances of the patient.

Monitoring
Table 59-3 lists the different lab tests used for monitoring of hemostasis and thrombosis.

ROTEM® Basics
Thromboelastography with ROTEM® is commonly used at TCH as point-of-care testing. ROTEM® includes 5 different tests: EXTEM, FIBTEM, INTEM, HEPTEM, and APTEM (Table 59-4). For each of the tests, a graph is depicted (Figure 59-1). Table 59-5 lists the different parameters provided and their interpretation.

Consultations
- **Arterial / Venous Thrombosis:** HAT Team
- **Stroke:** Neurology, HAT Team
- **ECMO / VAD:** Transfusion Medicine

Table 59-5. ROTEM® paremeters.

Parameter	Description
Clotting time (CT), secs	Time for a 2 mm clot to form. Measures initiation of clotting, thrombin formation, start of clot polymerization.
Clot formation time (CFT), secs	Time elapsed from 2 to 20 mm clot formation. Measures fibrin polymerization, stabilization with platelets, factor 8.
alpha-angle, degrees	Slope of CFT from CT. Small angle suggests low platelets or low fibrinogen. Large angle suggests clot stability, hypercoagulable state.
Max clot firmness (MCF), mm	Maximum amplitude prior to clot breakdown by fibrinolysis. Defines clot stability.
Max lysis (ML), %	% reduction of maximum clot amplitude by lysis at measurement end (1 h).

60 Intraoperative Hemostasis

Erin A. Gottlieb, Jun Teruya

The approach to intraoperative bleeding begins preoperatively with identification of the patient at risk for bleeding and continues into the intraoperative and postoperative periods.

Preoperative: Identification of the Patient at Risk for Bleeding

There are patient and surgical factors associated with bleeding risk. *Patient factors* include young age, low weight, cyanosis, polycythemia, preoperative anticoagulant/antiplatelet medications, history of VAD or ECMO support. *Surgical factors* include multiple reoperations, use of deep hypothermia, and extensive high-pressure suture lines. Acquired von Willebrand syndrome (AVWS) can increase the risk of bleeding. Risk factors for AVWS include lesions or conditions associated with high-shear stress such as pinhole VSD, severe aortic or pulmonary valve stenosis, ECMO, and VAD. If risk factors are present, preoperative testing for AVWS should take place. If the patient has AVWS, replacement of VWF with human (Humate-P®) or recombinant (Vonvendi®) product should be planned.

Pre-CPB

Prior to initiation of CPB, tranexamic acid (Table 60-1) or epsilon-aminocaproic acid (Amicar®) (Table 60-2) are used. The activated clotting time (ACT) is measured at baseline. For neonates and infants, the pump prime includes both PRBCs and FFP to avoid excessive dilution of red cells and coagulation factors.

Before Separation from CPB

Prior to separation from CPB, a ROTEM® is sent during rewarming (see Chapter 59). Only the HEPTEM® and FIBTEM® channels are run, using a real-time ROTEM® viewer. This allows for goal-directed transfusion of products.

Anticipate the need for platelets, cryoprecipitate, FFP, and PRBC from the Blood Bank, and/or fibrinogen concentrate, 4-factor (nonactivated) prothrombin complex

Table 60-1. Tranexamic acid dosing chart.[1]

Weight (kg)	Concentration of bolus (mg/mL)	Bolus after induction (mg/kg)	CPB prime bolus (mg)[2]	Infusion (mg/kg/hr)[3]
<5	10	10	10	2.5
6-25	10	10	10	2
26-50	100	10	20	2
>50	100	5	20	5

[1] For children with a history of seizures, avoid the use of tranexamic acid after discussion with other team members.
[2] Please note that the CPB prime bolus is NOT weight-based.
[3] For children with creatinine >2 mg/dL, decrease the infusion rate by 50%.

Table 60-2. Epsilon-aminocaproic acid (Amicar®) dosing chart.

Age or Weight[1]	Concentration of bolus (mg/mL)	Bolus after induction	CPB prime bolus	Infusion
Age < 30 days	250	40 mg/kg	30 mg	40 mg/kg/hr
Age ≥ 30 days up to 50 kg	250	75 mg/kg	75 mg/kg	75 mg/kg/hr
> 50 kg	250	75 mg/kg up to a maximum of 5 g	5 g	1 g/hr

[1] Please note that dosing regimens are quite different based on age group and higher body weight (fixed pump bolus for some, not weight-based for larger patients).

concentrate (Kcentra®), and recombinant activated factor 7 from Pharmacy. Pharmacologic factors are not mixed or prepared until the decision is made to give them.

After CPB

Heparin is reversed with 1-1.3 mg of protamine per 100 U of pre-CPB heparin bolus. An ACT should be measured to assess whether ACT has returned to baseline.

There are 2 approaches used at TCH for intraoperative hemostasis:
- **ROTEM®-based approach**
  - Observe the surgical field and discuss whether the patient appears to be bleeding.
  - Use the ROTEM® obtained during rewarming to guide transfusion.
  - If the hematocrit is less than ideal due to dilution with clotting factors, transfusion of PRBC may be necessary.
- **Traditional approach**
  - Observe the field and discuss whether the patient appears to be bleeding.
  - Give platelets (10 mL/kg) as a first line treatment and cryoprecipitate (1 unit/5 kg of body weight) as the second line. If bleeding continues, may give another round of platelets (10 mL/kg). If bleeding continues, consider FFP or prothrombin-complex concentrate (e.g., Kcentra®), or recombinant activated factor 7.
  - If the hematocrit is less than ideal due to dilution with clotting factors, transfusion of PRBC may be necessary.

Postoperative Period

Communication to the CICU regarding the extent of bleeding, blood products given, tests run, and pharmacologic factors given is mandatory. Poor communication can lead to undertreatment or overtreatment of coagulopathy, which can have catastrophic results.

If bleeding continues in the postoperative period, diagnosis and treatment should continue. Strategies include:
- **Recheck ACT.** If ACT is higher than baseline, this suggests heparin rebound effect, and additional protamine may be necessary.
- **Check other labs** including PT, PTT, INR, platelet count, fibrinogen, ROTEM® to identify which products or factors are needed.
- If all labs are normal, consider the need for surgical reexploration (see Chapter 76).

61 Discharge Education after Congenital Heart Surgery

Meghan Anderson, Amy Hemingway, Antonio R. Mott

Discharge teaching after CHS is usually provided to the patients and families by the surgical nurses and NPs.

Activity Restrictions

The sternum takes 6-8 weeks to completely heal after surgery. During this time, patients should observe "sternal precautions" in efforts to avoid injury to their chest.

In the infant population, our goal is to allow patients to continue their developmental milestones. Infants should avoid forced tummy time for 6 weeks after surgery, while the sternum is healing. However, patients are not restricted from rolling over or crawling if they are developmentally able to perform these activities. Infants should not be picked up under their arms, but rather "scooped" after surgery.

For toddler and school age patients, the focus of sternal precautions is to avoid activities in which a fall or injury to the chest could occur. These activities include riding bicycles, organized contact sports, playing on playground equipment, jumping on a trampoline, etc. Similar to the infant population, toddlers should be "scooped" and not picked up under the arms after surgery.

Adolescent and adult patients should avoid contact sports for 6-8 weeks. Additionally, patients should avoid pushing, pulling, lifting objects over 5 pounds, and repetitive movements, such as throwing a ball, for 6 weeks following surgery. Patients are also instructed to avoid wearing backpacks for 12 weeks and avoid sexual activity for 6 weeks following surgery. Due to the potential injury caused from deployment of air bags, patients are instructed not to drive or ride on the front seat of a car for 6 weeks after surgery. Adolescent females should wear support bras and avoid bras with underwire until the incision is well healed.

Wound Care

Median sternotomy and thoracotomy incisions are closed using multiple layers of stitches. The most superficial layer of skin is covered with Dermabond® or Steri-Strips™, depending on surgeon's preference. While the incision is healing, the goal of wound care is to keep the incision clean and dry. Patients with Steri-Strips™ over their incision will have a sterile dressing placed in the OR. This dressing will be removed on postoperative day (POD) 2 and the Steri-Strips™ covering the incision should be painted twice a day using Betadine® swabs. If Steri-Strips™ are used, they should fall off on POD 7-14, depending on wound healing and patient age (i.e., Steri-Strips™ are left in place longer for neonates and transplant patients). Patients will have their subcuticular (PDS®, Vicryl®, or Monocryl®) stitches removed on POD 7-14 depending on type, location, and other factors such as immune or nutritional status. After the subcuticular sutures have been removed (POD 7-14), patients can wash the incision with antibacterial soap and water. Chest tube stitches will be removed 5-7 days after the chest tube is removed.

If Dermabond® is used to close the incision, it will typically stay in place for 7-14 days. Once the Dermabond® has fallen off, the incision should be washed with antibacterial soap and water. Due to the potential for differential tanning, the wound should be kept out of the sun for 1 year.

Bathing

Patients may take modified baths and showers once their chest tubes have been removed. They should avoid submerging the surgical incision underwater, the shower head should be directed toward the patient's back, and the incision should be kept as dry as possible. After all sutures have been removed, patients may shower/bathe and discontinue cleaning the incision with Betadine®. Younger patients may take a sponge bath using similar precautions to keep the incision dry. Patients should refrain from submerging the surgical incision and chest tube sites under water for 4-6 weeks after surgery. Patients should also refrain from applying creams, ointments, and lotions to their surgical incisions until the incision is well healed.

Avoiding Infections

Patients should be counseled on the importance of avoiding infections in the postoperative period. They should be mindful of avoiding large crowds, particularly during cold and flu season, in efforts to avoid infectious contacts. Families are encouraged to use antibacterial hand sanitizer at home to decrease the spread of germs. Patients who are due for scheduled immunizations should avoid these for 6 weeks after surgery. However, patients may receive the influenza virus and RSV vaccines during this time period.

Follow-Up Care

Patients should follow up in the CHS clinic 1 week after hospital discharge. Patients from outside of the Houston area should stay locally (1 hour from the hospital) for at least 1 week after discharge from the hospital, until their postoperative appointment with the CHS team. The rationale for patients staying locally in the immediate postoperative period is for the CHS team to monitor for potential postoperative complications such as accumulation of pleural fluid or development of a pericardial effusion. Additionally, this time is used to assess wound healing and remove any remaining stitches prior to the patients returning home. Patients should follow up with their cardiologist 2-4 weeks after surgery and this appointment should be made during their inpatient hospitalization.

62 Child Life

Katie Persha, Sara H. Reynolds

Visiting the hospital can be a challenging and frightening experience for a child and their family. The Heart Center at TCH has Certified Child Life Specialists (CCLS) available to help reduce fear and anxiety that come when facing hospitalization and medical interventions. Child life specialists are available to provide services in all areas of the Heart Center and work as part of the multidisciplinary team to provide developmentally appropriate therapeutic interventions.

Services and programming vary based upon a patient's age, diagnosis, and coping needs. Because of the chronic nature of CHD, the Child Life team has experience in supporting patients from birth to adulthood, as well as siblings and other important members of a patient's life. The team supports the infant population by promoting bonding and attachment with parents as well as providing appropriate stimulation and play to help meet developmental milestones while in the hospital environment. Additionally, child life specialists are able to provide education to both parents and siblings on supporting and promoting normal growth and development. To support older patients, child life specialists are available to provide developmentally appropriate education and preparation for medical tests and procedures, surgeries, and diagnoses. The specialists work with the goal to clarify misconceptions and empower patients with appropriate knowledge and understanding, therefore helping to reduce fear and anxiety. Typical interventions include preoperative tours of the Heart Center before surgery, supporting patients before and during procedures, preparation for procedures using photo preparation books and developmentally appropriate terms, and diagnosis-specific education.

The Child Life team strives to normalize the hospital environment and create positive experiences for patients and their families throughout their time in the Heart Center. The team works with patients and families to ensure that the holidays and milestones most important to them are celebrated while in the hospital setting. The team also encourages developmentally appropriate play to patients throughout the Heart Center to promote normalization throughout a patient's hospitalization.

Child life specialists in the Heart Center are experienced in working with CHD patients across their lifespan, including providing comfort and support during the end of life. They are available to provide appropriate support and education to siblings about death and have materials/resources for parents to utilize with siblings of all ages. Our child life specialists work with the patient and family to assess how we can honor their child's legacy in a meaningful way.

The Heart Center also has a variety of other creative arts professionals available who collaborate with child life specialists to provide psychosocial support to patients and families. Assisted animal therapy, art therapy, and music therapy all provide services to the Heart Center.

Music Therapy

Music therapy can provide support for hospitalized children in a variety of ways through individualized and group sessions. Individual music therapy services are available for

Heart Center patients on a consult basis. Music therapy is effective in managing pain, decreasing agitation, providing support and structure during procedures, facilitating bonding, increasing relaxation, providing nonverbal outlets for self-expression, and enhancing quality of life. Music therapy is uniquely equipped to meet the needs of medically fragile infants by providing regulated multisensory stimulation. Music therapy groups are offered on the acute cardiology floors with a goal to provide a space for appropriate stimulation and socialization for our infant population.

Art Therapy

The art therapist within the Heart Center uses the expressive power of art to support the individualized needs of children and their families throughout hospitalization. Art therapy offers creative tools and interventions that aim to achieve a variety of goals, including providing opportunities for creativity and self-expression, promoting relaxation and pain management, increasing positive self-esteem and resilience, developing healthy problem-solving and adaptive skills, fostering peer support and a sense of community in the medical environment, and facilitating legacy building and memory making. Both group and individual art therapy sessions are provided to patients and families throughout the Heart Center on a consult basis.

Assisted Animal Therapy

The TCH Pawsitive Play Program has a facility dog dedicated to the Legacy Tower that is available to work with our patients and families in the Heart Center. The dog and its handler, a child life specialist, help normalize the hospital setting, meet specific goals, and enhance the emotional well-being of our patients and families. Our facility dog and handler can be consulted by a patient's child life specialist for individual bedside visits. In addition to individualized services, Pawsitive Play provides a regularly scheduled "Bow Wow Hour" in the cardiac progressive care unit (CPCU) playroom open to all patients and families.

63 The Emotional and Spiritual Components of Congenital Heart Disease

Thomas P. Sharon

Caring for patients with CHD involves caring for the whole person and their family and caregivers. This includes the physical, emotional, and spiritual elements of their beings. It is vital that who they are and will be is not only shaped by the grief and trauma that they will overcome under our care.

Grief is an inherent element of CHD. It is the emotional and spiritual factor in the disease and is as real as the physical illness itself. How the family and the patient are able to cope with their grief directly impacts the physical treatments and care that can be provided, as well as the quality of life or death that the patient and family will experience. Grief is not a linear process. It is cyclical, and when experienced, becomes part of a human's being to the extent that it impacts the physical, emotional, and spiritual elements of the person. CHD is complex because it may become an inherent element of who the patient is and will be for the rest of their life.

Chaplains are trained to recognize the grief from past experiences and how that is impacting the grief and coping within the current manifestation of it in themselves, patients, families and all levels of care providers.

The Family Factor

Parents and families are changed by their child's disease. Their view of themselves, life, their family, the world, and the Divine is not only forever changed but it is continually evolving, and they are struggling with how to cope with a new and fluid state of being. How they are able to cope will directly relate to the care they provide for the patient and the care they will allow for themselves.

The first round of grief comes the moment the family receives the diagnosis. This is where they begin the journey of round after round of acceptance. Acceptance that their baby or child has CHD, that their child will require medical treatments that often cause suffering to sustain life or an acceptable quality of life, that they have to work with medical professionals to make decisions that impact the rest of their child's life, and that their life and that of their other children will forever be changed.

The stages of grief, as the family moves through denial, anger, guilt, blame, bargaining, and acceptance, occur throughout the hospital admission, future admissions, once they discharge, and throughout the lives of CHD families. Because of how these changes have impacted the parents and family, the person that the physicians and caregivers face during the initial admission and into future clinic visits and admissions will also change. This is often subtle but can be profound. It will vary between each parent and can cause conflicts between the parent or family member who is present with the patient throughout the admission and the family members who are not. The parent or family members not present are not only struggling to understand the status and plan of care with which the parent at bedside continually lives, they are also struggling to understand this new person that the parent living the admission has become.

These changes manifest most vividly during a new diagnosis and changes in plan of

63. THE EMOTIONAL AND SPIRITUAL COMPONENTS OF CONGENITAL HEART DISEASE

care, especially those involving surgical procedures, codes, patient setbacks, and the point where there are no further viable medical options for the patient. As parents and families experience the suffering inherent with their child's disease, they will sometimes reach the point that they feel the emotional costs to the patient, themselves, and/or their family outweigh the physical benefits of continuing the patient's life. Parents will at times refuse surgical or treatment options or even request a move to withdraw of life sustaining therapies (WOLST). This can present as the parents saying they want to "leave it to God" or "let God make the decision" because they no longer have the emotional reserves to make decisions that cause the patient's continued suffering. It can also present in the parents' abandonment of the patient on various levels and/or refusal to consent to vital treatment needs for the patient. This is often the result of a lack of effective processing of the grief residue that accumulates during the patient's admission. The level at which the residue reaches critical mass varies significantly with each person depending on their past experiences and coping needs and resources.

It is the fundamental role of the chaplain to assess the physical, emotional, relational, and spiritual needs and resources of the family and patients, and coordinate the supports needed. Therefore, the chaplains are one of the hospital's vital resources in working with families to process their grief and trauma residue so it does not reach critical mass at the most significant points in the patient's care. On-call chaplains can help but the unit chaplains build the relationships essential for parents and families to process and work through their distress at the points that they have the emotional and physical strength to do so. Clinicians are a vital part of this by initiating a consult with the chaplain whenever they note emotional distress or a low affect with parents and family. It is also helpful to have the chaplain present during family meetings to discuss a new diagnosis, changes in the plan of care, or other news that are not within the scope of expectations of the parents. These interactions should not be limited to code status changes or end-of-life planning, but throughout the entire hospitalization.

An important time to also involve the chaplain is when patients move out of the CICU and start preparing for discharge, as many parents and families have continued to cope throughout the patient's admission with a certain level of denial and refusal. Going home is not only frightening because of the complexity of care that the patient requires but also for how they will return to their partner, children, family, friends, and life itself, as this new person they have become. Because of the relationships and the inherent cultural status of the chaplain as a confidential outlet who is also removed from their home resources and supports, they will often share their deeper struggles with the chaplain when they are unwilling to do so with other psychosocial supports or their family or clergy.

When family's grief reaches its apex is of course if the child dies. It is at this point above all others that the relationships the family has built with the chaplain, social worker, and child-life specialist become vital as the primary emotional and spiritual resources for most – but not all – families. The anticipatory grief amplifies as the clinical team and physicians have the family meetings leading up to the WOLST or amid a code crisis leading to death. If a family meeting is held for end-of-life discussions, a premeeting is very beneficial. The attending physician leads the meeting with the chaplain, social worker, and child life specialist to review family dynamics, grief assessments and meaningful coping resources, and a postmeeting plan for family support. The postmeeting plan provides an essential framework for the transition from anticipatory grief to end-of life-grief. When possible, the chaplain should be available during or immediately after the family meeting to plan for spiritual and emotional supports that are meaningful for the family.

The chaplain has access to a wide variety of community clergy to meet the requirements of almost all faith traditions or can make the contact with the family clergy to be present in the way that the family requests. The chaplain is also trained to not let the cultural expectations within any faith tradition limit the supports offered and provided to families. The chaplain can normalize the grief, family and cultural dynamics so the grief does not spiral into a negative environment. Therefore, the chaplain is present at TCH for all codes and a referral is made for the chaplain to be present prior to and at the time of death. The chaplain will also assist the nursing staff with escorting large family groups in and out of the CICU at the time of death and out of the room and hospital after death. The chaplain should also be present prior to the family leaving the hospital after their child's death. This is a final point of closure for families who may have spent months, if not years, in the hospital, and often have spent the patient's lifetime there.

The Patient Factor

Grief for patients comes in different forms and ways based on their developmental status. Infants are in the trust stage and if the only ones in their realm of existential reality cause pain and trauma, the chaplain provides a presence who does not inflict pain. There is also a dynamic in which the peace and release of tension that the parents feel when the chaplain visits are felt by the patient.

The chaplain can also provide the consistency of presence needed to establish the bond of trust that is vital with teenagers before they are willing to become vulnerable and share their fears, hopes, and grief over their losses. The teen will begin to experience anticipatory grief as their friends make plans for adulthood and they face the limitations inherent to their illness. They feel different and isolated from friends, which creates levels of loss of their community identity, a fundamental coping need for teens. In addition to the cognitive developmental phases that teens go through, there are also faith maturation challenges for the spiritual essence of the patient. There is an inherent progression in the late teens to early adulthood from the "Synthetic-Conventional" faith stage to the "Individuative-Reflective" faith stage (Fowler 1995). They will move past the values and belief systems of their family and peers and begin to question and redevelop their value system as their faith matures and becomes their own. This stage can leave them with a sense of uncertainty with regard to the faith and value system coping resources. Teens are often not comfortable sharing these faith struggles with their parents or other clergy because some of their struggles are deeply seeded in these relationships. They will often share these struggles with a chaplain who maintains the element of anonymity from their home context and confidentiality that they have come to expect.

The chaplain can also be a bridge between the family and patient at times of life and health transitions, and pending death. They can encourage family members to speak to patients who are intubated or dying so they have the comfort of their presence at the most critical time in their life.

The time to make a referral to the chaplain is when patients present with a low affect, are struggling with compliance with their plan of care, are in distress, have received a new diagnosis or change in plan of care, prior to discharge, and when there has been a code change, code, or pending death. The other nonclinical time for a chaplain referral is when there is a change in the patient's family system or structure.

The Clinician Factor

Physicians and other clinicians also experience profound grief. It is vital that the humanity of everyone caring for these children is accepted and the impacts validated. The residue needs to be processed in positive, effective ways to avoid burnout or the loss of quality of life. As the chaplain walks alongside the physicians and clinicians, there is an element of the physician healing themselves because those relationships that are meaningful to the patients and families are also established with and for them. The chaplain will make themselves present immediately after codes, setbacks, and deaths, but they are also present as a confidential support for them. The TCH Heart Center has established a Work/Life Balance Committee which is developing meaningful outlets for the individual, and TCH has created a Physicians' Well-Being Committee which continues to expand the resources available for restoration. This begins with acceptance of the cycles of grief inherent to caring for congenital heart patients in the same way it does for the patients and families. Denial seems to be the easy path, and while it has a place in grief and coping, it is as destructive for the physicians and clinicians as it is for the patient and family if they do not move to acceptance and action toward restoration.

Suggested Readings

Fowler, JW. Stages of Faith: The Psychology of Human Development and the Quest for Meaning. HarperOne; 1995.

V. Lines, Tubes, and Monitors

64 Endotracheal Intubation

Stuart R. Hall

Indications

Intubation of the critically ill patient has several key indications, the foremost of which is maintenance of a secure airway and providing optimal gas exchange during and following procedures, and at times of actual or potential instability. Intubation is the only practical way to deliver high inspired oxygen concentrations, with or without the use of iNO. Patients may be admitted to the CICU from the OR with an ETT still in place, may be transferred from another institution with an ETT, or may need to be intubated while in the CICU.

Procedure and Other Considerations

Institutional practice in the OR is to intubate smaller children (neonates, infants, and children less than approximately 30 kg) nasally, primarily to facilitate the use of TEE so that the probe and ETT do not share the mouth under the drapes where loss of the airway would be challenging to manage. In the CICU, nasal ETTs are considered by most to provide a more stable and consistent tube position with a lower risk of dislodgement. In an emergency situation however, it is usually faster to secure the airway orally.

Whenever a patient needs intubation in nonemergent situations, it is customary to obtain informed consent from the parents. Make sure to have working laryngoscope blades and handles available. Appropriately sized endotracheal tubes should be available. One tube should be the predicted size for the patient and extra tubes should be one half-size larger and one half-size smaller. Uncuffed tubes are generally not used, except perhaps in the case of very small infants in whom a 3.5 mm cuffed tube will not fit. A 3 mm ETT has an exceedingly narrow lumen which makes pulmonary toilet a challenge: some choose to use 3.5 mm uncuffed tubes over 3 mm cuffed tubes for that reason. Nasal intubations can be challenging.

Much has been written about predicting what size of ETT a child will need: in fact, for every formula, you can easily find the paper disproving it. Generally speaking, full-term neonates will need a 3.5 mm cuffed tube. Larger infants (6 months – 1 year) a 4 mm cuffed, toddlers and small children a 4.5 mm cuffed, with 8-year olds taking 5 or 5.5 mm cuffed tubes. Use whatever formula you and your attending prefer, and be prepared to change the tube size if it will not pass easily (or if it seems the tube is visually very small relative to the glottis). Tube depth for a nasal ETT can be estimated by 3 times the inner diameter of the tube; under direct vision, ensure the cuff has passed the vocal cords and do not push the tube in as far as it will go. If you are using a stylet, remove the stylet before passing the tube much past the vocal cords as an ETT rendered rigid by a stylet can puncture the trachea.

Sedation for endotracheal intubation can be accomplished in many ways. If the patient is appropriately fasted (6 hours for solid food, 4 hours for breast milk, 2 hours for clears), a gentle induction with titrated doses of midazolam (0.1 mg/kg) and fentanyl (1-2 mcg/kg) works well, followed by either vecuronium (0.1 mg/kg) or rocuronium

64. ENDOTRACHEAL INTUBATION

(0.5-1 mg/kg). Remember that in patients with severely compromised hemodynamics, it can take minutes to see any effect from sedatives or neuromuscular blockade, and it is important to be patient. Assist the patient's ventilation using bag-mask ventilation (with a Jackson-Rees "anesthesia" circuit or an Ambu® Bag) as indicated. Nominally, an intubating dose of vecuronium can take 3-4 minutes to become effective, while rocuronium (1 mg/kg) takes 30-60 seconds to work, with all of these times extended when a patient's circulation time is long. Once the airway has been secured with a tube, disposable CO_2 detectors are available to confirm tube placement, as well as auscultation and CXR.

At TCH, there is an anesthesiologist and a CRNA in the hospital 24/7, and therefore, in situations where the patient is unstable or has a difficult airway, someone is always available to help with intubation. Institutional policy dictates that after 2 attempts at intubation, Anesthesia should be called to help with securing the airway. In particularly sick and unstable patients, many attendings will call the CV anesthesiologist on-call to assist with sedation and intubation. If the patient is very sick and unstable, it is appropriate for the most skilled individual available to perform an intubation.

65 Central Venous Catheters

Patricia Bastero, Stuart R. Hall, Carlos M. Mery, Cynthia Sturrock

A central venous catheter is useful for diagnostic and therapeutic purposes, and is one of the most common lines used in patients with CHD.

Indications
- Administration of inotropic support
- Fluid resuscitation
- Assessment of central venous pressures and fluid status
- Assessment of mixed venous oxygen saturation

Insertion Technique and General Considerations

Central venous access can be achieved through different routes. The most common include the IJ veins, subclavian veins, femoral veins, or directly into the atria.

When central venous access is indicated, a first question is how many lumens are actually needed. Commonly, central lines have 1, 2, or 3 lumens. Double-lumen lines are the most common; the risk of central line-associated bloodstream infection (CLABSI) increases with the number of lumens present.

Placement should be performed with the utmost attention to sterile technique with the routine use of "bundles". TCH has a central line placement kit available in the procedure carts. The kit includes all of the equipment needed to place a line except the line itself, gloves, and the patient's drape (small vs. large). The use of the central line insertion checklist (also available in the kit) and CLABSI prevention bundle is important (Table 65-1).

Institutional practice is to avoid the IJ in patients <5 kg due to the length of available lines and the potentially major implications for the patient and subsequent surgeries of a thrombosed neck vein or SVC. In infants <5 kg, femoral venous cannulation is preferred. Larger patients going toward the single-ventricle pathway who rely (or will rely) on IJ flow as a source of pulmonary blood flow, particularly during the bidirectional Glenn phase, have no real "central" access from the upper body. In these patients, avoiding the IJ is advisable. In patients with a Fontan circulation, there is no difference between femoral and IJ access (since all veins lead to the lungs, not the heart), so in those patients either site may be appropriate.

Central lines should not routinely be used for rapid infusion of volume or blood products due to the limited caliber of the lumens (particularly of smaller lines) limiting the speed of infusion, and to the increased risk of CLABSI if blood products are infused. We therefore recommend that the smallest caliber line appropriate for the patient is selected. Generally speaking, in neonates, a 4 Fr, 12 cm double-lumen femoral catheter is appropriate. A 4 Fr catheter will work for most children, and a 5 Fr catheter is adequate for older school-age children and adolescents.

In many patients, even up to adult sizes, large-bore peripheral IV access will allow for more rapid infusion of volume than one lumen of a central line. There are large (i.e., 8 Fr,

Table 65-1. Central line insertion checklist and central line-associated bloodstream infection (CLABSI) prevention bundle.

Central Line Insertion Checklist
Patient and family education
• Patient and family educated about central line-associated bloodstream infection and prevention practices prior to line placement.
Hand hygiene
• Personnel with patient contact: hand hygiene prior to line placement.
Maximum sterile barrier precautions
• Personnel with field contact: sterile gown, sterile gloves, hat, and mask. • Personnel within 3 feet of the procedure don hat and mask. • Use of a head-to-toe body drape for the procedure
Chlorhexidine-based antiseptic
• Use of a chlorhexidine based antiseptic for skin preparation unless contraindicated (e.g. patient <60 days old, allergy to chlorhexidine)
Site selection
• Avoid femoral line placement in the older adolescent or adult when possible unless medical conditions warrant its use.

CLABSI Prevention Bundle Elements
Central line maintenance bundle
• Necessity of line discussed on daily rounds and document as "Y" (Yes) on the Lines/Drains/Airways (LDA) Flowsheet • Dressing clean, dry, and intact *always* • Dressing labeled (time + dated) • Dressing changed every 7 days/as needed unless Neo-PICC • Tubing labeled (time + dated) • Proper hand hygiene performed • Gloves worn for all tubing and connector entries • Cap connection scrubbed with alcohol 15:15 • Sterile cap changed per protocol (usually every 4 days with tubing)
Central line hygiene protocol

• Chlorhexidine bath daily per protocol and documented
   - 2 wipes for <10kg
   - 4 wipes for 10-30kg
   - 6 wipes for >30kg
   - NOT for patient's <2 months of age
• Document refusal
• Chlorhexidine info sheet given to family
• Oral care twice daily and documented
• Linen changed daily
• Clean environment of care (e.g., free of clutter, discarding of leftover food, bed changed every 30 days)

PART V. LINES, TUBES AND MONITORS

and resuscitation, but large lines are usually only appropriate for patients close to adult size.

Catheter depth can be approximated using the patient's height. Divide the height by 10 and subtract 1 if the patient is <100 cm tall or use 2 cm for patients >100 cm. This number approximates the depth of insertion for an IJ catheter's tip to reach approximately the SVC-RA junction. For femoral lines, even a 12 cm line will not reach the atrium of a term neonate, so a 4 Fr, 12 cm catheter is appropriate for most infants. The smallest venous catheter readily available is a 3 Fr, 8 cm single-lumen catheter.

Ultrasound guidance is recommended for central-line placements. Be sure to use a sterile sheath for the ultrasound probe, and have someone available to help with the controls on the ultrasound machine. Lines are placed with sterile Seldinger technique. Ultrasound guidance is exactly that: guidance. Identify landmarks before prepping the patient, including palpation of nearby arteries, to orient yourself to the patient's anatomy. Identify the vein to be cannulated, as well as other regional landmarks, before attempting to cannulate any vessels. In code situations, some experienced providers may choose to use landmarks and pulses to find veins for cannulation, but if time allows, current standard of care is to visualize the vein on ultrasound before placement.

In patients who will need long-term access, consider scheduling the patient for placement of a PICC line. For most patients, this must be done in the IR suites but on occasions, particularly if the patient is too unstable to be safely transported, the IR team may come to the bedside to place a PICC. The timing of PICC-line requests needs to be carefully considered: these are "elective" procedures that are usually done on a weekday as part of a routine list. In an emergency, conventional central lines should instead be placed.

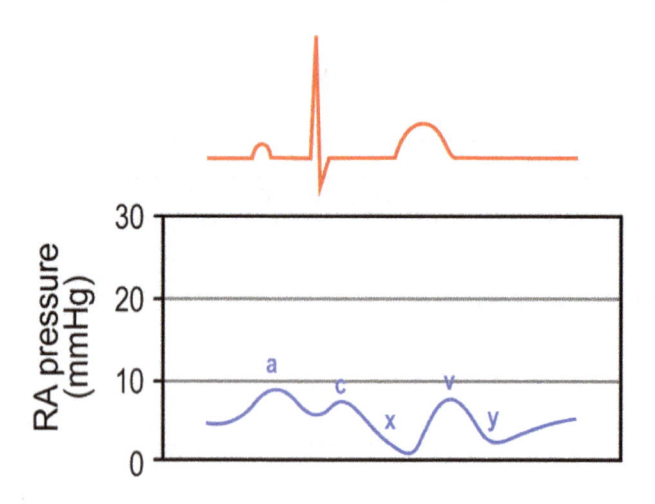

Figure 65-1. Right atrial / CVP tracing (see text for details).

65. CENTRAL VENOUS CATHETERS

Table 65-2. Changes in CVP under different conditions.

Lesion	CVP
RV dysfunction	↑
RV hypertrophy	↑
Tricuspid stenosis or regurgitation	↑
Volume overload	↑
LV-to-RA shunt	↑
AV disassociation	↑
Tachyarrhythmias	↑
Tamponade	↑
Artifact	↑ or ↓
Hypovolemia	↓

CLABSI Prevention

The prevention of CLABSIs is a key responsibility of the clinicians, and this is a true *team effort* that requires adherence to protocols, empowerment of nurses, and regular audit and review. Methods useful for infection prevention include, but are not limited to, meticulous hand technique when manipulating lines, keeping central line dressings intact, cleaning all entry ports prior to access, and holding other team members accountable to follow all elements of the CLABSI prevention bundle (Table 65-1). The incorporation of best practices and collaboration with other members of the patient's multidisciplinary team, including Infection Control, the Vascular Access Team, and family members, also contribute to safe line maintenance.

Interpretation

CVP is an indicator of RV filling pressures and in the normal healthy circulation, measures from 2 to 6mmHg. However, even though it is a proxy of volume status, it may not correlate properly with left ventricular end-diastolic pressure (LVEDP) in the setting of cardiac or respiratory disease. CVP can be affected by RV compliance, which itself can be aletered by changes in intrathoracic pressure, myocardial disease, and pericardial disease. As such, the response of CVP to fluid administration can be used to infer RV compliance. Table 65-2 depicts the changes seen in RA pressure or CVP with different conditions.

There is a fair amount of information that can be obtained from the RA or CVP tracing (Figure 65-1). The *a* wave represents the atrial contraction (coincides with the p wave in ECG). The *c* wave represents the AV valve propulsion toward the atria with ventricular contraction (coincides with the QRS in ECG). The *x'* descent shows the AV valve pulled downward at end-ventricular contraction. The *v* wave represents atrial filling (end of the T wave on ECG). The *y* descent shows the AV valve opening on ventricular diastole.

Assessment of the actual tracing can be useful in certain conditions:
- Arrhythmias (patients with AV dissociation will have cannon *a* waves)
- Tricuspid valve disease (patients with tricuspid regurgitation will have tall systolic *c-v* waves)
- Tamponade (all pressures are elevated without a *y* wave)

66 Left-Atrial Lines

Patricia Bastero, Carlos M. Mery, Virginia Smith

Left-atrial (LA) lines can be helpful in the management of postoperative patients. The LA pressure (LAP) provides a more accurate measurement of volume status or load, and LV end-diastolic pressure (LVEDP) than CVP.

Indications
- Evaluation of intravascular volume status in cases of altered RV compliance or pulmonary disease
- Postoperative assessment of LV performance
- Assessment of left AV valve disease (regurgitation or stenosis)

Insertion Technique and General Considerations

In general, LA lines are placed in the majority of newborns undergoing complex repairs and can be useful in patients undergoing tetralogy of Fallot repairs (due to the risk of RV diastolic dysfunction), patients with marginal left-sided structures, and those undergoing repair of complete AV septal defects.

LA lines are placed in the OR at the time of repair. They are inserted during CPB and are generally placed through the LA appendage. A small incision is created in the appendage, the line is placed, and secured with a pursestring around the appendage, a fine suture holding the line in place, and a rubber band around the appendage to avoid bleeding upon removal. In some situations, such as after heart transplants, the line is placed directly through the LA sutureline. These lines may be more prone to bleeding upon removal given the absence of the rubber band around the appendage.

In the CICU, LA line tubing should be inspected for the presence of air bubbles hourly, or more frequently, in order to avoid systemic air embolism. Removal of air bubbles should only be performed by appropriately-trained nurses or medical staff. Transducers should be leveled and zeroed at the phlebostatic axis once per shift or when there is a sudden change in the reading. Fluid boluses should not be given through this line and a continuous infusion of heparinized saline (1 U/mL) should be infused through it to maintain patency.

Interpretation

LAP normal values range from to 4 to 10 mmHg. In the healthy heart with normal RV function, the LAP is usually 1 to 2 mm Hg higher than RA pressure. Values for LAP are often elevated in postoperative patients (8-10 mm Hg). Table 66-1 shows variations in LAP seen in different conditions.

Similar to RA pressure, LA waveform analysis can be helpful (Figure 66-1). The *a* wave represents the atrial contraction (coincides with the p wave in ECG). The *c* wave represents the AV valve propulsion toward the atria with ventricular contraction (coincides with the QRS in ECG). The *x'* descent relates to the descent of the AV valve

PART V. LINES, TUBES AND MONITORS

Table 66-1. Changes in LAP in different conditions.

Lesion	CVP
Mitral stenosis or regurgitation	↑
Cardiogenic pulmonary edema	↑
LV dysfunction	↑
LV hypertrophy	↑
Left-to-right shunt	↑
Tachyarrhythmias	↑
Volume overload	↑
Tamponade	↑
Hypovolemia	↓
Pulmonary hypertension	↓
Permeability pulmonary edema	N
Artifact	↑ or ↓

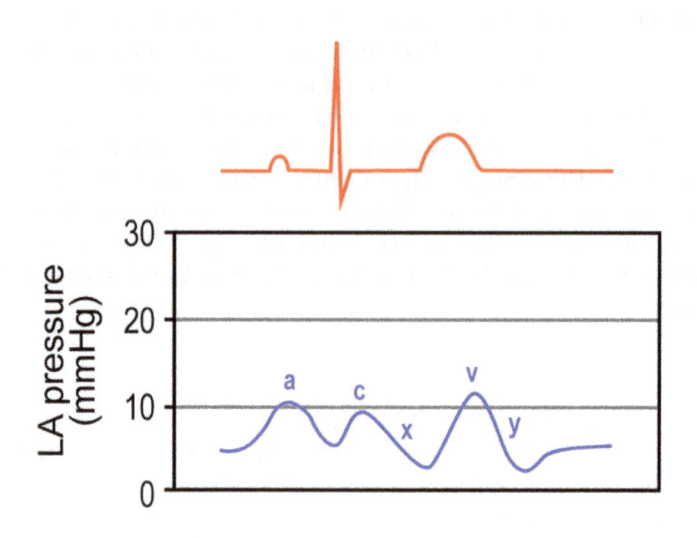

Figure 66-1. Left atrial pressure tracing (see text for details).

at end-ventricular contraction. The v wave represents atrial filling (end of the T wave on ECG). The y descent shows the AV valve opening and ventricular diastole.

Removal

Removal of the LA line is performed in the CICU by the surgical NPs. Due to the possibility of bleeding and emergent intervention, patients are kept NPO for 4-6 hours and the removal is only performed while there is a CVOR surgical team in house. Heparin must be turned off 4-6 hours prior to removal. PRBCs are made available at the bedside and platelet count and coagulation parameters are measured prior to removal. If the platelet count is <50,000-100,000 /mcL, a platelet transfusion may be indicated before removal (after discussion with the surgical attending).

The securing stitches are removed and the line is slowly pulled out in increments until a slight snap indicates that the line has been dislodged from the appendage. The line is then removed. Once the line is removed, if there is some bleeding through the tunnel, the area is dabbed with a gauze until the bleeding stops. No pressure is applied due to the risk of retaining blood in the mediastinum and causing tamponade. If the bleeding is significant, doesn't slow down, or there are hemodynamic changes, emergent intervention is indicated.

Most patients with LA lines will still have a mediastinal chest tube in place. This tube should be patent and the output monitored before and after line removal. Changes in the amount or type of drainage should be reported to the physician team immediately. Vital signs are monitored closely after removal: every 15 min for a minimum of 1 hour and then per unit policy. PRBCs should be kept at the bedside for at least one hour after removal.

67 Chest Tubes

Ziyad M. Binsalamah, Amy G. Hemingway, Miranda A. Rodrigues

Chest tubes are used to drain the pericardial and pleural spaces of air, blood, or fluid, and allow for expansion of the lungs. They are inserted in the OR at the end of surgery, the procedure room, or at the bedside in the CICU. Patients in the ICU may also require chest tubes to be inserted at the bedside under the supervision of the CICU team. Patients located in the acute care areas requiring chest tube placement will either be transferred to the CICU or to the procedure room with CV anesthesia for the procedure.

General Considerations

The chest-tube system is composed of two parts: chest tube and the container system (Atrium™).

There are 4 different types of chest tubes used at TCH (Figure 67-1):

- **Pigtails** (Fuhrman Pleural Drainage Set, Cook Medical, Bloomington, IN, USA): available in 3 sizes (5 Fr, 8.5 Fr, and 12 Fr)
- **Blake™ drains** (Ethicon, Somerville, NJ, USA): available in different sizes (10 Fr, 15 Fr, 19 Fr, and 24 Fr)
- **Yellow rubber drains** (Bard Urethral catheters, Covington, GA, USA): available in 2 sizes (12 Fr and 14 Fr)
- **Argyle™ chest tubes** that are used in the operating room (PVC Thoracic Catheters, Atrium Medical, Hudson, NH, USA) or inserted at the bedside (Thal-Quick Chest Tube, Cook Medical, Bloomington, IN, USA): available in different sizes from 12 Fr to 36Fr

Blake™ drains can be connected to either an Atrium™ or a plastic bulb, while pigtails, yellow rubber drains, and Argyle™ tubes can only be connected to the Atrium™.

The Atrium™ (Figure 67-2) is composed of 3 chambers:

- **Drainage collection chamber**: collects the fluid drained from the pleural or mediastinal space.
- **Water-seal chamber** (filled with sterile water to 2 cm): avoids air from entering the pleural/mediastinal space.
- **Suction-control chamber:** the level of suction depends on the level of water in the system (5, 10, 15, or 20 cmH_2O) and *not the external suction source* unless there is no built-in regulator into the chest-tube system. Increasing suction beyond gentle bubbling will not increase the suction pressure but will increase the rate of evaporation.

Insertion Technique

The insertion a chest tube during surgery is done under direct visualization with the chest open. Insertion of a chest tube outside the OR requires certain equipment to be available:

- Chest tube set
- Atrium™
- Suction source and tubing
- 1% lidocaine

67. CHEST TUBES

- 20 mL syringe
- No. 11 blade
- Silk suture
- Needle driver
- Sterile towels

The 2 types of chest tubes that can be inserted at the beside are pigtails and Argyle™ chest tubes. The CICU prefers placing pigtails as they are easy to insert and less painful than the Argyle™ chest tubes. However, the largest pigtail available is a 12 Fr. In general, the chest tube size commonly used in patients based on weight is:
- <2.5 kg: 5 Fr pigtail
- >2.5 kg and <40 kg: 8.5 Fr pigtails
- >40 kg: 12 Fr pigtail or 14 Fr Argyle™ chest tube (bigger sizes may be used for larger patients).

If there is a suspicion of hemothorax, a larger chest tube may be required.

The steps for chest tube insertion are:
1. Obtain informed consent from the parents.
2. Gather all the necessary equipment (see above) and prepare the Atrium™.
3. Confirm the side for insertion by displaying the latest CXR.
4. Time-out with all personnel (as per TCH protocol).
5. Position the patient in a way that the affected side is slightly elevated. The arm on the affected side should be abducted, externally rotated, and secured to the bed.
6. The affected side is prepped and draped (from medial to the nipple, to beyond the posterior axillary line).
7. Locate the fifth intercostal space (usually the space below the nipple line in children) and identify the corresponding site at the anterior axillary line (be sure to avoid breast tissue).
8. Infiltrate the skin, subcutaneous tissue, periosteum, and pleura with 1% lidocaine. It is useful to use the anesthetic needle to enter the pleural space and confirm that air or fluid is present. Remember that the intercostal neurovascular bundle travels below each rib so the insertion should be aimed to just above the underlying rib.
9. Make a 2 mm skin incision using the No. 11 blade.
10. Using the Seldinger technique (needle, guidewire, dilator, chest tube), insert the pigtail above the rib. Pigtails do not have marks; make sure that you measure the pigtail and decide how far to insert it beforehand.
11. Connect the pigtail to the Atrium™ and secure it to the skin using a silk suture.
12. Perform a CXR to confirm proper positioning of the chest tube.

Assessment and Management

Chest-tube patency is maintained by stripping the tube every 15 minutes for one hour after surgery, then every hour while in the CICU, and every 4 hours while on acute care floors. The chest tube unit and all tubing should be below the patient's chest level to facilitate drainage. Tubing should have no kinks or obstructions that may inhibit drainage and should be anchored to the patient's skin to prevent dislodgement of the

PART V. LINES, TUBES AND MONITORS

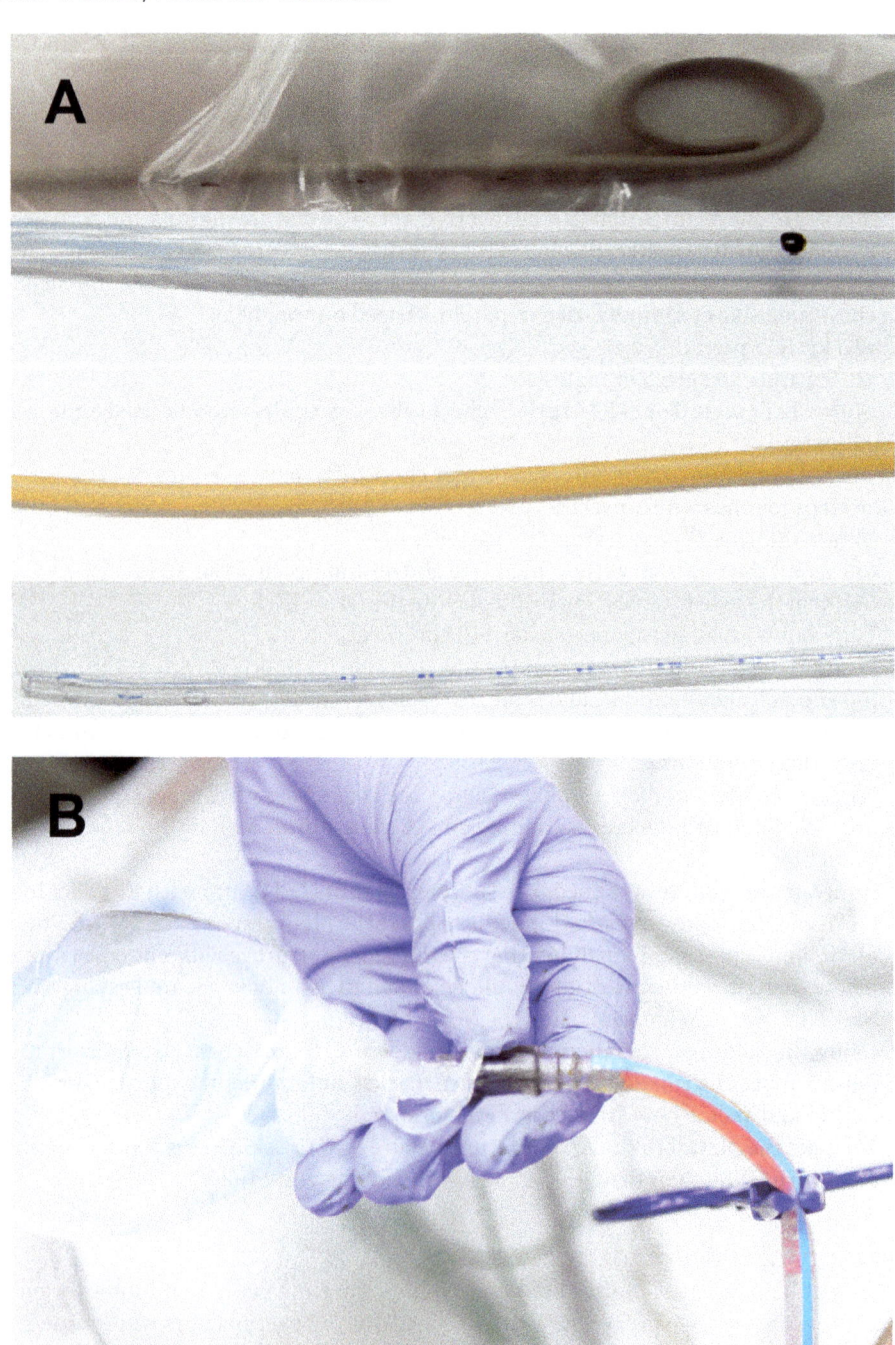

Figure 67-1. A) Types of chest tubes in descending order: pigtail, Blake™ drain, yellow rubber tube, and Argyle™ chest tube. B) Blake™ drain connected to a bulb.

67. CHEST TUBES

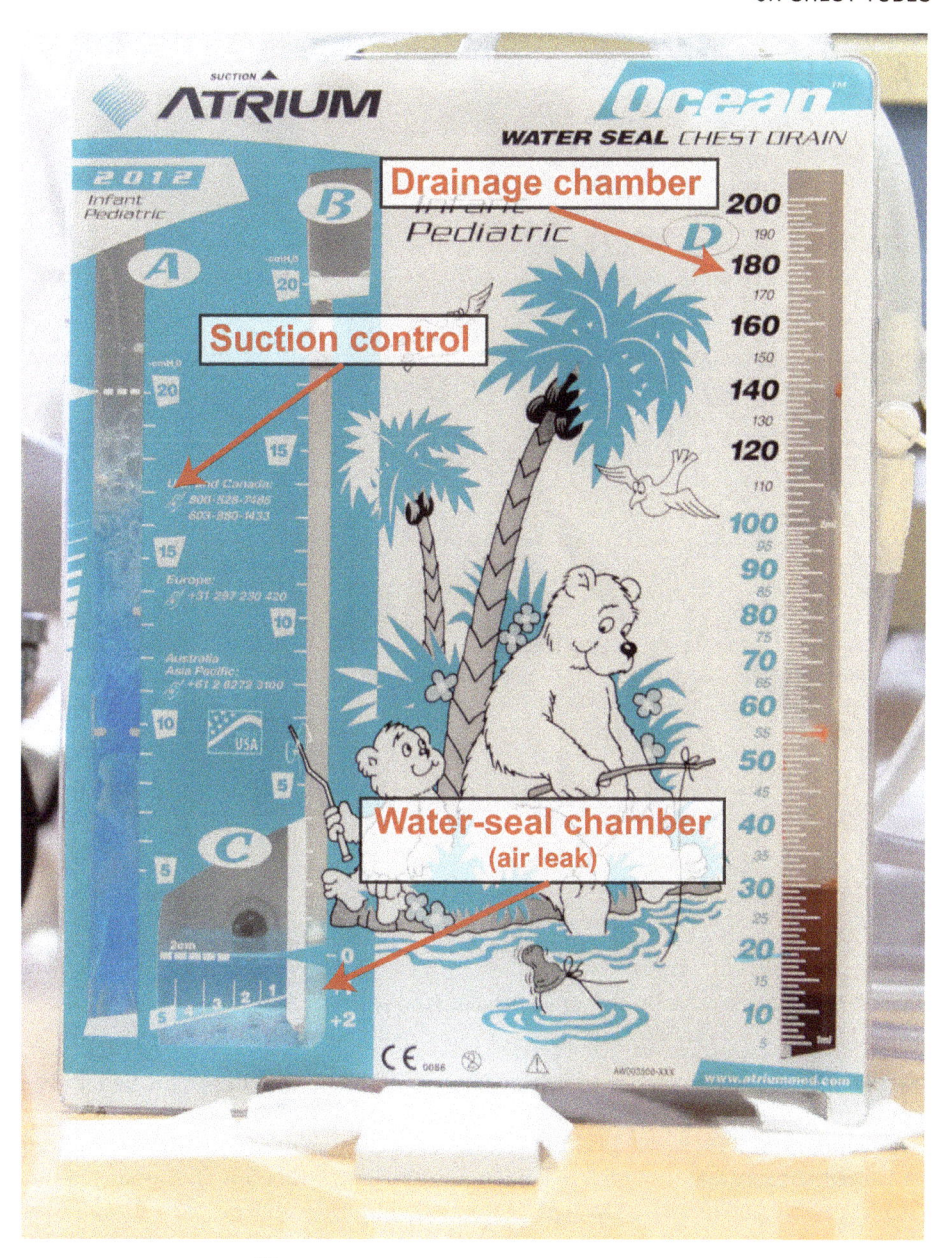

Figure 67-2. The Atrium™ and its components.

PART V. LINES, TUBES AND MONITORS

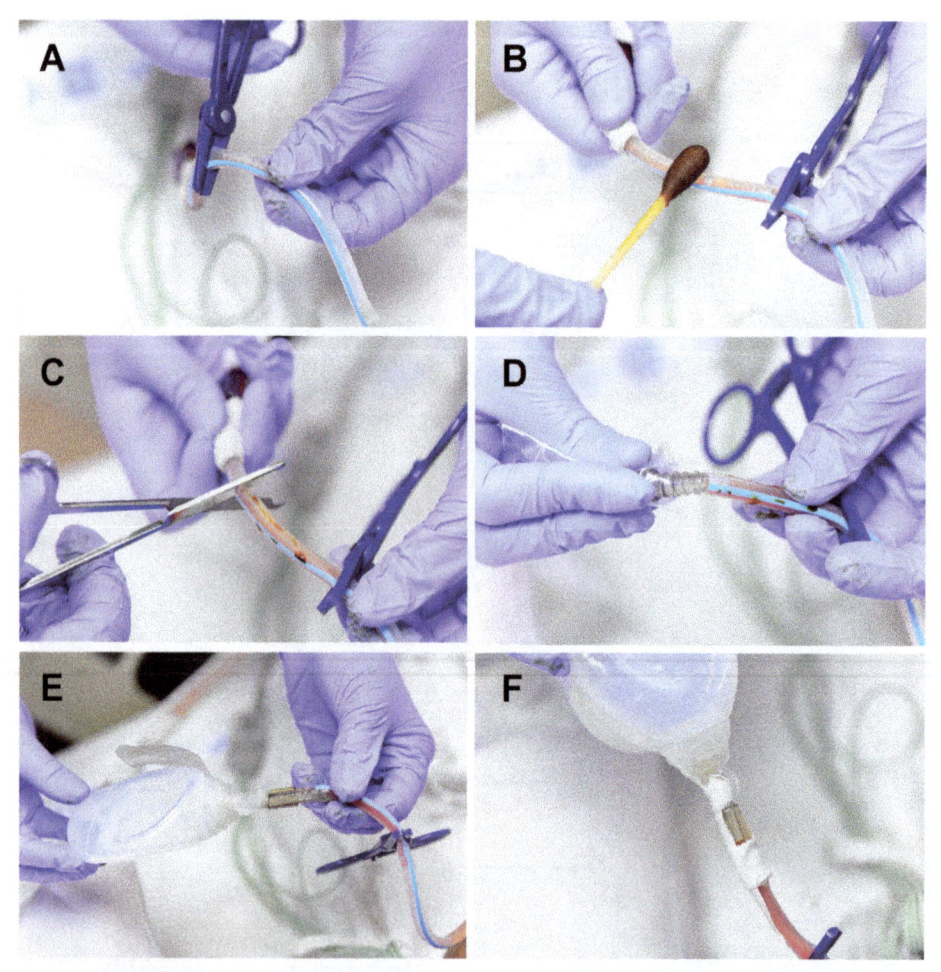

Figure 67-3. Steps to put a Blake™ drain to bulb (see text).

drain. The unit must be securely positioned on its stand or hanging on the bed. Bulbs should be secured to the patient's clothing.

The amount of fluid in the drainage chamber is documented every hour. Medical staff should be notified if there is a sudden increase in the amount of drainage, if the output is >2 mL/kg/hr, there is a significant acute decrease in chest tube output, or if there are any changes in the color or type of the drainage. The chest tube site should be assessed and the dressing should be changed every day or as needed. Blake™ drains have a black dot that should be at the skin level. Argyle™ tubes have a centimeter mark at the skin. This should be documented daily to verify tube position.

Sometimes, if the drainage of the chest tube is not significant and there is no pneumothorax, a Blake™ chest tube may be connected to a bulb instead of an Atrium™. To connect to a bulb, follow these steps (Figure 67-3):

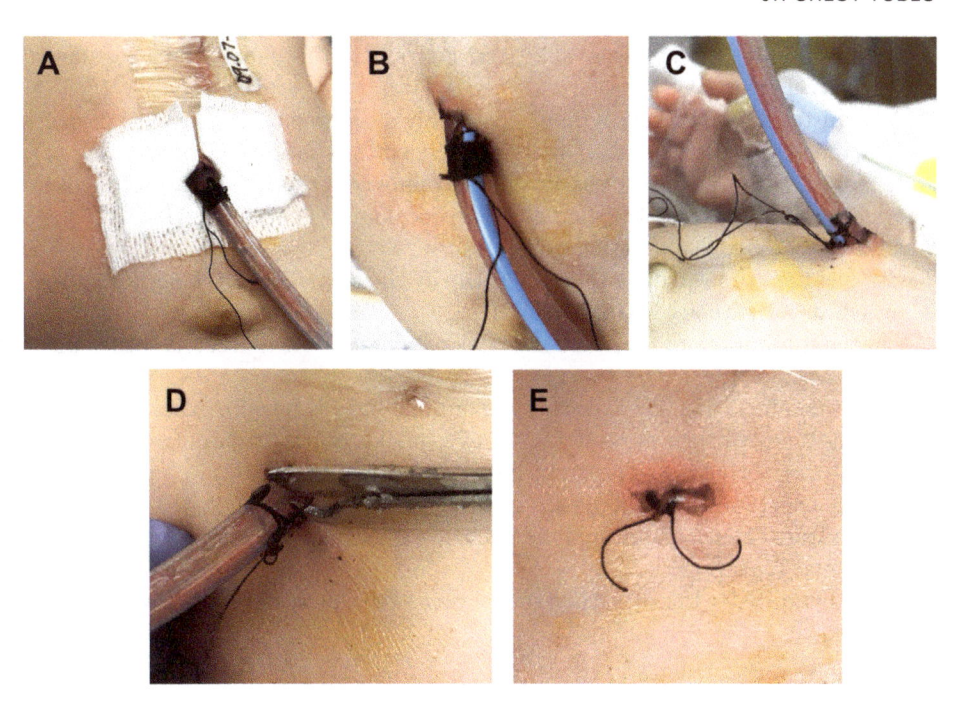

Figure 67-4. Steps for chest tube removal (see text).

1. Gather the necessary supplies (plastic clamps, Betadine® swabs, suture-removal kit, connector for the bulb, plastic bulb, tape).
2. Clamp the tube a few centimeters close to its end (Panel A).
3. Clean the tube distal to the clamp with a Betadine® swab (Panel B).
4. Using sterile scissors from a suture removal kit, divide the tube at the clean site (Panel C).
5. Insert the connector for the bulb (Panel D).
6. Insert the bulb into the connector, apply pressure to the bulb, and while holding the pressure, close the bulb to keep the suction applied (Panel E).
7. Apply tape to secure the bulb in place (Panel F).
8. Remove the clamp.

Chest-Tube Removal

Once the patient does not need the chest tube anymore (see Chapters 78 and 80 for guidelines used in chest tube removal), the chest tube is removed. The patient does not need to be NPO before chest tube removal. The steps for chest tube removal (Figure 67-4) are:

1. Confirm that the chest tube is ready to be removed, including review of the most recent CXR.

2. Gather supplies: suture removal kit, 2x2 gauze, Vaseline gauze, and a Tegaderm occlusive dressing.
3. Administer pain medication (most commonly morphine 0.1 mg/kg/dose prior to tube removal; if no IV access, Hycet or equivalent can be administered).
4. Remove dressing (avoid the use of adhesive remover as this will make it difficult to apply an occlusive dressing should that be necessary) (Panels A and B)
5. Take the chest tube off suction .
6. Unravel the purse string suture and identify the stay suture (triangular suture attaching chest tube to skin) (Panel C).
7. Cut the stay suture and then use the hook of your scissors to free the suture from the skin (Panel D).
8. Once the tube is free, try to coordinate pulling of the tube with exhalation while keeping tension on the purse string sutures; quickly pull the tube out and tie down the suture to bring the edges of the insertion site together (Panel E).
9. Obtain a portable stat CXR to exclude a pneumothorax.
10. If the suture does not hold, apply an occlusive dressing with Vaseline gauze, a 2x2 gauze and Tegaderm™.
11. Apply Betadine® to the chest tube suture twice a day (unless an occlusive dressing is in place).

68 Peritoneal Dialysis

Ziyad M. Binsalamah, Ayse Akcan-Arikan, Heather A. Dickerson

Acute kidney injury (AKI) is a well-known complication after CHS. Risk factors that may have an influence on the development of AKI postoperatively include younger age (particularly neonates), CPB duration, cross-clamp time, the use of circulatory arrest, and LCOS. It is not uncommon for patients with severe AKI to require renal replacement therapy (RRT) postoperatively; the modality of choice usually depends on the patient's age. For patients <4 years of age, our preference is to use peritoneal dialysis (PD) as a mean for RRT.

In addition, at TCH, PD catheters are routinely placed and often used for maintenance of fluid balance in most complex neonatal (and some infant) cardiac procedures. Low-volume continuous manual PD is generally safe and achieves fluid removal without compromising the limited vascular access in children. The use of PD delays the use of diuretics in these patients that may have compromised renal function and lessens the electrolyte disturbances seen with the use of diuretics. By improving the acid-base derangements and fluid removal, it may also improve hemodynamics by decreasing inotropic support and filling pressures.

General Considerations

In general, most neonates and some young infants (<6 months of age) who undergo open heart surgery with the use of CPB will have a temporary PD catheter placed to aid in the immediate postoperative fluid management as we try to avoid the use of diuretics in the first 24 hours postoperatively. Older infants (>6 months of age) who undergo complex heart surgieries (unifocalization, Rastelli procedure, repair of combined tetralogy of Fallot and AV septal defect) may also have a PD catheter placed intraoperatively at the discretion of the surgeon.

Insertion Technique

For PD at TCH, we place the straight temporary Tenckhoff catheter (Argyle™, Covidien, Mansfield, MA, USA) (Figure 68-1). The catheter is available in 4 lengths: 31 cm (used for patients <2.5 kg), 37 cm (for patients >2.5 kg and <6 kg), and 41 and 46 cm (for larger children).

The PD catheter is inserted at the end of the surgery, after assuring hemostasis and just before closing the sternum. A transverse midline supraumbilical incision is made. Two simple silk sutures are placed at each end of the incision to fix the catheter to the skin. Two additional silk sutures are placed as vertical mattress sutures within the skin incision. Those sutures will later be used after removing the PD catheter to close the skin incision. The peritoneum is accessed through the median sternotomy incision just above the diaphragm and a small opening is created using electrocautery. A small right-angled instrument is used to perforate the abdominal fascia just underneath the previously placed supraumbilical incision. The PD catheter is then placed in the abdominal cavity under direct vision. The optimal course of the catheter is when

PART V. LINES, TUBES AND MONITORS

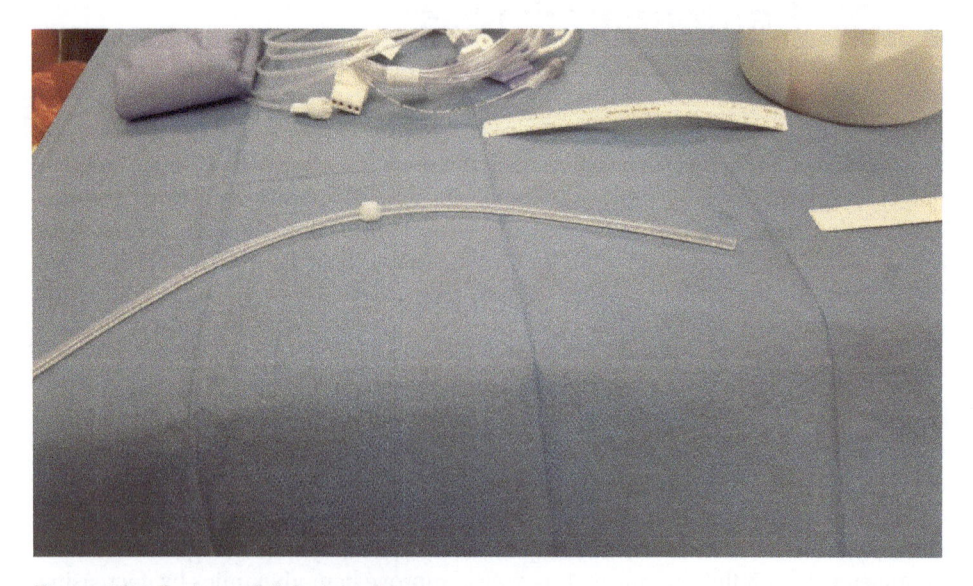

Figure 68-1. Peritoneal dialysis catheter.

the tip faces the left or right lower abdominal quadrants (LLQ or RLQ), the so-called "gutter" (Figure 68-2).

In some situations, a PD catheter may need to be placed postoperatively. In this case, the sternotomy is not reopened, but rather, a longitudinal sub- or supraumbilical incision is performed, the fascia is opened with electrocautery, and the PD catheter is inserted over a metal stylet and directed to the LLQ. A pursestring is placed in the fascia using a Vicryl suture to prevent leaking of the peritoneal fluid around the catheter. This type of catheter is referred to as a surgical PD as it is performed at the bedside with the aid of the OR team. The fascia needs to be closed with a suture after removing the PD, whereas for those PD catheters placed intraoperatively, the small fascial inicision is left alone.

Management

PD is prescribed by the nephrologists for either early postoperative fluid management (as identified by the surgical and CICU teams) or severe AKI. Low-volume continuous PD (dwell volume of 10 mL/kg) cycled each hour utilizing the Gesco® system is the choice at TCH. The renal acute dialysis nurse is responsible for the setup, which should be changed at 72 hour intervals. Dianeal® 1.5% with routine addition of heparin 200 U/L and potassium chloride 2 mEq/L is the starting prescription. Heparin aids in dissolution of fibrin clots and low potassium avoids the need for IV potassium runs due to dialytic losses. Typical cycles are fast fill (5 minutes) and drain (10 minutes) with 45-minute dwells. A Buretrol® infusion device is used for accurate measurement of dwell volumes. A warming blanket is utilized as an external warming device as part of the Gesco® setup to avoid temperature swings. If more aggressive ultrafiltration is desired, the glucose concentration of the dialysate can be carefully increased using commercially available Dianeal® solutions with the nephrologists' order (dialysate solution concentration ranges

68. PERITONEAL DIALYSIS

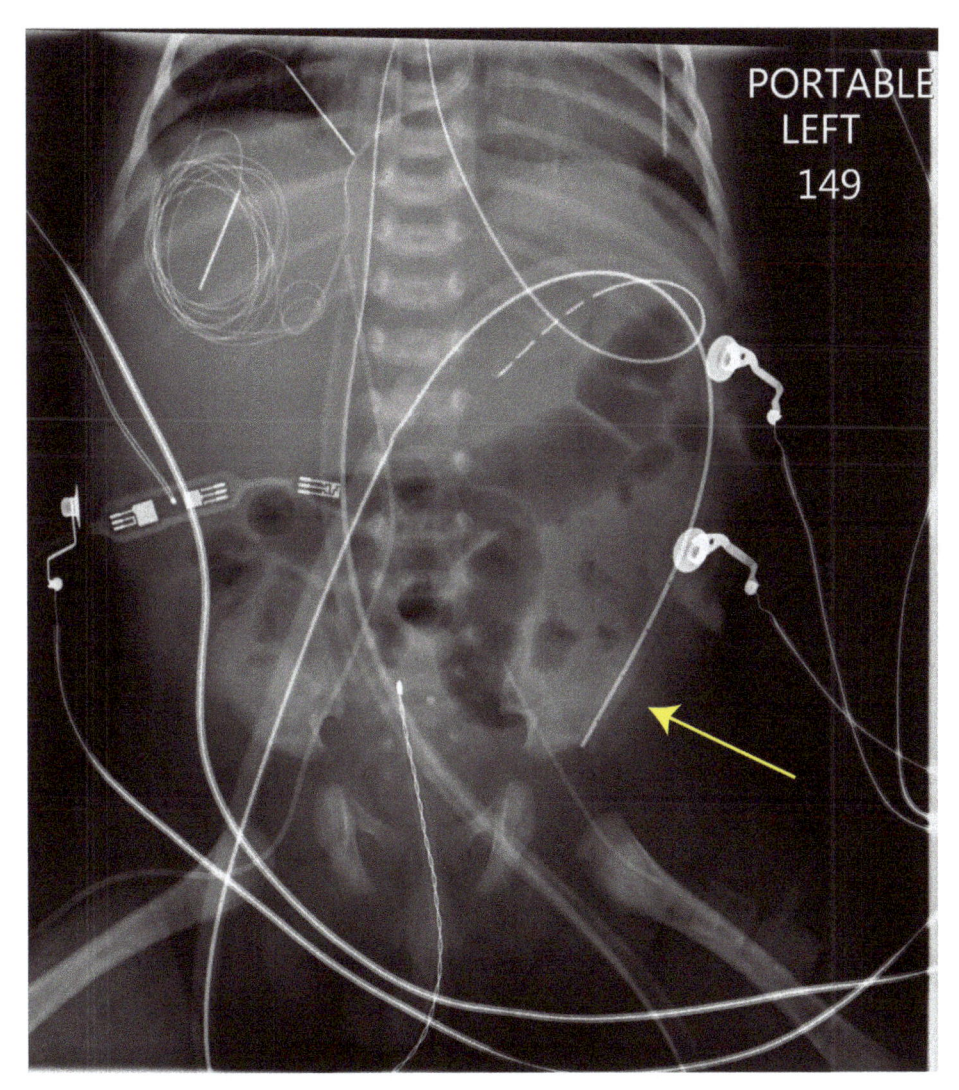

Figure 68-2. Ideal position of a peritoneal dialysis catheter.

from 1.5% to 4.5%). Ensuring a serum albumin concentration above 2.5 g/dL usually assists with fluid removal in selected patients.

Malfunctioning of the PD catheter in the form of fluid retention can be seen and position changes might help with drainage. In some cases, malfunction is due to omental entrapment and usually requires replacement of the catheter at the bedside by the surgical team. Replacement of the catheter is performed under sterile conditions by removing the old catheter and placing a new one using a metal stylet to guide it to the LLQ. Retention within the first few cycles might be due to relative intravascular depletion following intraoperative ultrafiltration during CPB and might require PD to be put on hold until the intravascular volume is restored.

Other complications related to PD include an intrathoracic communication between the peritoneum and the mediastinum, leading to leakage of peritoneal fluid through the chest tubes. If there is a suspicion, the chest tube drainage may be checked for glucose and if positive, the PD catheter should be placed to drain. Leakage at the exit site of the PD may increase the risk of infection and may require to put the PD on hold for 24 hours. Although very rare, whenever the PD effluent appears cloudy, it should be sent for cell count and culture to rule out PD-related peritonitis. Withdrawal of fluid for culture should be done by the dialysis nurses.

PD-Catheter Removal
Once the patient's postoperative status is stable (usually after 24-48 hours postoperatively), the patient may be given furosemide to encourage diuresis. If there is adequate urine output or when patients with AKI have recovered renal function, the PD catheter is placed to drain. In general, the PD should be placed to drain for at least 8-12 hours with an output of less than 2 mL/kg/hr before removing it. PD removal is done at the bedside by the surgical team under strict sterile technique and with adequate sedation to prevent omental herniation. The patient is made NPO for a minimum of 4 hours (depending on the type of enteral nutrition) before PD removal. This is particularly important if the patient is already extubated, as the patient may need to be reintubated to reduce the omentum back into the abdominal cavity if it herniates during catheter removal.

69 Near-Infrared Spectroscopy

Nancy S. Ghanayem, Ken Brady, Ronald A. Bronicki

Near-infrared spectroscopy (NIRS) provides a continuous noninvasive assessment of regional hemoglobin oxygen saturation (rSO_2) in the deep tissue beneath the probe. NIRS provides an estimation of the regional oxygen supply-demand relationship, or oxygen economy in the brain. Continuous, real-time changes in rSO_2 reflect changes either in metabolic demand or oxygen supply, the latter being a function of cardiac output, arterial oxygen content, and total and regional vascular resistance.

In order to apply this technology, it is important to have knowledge of normal rSO_2 values in healthy patients, as well as knowledge of baseline and potentially abnormal values in patients with underlying vulnerable physiology. The baseline cerebral rSO_2 values of healthy children and children with acyanotic heart disease are similar to adults, with an arterial saturation (SaO_2) – cerebral rSO_2 difference of approximately 30%. Cerebral and somatic rSO_2 values in healthy neonates with normal SaO_2 have been shown to have an SaO_2 – cerebral rSO_2 difference of 20-25% and an SaO_2 – somatic rSO_2 difference of 10-15%, reflecting higher oxygen extraction across the cerebral bed compared to the renal-somatic bed. Pediatric patients with left-to-right shunts, regardless of whether they have cyanosis or not, have lower baseline cerebral rSO_2, with SaO_2 – cerebral rSO_2 differences of 40% compared to those without left-to-right shunts, regardless of SaO_2.

Several prospective observational studies have evaluated the relationship of multi-site NIRS and mixed-venous oxygen saturation (SvO_2), or indicators of anaerobic metabolism, in infants and children. Cerebral and somatic rSO_2 are loosely related with SvO_2, but more closely related when considered together.

Differences in cerebral and somatic rSO_2 of less than 10% have been shown to predict anaerobic metabolism in infants with hypoplastic left heart syndrome (HLHS). Following the Norwood procedure, somatic rSO_2 <60% and a cerebral-somatic rSO_2 difference approaching zero during the first 48 postoperative hours is associated with predicted biochemical shock, complications, and longer ICU length of stay. Intraoperative and early postoperative cerebral desaturations have also been found to correlate with worse neurodevelopment outcomes in 1-year-old and preschool-aged children.

Intraoperative and postoperative cerebral NIRS monitoring is routine practice within the CVOR and CICU. Two-site NIRS monitoring of cerebral and somatic tissue beds is becoming standard in the CICU in infants and small children. Based on best-available evidence, physiologic targets would include a cerebral NIRS >45% in all patients, but one would expect a SaO_2 – cerebral rSO_2 difference <40% in fully saturated healthy patients. Optimal somatic NIRS is 20% lower than SaO_2 and ideally exceed cerebral NIRS by more than 10%.

70 Feeding Tubes

Patricia Bastero

Feeding tubes are widely used to administer and supplement enteral nutrition.

Indications
- Early enteral nutrition in mechanically-ventilated patients
- Administration of enteral nutrition in patients that cannot eat by mouth (e.g., risk of aspiration)
- Increase and optimize caloric intake in patients not taking enough PO

General Considerations
There are different types of enteric tubes in the market. The tubes that are used for feeding purposes are made out of polyurethane and soften at body temperature. Salem-sump (double-lumen) gastric tubes are made out of hard plastic (polyvinyl chloride, PVC) and are only used for gastric decompression. These should be removed as soon as possible once active decompression is no longer indicated and should not be routinely used for feeding.

Feeding tubes can be placed either *gastric* (nasogastric or orogastric) or *postpyloric* (terminating in the duodenum or the jejunum). Postpyloric tubes are used in patients that suffer from significant GERD, those that are at risk for aspiration due to vocal cord paresis or poor gag and cough reflexes, and patients with pancreatitis.

Gastric feeds can be provided in bolus or continuously. Postpyloric feeds must be run continuously.

Feeding tubes come in different sizes. In general, we use a 5 or 6 Fr tube for neonates, a 6 or 8 Fr tube for children, and a 10 or 12 Fr tube for adolescents and adults.

Feeding tubes can also be surgically placed (e.g., gastrostomy) in those patients expected to have long-term difficulties with optimal PO feeding (see Chapter 58).

Insertion Technique
Feeding tubes can be inserted either orally or nasally. Nasal insertion is more comfortable for patients. However, nasal placement can interfere with noninvasive positive mechanical ventilation devices, especially in neonates and infants requiring HFNC.

The steps for placement of a feeding tube are:
1. Wash your hands and put on gloves.
2. Position the patient supine with the head of the bed between 15° and 30° of elevation. The face should be centered and the neck slightly flexed.
3. Measure the length from the edge of the mouth (oral) or nares (nasal) to either the tip of the ear lobe and the xiphoid process (gastric), or the ear lobe, xiphoid process, and lateral border of the ribs (postpyloric). Marks can be made on the feeding tube to reflect the different positions.

4. Prebend the tube to reflect the curvature of the inferior aspect of the nasopharnx or oropharynx for nasal and oral tubes, respectively.
5. Apply gel or any water-soluble lubricant to the tip of the tube to facilitate its insertion and minimize the risk of trauma.
6. For orally inserted tubes, a tongue depressor might be useful.
7. Insertion of the tube:
- **Gastric tubes:**
  - Insert the tube and stop at the distance measured earlier.
  - Place the stethoscope on the stomach area, push air with a syringe, and listen for that air entering the stomach.
  - Good position should be verified by hearing the rush of air, followed by confirmation with a CXR.
  - Take the wire out (if present) and tape the tube to the patient's face.
  - For older patients, it is helpful to ask them to swallow while placing the tube.
- **Postpyloric tubes:**
  - These tubes can be placed at the bedside using a "blind" technique, or the Cortrak® guide, or can be placed under fluoroscopy in the IR suite.
  - If possible, put the patient on right lateral decubitus.
  - Introduce the feeding tube slowly. Once you have passed the gastric mark, start instilling air with a syringe. The tube is close to the pylorus when the air is heard on the right upper quadrant. Continue to slowly advance the tube while instilling air (5-10 mL). Once the tube reaches the duodenum, the rush of air heard on the abdomen changes to a higher tone and it is not possible to aspirate the total amount of air introduced.
  - Position can be confirmed by obtaining a sample from the tube with an alkaline pH. Position must be confirmed with a CXR as well.
  - Take the wire out and tape the tube to the patient's face.
  - The use of 0.1 mg/kg of IV metoclopramide 10 minutes before inserting the postpyloric tube might help with gastric motility and tube placement.

VI. Postoperative Scenarios

71 Low Cardiac Output Syndrome

Natasha Afonso, Heather A. Dickerson

Low cardiac output syndrome (LCOS) or state refers to the clincial manifestations of the reduction in cardiac output, usually following CPB. The key to managing LCOS is early identification and rapid management of reversible causes in order to prevent perioperative morbidity and mortality. Generally, LCOS occurs 6-12 hours after CPB.

Diagnosis

The diagnosis is made by the identification of signs and symptoms that reflect decreased oxygen delivery to tissues. Multiple signs and monitoring modalities are available in order to diagnose LCOS and provide timely intervention:
- Tachycardia
- Decreased capillary refill or peripheral perfusion
- Metabolic acidosis
- Elevated (>2 mmol/L) or rising lactate levels
- Increased core-to-toe temperature gradient
- Increased arterial CO_2 to $ETCO_2$ gradient
- Decreased urine output
- Decreased differential between cerebral and somatic rSO_2 by NIRS (see Chapter 69) can be a sign of redistribution of perfusion away from the somatic circulation – an indicator of worsening cardiac output
- Overall decrease in cerebral or somatic rSO_2 (NIRS), or widening of the arterial – central venous saturation difference. The oxygen-extraction ratio (O_2ER) is very helpful as a marker of oxygen delivery (Table 71-1):

$$O_2ER = \text{Oxygen Consumption } (VO_2) / \text{Oxygen Delivery } (DO_2)$$

$$= (SaO_2 - SvO_2) / SaO_2$$

Hypotension may be seen with LCOS although it is a late finding given the ability of most children to compensate for their shock state by increasing their SVR. Additional monitoring via intra-atrial lines can provide important information and feedback regarding causes and response to interventions. A postoperative patient requires diligent monitoring and frequent reassessment as data trends can be very informative. It

Table 71-1. Interpretation of mixed-venous saturation and oxygen-extraction ratio.

SvO_2	O_2ER	Interpretation
>75%	<25%	Normal
50 to 75%	25 to 50%	Increased extraction
25 to 50%	50 to 75%	Increased lactate, cellular dysfunction
<25%	>75%	Shock, cell death

O_2ER: oxygen-extraction ratio, SvO_2: mixed-venous oxygen saturation.

71. LOW CARDIAC OUTPUT SYNDROME

Table 71-2. Strategies for diagnosis and treatment of LCOS.

CVP/RAP	LAP	Transpulmonary gradient	Etiology	Treatment
Decreased	Decreased	Normal	Hypovolemia	Give volume
Increased	Normal	Increased	Increased PVR	Ventilation, O_2, iNO, sedation/neuromuscular blockade
Increased	Increased	Normal	Ventricular dysfunction AVVR Tamponade/PCE Lack of AV synchrony	Inotropes Afterload reduction Drainage of PCE Pacing

AV: atrioventricular, AVVR: atrioventricular valve regurgitation, CVP: central venous pressure, iNO: inhaled nitric oxide, LAP: left atrial pressure, PCE: pericardial effusion, PVR: pulmonary vascular resistance, RAP: right atrial pressure.

is important to also consider if additional monitoring methods (e.g., PiCCO® catheter) are needed to help in the early identification and management of LCOS. An echocardiogram is helpful to assess cardiac function, AV valve regurgitation, pericardial effusion (PCE), and assess for any residual defects. Late findings of LCOS include an increase in creatinine, elevation in liver enzymes, and other signs of poor tissue perfusion, and ultimately - shock and cardiac arrest. Table 71-2 provides an overview of diagnosis and management of LCOS.

Management
The goal in treating a patient with LCOS is to optimize systemic oxygen delivery through careful interventions in order to improve the relationship between oxygen supply and demand. Important goals in the management of LCOS are to:
- **Optimize preload.** Preload can be inadequate due to blood loss, fluid shifts related to CPB or changes in ventricular compliance. If hypovolemic, volume replacement should occur with 5% albumin or normal saline boluses. Judicious aliquots of fluid (5-10 mL/kg) should be used and the physiologic response assessed after each bolus. The lack of a response suggests that additional volume can cause harm by increasing filling pressures and increasing oxygen demand.
- **Optimize hemoglobin.** If bleeding, replace blood products as necessary to normalize coagulation factors and replace lost blood volume. Monitor chest-tube output closely. While replacing volume, it is imperative to closely monitor filling pressures.
- **Increasing systolic function using inotropic support.** Milrinone and epinephrine can help support cardiac output by increasing contractility. Exercise caution with milrinone in patients with renal injury as accumulation of milrinone can occur and cause hypotension. Epinephrine also can increase myocardial oxygen demand and increase the propensity for tachyarrhythmias. Calcium is especially important in neonatal hearts since they are dependent on extracellular calcium for

contractility, but levels should not be driven to supraphysiologic values as this can cause significant harm and ultimately, myocardial necrosis. Remember to assess for hypocalcemia in patients with DiGeorge syndrome, on amiodarone, and after blood transfusions as the citrate in blood products can bind calcium and cause hypocalcemia.
- **Control afterload.** Milrinone has the added benefit of reducing both SVR and PVR. If SVR is elevated, the patient may require nitroprusside or nicardipine as additional vasodilators to improve perfusion and oxygen delivery. In contrast, if SVR is low and the patient is vasoplegic, vasopressin, norepinephrine, or phenylepinephrine can be used to increase SVR. However, in patients with impaired ventricular function, increasing SVR can reduce cardiac output.
- **Consider adrenal and/or thyroid** dysfunction in persistent hypotension refractory to catecholamines. For adrenal insufficiency, start hydrocortisone 100 mg/m^2/day divided every 6 hours. It can be helpful to send a cortisol-stimulation test first or a random cortisol level if time permits though even patients with "adequate" levels often respond to hydrocortisone dosing with improved hemodynamics. For thyroid dysfunction, a triiodothyronine (T3) infusion can be started (general dosing: 0.05-0.15 mcg/kg/hr).
- **Positive pressure ventilation.** Full ventilator support may be necessary to reduce the workload of the respiratory muscles and improve cardiac output. This strategy can be especially helpful in patients with decreased LV function. Care is taken to avoid overdistension/ventilation with increased tidal volumes as this can impede RV output and/or increase PVR. Goal ventilation is at functional residual capacity.
- **Sedation and pain control to minimize oxygen demand** and avoid patient agitation or asynchrony with the ventilator. Neuromuscular blockade can also be used in this setting.
- **Assess for cardiac tamponade.** PCEs can be seen after cardiac surgery and require immediate recognition and management. Hemodynamic changes with cardiac tamponade are usually associated with an elevation in the right- and left-ventricular filling pressures due to external compression. A significant PCE should be considered in a patient with a chest tube with rapidly diminishing drainage and progressively low cardiac output. Immediate attempts should be made to strip the chest tube, provide volume to overcome the tamponade effect, and if necessary, surgical exploration and drainage. An echocardiogram can be helpful in making the diagnosis and should not only evaluate for circumferential but also localized effusions as these can also compromise filling and cardiac output.
- **Ensure AV synchrony.** Ensure that the patient is in sinus rhythm to maximize cardiac output. The patient may require atrial pacing for junctional bradycardia or to overdrive-pace JET if needed to support hemodynamics.
- **Consider reopening the chest** to allow for better filling and cardiac output. Remember that tamponade physiology can occur secondary to edema of the myocardium without significant effusion.
- **Consider mechanical circulatory support** in extreme circumstances if medical treatment strategies are not successful in managing the LCOS state.

72 Cardiopulmonary Arrest

Aarti Bavare, Patricia Bastero, Iki Adachi

Cardiac arrest is a pathologic state characterized by loss of effective circulation. Return of spontaneous circulation and survival after in-hospital cardiac arrest varies considerably (0-60%). The outcomes are dependent on the cause of arrest and treatment provided during and after the arrest. Morbidity, especially neurologic sequelae, are frequent in survivors. Cardiac arrest occurs due to impaired myocardial performance resulting in a nonperfusing rhythm, whether it is pulseless electrical activity, asystole, ventricular tachycardia, or ventricular fibrillation. Usually, the preceding conditions are primary cardiac abnormalities or cardiac compromise due to respiratory, neurologic, or metabolic abnormalities.

Diagnosis

Manifesting signs of cardiac arrest include pulselessness, apnea, and loss of consciousness. If invasive monitoring is available, cardiac arrest can be promptly recognized by loss of the arterial waveform and/or rapid fall in end-tidal CO_2. Continuous monitoring with ECG, ST-segment variability, invasive and noninvasive BP, NIRS, and blood gas analysis are performed for all patients with critical cardiac disease at TCH. In most cases, impending cardiac and/or respiratory collapse can be recognized with these monitoring instruments and appropriate interventions can be performed to prevent cardiac arrest.

Management

Anticipation and Prevention

The vast majority of cardiac arrests in cardiac patients occur in those who are deemed "high-risk". It is rare for patients without significant risk factors to unexpectedly develop cardiac arrest. The high-risk population includes patients with: single-ventricle physiology, particularly shunt-dependent circulation (e.g., after the Norwood operation); coronary insufficiency (e.g., patients with supravalvar aortic stenosis associated with Williams syndrome or posttransplant coronary vasculopathy); pulmonary hypertension; ventricular arrhythmia syndromes; or acute or acute-on-chronic heart failure. Fresh postoperative patients with marginal circulation despite high-dose inotropic support are also at substantial risk for acute decompensation.

The prevalence of cardiac arrest at TCH is 2% of all CICU encounters, which is lower than that reported by other centers to the Pediatric Cardiac Critical Care Consortium (PC4). Certain pragmatic preventive strategies that potentially contribute to lower arrest rates in the CICU at TCH include cohorting of high-acuity patients, high use of noninvasive and invasive monitoring, preparedness with emergency medications at the bedside, and effective multidisciplinary communication. As soon as the first signs of inadequate cardiorespiratory function are discovered, increased monitoring (if not already present) and critical therapies to optimize cardiac function, improve end-organ oxygen delivery, and minimize oxygen consumption are instituted. If the patient is not

PART VI. POSTOPERATIVE SCENARIOS

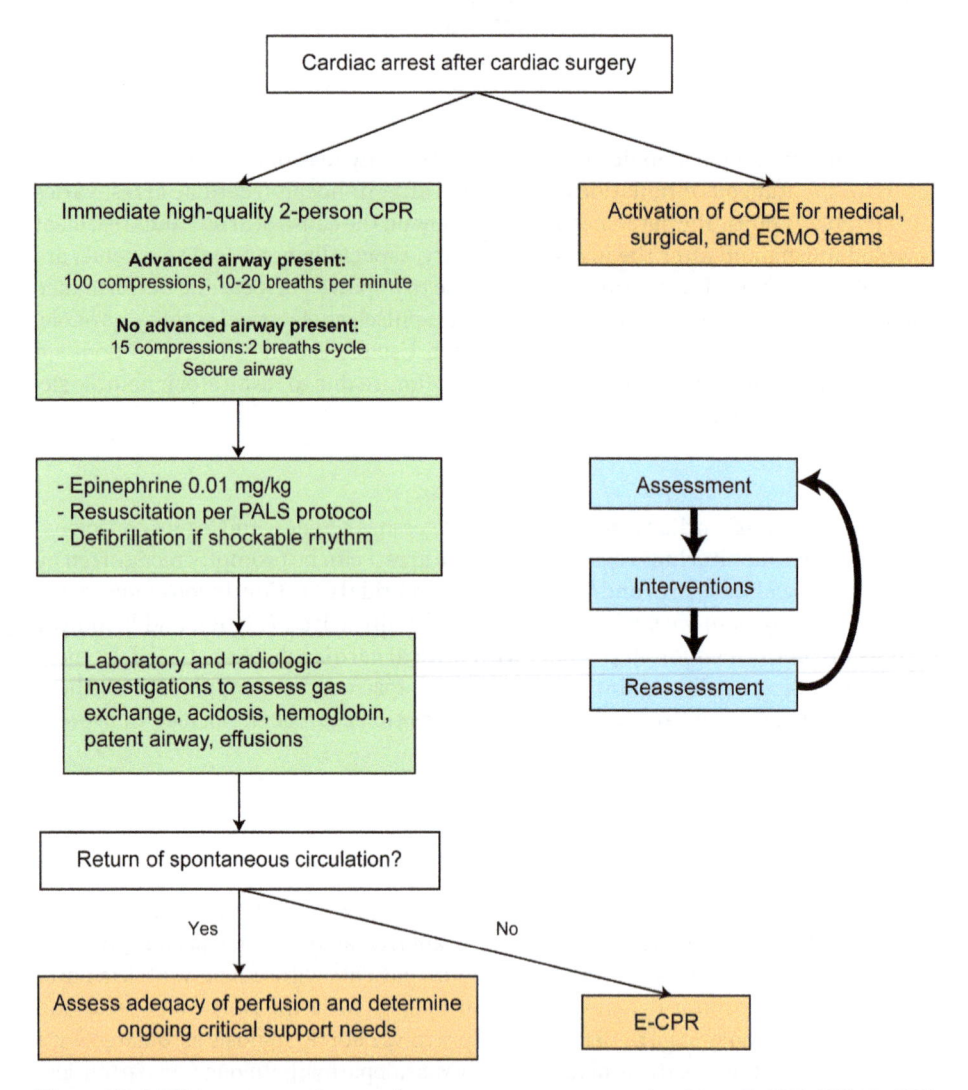

Figure 72-1. TCH postoperative cardiac arrest management algorithm. E-CPR: ECMO-CPR, PALS: Pediatric Advanced Life Support.

in the CICU, a rapid-response or code-response team (critical care nurse, respiratory therapist, and a physician) is activated to initiate critical therapies and facilitate safe transfer to the ICU.

The objective of prevention is to optimize oxygen delivery (DO_2) and diagnose the leading cause for deterioration as soon as possible, in order to initiate specific therapies. In order to improve DO_2, inotropic and ventilatory support are established; oxygen-carrying capacity (hemoglobin levels), preload and SVR are optimized; and oxygen consumption (VO_2) is minimized by controlling temperature, pain, and in

72. CARDIOPULMONARY ARREST

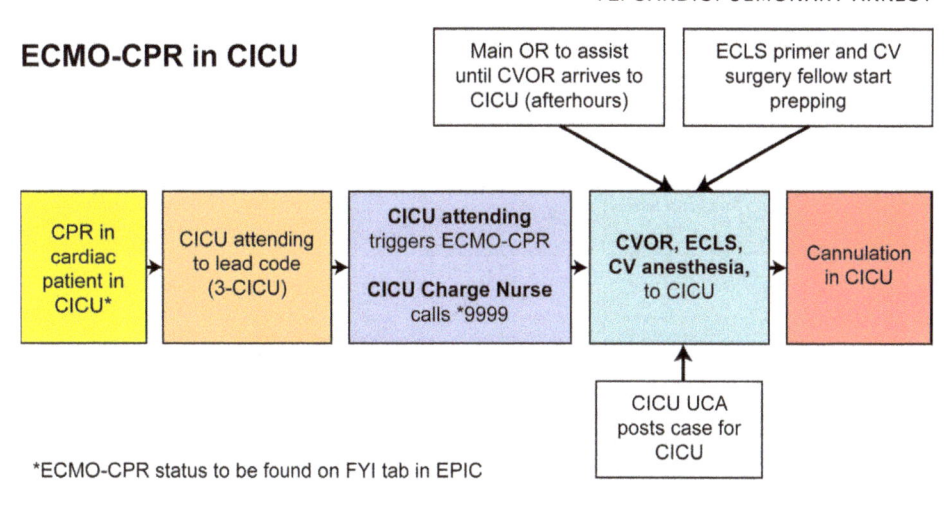

ECMO-CPR in CICU

Figure 72-2. TCH algorithm for ECMO-CPR activation in the CICU. UCA: unit clerk associate.

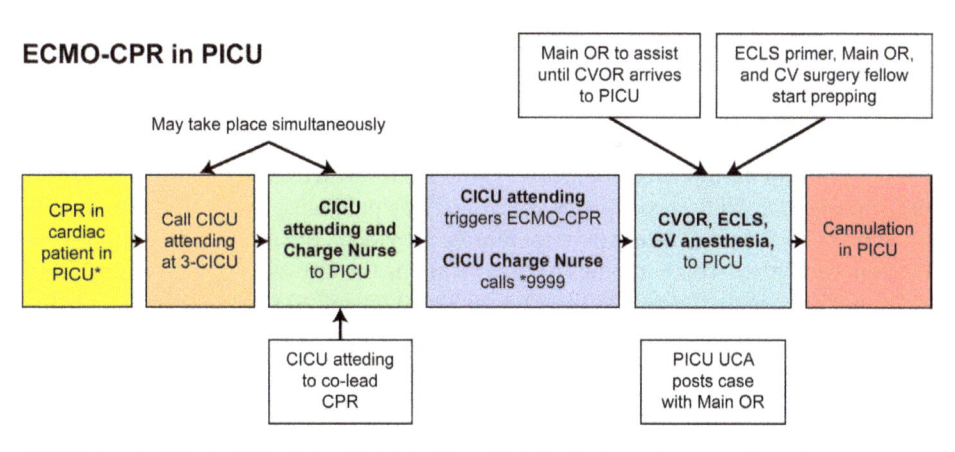

ECMO-CPR in PICU

Figure 72-3. TCH algorithm for ECMO-CPR activation in the PICU. UCA: unit clerk associate.

certain instances, sedating the patient. To guide interventions, central venous and arterial accesses are established, and laboratory tests are obtained (gas exchange, acid-base balance, electrolyte measurements, hematocrit and cell counts, and blood type and cross-match). The respiratory function is assisted by invasive ventilation. Cardiac preload, contractility, and afterload are optimized. Inotropic agents are used to maintain adequate coronary and systemic perfusion. An epinephrine drip and epinephrine "spritzers" (0.1 mg/mL of epinephrine diluted to yield a 0.01 mg/mL "spritzer") are oftentimes used in response to hypotension. The goal of treatment is to maintain adequate *perfusion* (i.e., cardiac output) and not necessarily to maintain a certain BP. Hematocrit and SaO_2 are optimized. Hypoglycemia and/or hypocalcemia are corrected.

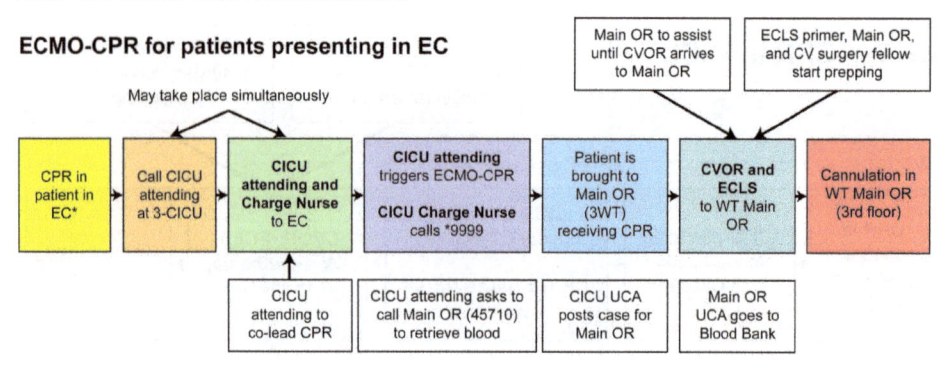

PART VI. POSTOPERATIVE SCENARIOS

ECMO-CPR for patients presenting in EC

Figure 72-4. TCH algorithm for ECMO-CPR activation for patients in the emergency room. EC: emergency center, UCA: unit clerk associate.

In the setting of limited cardiac output, metabolic demands are decreased by fever control, sedation and/or chemical paralysis, parenteral nutrition, etc. to minimize VO_2.

Multidisciplinary communication and regular updates of changes in patients' clinical condition is conducted. Families are kept updated of the clinical course and their input regarding the resuscitation wishes of the patient are solicited.

Resuscitation During Cardiac Arrest

In the event that cardiac arrest ensues or when cardiac arrest is the initial presentation, high-quality CPR according to the guidelines published by the AHA (Pediatric Advanced Life Support, PALS) is immediately provided. The important components that translate into better outcomes include reducing the duration of cardiopulmonary arrest and improving the quality of CPR provided. Figure 72-1 shows the algorithm for management of cardiac arrest in postoperative patients at TCH.

The use of adrenergic agents such as epinephrine produces intense systemic vasoconstriction and elevated aortic diastolic pressures to facilitate coronary and cerebral blood flow during CPR, while redirecting flow away from other organs. Investigations and management are tailored to achieve reversal of cardiac or extracardiac inciting pathologies.

When return of spontaneous circulation (ROSC) is not achieved with medical therapy, or the perfusion is deemed to be inadequate, the ultimate mode of support is venoarterial ECMO, if indicated (see Chapter 43). In general, patients with acute and reversible conditions are ECMO candidates unless otherwise stated, while careful consideration is necessary in those with chronic conditions who may not have a valid "exit" strategy. A preemptive discussion before cardiac arrest regarding ECMO candidacy is important for patients who are deemed "high-risk".

The procedure for activation of ECMO-CPR for patients in the CICU, PICU, and for patients in the emergency room is illustrated on Figure 72-2, Figure 72-3, and Figure 72-4, respectively.

Postcardiac-Arrest Syndrome
Postcardiac-arrest syndrome is a multiorgan disease characterized by organ injury during and after reperfusion. The syndrome is the result of ischemia followed by reperfusion injury. It combines the effects of the primary disease that led to the arrest, myocardial dysfunction, high risk for cerebral injury secondary to microcirculatory insult with neuronal death and apoptosis, and systemic inflammatory response. The longer the hypoperfusion time, the more severe the secondary injuries.

Management After Cardiac Arrest
Postcardiac-arrest management includes invasive monitoring and investigations to ensure optimal gas exchange (aim for normocapnia), resolution of acidosis (prevent hypotension), adequate oxygenation (prevent hyperoxia), nutrient delivery (aim for normoglycemia), and maintain normothermia. At present, there is no evidence to support the use of deliberate hypothermia for inhospital cardiac arrest.

73 Supraventricular Tachycardia

Mubbasheer Ahmed, Caridad M. de la Uz

Supraventricular tachycardia (SVT) is a tachyarrhythmia originating above the ventricular tissue, which requires involvement of the atrium or AV-nodal tissue. It is the most common tachyarrhythmia in the pediatric population, with an incidence of 0.1-0.4%. Most patients present before 2 months of age and approximately 80% have structurally normal hearts. SVT can also complicate the postoperative state of patients after CHS. There are 2 distinct mechanisms that cause SVT:
- **Reentry.** Most common etiology (>90%). It is caused by an electrical circuit within the atrium.
  - Atrial flutter due to reentrant circuit within the atrium
  - AV reentrant tachycardia (AVRT) due to a pre excitation accessory pathway (e.g., Wolff-Parkinson-White syndrome)
  - AV nodal reentrant tachycardia (AVNRT) via a slow pathway within the AV-nodal tissue
- **Automaticity.** Caused by a focus of enhanced automaticity in the heart. Atrial ectopic tachycardia (AET) implies that the focus is within the atrial tissue.

Diagnosis
The presenting symptoms in infants include lethargy, agitation, poor feeding, and pallor. Older children may present with palpitations, chest discomfort, syncope, or difficulty breathing. Postoperative patients that are being monitored will be identified by a change in their ECG.

The ECG findings on SVT include:
- Narrow QRS complex similar to sinus (most common), although antidromic SVT and SVT with a bundle-branch block can present as a wide-QRS tachycardia and may mimic ventricular tachycardia (VT)
- P waves are present, but frequently not visible on ECG as they are often buried in the terminal portion of the QRS
- In reentrant SVT, the onset and termination is abrupt and the rate is minimally variable
- Atrial tachycardia demonstrates a warm-up and cool-down of the rate and may have more R-R variability
- AV ratio is 1:1 (if AV dissociation is noted, this rules out SVT)

Management
For atrial flutter, adenosine may be given for diagnostic purposes, but will not terminate the flutter. Treat with synchronized cardioversion or atrial overdrive pacing or transesophageal pacing.

Unstable reentrant SVT (shock, hypotension, impaired mental status) requires rapid termination of the arrhythmia with synchronized cardioversion starting at 0.5 J/kg.

For stable reentrant SVT, vagal maneuvers and chemical cardioversion can be

73. SUPRAVENTRICULAR TACHYCARDIA

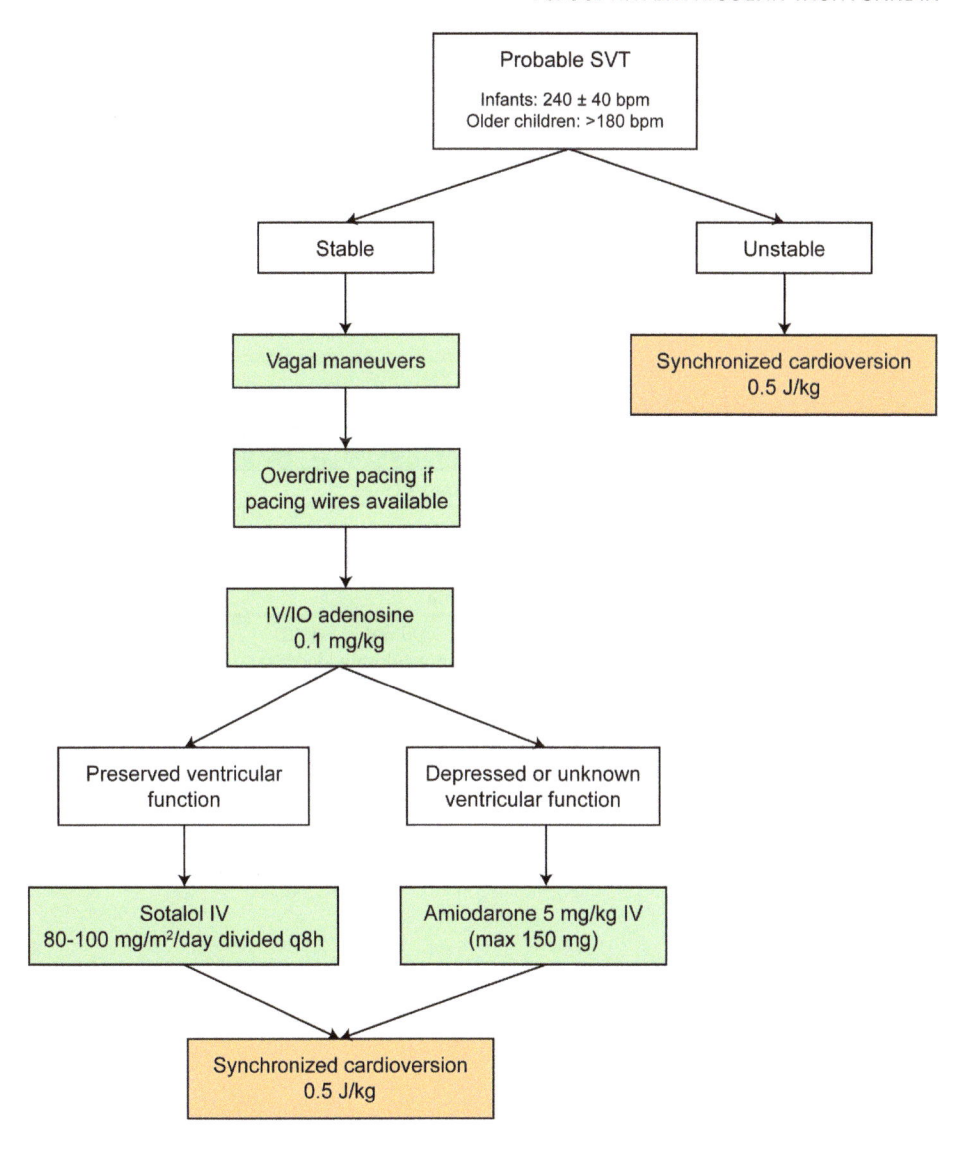

Figure 73-1. Algorithm for management of SVT.

attempted. Reentrant SVT uses the AV node as its anterograde or retrograde limb most of the time and can thus be classified as AV-node dependent. Therapeutic interventions focus on influencing AV-nodal conduction and refractory period, or causing a transient AV-nodal block. Vagal maneuvers cause a delay in AV-nodal conduction. These maneuvers include Valsalva maneuvers (bearing down), blowing in an occluded straw, or ice over the nasal bridge and forehead for approximately 10 seconds. If vagal

475

maneuvers fail, adenosine is the first-line chemical intervention with a success rate >85%. Given the short half-life of adenosine (<2 seconds), a rapid push administration in the most central venous structure is necessary for effectiveness. The initial dose is 0.1 mg/kg followed by 0.2 mg/kg, with a maximum dose of 12 mg. When administering adenosine in postoperative patients, consider what the most direct vascular route to the heart is prior to obtaining access. In heart transplant patients, the denervated heart can respond with prolonged asystole to normal doses of adenosine; lower doses of adenosine must be used.

Figure 73-1 shows the algorithm for treatment of SVT. Table 73-1 lists the medications that can be used for treatment of SVT and their dosages.

Table 73-1. Medications and dosages used for management of SVT.

Drug	Dose
Adenosine (IV/IO)	0.1 – 0.3 mg/kg (max 12 mg)
Amiodarone (IV/PO)	5 mg/kg (max 300 mg)
Digoxin (IV)	Initial 15-30 mcg/kg/day divided TID
Esmolol (IV)	50-300 mcg/kg/min
Flecainide (PO)	Neonates: 2-6 mg/kg/day divided BID Infants: 50-200 mg/m^2/day divided BID
Nadolol (PO)	0.5-1 mg/kg QD
Procainamide (IV)	Load: 10-15 mg/kg over 30-60 min Continuous infusion: 20-80 mcg/kg/min
Propranolol (PO)	1-4 mg/kg/day divided Q6-8H
Sotalol (IV/PO)	PO: 50 mg/m^2/day divided Q8H IV: 80-100 mg/m^2/day divided Q8H

74 Junctional Ectopic Tachycardia

Caridad M. de la Uz, Rocky Tsang, Lara S. Shekerdemian

Junctional ectopic tachycardia (JET) is a tachyarrhythmia arising from abnormal automaticity in the area of the AV junction (AV node/His bundle region), and may cause hemodynamic compromise. It is one of the most common arrhythmias in children, with a reported incidence of up to 8% in patients undergoing cardiac surgery.

JET typically occurs in the immediate postoperative period after congenital heart surgical procedures that involve manipulation of the crux of the heart. Risk factors include: long cross-clamp or bypass time, surgery involving the ventricular septum or significant traction on the heart, need for inotropic support, hypomagnesemia, and young age.

Diagnosis

On ECG, JET presents as a tachyarrhythmia with the QRS morphology being the same as the sinus QRS morphology. The P waves are absent preceding the QRS. One may see retrograde P waves, possibly buried within the terminal portion of the QRS, and AV dissociation with occasional sinus capture beats.

An atrial electrogram performed via temporary pacing wires permits the detection of P waves that are buried within the QRS (Figure 74-1). Hemodynamic monitoring of CVP simultaneously with ECG allows for identification of cannon "a" waves (Figure 74-2), consistent with AV dyssynchrony. These represent an increased pressure in the RA when the RA contracts against a closed tricuspid valve (also seen in ventricular tachycardia, complete AV block, pulmonary hypertension, and pacemaker syndrome). The administration of adenosine may cause AV dissociation, but will not terminate JET.

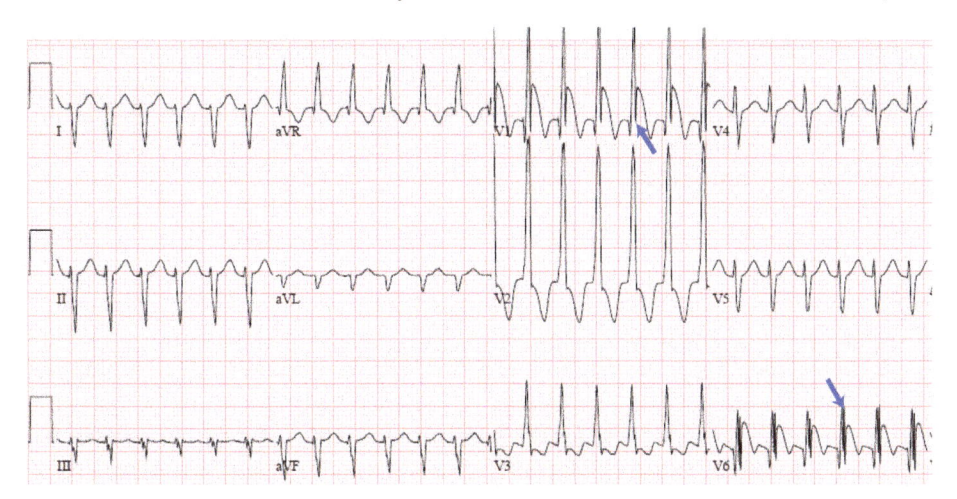

Figure 74-1. Atrial electrogram performed via leads V1 and V6 in a patient with JET. The electrical signals (arrows) noted in the latter portion of the QRS identify retrograde P waves buried in the QRS complex.

PART VI. POSTOPERATIVE SCENARIOS

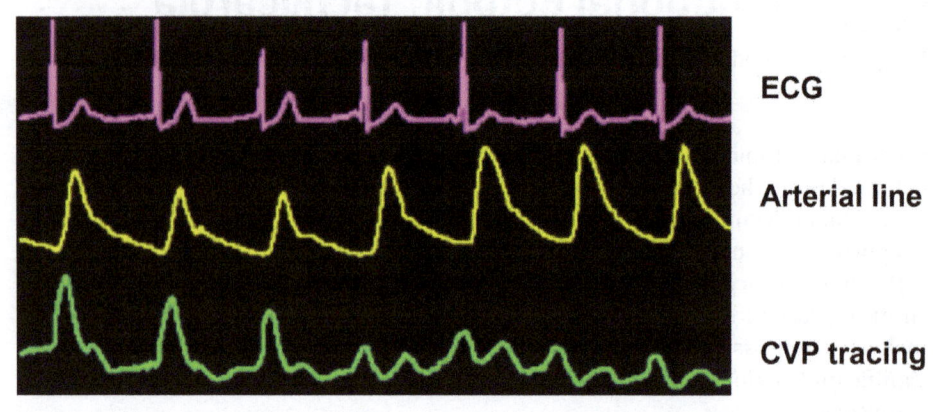

Figure 74-2. ECG, arterial line, and CVP tracings in a patient converting from junctional rhythm to sinus rhythm. Note the "cannon A waves" (first three beats) in the CVP tracing consistent with AV dyssynchrony when patient is in junctional rhythm. Note the return of the P wave in the ECG tracing and the corresponding loss of cannon A waves in the subsequent four beats of the CVP tracing. Adapted from Tsang R. Hemodynamic monitoring in the cardiac intensive care unit. Congenital Heart Disease 2013; 8:568-575, with permission.

Management

The goal of managing postoperative JET can be either to eliminate the tachyarrhythmia or to control the JET rate so hemodynamic stability is achieved. Conservative measures include cooling the patient (no lower than 33 °C), sedation (to decrease endogenous catecholamines), weaning inotropes, and correcting electrolyte derangements and hypovolemia. More aggressive interventions include:

- **Overdrive pacing.** Atrial overdrive pacing in AAI mode (if AV conduction is intact) or DDD mode (if AV block is present) at a rate above the intrinsic junctional rate may be performed. This will provide AV synchrony. If the JET rate is excessively rapid, atrial overdrive pacing at faster rates may be possible, but may not result in hemodynamic improvement due to limited filling time during rapid atrial pacing. **Warning:** rapid atrial pacing via a temporary pacemaker with poor atrial sensing can lead to atrial fibrillation.
- **Antiarrhythmics.**
  - *Esmolol* may be considered in patients whose ventricular function is preserved and who are not on high doses of inotropes, although success of conversion is low.
  - *Amiodarone.* The recommended dose is a one-time IV bolus of 5 mg/kg to be given over 1-2 hours. However, due to the potential cardiodepressant effects of amiodarone, in particular in neonates and young infants, it is preferable to slowly administer smaller boluses (1-2 mg/kg at a time over 30-60 min) until effect. Another 5 mg/kg bolus may be repeated if the first bolus fails to control the rhythm or decrease the rate of the tachycardia enough to improve hemodynamics. CaCl or Ca gluconate should be administered prior to amiodarone administration to mitigate risk of cardiovascular collapse from IV amiodarone. Frequently, a single dose of IV amiodarone is sufficient to convert postoperative

JET. An amiodarone drip (5-20 mg/kg/day IV) may be initiated if there is persistent arrhythmia with hemodynamic compromise after bolus dose administration. If using a drip, calcium levels and QTc should be monitored daily.
  - *IV Sotalol.* There is limited data on the use of sotalol for JET. In situations where this is being considered, it is recommended to consult the electrophysiology (EP) service first. This drug should be used in patients with, at most, moderately depressed function. Administer 1 mg/kg IV over one hour; the bolus may be repeated once. Monitor the QTc.
  - *Procainamide.* 3-6 mg/kg/dose over 5 minutes, not to exceed 100 mg/dose. Procainamide levels are not available at TCH, and its administration should not be considered without the input of the EP service.
- **ECMO.** Patients with intractable, hemodynamically significant JET that is refractory to standard medical and pharmacological interventions, may require ECMO support.

The majority of postoperative JET resolves within 36 hours of surgery and does not require further treatment beyond the immediate postoperative period.

75 Complete Atrioventricular Block

Jeffrey J. Kim, Iki Adachi

Complete AV block, known as third-degree heart block, occurs when electrical signals that trigger cardiac contraction are completely blocked between the atria and the ventricles. This is characterized by total failure of atrial impulses to be conducted to the ventricles, and there is complete dissociation between atrial and ventricular depolarization, typically followed by a junctional escape rhythm. Certain forms of CHD are at increased risk of intrinsic AV block, including patients with congenitally corrected transposition (ccTGA) and those with left-atrial isomerism. AV block can also be acquired postoperatively as a complication from surgical damage to the compact AV node or bundle of His. Surgeries most commonly associated with postoperative AV block include repair of AV septal defect, VSD closure, subaortic tissue resection, and surgical intervention on patients with ccTGA. In postoperative cases, recovery of AV conduction can occur, usually within the first 10 postoperative days.

Diagnosis

The diagnosis of complete AV block is typically made on rhythm evaluation, including telemetry and 12-lead ECG. These evaluations show that all atrial impulses that should conduct to the ventricle fail to do so (Figure 75-1), and the P waves are thus dissociated from the QRS complexes (more P waves than QRS).

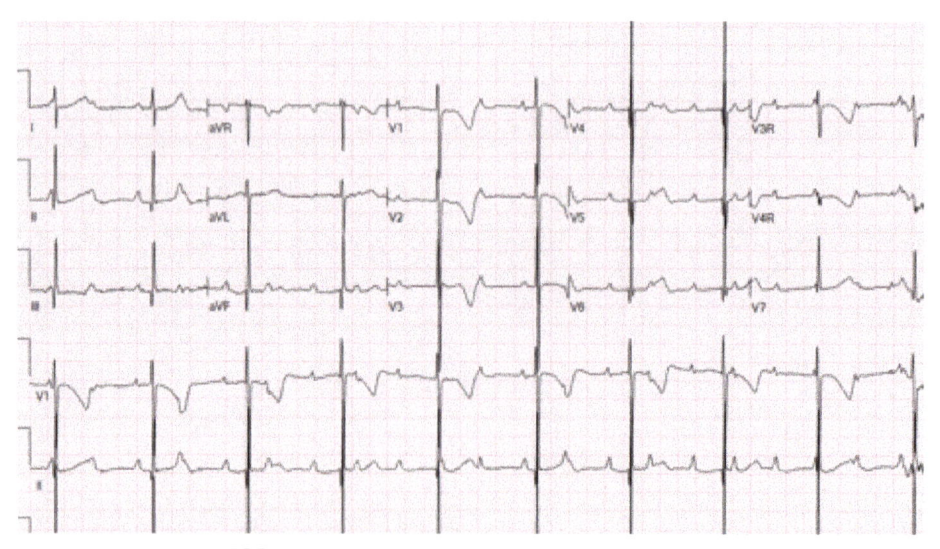

Figure 75-1. 15-lead ECG showing complete AV block with AV dissociation and junctional escape rhythm. All atrial impulses that should conduct to the ventricles fail to do so, and there are more P waves than QRS complexes.

Management

Acute treatment options for AV block are dependent on hemodynamic sequelae of bradycardia. If the junctional escape rhythm is of adequate rate to support stable hemodynamics, urgent treatment may not be necessary. If acute treatment is deemed necessary, several options can be considered based on the scenario:

- **Pharmacotherapy.** Medications such as isoproterenol or epinephrine can be used to increase the junctional escape rate.
- **Transcutaneous pacing.** External pacing utilizing pacing pads and an external unit can be used emergently if necessary. This should only be considered a temporary means.
- **Cardiac pacing via temporary pacing wires.** If postoperative external pacing wires are available, this may provide the most stable means of acute therapy. In AV block, atrial pacing alone will not be beneficial, thus the mode of temporary pacing should be programmed to DDD or VVI (See Chapter 41). Pacing settings and capture/sensing thresholds should be interrogated on a daily basis.
- **Transvenous pacing.** If temporary pacing wires are not available, insertion of a temporary pacing catheter into the ventricle with subsequent ventricular pacing can be used.

Ultimately, long-term care of postoperative AV block would hinge on a decision to implant a permanent pacemaker. Before a decision is made on permanent pacing however, a period of observation for recovery is warranted. Implantation of a pacemaker is generally indicated in patients who have not recovered AV conduction within 10 days after surgical intervention, although a small subset of patients have been shown to have late recovery. ACC/AHA/HRS guidelines for device-based therapy of cardiac rhythm abnormalities are available (Epstein et al. 2008, Brignole et al. 2013).

Suggested Readings

Brignole M, Auricchio A, Baron-Esquivias G, et al. 2013 ESC Guidelines on cardiac pacing and cardiac resynchronization therapy: the Task Force on cardiac pacing and resynchronization therapy of the European Society of Cardiology (ESC). Developed in collaboration with the European Heart Rhythm Association (EHRA). Eur Heart J. 2013;34:2281-2329.

Epstein AE, DiMarco JP, Ellenbogen KA, et al. ACC/AHA/HRS 2008 Guidelines for Device-Based Therapy of Cardiac Rhythm Abnormalities: a report of the American College of Cardiology/American Heart Association Task Force on Practice Guidelines (Writing Committee to Revise the ACC/AHA/NASPE 2002 Guideline Update for Implantation of Cardiac Pacemakers and Antiarrhythmia Devices) developed in collaboration with the American Association for Thoracic Surgery and Society of Thoracic Surgeons. J Am Coll Cardiol. 2008;51:e1-62.

76 Postoperative Bleeding

Erin A. Gottlieb, Justin Elhoff, Ziyad M. Binsalamah

Bleeding following a surgical procedure can be classified into 3 main categories: early, delayed, and late bleeding. Early bleeding is basically a continuation of bleeding from the OR. Delayed bleeding occurs few hours after the patient's arrival to the CICU, while late bleeding occurs a few days or weeks after surgery, and usually manifests as pleural or pericardial effusion.

Clear and consistent communication between the surgical, anesthesia, and critical care teams is paramount in preparation for and prevention of significant bleeding complications in the cardiac surgical patient. Signout of postoperative patients to the critical care team includes a comprehensive report on the extent of bleeding in the OR, as well as results of all analyses performed and products/factor concentrates administered prior to arrival to the CICU. Following arrival to the CICU, basic coagulation studies (PT/INR, PTT, and platelet count) are checked, and in the absence of significant bleeding (chest-tube output <1 mL/kg/hr), these studies are checked daily until normalization. Additionally, basic coagulation studies and platelet count are checked prior to removal of any intracardiac lines or transcutaneous pacing wires.

Diagnosis

The ICU team, starting with the nursing staff, must remain acutely aware of significant postoperative bleeding. Chest-tube output >1 mL/kg/hr but <2 mL/kg/hr merits close observation. Chest-tube output surpassing 2 mL/kg/hr of frank bloody output warrants discussion with the surgical team and consideration of further laboratory evaluation for coagulopathy, including ROTEM® analysis and evaluation for a drop in hematocrit.

In certain instances, the chest-tube output may be relatively insignificant (<1 mL/kg/hr) but a drop in hematocrit or a change in hemodynamic or respiratory status should raise concern for accumulation of blood within the thorax or mediastinum. In these instances, investigation for a potential source of bleeding is warranted, starting with a CXR and potentially echocardiogram.

Management

Coagulopathy is addressed utilizing the same strategy as is used in the OR (see Chapter 60 for guidelines utilized). PRBCs are administered as necessary based on a patient's hemodynamic status and the degree of decrease in hematocrit noted.

In all scenarios, assessment of the nature of chest-tube output is of utmost importance. As a general rule, dark bloody output is most consistent with a venous source of bleeding which, if not excessive, is likely to cease with correction of any coagulation abnormalities. On the other hand, bright red blood typically signifies an arterial source of bleeding which is unlikely to be successfully managed medically and will need to be dealt with in the OR.

Any bleeding that is associated with hemodynamic instability should be dealt with promptly by calling the surgical team for emergent chest exploration at the bedside in the CICU.

77 Chylothorax

Saul Flores, Antonio G. Cabrera, Kimberly Krauklis, Timothy J. Humlicek, Carlos M. Mery

Chylothorax is defined as the drainage of lymphatic fluid into the chest cavity (mediastinum and pleural spaces). Chylothorax can occur after CHS due to traumatic disruption of lymph nodes or lymphatic channels. It can also be due to increased CVP and overall venous pressures, particularly in patients with a palliated single ventricle, or due to obstruction of the SVC or the left-upper-extremity/neck veins where the thoracic duct drains. It is associated with significant morbidity and mortality due to malnutrition (loss of protein and fat) and immunosuppression (loss of immunoglobulins). Risk factors for the development of chylothorax after CHS include younger age, genetic syndromes, type of cardiac procedure, and neck or upper-extremity vein thrombosis. The TCH algorithm for diagnosis and management of chylothorax is illustrated in Figure 77-1.

Diagnosis

The diagnosis of postoperative chylothorax is typically triggered by the evidence of high chest-tube output (>5 mL/kg/d) in a patient after postoperative day 4. The chest-tube output tends to be whitish due to the presence of long-chain fatty acids and chylomicrons. In addition, chylothorax should be suspected with the new development of a pleural effusion or increasing chest-tube output in patients after high-risk procedures (e.g., aortic arch repair, Fontan procedure) and in patients with significant RV dysfunction.

A sample of the chest-tube fluid is sent for histochemistry and cell count. The presence of >110 mg/dL triglycerides or >70% lymphocytes confirms the diagnosis. It is important to take into account the oral-intake status of the patient, as it can change the fluid appearance (to a "milky" appearance) and the triglyceride concentration. For instance, the chylous fluid will have a high triglyceride concentration if the patient had already established enteral nutrition, whereas in the fasting patient, the concentration may be low and the fluid may look serous. If inconclusive, lipoprotein electrophoresis may be ordered; the presence of chylomicrons in the pleural fluid confirms the diagnosis.

The potential etiology of chylothorax may be assessed by echocardiography and ultrasonography. The presence of central-venous hypertension can lead to impairment of lymphatic drainage. Assessment by echocardiogram of right heart function and neck, thoracic, and upper extremity venous structures for line-related thrombosis or venous obstruction should be performed, as they could be correctable.

Management

Surgical reexploration may be considered in patients with very high chest-tube output, especially in those that underwent a thoracotomy since disruption of a major lymphatic channel is the most plausible cause. Otherwise, the initial treatment strategy is the institution of a chylothorax diet (<5 g of fat per day). Neonates and infants are placed on a low-fat formula such as Enfaport™ (only formula that contains essential fatty acids), Portagen®, Vivonex® Pediatric, or Tolerex®.

If patients fail to improve after initiation of a chylothorax diet, a trial of NPO/TPN is

PART VI. POSTOPERATIVE SCENARIOS

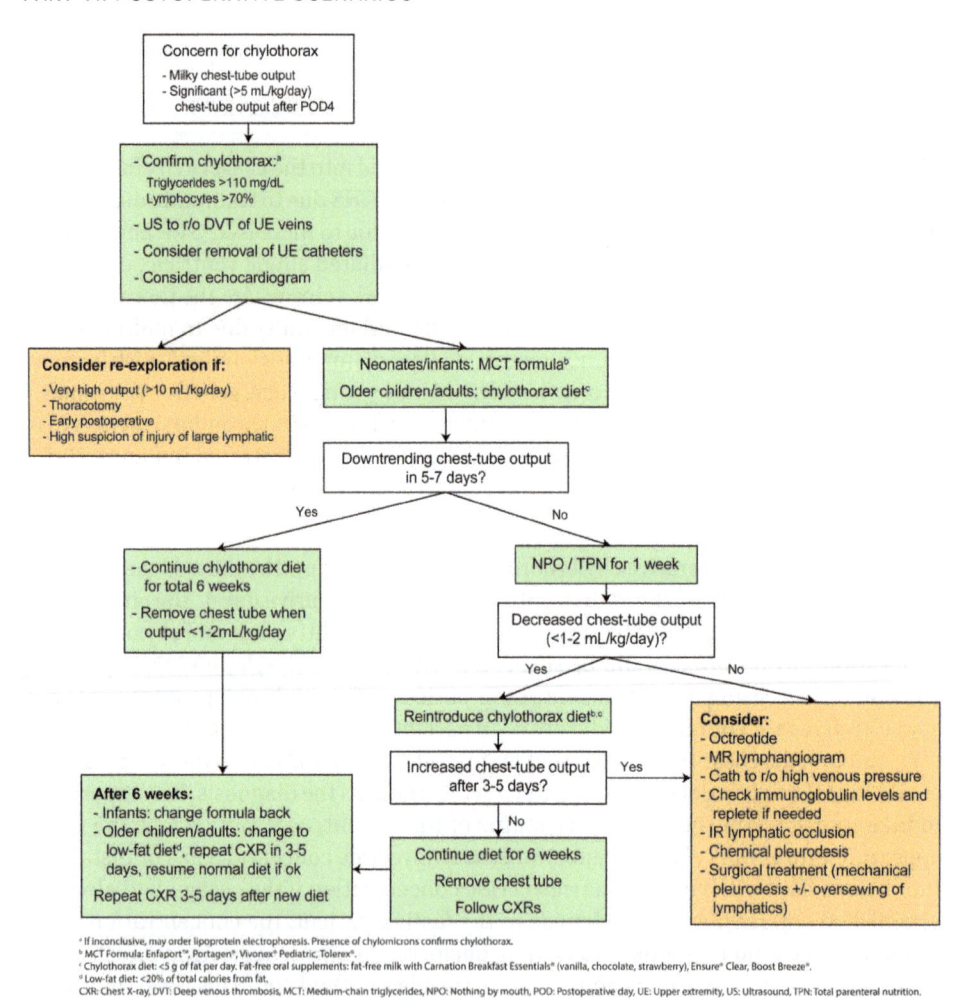

Figure 77-1. Algorithm for diagnosis and management of chylothorax.

warranted. If the trial fails, other strategies may include the use of octreotide, further workup such as MRI lymphangiogram or cardiac catheterization, lymphatic occlusion by IR, chemical pleurodesis, or surgical treatment (mechanical pleurodesis and possible oversewing of lymphatic channels).

Chemical Pleurodesis

The drug of choice at TCH for chemical pleurodesis is doxycycline. Table 77-1 describes the dosage of doxycycline used for pleurodesis. Compounding is performed by Pharmacy. The procedure is as follows:

1. Premedication with appropriate analgesics and anxiolytics and discontinuation of all anti-inflammatory medications.

2. Instill mixture into pigtail or chest tube slowly while monitoring patient's tolerance. Clamp the chest tube.
3. Reposition the patient every 20 minutes for 2 hours.
4. Remove/aspirate the mixture from the pigtail or chest tube at the end of 2 hours.
5. Reconnect the pigtail or chest tube to a new sterile collection system.
6. Obtain CXR.
7. Continue analgesics.
8. Document procedure.
9. Repeat CXR the following day.

Chemical pleurodesis can cause a significant postprocedural inflammatory reaction with worsening of lung compliance, fevers and increased WBC count that can mimic sepsis.

Table 77-1. Dosage of doxycycline for chemical pleurodesis.

Weight	Total volume (normal saline)	Dosage
≤12.5 kg	40 mL	20 mg/kg doxycycline (10 mg/mL), 0.5 mL of 2% lidocaine (max 3 mg/kg)
12.5-25 kg	50 mL	20 mg/kg doxycycline (10 mg/mL), 1 mL of 2% lidocaine
25-50 kg	60 mL	500 mg doxycycline (10 mg/mL), 1.5 mL of 2% lidocaine
>50 kg	120 mL	1000 mg doxycycline (10 mg/mL), 3 mL of 2% lidocaine

Suggested Reading

Mery CM, Moffett BS, Khan MS, et al. Incidence and treatment of chylothorax after cardiac surgery in children: analysis of a large multi-institution database. J Thorac Cardiovasc Surg 2014;147:678-686.

78 Pneumothorax

Fabio Savorgnan, Ziyad M. Binsalamah, Paul A. Checchia

Pneumothorax is the accumulation of air between the visceral and parietal pleurae in the chest. This accumulation of air can lead to compression of the intrathoracic structures. Compression and collapse of the lung can lead to respiratory failure. Compression of cardiovascular structures can lead to obstructive shock and hemodynamic collapse. When this happens, the pneumothorax is known as a tension pneumothorax. The most frequent causes of pneumothorax in the CICU are *barotrauma* from mechanical ventilation with high pressure in an injured lung or aggressive bagging, and *air entrapment* after removal of a chest tube.

Diagnosis

Clinical manifestations of a pneumothorax in the CICU vary from an incidental finding on a CXR, to different degrees of respiratory distress with tachypnea, accessory muscle usage, shortness of breath, chest pain and/or decrease in SaO_2, to significant hemodynamic instability and impending cardiorespiratory arrest. On auscultation, one can find asymmetric breath sounds. If the patient's condition permits, a CXR is indicated to confirm the diagnosis (Figure 78-1).

Treatment

The decision to intervene on a patient with a pneumothorax is dictated by the patient's clinical condition and the circumstances surrounding the pneumothorax. Asymptomatic patients with a small pneumothorax (when air occupies <25% of the lung space) may be observed and closely monitored with serial CXRs. Similarly, patients with pneumothoraces caused by air entrapment from removal of a chest tube may be observed since these pneumothoraces tend to resolve spontaneously and rarely cause significant symptoms. If the decision is made to observe a patient with a pneumothorax, serial CXRs are mandatory, especially in patients that are mechanically ventilated as the pneumothorax can rapidly expand. Patients with a life-threatening clinical condition will require emergent intervention.

The treatment of a pneumothorax is decompression of the extrapleural air, usually by insertion of a chest tube. Under urgent circumstances, needle decompression can be utilized for rapid stabilization prior to insertion of a chest tube. See Chapter 67 for information about the different types of chest tubes and how to insert them.

Assessing air leaks after chest tube insertion is critical. Air bubbles in the water-seal chamber indicate the presence of an air leak, which can arise from a parenchymal injury, a leak around the tube, or a leak in the tube-system itself. It is incumbent on the clinician to differentiate these different sources of air in the bubble chamber.

Despite the presence of numerical divisions in the water-seal chamber, it is difficult to accurately quantify the degree of an air leak. In general, air leaks tend to resolve with time. It usually takes 2 to 5 days for small intermittent air leaks to disappear, but it may take longer for more significant air leaks. Once the air leak disappears and there are

78. PNEUMOTHORAX

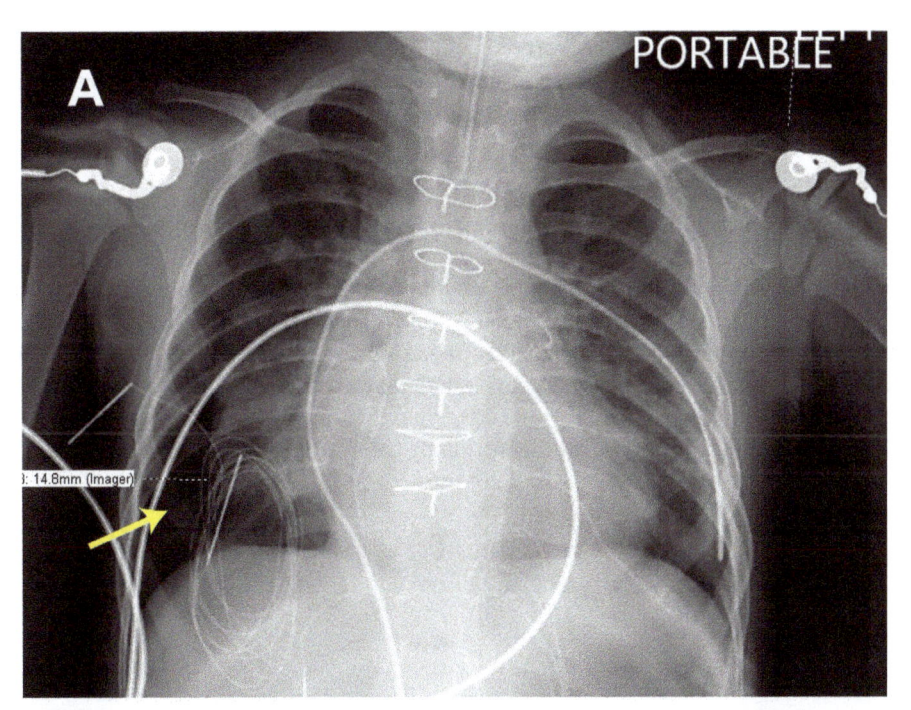

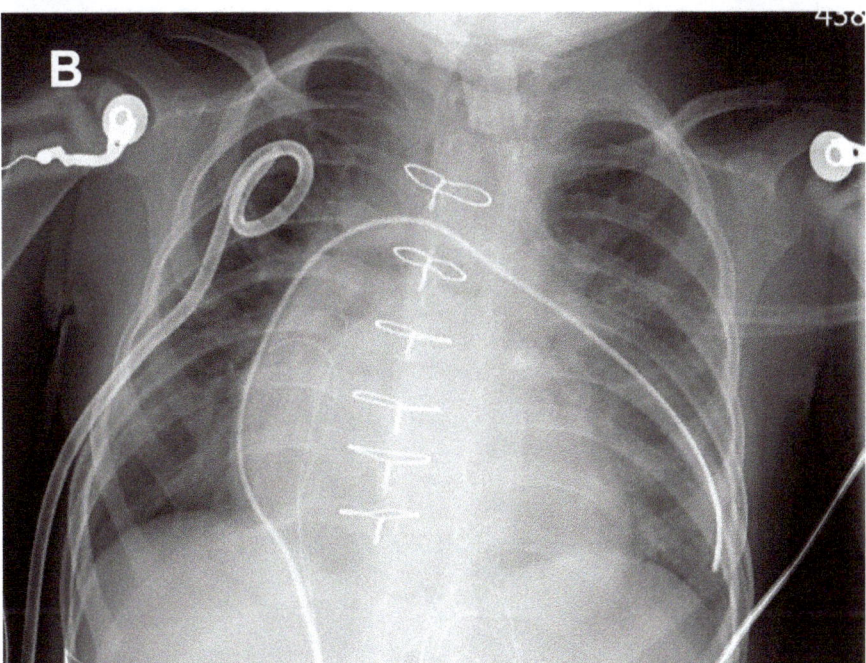

Figure 78-1. A) CXR of a patient with a large pneumothorax (arrow). B) CXR of the same patient after insertion of a pigtail chest tube.

487

no air bubbles visualized in the water-seal chamber, a water-seal trial is performed. For this, obtain a baseline CXR, discontinue the suction from the system, and repeat a CXR 4 hours later. If there is no pneumothorax or a small pneumothorax is stable from baseline, the chest tube is removed.

Relative Contraindications to Placement of a Chest Tube

There are no contraindications to the insertion of a chest tube if the patient's clinical condition is deteriorating. However, if the patient's clinical condition allows, then any significant coagulopathy and thrombocytopenia should be corrected. In general, correct the parameters to an INR <1.5 and platelet count >50,000 /mcL. If possible, avoid areas with local infection when placing a chest tube. Additionally, the practitioner should be aware of anatomical variations (e.g., cardiomegaly, dextrocardia) and situations with potentially large collaterals (e.g., cyanotic lesions) that may make chest-tube insertion more challenging and may warrant insertion by the cardiac surgeon.

79 Pulmonary Hypertension

Ryan D. Coleman, Corey Chartan, Heather A. Dickerson

Pulmonary hypertension (PH) in the CICU is a common phenomenon, both in the preoperative and postoperative periods. PH is traditionally defined as a mean PA pressure ≥25 mmHg and a PVR ≥3 Wood units/m². It is important, however, to understand the etiology of the PH in order to best address it (Table 79-1).

Diagnosis

PH crises are the result of acute RV failure secondary to an abrupt rise in PVR. It is important to distinguish true acute RV failure resulting from an acute rise in PVR versus an acute rise in PVR that may cause systemic hypoxemia with some potential hemodynamic instability but with a normally functioning RV. The pathophysiology and manifestations of a PH crisis can be seen in Figure 79-1.

The defects that are at highest risk for a PH crisis postoperatively include truncus arteriosus, cor triatriatum, total anomalous pulmonary venous return (especially when obstructed), large PDA, AV septal defect (particularly in older patients with Down syndrome), and transposition of the great arteries.

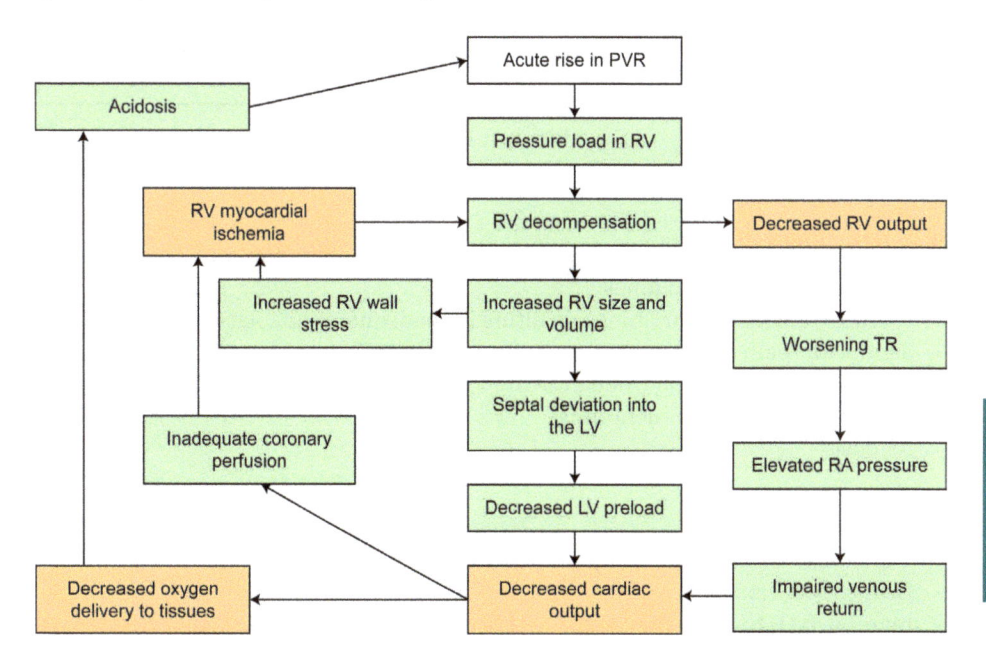

Figure 79-1. Pathophysiology of a PH crisis. LV: left ventricle, PVR: pulmonary vascular resistance, RV: right ventricle, TR: tricuspid regurgitation.

Table 79-1. Different etiologies and management of PH

	Mechanism	Common examples	Basic management
Increased pulmonary blood flow	Increased cardiac output	Vein of Galen malformation	Control flow through malformation Inhaled nitric oxide
	Systemic-to-pulmonary shunts	PDA VSD AVSD	Diuresis Agents to lower SVR (ACE-inhibitors) to decrease shunting
Increased precapillary resistance	Constriction	Hypoxemia BMPR2 mutation	Systemic pulmonary vasodilators
	Obstruction	Pulmonary embolism	Obstruction relief Anticoagulation
	Abnormal development or destruction of vasculature	Bronchopulmonary dysplasia Connective tissue diseases	Systemic pulmonary vasodilators Optimize ventilator strategy Tight fluid management
Increased postcapillary resistance	Pulmonary venous abnormalities	Pulmonary vein stenosis Pulmonary veno-occlusive disease	Relief of obstruction Tight fluid management Consider sildenafil in post-intervention period
	Left-sided heart disease	Mitral valve stenosis Shone's complex	Relief of left-sided obstruction Tight fluid management Careful use of sildenafil in post-intervention period Beta-blockers

ACE: angiotensin-converting enzyme, AVSD: atrioventricular septal defect, PDA: patent ductus arteriosus, VSD: ventricular septal defect, SVR: systemic vascular resistance.

The most common triggers of PH crises are:
- Suboptimal ventilation resulting in hypercarbia and/or hypoxemia
  - Inadequate tidal volumes
  - Incorrect inspiratory times resulting in inadequate exhablation
- Significant pain and/or agitation
  - Inadequate sedation while intubated
  - Endotracheal tube suctioning
- Acidosis

Management

A PH crisis can be managed using the following interventions:
- Deepen sedation and paralysis
- Increase FiO_2 to 1.0
- Decrease pCO_2 to normal to low-normal values
- Initiate iNO at 20 ppm if not already being used
- Inhaled iloprost (0.5-1 mcg/kg/dose)
- Sodium bicarbonate (1 mEq/kg) to improve any acidosis
- Calcium chloride (20 mg/kg) to improve myocardial contractility

79. PULMONARY HYPERTENSION

Table 79-2. Common PH medications and doses

Drug	Class	Dose	Important points
Sildenafil PO	PDE-5	1 mg/kg PO <12 mo: q6h >12 mo: q8h	Start with low dosing and gradually increase as hemodynamics tolerate
Sildenafil IV	PDE-5	0.5 mg/kg IV <12 mo: q6h >12 mo: q8h	Start with low dosing and gradually increase as hemodynamics tolerate; tend to see hypotension ~30 minutes after dose given
Bosentan PO	ERA - dual ETA/ETB	1-2 mg/kg PO q12h	Monitor LFTs monthly Can have GI side-effects Do not use if underlying hepatic dysfunction
Epoprostenol IV (Veletri®)	Prostanoids	Starting dose: 2 ng/kg/min	Major side effects: headache, nausea/vomiting, hypotension Can be kept at room temperature 1/2-life: 4-6 min
Treprostinil SQ or IV (Remodulin®)	Prostanoids	Starting dose: 2 ng/kg/min	1/2-life: 4-5 hrs Stable at room temperature
Iloprost INH	Prostanoids	0.25-1 mcg/kg q3 hrs	Can cause flushing/headache Can cause bronchospasm

ERA: endothelin receptor antagonists, ETA: endothelin receptor A, ETB: endothelin receptor B, GI: gastrointestinal, INH: inhaled, IV: intravenous, LFT: liver function test, PDE-5: phosphodiesterase-5 inhibitors, PO: per os (oral), SQ: subcutaneous.

- Small boluses of epinephrine (0.01 mg/kg diluted in 10 mL of normal saline) to improve cardiac output without a concomitant rise in PVR
- Vasopressin (0.01-0.04 U/kg/hr) to aid in shifting the interventricular septum towards the appropriate position

Table 79-2 lists some of the most common PH medications and doses.

Special Considerations

For patients with small left-sided structures (e.g., Shone's complex, transposition of the great arteries after an arterial switch operation, total anomalous pulmonary venous return after repair), volume administration can precipitate an acute rise in PVR due to the small left-sided structures in combination with diastolic dysfunction. Monitor the LA pressure closely while giving fluid boluses and use small aliquots of volume.

In single-ventricle patients, a PVR <2 Wood units/m^2 is ideal prior to proceeding with Fontan completion. If PVR is higher, consider adding enteral pulmonary vasodilators and repeating the cardiac catheterization several months later to reassess PVR. In patients with a bidirectional Glenn and PH that present with worsening cyanosis, it is important to rule out the presence of decompressing veins (from the upper to the lower body) that may need to be addressed.

80 Pleural Effusion

Parag Jain, Antonio R. Mott, Ziyad M. Binsalamah

Pleural effusion refers to abnormal and excessive collection of fluid in the pleural space. This can happen due to either excess production or decreased absorption. There are 4 major types of pleural effusions:
- **Transudative.** Most common form of effusion after CHS. Occurs as a result of imbalance between Starling forces (capillary hydrostatic pressure > oncotic pressure).
- **Exudative.** Caused by inflammation of the lung or pleura, resulting in increased capillary permeability. Relatively uncommon after cardiac surgery.
- **Chylous.** Effusion which has high fat content and usually manifests after initiation of enteral feeding postoperatively (see Chapter 77).
- **Hemothorax.** Bleeding should be considered in early postoperative patients.

Diagnosis

Clinically, patients may have signs of increased work of breathing, use of accessory breathing muscles, or oxygen desaturations. Large effusions, and particularly rapid accumulations, may result in significant hemodynamic instability in addition to respiratory impairment. Auscultation of the respective lung field will reveal decreased air entry. Definitive diagnosis is often made with help of imaging.

Findings on CXR vary depending on the extent of the effusion. A CXR will often reveal opacification of lung fields, especially obliteration of the costophrenic and cardiophrenic angles (Figure 80-1). Moderate-to-large effusions can lead to collapse of nearby lung segments. A decubitus CXR often shows layering of the fluid and can help differentiate simple (nonseptated) from complex (septated) effusions.

Ultrasound imaging may be used to evaluate the extent of the effusion and to differentiate between simple and complex effusions. CT scan is often regarded as the gold standard for diagnosis, but is rarely required.

Management

Some effusions, particularly in the early postoperative period when there is overall fluid overload, can be managed medically with diuretics. We usually use furosemide 1 mg/kg/dose Q8h or Q6h IV as our first line therapy.

Moderate-to-large effusions or effusions with significant clinical symptoms often require insertion of a chest tube (Figure 80-2) (see Chapter 67). If hemothorax is suspected, surgical intervention may be required. Complex effusions may need chest-tube placement by IR with lysis of adhesions using tissue plasminogen activator (tPA). The use of tPA is contraindicated in the fresh postoperative patient (less than one month after surgery).

The chest tube is removed when the drainage is serous or serosanguineous and is <2.5 mL/kg/day. For patients with bloody or chylous drainage, the chest tube is usually left until the drainage is <1 mL/kg/day. The patient does not need to be NPO before chest tube removal. See Chapter 67 for details on chest tube removal.

80. PLEURAL EFFUSION

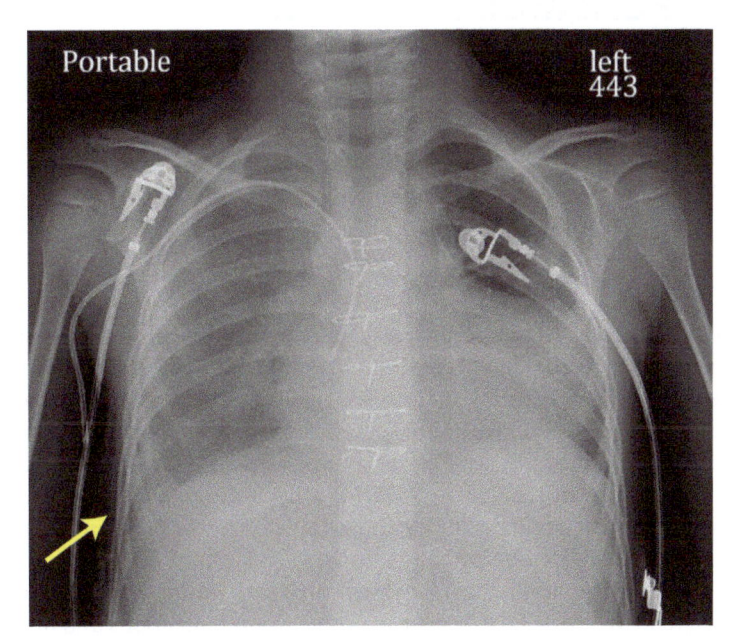

Figure 80-1. A CXR showing a moderate right-sided pleural effusion (arrow).

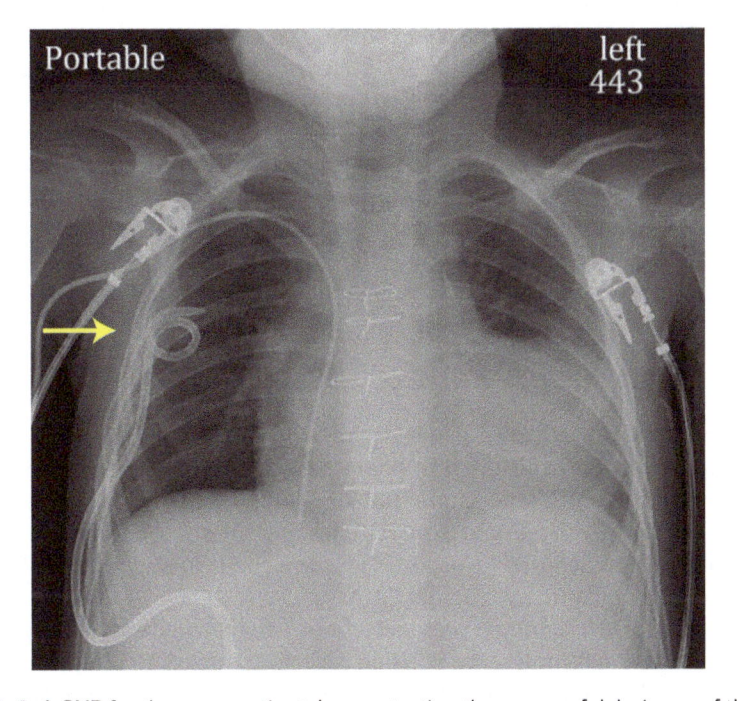

Figure 80-2. A CXR for the same patient demonstrating the successful drainage of the right-sided pleural effusion after the insertion of a pigtail chest tube (arrow).

493

81 Pericardial Effusion

Alan F. Riley, Aimee Liou

Pericardial effusions are commonly encountered in the postoperative period. Their clinical impact depends on multiple factors including etiology, rapidity of accumulation, and response to medical therapy.

Diagnosis

In the immediate postoperative period, pericardial effusions can be the result of uncontrolled bleeding. Due to the short-term limited compliance of the pericardial sac, even a small localized effusion rapidly accumulating within the pericardium can result in tamponade. Unexpected poor cardiac output, tachycardia, and/or rising and equalizing atrial pressures in the postoperative period should raise concerns for a pericardial effusion. Even with reassuring CXR, urgent bedside echocardiography should be performed if there are any clinical concerns for a pericardial effusion or tamponade, since small postoperative effusions can be hemodynamically significant. Close attention should be paid by the sonographer to visualize the entire pericardial space, particularly the posterior, dependent areas. Rarely, postoperative wound infections and mediastinitis can be associated with pericardial effusions.

Delayed presentation of a new pericardial effusion raises the clinical suspicion for postcardiotomy syndrome (PCS), which can present in patients after 1 week postoperatively. PCS can complicate the later course after relatively low-risk cardiac operations including ASD repairs. It is likely a systemic autoimmune reaction and can be associated with fever, fatigue, irritability, and anorexia. PCS should be considered in all postoperative patients with delayed systemic symptoms, pericardial friction rubs, and/or diffuse ST-segment elevation on postoperative ECG. An echocardiogram and a posteroanterior and lateral CXR are routinely scheduled prior to hospital discharge. A CXR is repeated during the initial postoperative visit in order to assess for delayed pericardial effusions in asymptomatic patients. Tamponade is rarely seen in PCS, but the effusions can be large and become hemodynamically significant, particularly if hypovolemia is present.

Management

The treatment of pericardial effusions depends on the etiology, timing, and clinical presentation. Hemodynamically significant pericardial effusions in the immediate perioperative period with inadequate drainage from the current chest tubes require immediate surgical drainage and exploration, sometimes at the bedside in the CICU. Pericardial effusions believed to be potentially infectious in origin should be drained and treated with systemic antimicrobials.

For patients with PCS and no evidence of tamponade, medical therapy is usually the first line of therapy, unless the effusion is very large. Non-steroidal anti-inflammatory drugs (NSAIDs) (ibuprofen 10 mg/kg every 6 or 8 hours, or high-dose aspirin if <6 months old) and diuretics are recommended; prednisone is used on occasion as a last

81. PERICARDIAL EFFUSION

resort for recurrent or refractory cases. Overdiuresis should be avoided as it can precipitate tamponade physiology. Hospital readmission may be necessary for monitoring during initiation of diuretics in large or potentially hemodynamically significant late pericardial effusions. NSAIDs should be continued for at least 2 weeks in medically responsive patients; tapering of dose is usually advisable. Medically refractory patients or those with large hemodynamically significant late pericardial effusions are referred for drainage, either via transcutaneous approach in the cardiac catheterization lab or via surgical approach.

VII. Appendices

A Drugs

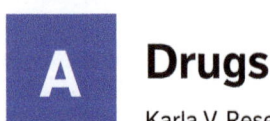

Karla V. Resendiz, Timothy J. Humlicek, Brady S. Moffett

Vasoactive Medications

Amlodipine
Mechanism of action: Calcium-channel blocker (dihydropyridine); vasodilation of vascular and coronary smooth muscle.
Indications: Treatment of hypertension.
Contraindications: Hypersensitivity to amlodipine or other dihydropyridines. Severe hypotension.
Dosage:
- Children (1-5 years): 0.05-0.1 mg/kg daily, initial dose not to exceed 2.5 mg. Titrate weekly to a maximum dose of 10 mg/day.
- Children (6-17 years): 0.05 mg/kg/day, initial dose not to exceed 2.5-5 mg. Titrate weekly to a maximum dose of 20 mg/day.
- Adults: 2.5-5 mg po daily. Titrate weekly to a maximum dose of 10 mg/day.

Adjustment for kidney / liver dysfunction: Start at lower doses in hepatic impairment.
PK/PD: Onset for hypertensive effects ~24-72 hrs. Half-life 30-50 hours, longer in hepatic disease.
Common adverse events: Peripheral edema (15-30%).
Administration:
- Oral suspension: 1 mg/mL (compounded).
- Tablets: 2.5, 5, 10 mg.

Other: Peripheral edema may occur 2-3 weeks after therapy initiation.

Captopril
Mechanism of action: Angiotensin-converting enzyme (ACE)-inhibitor; prevents conversion of angiotensin I to angiotensin II, overall increase in renin activity and decrease in aldosterone.
Indications: Treatment of hypertension, CHF.
Contraindications: Hypersensitivity to captopril or other ACE-inhibitors.
Dosage:
- Full-term neonate: 0.05 mg/kg/dose q8-24h. Titrate to max: 0.5 mg/kg/dose q6h.
- Infants: 0.1 mg/kg q8-12h, titrate by 0.1 mg/kg/dose to a max of 6 mg/kg/day in 3-4 divided doses.
- Children: 0.3 mg/kg/dose q8h, initial dose not to exceed 6.25 mg. Titrate to a max of 6 mg/kg/day in 3 divided doses, max 50 mg TID.
- Adults: 25 mg po q8h, titrate weekly by 12.5-25 mg per dose. Max: 50 mg TID.
- Heart failure (afterload reduction): Start patients at lower doses compared to hypertension dosing to prevent symptomatic hypotension.

Adjustment for kidney / liver dysfunction:
- eCrCl 10-50 mL/min: Decrease usual dose by 25%.
- eCrCl <10 mL/min: Decrease usual dose by 50%.

PK/PD: Onset of action ~15 minutes, peak effect: 1-2 hrs after dose. Half-life in children ~1.5 hrs, infants and heart failure patients have longer half-lives.
Common adverse events: Hyperkalemia (11%), hypotension, cough, increased creatinine.
Administration:
- Oral suspension: 1 mg/mL (compounded).
- Tablets: 12.5, **25**, 50, 100 mg.

Other: Do not use in pregnant patients; consider labetalol, methyldopa, or nifedipine instead. instead. Hypotension may occur with general anesthesia; perioperative discontinuation is controversial. Angioedema can occur at any time; patients with history of idiopathic or familial angioedema, heart failure, female or black patients may be at higher risk.

Clonidine
Mechanism of action: Stimulates alpha2-adrenoceptors in the brain stem resulting in decreased CNS sympathetic outflow and thus leading to decreased PVR, decreased renal-vascular resistance, lower heart rate, and lower BP.
Indications: Hypertension, opioid-withdrawal prevention.
Contraindications: hypersensitivity, bradycardia.
Dosage:
- Neonates and infants:
  - Opioid-withdrawal syndrome: IV/PO: 1-2 mcg/kg/dose every 6-8 hours.
- Children:
  - Hypertension (PO): Initial 5-10 mcg/kg/day in divided doses every 8-12 hours; increase gradually, if needed, to 5-25 mcg/kg/day in divided doses every 6 hours; maximum dose: 0.9 mg/day.
  - Opioid-withdrawal syndrome (IV/PO): 1-2 mcg/kg/dose every 6-8 hours (maximum: 30 mcg/dose).
  - Transdermal: May switch to transdermal patch after stable oral dose has been achieved. Use transdermal doses approximately equivalent to the total oral daily dose.

Adjustment for kidney / liver dysfunction: Monitor for increased adverse effects in renal dysfunction.
PK/PD: Patch will reach steady state in 3 days. Extensive hepatic metabolism to inactive metabolites. Half-life in children ~6 hrs, longer in renal impairment or with patch use. Time to peak 1-3 hours (oral), 3 days (patch).
Common adverse events: Hypotension, increased sedation, constipation.
Administration: Do not cut transdermal patches; for partial doses, apply occlusive tape to active side of patch.
Other: Remove patch prior to MRI to prevent burns. For IV formulation, dedicated central line is preferred.

Enalapril
Mechanism of action: ACE-inhibitor; prevents conversion of angiotensin I to angiotensin II, overall increase in renin activity and decrease in aldosterone.
Indications: Hypertension, CHF, asymptomatic LV dysfunction.
Contraindications: Hypersensitivity to enalapril or other ACE-inhibitors.

Dosage for hypertension:
- Full-term neonate: Initial 0.05 mg/kg/day q24h. Titrate to max: 0.27 mg/kg/day div q12h.
- Infants, children, adolescents: 0.08 mg/kg q24h, max initial dose 5 mg. Adjust to 0.6 mg/kg/day, max: 40 mg/day.
- Adults: Initial dose 2.5 mg/DAY, max: 40 mg/DAY divided in 1-2 doses.

Dosage for heart failure (afterload reduction):
- Infants, children, adolescents: 0.1 mg/kg/DAY divided in 1-2 doses. Usual max dose: 0.5 mg/kg/DAY.
- Adults: 2.5 mg BID, increase as tolerated. Usually, 20 mg/DAY div q12h.

Adjustment for kidney / liver dysfunction:
- eCrCl 10-50 mL/min: Decrease usual dose by 25%.
- eCrCl <10 mL/min: Decrease usual dose by 50%.

PK/PD: Prodrug, hepatic metabolism to active drug enalaprilat. Onset of action ~1 hour, peak effect 4-6 hrs after dose. Duration 12-24 hrs. Half-life in children ~3 hrs; infants and CHF patients have longer half-lives.

Common adverse events: Increased creatinine (20%), hyperkalemia, hypotension, cough.

Administration:
- Oral solution: 1 mg/mL (commercially available).
- Tablets: 2.5, 5, 10, 20 mg.

Other: Do not use in pregnant patients; consider labetalol, methyldopa, or nifedipine. Hypotension may occur with general anesthesia and CPB; perioperative discontinuation should be considered on a case-by-case basis. Angioedema can occur at any time; patients with history of idiopathic or familial angioedema, CHF, female or black patients may be at higher risk.

Enalaprilat

Mechanism of action: ACE-inhibitor; prevents conversion of angiotensin I to angiotensin II, overall increase in renin activity and decrease in aldosterone.

Indications: Treatment of hypertension when oral therapy is not practical.

Contraindications: Hypersensitivity to enalapril/enalaprilat or other ACE-inhibitors.

Dosage:
- Neonate: 5-10 mcg/kg/dose IV q8-24h.
- Infants and children: 5-10 mcg/kg/dose every 8-24h, max dose 1.25 mg.
- Adolescents and adults: 0.625-1.25 mg every 6 hours.

Adjustment for kidney / liver dysfunction:
- eCrCl 10-50 mL/min: Decrease usual dose by 25%.
- eCrCl <10 mL/min: Decrease usual dose by 50%.

PK/PD: Onset of action ~15 minutes, peak effect 1-4 hrs. Duration ~6 hours. Half-life in children ~11 hrs.

Common adverse events: Increased creatinine (20%) hyperkalemia, hypotension, headache.

Administration: Injection 0.025 mg/mL (diluted) and 1.25 mg/mL (undiluted).

Other: Do not use in pregnant patients; consider labetalol, methyldopa, or nifedipine. Hypotension may occur with general anesthesia and CPB; perioperative discontinuation should be considered on a case-by-case basis. Angioedema can occur at any time; patients with history of idiopathic or familial angioedema, CHF, female or black patients may be at higher risk.

Hydralazine

Mechanism of action: Arterial vasodilator via multiple pathways.

Indications: Severe essential hypertension.

Contraindications: Hypersensitivity to hydralazine; coronary artery disease, mitral valve rheumatic heart disease.

Dosage:
- Neonates (PO, IM, IV): 0.1-0.5 mg/kg q3-6h as needed for BP control. Use of dilution may be needed.
- Infants and children:
  - PO: 0.75-0.1 mg/kg/DAY divided q6h, initial dose not to exceed 25 mg.
  - IV/IM: 0.1 mg/kg/dose q4-6h prn severe hypertension, initial dose not to exceed 20 mg.
- Adults:
  - PO: Start 10 mg 4x/day, titrate by 10-25 mg to a daily max of 300 mg.
  - IV/IM: 10-20 mg q4-6h prn severe hypertension, not to exceed 40 mg/dose.

Adjustment for kidney / liver dysfunction:
- eCrCl 10-50 mL/min: Decrease usual dose by 25% and administer q8h.
- eCrCl <10 mL/min: Decrease usual dose by 50%; administer q12-24h based on acetylator status.

PK/PD: Onset of action (IV) 10-80 minutes. Duration up to 12 hours depending on patient-specific hepatic acetylation. Half-life 3-7 hours.

Common adverse events: Angina, hypotension, thrombocytopenia (IV).

Administration:
- Oral Suspension: 1 mg/mL (compounded)
- Tablet: 10, 25, 50, 100 mg
- IV: 0.2 mg/mL (diluted), 20 mg/mL (undiluted)

Other: May be associated with vasculitis when used in combination with iodine-containing IV contrast, avoid combination when possible. Higher doses or patients with renal dysfunction may be at higher risk.

Lisinopril

Mechanism of action: ACE-inhibitor; prevents conversion of angiotensin I to angiotensin II, overall increase in renin activity and decrease in aldosterone.

Indications: Treatment of hypertension, CHF.

Contraindications: Hypersensitivity to or angioedema as result of lisinopril or other ACE-inhibitors.

Dosage:
- Hypertension (patients >6 years of age): 0.07-0.1 mg/kg daily, initial dose not to exceed 5 mg. Titrate weekly to a maximum dose of 0.6 mg/kg/day or 40 mg/day.
- Heart failure (adjunct): Start patients at 50% usual hypertension dose to prevent symptomatic hypotension.

Adjustment for kidney / liver dysfunction:
- eCrCl 10-50 mL/min/decrease usual dose by 50%.

- eCrCl <10 mL/min/decrease usual dose by 75%.

PK/PD: Onset of action ~1 hour, peak effect: ~6 hrs. Duration 24 hrs. Half-life ~12 hrs.

Common adverse events: Increased creatinine, hyperkalemia, hypotension, dizziness.

Administration:
- Oral solution: 1 mg/mL, commercially available.
- Tablet: 5, 10, 20 mg

Other: Do not use in pregnant patients; consider labetalol, methyldopa, or nifedipine. Hypotension may occur with general anesthesia and CPB; perioperative discontinuation should be considered on a case-by-case basis. Angioedema can occur at any time; patients with history of idiopathic or familial angioedema, CHF, female or black patients may be at higher risk.

Milrinone

Mechanism of action: Phosphodiesterase inhibitor in cardiac and vascular tissue, resulting in vasodilation and inotropic effects with little chronotropy. Lusotropic effects have also been observed.

Indications: Inotropic support.

Contraindications: Hypersensitivity.

Dosage: 0.375 to 0.75 mcg/kg/min continuous infusion.

Adjustment for kidney / liver dysfunction:

eCrCl (mL/min)	Starting dose (mcg/kg/min)		
>50	0.375	0.5	0.75
50	0.25	0.375	0.5
40	0.125	0.25	0.375
30	0.0625	0.125	0.25
20	Consider alternative therapy	0.0625	0.125
10	Consider alternative therapy		0.0625
5	Consider alternative therapy		

PK/PD: Onset 5 to 15 minutes. Half-life in children 1.8 to 3.1 hours; adults 2.3 hours. Metabolism: Hepatic via cytochrome P450 3A4. Elimination: Primarily urine (83%).

Common adverse events: Ventricular and atrial arrhythmias (ectopy, tachycardia).

Administration: IV - 0.2 mg/mL usual concentration; 0.8 mg/mL via central line.

Other: If given in combination with plasmapheresis, dose should be given after session, ideally with 24 hours between dose and the next scheduled session.

Nicardipine

Mechanism of action: Calcium-channel blocker (dihydropyridine); vasodilation of vascular and coronary smooth muscle.

Indications: Treatment of hypertension when oral therapy is not practical.

Contraindications: Hypersensitivity to nicardipine or other dihydropyridines; advanced aortic stenosis / risk of ischemia due to decreased coronary perfusion.

Dosage:
- Neonates: 0.5 mcg/kg/min; limited data available.
- Infants, children, adolescents: 0.5-1 mcg/kg/min. Titrate by 0.5-1 mcg/kg/min q15-30min, max: 5 mcg/kg/min.
- Adults: 5 mg/hr, titrate by 2.5 mg/hr, max 15 mg/hr.

Adjustment for kidney / liver dysfunction: Patients with hepatic or dysfunction may require lower doses, monitor closely, titrate to effect.

PK/PD: Rapid onset, peak effect ~45 minutes. Extensive, saturable, hepatic metabolism. Urine excretion (50% metabolites).

Common adverse events: Flushing (6-10%), pedal edema (7-8%), angina (dose dependent), hypotension, headache.

Administration: Injection 0.1 mg/mL, 0.5 mg/mL, central line preferred.

Other: Oral formulations not available at TCH.

Nitroprusside

Mechanism of action: Peripheral vasodilation by direct action on venous and arterial smooth muscle.

Indications: Treatment of hypertensive crisis

Contraindications: Avoid in patients at risk for hypotension: compensatory hypertension, concomitant use with sildenafil/tadalafil.

Dosage: 0.5 mcg/kg/min, titrate by 0.5-1 mcg/kg/min q5min. Usual dose 2-3 mcg/kg/min, not to exceed 10 mcg/kg/min. To avoid cyanide toxicity, limit high-dose infusions to no longer than 10 minutes.

Adjustment for kidney / liver dysfunction: Renal dysfunction increases risk of toxicity.
- eCrCl 10-30 mL/min: Limit infusion to <3 mcg/kg/min.
- eCrCl <10 mL/min: Avoid when possible, do not exceed 1 mcg/kg/min.
- Hepatic dysfunction: Use with caution, increased risk of toxicity.

PK/PD: Rapid onset of action, ~2 min. Duration of hypotensive effects ~10 min. Half-life of toxic metabolite: ~3 days (may be ~9 days in renal failure).

Common adverse events: hypotension, cyanide toxicity (metabolic acidosis, increased thiocyanate).

Administration: Sodium thiosulfate should be added to all infusions, especially in: renal dysfunction, doses >3 mcg/kg/min for >3 days. Protect solution from light, not necessary to wrap administration set or IV tubing.

Other: High-cost medication ($500-1000 per day). Monitor thiocyanate, methemoglobin as needed.

Antiarrhythmics

Amiodarone
Mechanism of action: Class III antiarrhythmic (alpha- and beta-blocking properties), affects Na+, K+, and Ca++ channels, increases action potential and increases refractory period in myocardial tissue; decreases AV conduction and sinus node function.
Indications: Ventricular tachycardia, ventricular fibrillation, supraventricular tachycardia.
Contraindications: Hypersensitivity to iodine.
Dosage:
- Children (IV): 5 mg/kg, max 300 mg IV push. Additional 5 mg/kg boluses (max 150 mg) may be given to a total daily max of 25 mg/kg or 2.2 g/day. Long-term (IV): Load 10-20 mg/kg/day via continuous infusion for 10-14 days, followed by maintenance dose of 10-15 mg/kg/DAY. For JET in newborns and infants, slowly administer boluses of 1-5 mg/kg at a time until effect to avoid decreased ventricular function.
- Children (PO): Load 10-20 mg/kg/DAY divided q12-24h for 10 days or until arrhythmia control; then decrease to 5-10 mg/kg/DAY given daily for several weeks; decrease dose to lowest effective level, usually 2.5-5 mg/kg/DAY.
- Adults (IV): Load 150 mg over 10 min, followed by 360 mg over 6 hr. Give supplemental boluses of 150 mg over 10 min for breakthrough ventricular fibrillation or hemodynamically unstable ventricular tachycardia. Maintenance 540 mg administered over the next 18 hrs; then maintenance dose of 0.5 mg/min.
- Adults (PO): 800-1600 mg/day in 1-2 doses for 1-3 weeks, then 600-800 mg/DAY in 1-2 doses for 1 month, then 400 mg/day or lowest effective dose.
- Lower doses are recommended for supraventricular arrhythmias.

Adjustment for kidney / liver dysfunction: None.
PK/PD: Onset: Oral 2 days to 3 weeks; IV within hours. Peak 1 week to 5 months. Duration after discontinuation variable (2 weeks to months). Absorption: Oral slow and variable; bioavailability ~50%; peak oral 3-7 hrs; protein binding (96%). Metabolism: Hepatic via CYP2C8 and 3A4 to active metabolite; possible enterohepatic recirculation. Excretion: Feces and urine.
Adverse events: QTc prolongation, hepatotoxicity, thyroid dysfunction, corneal deposits (long-term), pulmonary fibrosis, skin sensitivity/skin color changes, hypotension with IV.
Administration:
- Oral: Give with food.
- IV: Use in-line filter. Infusions should be prepared in non-DEHP containers and all tubing at TCH is DEHP-free. Administer bolus undiluted for pulseless ventricular tachycardia/fibrillation.

Other: Serum levels do not correlate with efficacy. Drug-drug interactions are common. Administer with care in newborns due to potential for decreased function; administer slowly.

Atenolol
Mechanism of action: Competitively blocks response to beta-adrenergic stimulation, selectively blocks beta1-receptors with little or no effect on beta2 except at high doses.
Indications: ventricular tachycardia, supraventricular tachycardia, hypertension.
Contraindications: bradycardia, decompensated CHF.
Dosage:
- Arrhythmias:
  - Long-QT syndrome: Initial 0.5-1 mg/kg/DAY given divided q12-24h; usual dose: 1.4 ± 0.5 mg/kg/DAY.
  - Supraventricular tachycardia: 0.5-1 mg/kg/DAY divided q12-24h; max 1.4 mg/kg/DAY.
- Hypertension:
  - Children: 0.5-1 mg/kg/DAY divided q12-24h; usual range: 0.5-1.5 mg/kg/DAY; max dose 2 mg/kg/DAY (do not exceed adult maximum dose of 100 mg/DAY).
  - Adults: 25-50 mg once daily; max dose 100 mg once daily.

Adjustment for kidney / liver dysfunction:
- eCrCl 30-50 mL/min: Administer daily; max 1 mg/kg/DOSE or 50 mg.
- eCrCl <30 mL/min: Administer every other day; max 1 mg/kg/DOSE or 50 mg.

PK/PD: Onset of action ≤1 hour; peak effect 2 to 4 hours. Duration 12 to 24 hours, prolonged with renal impairment. Absorption rapid, incomplete (~50%); time to peak in plasma 2 to 4 hours. Distribution: Low lipophilicity; does not cross blood-brain barrier; protein binding 6% to 16%. Metabolism: Limited hepatic. Excretion: Feces (50%); urine (40% as unchanged drug).
Common adverse events:
- Cardiovascular: Bradycardia (persistent), cardiac failure, chest pain, cold extremities, complete AV block, edema, hypotension, Raynaud phenomenon, second degree AV block.
- Central nervous system: Confusion, decreased mental acuity, depression, dizziness, fatigue, headache, insomnia, lethargy, nightmares.

Administration: Oral. May be administered without regard to food.
Other: Suspension of 2 mg/mL is compounded.

Carvedilol
Mechanism of action: Nonselective inhibitor of alpha1-, beta1-, and beta2-receptors.
Indications: Heart failure.
Contraindications: Bradycardia, heart block, decompensated heart failure.
Dosage: Initial 0.025-0.05 mg/kg (max initial 3.125 mg) twice daily. Titrate every 1-2 weeks to 0.2 mg/kg (max 0.4 mg/kg or 25 mg) twice daily.
Adjustment for kidney / liver dysfunction: No adjustment is necessary for renal impairment. However, children <3.5 years may need thrice daily dosing due to higher elimination.
PK/PD: Onset: 30-60 minutes with peak at 1-2 hours. Half-life: ~2.2-3.6 hours in infants, children, and adolescents; 7-10 hours in adults. Absorption: Rapid and well absorbed. Metabolism: Hepatic via multiple cytochrome P450 enzymes; major pathway is CYP2D6. Elimination: feces and urine.
Common adverse events: Bradycardia, hypotension.
Administration: Oral.
Other: Compounded suspension of 0.1 and 1.67 mg/mL; tablets 3.125 mg and 6.25 mg.

Digoxin
Mechanism of action:
- Heart failure: Inhibition of the sodium/potassium ATPase pump in myocardial cells results in a transient increase in intracellular Na+, which in turn promotes Ca++ influx via the sodium-calcium exchange pump leading to increased contractility.
- Supraventricular arrhythmias: Direct suppression of the AV node conduction to increase effective refractory period and decrease conduction velocity - positive inotropic effect, enhanced vagal tone, and decreased ventricular rate to fast atrial arrhythmias.

Indications: Heart Failure, tachyarrhythmias.
Contraindications: Ventricular fibrillation, Wolff-Parkinson-White.
Dosage: 5-10 mcg/kg/day given once to twice daily.
Adjustment for kidney / liver dysfunction:
- eCrCl 30-50 mL/min: Administer 75% of normal dose at normal intervals.
- eCrCl 10-29 mL/min: Administer 50% of normal dose at normal intervals or administer normal dose every 36 hours.
- eCrCl <10 mL/min: Administer 25% of normal dose at normal intervals or administer normal dose every 48 hours.

PK/PD: Onset of action: Oral 1-2 hours; IV 5-60 minutes. Peak effect: Oral 2-8 hours; IV 1-6 hours. Duration: 3-4 days. Absorption: Elixir 70-85%; tablet 60-80%. Distribution: Patients with alterations in albumin, serum electrolytes, or thyroid hormones may have alterations in digoxin pharmacokinetics. Metabolism: Via intestinal bacteria. Half-life elimination: 38 hours. Excretion: Urine (50-70% as unchanged drug).
Common adverse events: Bradycardia, digoxin toxicity (arrhythmias, nausea / vomiting / anorexia, visual changes).
Administration: Oral.
Other: Serum digoxin levels are rarely useful in therapy. Patients can experience toxicity with normal concentrations. Caution should be taken to ensure appropriate dosing and preventing confusion with mcg and mg.

Esmolol
Mechanism of action: Class-II antiarrhythmic. Competitively blocks response to beta1-adrenergic stimulation with little or no effect on beta2-receptors.
Indications: Ventricular tachycardia, supraventricular tachycardia, hypertension.
Contraindications: Bradycardia.
Dosage:
- Hypertension (infants, children, and adolescents): Continuous IV infusion 100-500 mcg/kg/minute.
- Supraventricular tachycardia (children and adolescents): Limited data available. Initial IV bolus 100-500 mcg/kg over 1 minute followed by a continuous IV infusion; initial rate 25-100 mcg/kg/minute, titrate in 25-50 mcg/kg/minute increments; usual maintenance dose 50-500 mcg/kg/minute; doses up to 1,000 mcg/kg/minute have been reported.

Adjustment for kidney / liver dysfunction: None.
PK/PD: Onset of action: Beta-blockade IV 2-10 minutes (quickest when loading doses are administered). Duration of hemodynamic effects: 10-30 minutes; prolonged following higher cumulative doses, extended duration of use. Metabolism: In blood by red-blood-cell esterases. Half-life: 2.7-9 minutes. Excretion: Urine (~73-88% as acid metabolite, <2% unchanged drug).
Common adverse events: Bradycardia, hypotension, hypoglycemia.
Administration: Bolus doses may be given IV push over 1-2 minutes. Continuous infusion.
Other: Commercially available concentrations (10 mg/mL and 20 mg/mL).

Flecainide
Mechanism of action: Class-Ic antiarrhythmic; slows conduction in cardiac tissue by altering transport of ions across cell membranes.
Indications: Tachyarrhythmias.
Contraindications: Use in structural heart disease.
Dosage:
- Infants: 100-120 mg/m2/DAY divided every 8 hours; may increase to 200 mg/m2/DAY based on response and serum level.
- Children: 100-120 mg/m2/DAY divided every 12 hours, may be changed to same total daily dose divided every 8 hours; may increase to 200 mg/m2/DAY based on response and serum level.
- Adults: Initial 100 mg every 12 hours, increase by 50 mg increments every 12 hours; max dose 400 mg/DAY.

Adjustment for kidney / liver dysfunction: For children and adults with eCrCl ≤35 mL/min/decrease the usual dose by 25-50%.
PK/PD: Absorption: Oral, nearly complete; decreased when administered with milk. Half-life elimination: 8-29 hours, longer in infants. Time to peak, serum: ~3 hours (range 1-6 hours). Excretion: Urine 30%; feces 5%.
Common adverse events: Arrhythmias.
Administration: Suspension, oral 20 mg/mL (compounded). Administration with milk / feeds reduces bioavailability.
Other: Optimal sampling time - trough 1 hour prior to next maintenance dose. Optimal serum concentration 200-1000 ng/mL.

Lidocaine
Mechanism of action: Class-Ib antiarrhythmic, decreases automaticity and conduction velocity through sodium channel blockade.
Indications: Ventricular arrhythmias.
Contraindications: None.
Dosage:
- Pediatric:
  - IV: 1 mg/kg slowly over 2 minutes; maximum 100 mg/dose. Continuous IV infusion 20-50 mcg/kg/minute.
  - Endotracheally: 2-2.5 times the IV bolus dose; dilute in 3-5 mL NS or distilled water.
- Adults:
  - IV: 1-1.5 mg/kg slowly over 2 minutes; may repeat doses of 0.5-0.75 mg/kg every 5-10 minutes if needed; maximum total dose 3 mg/kg. Continuous IV infusion 1-4 mg/minute.
  - Endotracheally: 2-2.5 times the IV bolus dose; dilute in 10 mL NS or distilled water.

Adjustment for kidney / liver dysfunction: None, not dialyzable (0-5%).
PK/PD: Onset of action: Single bolus dose 45 to 90 seconds. Duration: 10-20 minutes. Metabolism: 90% hepatic; active metabolites monoethylglycinexylidide (MEGX) and glycinexylidide (GX) may accumulate in liver disease and cause toxicity. Half-life elimination: Biphasic, prolonged with CHF, liver disease, shock, severe renal disease; initial elimination 7-30 minutes; terminal elimination in infants/premature 3.2 hours; adults 1.5-2 hours. Excretion: Urine (<10% as unchanged drug, ~90% as metabolites).
Common adverse events: Arrhythmias, paresthesias.

Administration:
- Endotracheal (infants, children, adolescents): May administer dose undiluted, followed by flush with 5 mL of NS after administration or may further dilute prior to administration; follow with 5 assisted manual ventilations.
- Parenteral: Rapid IV push; can be given as continuous infusion.

Metoprolol
Mechanism of action: Selective inhibitor of beta1-adrenergic receptors.
Indications: CHF, hypertension, ventricular tachycardia and fibrillation.
Contraindications: Bradycardia, heart block, decompensated CHF.
Dosage:
- Oral (hypertension):
  - Children and Adolescents (1-17 years):
    · Tablets and suspension (immediate release, as tartrate): Initial 0.5-1 mg/kg twice daily; maximum 6 mg/kg/DAY (≤200 mg/DAY).
    · Tablets (extended release, as succinate), children ≥6 years: Initial 0.5 mg/kg once daily (max initial dose 50 mg/DAY); titrate to response (max 2 mg/kg/DAY or 200 mg/DAY).
  - Adults:
    · Tablets (tartrate): Initial 50 mg twice daily; increase weekly to desired effect; usual dose 100-450 mg/DAY.
    · Extended release tablets (succinate): Initial 25-100 mg/DAY once daily; max daily dose 400 mg.
- Oral (heart failure):
  - Children (tartrate): 0.1-0.2 mg/kg/dose BID; titrate to as tolerated to 0.5 mg/kg BID; max 1 mg/kg BID.
  - Adults (succinate): NYHA Class II heart failure: 12.5-25 mg daily; more severe CHF: 12.5 mg daily; may double the dose q2wks as tolerated; max 200 mg/DAY.
- IV (hypertension/ventricular rate control):
  - Adolescents and adults: Initial 1.25-5 mg q6-12h.

Adjustment for kidney / liver dysfunction: None.
PK/PD: Onset of action: Oral immediate release within 1 hour. Peak effect: Oral 1 to 2 hours; IV 20 minutes. Duration: Oral immediate release variable; extended release ~24 hours. Absorption: Rapid and complete. Metabolism: Extensively hepatic via CYP2D6; significant first-pass effect (~50%). Bioavailability: Immediate release ~40% to 50%; extended release 77% relative to immediate release. Half-life: Neonates 5-10 hrs; adults: 3-4 hours (7-9 hrs in poor CYP2D6 metabolizers or hepatic impairment). Excretion: Urine 95%.
Common adverse events: hypotension, bradycardia, hypoglycemia.
Administration: Metoprolol tartrate: administer with food. Metoprolol succinate: Do not chew, crush, or break.
Other: Suspension, oral: 10 mg/mL extemporaneously prepared. Available as tartrate (immediate release) and extended release (succinate).

Propranolol
Mechanism of action: Nonselective beta-blocker (class-II antiarrhythmic); competitively blocks response to beta1- and beta2-adrenergic stimulation resulting in lower HR, lower BP, lower myocardial contractility, and lower O_2 demand.
Indications: Supraventricular tachycardia, hypertension, prevention of hypercyanotic spells (tetralogy of Fallot).
Contraindications: bradycardia; decompensated CHF.
Dosage:
- Arrhythmias:
  - Neonates: Oral 0.25 mg/kg/dose q6-8hr; titrate slowly to max of 5 mg/kg/DAY. For IV needs, use a different medication.
  - Children: Oral 1 mg/kg/dose q6-8hr; usual dose 3-5 mg/kg/DAY. IV 0.01-0.1 mg/kg/dose over 10 min; repeat q6-8hrs prn; max dose: 1 mg (infants); 3 mg (children).
  - Adults: Oral initial 10-20 mg/dose every 6-8 hours; increase gradually; usual range 40-320 mg/DAY. IV 1 mg/dose slow; repeat q5min to a total of 5 mg.
- Hypertension: consider different beta-blocker.
- Tetralogy of Fallot spells (infants and children): Oral initial 0.25 mg/kg/dose every 6 hours (1 mg/kg/DAY); if ineffective within first week of therapy, may increase by 1 mg/kg/DAY every 24 hours to maximum of 5 mg/kg/DAY.

Adjustment for kidney / liver dysfunction: None.
PK/PD: Onset of action: Oral 1 to 2 hours. Duration: Immediate release 6 to 12 hours; extended-release formulations ~24 to 27 hours. Absorption: oral rapid and complete, ~25% reaches systemic circulation due to high first-pass metabolism; oral bioavailability may be increased in Down syndrome children; protein-rich foods increase bioavailability by ~50%. Metabolism: Extensive first-pass effect, hepatically metabolized to active and inactive compounds CYP1A2, but also CYP2D6. Half-life elimination: Neonates possible increased half-life; infants median 3.5 hours; children 3.9 to 6.4 hours; adults with immediate-release formulation 3 to 6 hours. Excretion: Metabolites are excreted primarily in urine (96% to 99%); <1% excreted in urine as unchanged drug.
Common adverse events: Hypotension, hypoglycemia, bradycardia.
Administration: Administer IV over 10 minutes; do not exceed 1 mg/minute.
Other: Both 4 mg/mL and 8 mg/mL oral solutions are commercially available.

Sotalol
Mechanism of action: Beta-blocker which contains both beta-blocking (Class II) and potassium channel-blocking (Class III) properties.
Indications: Supraventricular tachycardia, atrial fibrillation.
Contraindications: Bradycardia, heart block, congenital QT prolongation.
Dosage:
- Oral:
  - Infants: 80-200 mg/m2/DAY in divided doses every 8 hours.
  - Children: 80-200 mg/m2/DAY divided into 2 doses.
  - Adults: Initial 80 mg twice a day; may increase to 240-320 mg/DAY after evaluation (higher doses of 480-640 mg/day have been used).
- IV (note: the IV dose is 93.75% of the oral dose):
  - Infants: 75-187.5 mg/m^2/DAY in divided doses every 8 hours.
  - Children: 75-187.5 mg/m^2/DAY divided into 2 doses.
  - Adults: Initial 75 mg twice a day, may increase to 225-300 mg/DAY after evaluation; in most patients, a therapeutic response is obtained with 150-300 mg/DAY divided in 2-3 doses; patients with life-threatening refractory ventricular arrhythmias may require doses of 450-600 mg/DAY.

Adjustment for kidney / liver dysfunction:
- eCrCl >60 mL/min: Administer usual daily dose div q12h.
- eCrCl 30-60 mL/min: Administer 50% of usual daily dose q24h.
- eCrCl 10-30 mL/min: Administer every 36-48 hours.
- eCrCl <10 mL/min: Individualize dose, consider alternative agent.

PK/PD: Onset of action: Oral 1-2 hours; IV when administered over 5 minutes ~5-10 minutes. Bioavailability: Oral 90-100%. Half-life elimination: 8-12 hours, prolonged in patients with kidney dysfunction. Excretion: Urine (as unchanged drug).
Common adverse events (>5%): Hypotension, bradycardia, hypoglycemia, QT prolongation.
Administration: Available as tablets, commercially available solution, and IV.
Other: IV cost $1695.60 per vial.

Anticoagulants

Antithrombin (AT)
Mechanism of action: Inactivation of thrombin, plasmin, and factors IXa, Xa, XIa, and XIIa.
Indications: Antithrombin III deficiency (hereditary or iatrogenic due to heparin use).
Contraindications: None.
Dosage: Goal AT level 80-100%. Administer 50 mg/kg IV x1, consider rechecking AT level 2 hours after dose is administered.
Adjustment for kidney / liver dysfunction: None.
PK/PD: Plasma derived, half-life elimination 2-3 days. Half-life may be decreased following surgery, with hemorrhage, acute thrombosis, and/or during heparin administration.
Common adverse events (>5%): Bleeding, infusion site reactions.
Administration: IV over 15 minutes.
Other: Only use the human-derived product, the recombinant product has a shorter half-life.

Aspirin
Mechanism of action: Irreversible inhibitor of cyclooxygenase-1 and 2 (COX-1 and 2) enzymes.
Indications:
- Antiplatelet effects: Mechanical prosthetic heart valves.
- Primary prophylaxis: Blalock-Taussig-Thomas shunts, following Fontan surgery, VAD placement.
- Anti-inflammatory, antiplatelet: Kawasaki disease.

Contraindications: Hypersensitivity to NSAIDs; patients with asthma, rhinitis, and nasal polyps; children or teenagers with viral infections (risk of Reye syndrome).
Dosage:
- Children:
  - Antiplatelet effects: 3-5 mg/kg/DAY to 5-10 mg/kg/DAY given as a single daily dose.
  - Kawasaki disease: Oral 80-100 mg/kg/DAY div q6h for up to 14 days or until fever resolves for at least 48-72 hours; then 3-5 mg/kg/DAY once daily.
- Adults:
  - Transient ischemic attack (TIA): Oral initial 160-325 mg within 48 hours of stroke/TIA onset, then 75-100 mg once daily (often in combination with another antiplatelet agent).
  - Myocardial infarction prophylaxis: Oral initial 162-325 mg/DAY given on presentation, followed by a maintenance dose of 75-100 mg once daily.

Adjustment for kidney / liver dysfunction: Avoid use if eCrCl <10 mL/min. Dialyzable (50-100%). Avoid use in severe liver disease.
PK/PD: Onset: Immediate release (non-enteric-coated) within 1 hour; enteric-coated expected to be delayed. Peak: Immediate release ~1-2 hrs; enteric-coated 3-4 hours. Duration: Immediate release 4-6 hours; however, platelet inhibitory effects last the lifetime of the platelet (~10 days). Absorption: Immediate release is rapidly absorbed in stomach and upper intestine. Bioavailability 50-75%. Metabolism: Hydrolyzed to salicylate (active) by esterases in GI mucosa, red blood cells, synovial fluid, and blood; salicylate is primarily hepatically metabolized. Excretion: Urine.
Common adverse events: Bleeding. Thrombocytopenia.
Administration: Do not crush enteric-coated tablet. Give with food or water to minimize GI distress. Round doses to facilitate administration (e.g., half of 81 mg tablet).
Other: Avoid use of aspirin suspension due to short stability.

Bivalirudin (Angiomax)
Mechanism of action: Direct thrombin inhibitor of free and clot-bound thrombin without antithrombin mediator.
Indications: Primary treatment or prophylaxis of thrombosis or as substitute in patients with heparin-induced thrombocytopenia.
Dosage: IV initial dose 0.15-0.2 mg/kg/hour; adjust to PTT Hepzyme 1.5-2.5 times baseline value (approximately 50-80). When transitioning from heparin to bivalirudin, recommend stopping heparin for at least 30 minutes before starting bivalirudin. Clinical practice guidelines for maintenance of bivalirudin infusion (non-ECMO):

PTT Hepzyme	Hold?	Dose adjustment	Recheck PTT
<50	No	Increase 10% (nearest 0.01 mg/kg/hr)	2-3 hrs after dose change
50-80	No	No change	2-3 hrs, then daily
81-90	1 hr	Decrease 10% (nearest 0.01 mg/kg/hr)	2-3 hrs after dose change
>91	1 hr	Decrease 20% (nearest 0.01 mg/kg/hr)	2-3 hrs after dose change

Adjustment for kidney / liver dysfunction:
- eCrCl 30-60 mL/min: initial dose 0.08-0.1 mg/kg/hour (reduce baseline initial dose 25-40%).
- eCrCl <30 mL/min: 0.04-0.05 mg/kg/hour (reduce baseline initial dose 60-80%).
- Intermittent hemodialysis: 0.07 mg/kg/hour (reduce from baseline 25-40%).
- Continuous renal replacement therapy (CRRT): 0.03-0.07 mg/kg/hour (reduce from baseline 50-80%).

PK/PD: Onset of action: immediate. Metabolism: Via the reticuloendothelial system. Half-life elimination: 1-2 hours. Excretion: Urine.
Common adverse events: Bleeding.
Administration: IV infusion. Usual concentration: 0.5 mg/mL; 5 mg/mL also available.

Clopidogrel
Mechanism of action: Metabolized to an active metabolite which inhibits glycoprotein IIb/IIIa-mediated platelet aggregation. Inhibition is maintained for the life of the platelet.
Indications: Antiplatelet medication.
Contraindications: None.
Dosage:
- Children ≤24 months: 0.2 mg/kg PO daily.
- Children >24 months and adolescents: 0.2-0.3 mg/kg PO daily up to 0.5-1 mg/kg PO daily (maximum 75 mg daily). Higher doses (1-2 mg/kg/DAY) have been used in patients on VADs who have failed other anticoagulation strategies.

Adjustment for kidney / liver dysfunction: None.
PK/PD: Onset of antiplatelet effect: 1-2 days. Duration of antiplatelet effect: ~5 days. Half-life: ~6 hours. Absorption: Rapid and well absorbed. Metabolism: Hepatic via cytochrome P450 2C19 to active metabolite. Elimination: Urine (50%); feces (46%).
Common adverse events: Bleeding.
Administration: Oral.
Other: Compounded suspension of 5 mg/mL.

Enoxaparin
Mechanism of action: Inhibits Factors Xa and II.
Indications: Treatment or prophylaxis of thromboembolism.
Contraindications: Patients with history of heparin-induced thrombocytopenia (HIT).
Dosage:
- Standard dosage for treatment or prophylaxis:

Age	Treatment (subcutaneous)	Prophylaxis (subcutaneous)
<2 months	1.7 mg/kg q12h	0.75 mg/kg q12h
2mo-18yrs	1 mg/kg q12h	0.5 mg/kg q12h
Adults	1 mg/kg q12h	40 mg q24h

- Dosage titration based on antifactory Xa levels:

Antifactor Xa level	Dose titration	Time to repeat antifactor Xa level
<0.35 Units/mL	Increase by 25%	4 hrs after next dose
0.35-0.49 Units/mL	Increase by 10%	4 hrs after next dose
0.5-1 Unit/mL	Keep same dose	Next day, 1 wk later, the monthly (4 hrs after dose)
1.1-1.5 Units/mL	Decrease by 20%	Before next dose
1.6-2 Units/mL	Hold dose for 3 hrs and decrease by 30%	Before next dose, then 4 hrs after next dose
>2 Units/mL	Hold all doses until factor Xa level 0.5 Units/mL, then decrease by 40%	Before next dose and every 12 hrs until antifactor Xa level <0.5 Units/mL

Adjustment for kidney / liver dysfunction: If eCrCl <30 mL/min, reduce dose by 30% and monitor antifactory Xa levels closely.
PK/PD: Peak effect: 3-5 hours. Half-life: 4.5-7 hours. Duration: ~12 hours. Metabolism: Hepatic. Excretion: Urine (40% of dose as active and inactive fragments).
Common adverse events: Bleeding.
Administration: Subcutaneous. Do not rub injection site after subcutaneous administration as bruising may occur. For doses ≤10 mg, the 20 mg/mL concentration should be used. For doses >10 mg, the 100 mg/mL concentration should be used. Do not expel the air bubble from the syringe prior to injection (in order to avoid loss of drug).
Other: Accidental overdosage may be treated with protamine sulfate. 1 mg protamine sulfate neutralizes 1 mg enoxaparin.

Heparin (Unfractionated)

Mechanism of action: Potentiates the action of antithrombin and thereby inactivates thrombin (as well as activated coagulation factors IX, X, XI, XII, and plasmin) and prevents the conversion of fibrinogen to fibrin.
Indications: Treatment or prophylaxis of thrombosis.
Contraindications: Heparin-induced thrombocytopenia.
Dosage: Adjust dose according to factor Xa and PTT.
- Treatment of thrombosis:

Age	Bolus (max: 5000 Units)	Starting dose (max: 1000 units/hr)
<1 year	75 units/kg	20-28 units/kg/hr
≥1 year	75 units/kg	20 units/kg/hr
ECMO	100 units/kg	20-25 units/kg/hr
Notes: Do not bolus in patients with stroke, bleeding, or high-risk for bleeding (postsurgical).		

- Low-dose prophylaxis for shunt thrombosis: 6 Units/kg/hr with no dose titration.
- Dosage titration algorithm using PTT and heparin levels (low PTT with elevated heparin level is not possible):

PTT and heparin level	Actions
PTT>100 seconds, heparin level ≤0.7 Units/mL	1. Assess for coagulopathy: PT, PTT, fibrinogen, PTT hepzyme, bilirubin, and other testing 2. Correct coagulopathy 3. Manage unfractionated heparin per heparin level
PTT >130 seconds, heparin level >1 Unit/mL	1. Assess collection method 2. Repeat PTT and heparin level STAT 3. If correct, adjust per protocol
PTT and heparin level MATCH	1. Manage unfractionated heparin per protocol 2. May use PTT to adjust unfractionated heparin dose 3. Measure heparin level at least every 24 hours
PTT and/or heparin level subtherapeutic	1. Recheck infusion dose / rate calculation 2. Measure antithrombin and correct if <60% 3. Check factor VIII, fibrinogen, and bilirubin 4. Manage unfractionated heparin per heparin level

Adjustment for kidney / liver dysfunction: None, adjust to therapeutic PTT or Xa goals.
PK/PD: Onset of action: Immediate. Metabolism: Via the reticuloendothelial system. Half-life elimination: 1-2 hours. Excretion: Urine.
Common adverse events (>5%): Immunologically mediated heparin-induced thrombocytopenia (HIT).
Administration: IV infusion. Usual concentration: 100 units/mL.
Other: Overdosage may be treated with protamine sulfate.

Warfarin

Mechanism of action: Inhibition of vitamin K-dependent clotting factors (II, VII, IX, X) and procoagulant factors of protein C and S.
Indications: Thrombosis (treatment or prophylaxis).
Contraindications: Pregnancy.
Dosage:
- Loading dose:
  - Infants and children: Load 0.2 mg/kg (max dose 5 mg). If hepatic dysfunction or post-Fontan, load with 0.1 mg/kg.
  - Adults: Start 2-5 mg daily for 2 days, or 5-10 mg daily for 1-2 days.
  - **Loading dose adjustments for days 2-4:**

INR	Dose adjustment
1.1-1.4	Repeat the initial loading dose
1.5-3	50% of initial loading dose
3.1-3.5	25% of initial loading dose
>3.5	Hold until INR <3.5, then 50% less than loading dose
Note: If INR <1.5 after 2 doses, increase by 50%	

- **Maintenance (days 5 and beyond)** treatment, titrate to INR goal, usually 2-3, or 2.5-3.5:

Goal INR 2-3	
1.1-1.4	Increase by 20%
1.5-1.9	Increase by 10%
2-3	No change
3.1-3.5	Decrease by 10%
3.5-5	Hold one dose, recheck INR in 24 hrs. when INR <3.5, restart at 20% less
>5	Hold until INR <3.5

Goal INR 2.5-3.5	
1.1-1.9	Increase by 20%
2-2.4	Increase by 10%
2.5-3.5	No change
3.5-5	Hold one dose, recheck INR in 24 hrs. when INR <3.5, restart at 20% less
>5	Hold until INR <3.5

Adjustment for kidney / liver dysfunction: See loading dose.
PK/PD: Onset of anticoagulation: 24-72 hours. Peak effect: 5-7 days; INR may increase in 36-72 hours. Duration: 2-5 days. Absorption: Rapid, complete. Metabolism: Hepatic, primarily via CYP2C9; minor pathways include CYP2C8, 2C18, 2C19, 1A2, and 3A4. Genomic variants: Approximately 37% reduced clearance of S-warfarin in patients heterozygous for 2C9 (*1/*2 or *1/*3), and ~70% reduced in patients homozygous for reduced function alleles (*2/*2, *2/*3, or *3/*3). Excretion: Urine (92%, primarily as metabolites; minimal as unchanged drug).
Common adverse events: Bleeding. Rare but important or life-threatening: Gangrene of skin or other tissue, purple toe syndrome.
Administration: Oral. Warfarin is available in many tablet strengths, doses should be rounded to the nearest half-tablet size.
Other: Use with caution is patients <1 years old. Antidote: Vitamin K, fresh frozen plasma; KCentra. Patients should be counseled to remain consistent on diet, in particular in regards to foods / formulas that contain Vitamin K. Drug-drug interactions are common with prescription and over-the-counter medications.

Immunomodulators

(Rabbit) Antithymocyte Globulin (ATG, Thymoglobulin®)
Mechanism of action: Rabbit-derived polyclonal antibody against human T-cell antigens, causing destruction of T-cells.
Indications: Prevention or treatment of rejection in transplant recipients. ATG can be used in patients with acute kidney injury to delay tacrolimus initiation, when a patient is highly HLA sensitized, or if the transplant was ABO incompatible.
Contraindications: Hypersensitivity to rabbit proteins, active or chronic infections, history of serum sickness following infusion (relative contraindication).
Dosage:
- Induction: 1.5 mg/kg (patients≥50 kg, round to nearest 25 mg) every 24 hours for 3-5 days.
- Acute cellular rejection: 1.5 mg/kg (patients≥50 kg, round to nearest 25 mg) every 24 hours for 5-14 days.
- Adjustments based on white blood cell (WBC) count of platelet count:
  – If WBC 2,000-3,000 /mcL or platelet count 50,000-70,000 /mcL, reduce dose by 50%
  – If WBC <2,000 /mcL, platelet count <50,000 /mcL, or CD3+ T-cell count <25%, consider discontinuing ATG.

Adjustment for kidney / liver dysfunction: None.
PK/PD: Onset: Within 24 hours. Half-life: 2-3 days. Duration: Lymphopenia can persist up to 1-2 years, patients often return to baseline within 4-8 weeks.
Common adverse events: Infusion related reactions, leukopenia, and thrombocytopenia can be dose limiting. Cytokine-release syndrome is rare, but life threatening. Those with serum sickness often present with joint swelling/pain and unresponsive fevers.
Administration: IV 0.5 mg/mL. Central-line administration is preferred with premedication 30-60 minutes prior (acetaminophen, diphenhydramine, hydrocortisone/methylprednisolone). For patients with peripheral lines, various admixtures with hydrocortisone and heparin are available. Doses typically given over 6 hours for initial doses. Doses as fast as 4 hours or as slow as 24 hours can be given.

Azathioprine
Mechanism of action: Derivative of mercaptopurine; metabolites (mainly 6-thioguanine nucleotide metabolites) are incorporated into replicating DNA and halt replication, but is not specific for lymphocytes.
Contraindications: Hypersensitivity. Complete TPMT deficiency (intermediate deficiency may be able to take with reduced dosage).
Dosage (heart transplant): 1-3 PO mg/kg (typically initiate 1.5 mg/kg) daily.
Adjustment for kidney / liver dysfunction:
- eCrCl 10-50 mL/min: Administer 75% of dose.

- eCrCl <10 mL/min or hemodyalisis: Administer 50% of dose.

PK/PD: Half-life: ~2 hours. Absorption: Well absorbed. Metabolism: Glutathione S-transferase reduction to 6-MP in liver and GI tract; metabolism via 3 major pathways: hypoxanthine guanine to active metabolites, xanthine oxidase to inactive metabolites, and TMPT to inactive metabolites. Elimination: Primarily urine.

Common adverse events: Hematologic/oncologic (leukopenia, thrombocytopenia, and anemia) occur commonly and may be dose limiting; hepatotoxicity.

Administration: Tablets 50 and 100 mg (may be cut).

Other: Deficiency in TMPT or xanthine oxidase inhibitors (allopurinol) can increase active metabolites and side effects.

Bortezomib (Velcade®)

Mechanism of action: 26S proteasome inhibitor leading to cell cycle arrest in plasma cells, the main producer of antibodies.

Indications: Antibody-mediated rejection in solid-organ transplant recipients.

Contraindications: Hypersensitivities to boron, boric acid, or mannitol.

Dosage: 0.7 mg/m² at minimum every 72 hours for 4 doses. Typical doses of 1.3 mg/m² associated with increased high-grade non-hematological adverse effects.

Adjustment for kidney / liver dysfunction: For hepatic impairment, the package insert recommends dose adjustment when bilirubin >1.5 the upper limits of normal, or depending on grade of neuropathies observed.

PK/PD: Half-life: 9-15 hours with single dosing up to 40-193 hours with multiple dosing. Metabolism: Hepatic via cytochrome P450 2C19 and 3A4.

Common adverse events: Neuropathies can be severe and often show after multiple dosing. Thrombocytopenia, neutropenia, anemia, and leukopenia nadir around 11 days following start. Hypotension and heart failure have been reported.

Administration: IV over 3-5 seconds; subcutaneous administration may reduce neuropathies.

Other: No premedications required.

Cyclosporine Modified (Neoral®/Gengraf®)

Mechanism of action: Binds to cyclophilin and subsequent complex inhibits calcineurin. Interleukin-2 dependent activation of resting T-lymphocytes is inhibited.

Contraindications: None; consider delaying initiation post transplant in patients with acute kidney injury or patients receiving induction therapy with depleting agents (anti thymocyte globulin) or non depleting agents (basiliximab).

Dosage (heart transplant):
- Initial:
  - IV: 1 mg/kg/DAY as a continuous infusion.
  - Oral: 2-3 mg/kg twice daily.
- Goal troughs:
  - Months 1-3: 300-350 ng/mL.
  - Months 3-12: 250-300 ng/mL.
  - Months 13-36: 200-250 ng/mL.
  - Beyond 3 years: 150-200 ng/mL.
  - Concomitant Sirolimus: 75-125 ng/mL.

Adjustment for kidney / liver dysfunction: No adjustment is necessary, but consider altering goal troughs in renal dysfunction. Removal via dialysis is not expected. Patients with diarrheal illnesses may have reduce elimination (increased levels).

PK/PD: Half-life: ~8.4 hours. Absorption: Erratic and incomplete (30-43% depending on formulation); modified formulations have up to 30% increased absorption. Metabolism: Hepatic via cytochrome P450 3A4. Elimination: Primarily feces.

Common adverse events: Hirsutism, gingival hyperplasia, hypertension; acute and chronic renal insufficiency thought to be greater incidence than tacrolimus; transplant diabetes is reduced compared to tacrolimus.

Administration: Solution of 100 mg/mL. Capsules: 25 mg and 100 mg. Oral modified formulations (Neoral®/Gengraf®) have more stable inter- and intraindividual absorption compared to non-modified (SandImmune®). When converting from IV to oral utilize 1:3 total daily dose.

Other: Food does not alter extent of absorption.

Immune Globulin (IVIG, Gamunex®-C)

Mechanism of action: Replaces IgG antibodies against bacterial, viral, parasitic, and mycoplasma antigens. Immune modulatory actions mediated by binding Fc receptors and down regulation of B-cells.

Indications: Myocarditis, antibody-mediated rejection in transplant recipients.

Contraindications: Hypersensitivity to components of formulations. Certain formulations have higher anti-IgA causing hemolysis in some patients. While sucrose stabilizers have been linked to acute kidney injury, Gamunex®-C is not stabilized with sucrose.

Dosage (use ideal body weight to dose):
- Kawasaki: 2,000 mg/kg once.
- Myocarditis: 2,000 mg/kg given as divided doses over 2-5 days.
- Antibody-mediated rejection:
  - With plasmapheresis: 100 mg/kg following sessions and 1,000 mg/kg following final session.
  - Without plasmapheresis: 1,000-2,000 mg/kg once weekly.

Adjustment for kidney / liver dysfunction: None.

PK/PD: Half-life: 14-24 days. Duration: 3-4 weeks; faster metabolism linked with fever and infection.

Common adverse events: Infusion-related reactions related to rate of infusion; premedication with diphenhydramine and hydrocortisone/methylprednisolone recommended.

Administration:
- Non-Kawasaki disease indications: Start at 0.6 mL/kg/hour for 30 minutes; increase rate by 0.6 mL/kg/hour every 15 minutes, if tolerated, to a maximum rate of 4.8 mL/kg/hour until desired dose administered.
- Kawasaki disease: Start at 0.6 mL/kg/hour for 30 minutes, increase rate by 0.6 mL/kg/hour every 30 minutes for 2 additional titrations. If tolerated, infuse remaining volume over 8.5 hours so that total dose is infused over 10 hours.
- Other: Pharmacy will round dose based on the absolute dose to a maximum of 140 grams:
- Doses <3 grams: Rounded to nearest 100 mg/1 mL.
- Doses ≥3 and <15 grams: Nearest 1 gram/10 mL.
- Doses ≥15 and <57.5 grams: Nearest 5 grams/50 mL.

- Doses ≥57.5 grams: Nearest 10 grams/100 mL.

Mycophenolate Mofetil (Cellcept®) and Mycophenolate Sodium (Myfortic®)
Mechanism of action: Inhibits inosine monophosphate dehydrogenase, which is responsible for purine synthesis specifically in activated T- and B-lymphocytes. Result is reduced synthesis of T- and B-cells.
Contraindications: Hypersensitivity.
Dosage:
- Mycophenolate Mofetil (Cellcept®):
  - Heart transplant: IV/oral initial 20 mg/kg every 12 hours (max: 1500 mg/DOSE).
  - Lung transplant: IV/oral Initial: 700 (non-cystic fibrosis) or 900 (cystic fibrosis) mg/m² every 12 hours.
  - Goal mycophenolic acid troughs*: 1-3.5 mcg/mL.
- Mycophenolate Sodium (Myfortic®):
  - BSA <1.19 m²: not recommended.
  - BSA 1.19-1.58 m²: 540 mg twice daily.
  - BSA >1.58 m²: 720 mg twice daily.

*Therapeutic levels are not well established as troughs do not correlate well with overall exposure and thus prevention of rejection and adverse reactions.

Adjustment for kidney / liver dysfunction: No adjustment is necessary immediate posttransplant, but renal impairment does increase exposure to the active metabolite mycophenolic acid.
PK/PD: Half-life (mycophenolic acid): 13-18 hours. Absorption: Rapid and extensive; bioavailability of mycophenolate mofetil is ~80-94%; bioavailability of mycophenolate sodium is 72%. Metabolism: Hepatic via cytochrome P450 3A4. Elimination (mycophenolic acid): Primarily urine (87%); feces.
Common adverse events: Nausea, vomiting, and diarrhea can be dose limiting. Myfortic® (enteric release) may be an option for nausea/vomiting. Dose-adjust for low WBC count (<3000 /mcL) or neutrophil count (<1000 /mcL). Pure red-cell aplasia can also occur. Mycophenolate is a known teratogen and should be avoided in pregnant patients. Azathioprine (pregnancy category D) may not cross the placenta and could be a substitute.
Administration:
- IV: 6 mg/mL. Administer over 2 hours.
- Oral: 200 mg/mL solution; 250 mg capsules; 500 mg tablets. Myfortic® capsules 180 mg and 360 mg.

Other: Proton-pump inhibitors may reduce oral absorption.

PredniSONE/PrednisOLONE
Mechanism of action: Decreases inflammation by suppression of migration of leukocytes and reversal of capillary permeability; suppresses immune system by reducing activity and volume of lymphatic system.
Contraindications: Hypersensitivities to formulation components.
Dosage:
- Asthma: 0.5-1 mg/kg twice daily (up to 40-80 mg) twice daily for 3 to 10 days.
- Myocarditis: 0.5-1 mg/kg twice daily for 4-6 weeks, followed by a taper.
- Physiologic dosing: 2-2.5 mg/m²/DAY once daily or in divided doses.

Adjustment for kidney / liver dysfunction: None.
PK/PD: Half-life: 2-3 hours. Absorption: Rapid and well absorbed. Metabolism: Prednisone converted to prednisolone; prednisolone primarily undergoes glucuronidation. Elimination: Primarily urine.
Common adverse events: Hypertension, headaches, insomnia, Cushingoid syndrome, hyperglycemia, and adrenal suppression with chronic use.
Administration:
- PredniSONE
  - Tablets: 1, 2.5, 5, 10, 20, 50 mg.
  - Solution: 1 mg/mL.
- PrednisOLONE: Solution 3 mg/mL.

Other: Administer with meals or mild to decrease GI upset.

Rituximab (Rituxan®)
Mechanism of action: Anti-CD20 antibody binds to ubiquitous CD20 receptor on B-cells, causing destruction, limited activation of plasma cells, and reduced antibody production.
Indications: Antibody-mediated rejection in solid-organ transplant recipients.
Contraindications: Known type-1 hypersensitivity to murine-based proteins.
Dosage: 375 mg/m² once weekly for 1-4 doses.
Adjustment for kidney / liver dysfunction: None.
PK/PD: Half-life: 18-32 days. Duration: Up to 6-9 months B-cell depletion.
Common adverse events: Infusion reactions, lymphocytopenia, leukopenia, and neutropenia can occur. Associated with peripheral edema, hypertension, fatigue, and neuropathy.
Administration: IV (0.5 mg/mL). Initial rate of 1 mg/kg/hour (max 50 mg/hour) for first hour; increase rate by 1 mg/kg/hour (max 50 mg/hour) every 30 minutes as patient tolerates. Do not exceed 8 mg/kg.hour or 400 mg/hour.

Sirolimus (Rapamune®)
Mechanism of action: Binds to FKBP-12 and complex inhibits the mammalian target of rapamycin (mTOR) C1 subtype. T-cell proliferation is suppressed by stopping the cell cycle in the G1 phase. mTOR signaling is increased in specific cancers. Sirolimus also has effects of vascular- and platelet-derived growth factors.
Contraindications: Hypersensitivity or history of hereditary angioedema; angioedema risk is increased in patients on angiotensin-converting enzyme inhibitors, but not necessarily angiotensin-receptor blockers. Sirolimus affects wound healing and has been associated with lymphocele/fluid accumulation; use within 30 days of surgery is often avoided. Combination therapy with calcineurin inhibitors has been associated with increased risk of renal impairment.
Dosage:

- Heart transplant:
  - Maintenance dose: Initial: 0.5-1 mg/m² PO once daily (loading dose typically avoided). Not started immediately after transplant.
  - Goal troughs: 2-5 ng/mL in combination with calcineurin inhibitors.
- Pulmonary vein stenosis: Initial: 0.5 mg/m² PO once daily (loading dose unnecessary).

Adjustment for kidney / liver dysfunction: For hepatic impairment, reduce dosage 33-50% depending on estimated degree of liver dysfunction.

PK/PD: Half-life: 13.7 ± 6.2 hours in children; 46-78 (mean 62) hours in adults. Absorption: Solution 14%; tablets 27%. Metabolism: Hepatic via cytochrome P450 3A4. Elimination: Feces (91%).

Common adverse events: Delayed wound healing, mouth ulceration, anemia, and hyperlipidemias are concerns of chronic use. Nephrotoxicity is increased in combination with calcineurin inhibitors. Proteinuria and nephrotic syndrome have been observed in some populations.

Administration:
- Solution: 1 mg/mL.
- Tablets: 0.5, 1, 2 mg.

Other: Avoid perioperative use in transplant patients. Bronchial anastomotic dehiscence, hepatic artery thrombosis, and increased pericardial effusion have been observed in lung, liver, and heart transplants, respectively.

Tacrolimus (Prograf®)

Mechanism of action: Binds to FKBP-12 and subsequent complex inhibits calcineurin. Subsequently interleukin-2-dependent activation of resting T-lymphocytes is inhibited.

Contraindications: None; consider delaying initiation post-transplant in patients with acute kidney injury or patients receiving induction therapy with depleting agents (antithymocyte globulin) or non depleting agents (basiliximab).

Dosage:
- Initial: 0.08 mg/kg PO twice daily.
- Goal troughs:
  - Months 0-12: 10-12 ng/mL.
  - Years 1-3: 8-10 ng/mL.
  - Beyond 3 years: 6-8 ng/mL.
  - Concomitant Sirolimus: 4-8 ng/mL.
- Lung-transplant goal trough (months 1-3): 12-15 ng/mL.

Adjustment for kidney / liver dysfunction: No adjustment is necessary, but consider altering goal troughs in kidney dysfunction. Removal via dialysis is not expected. Patients with diarrheal illnesses may have reduce elimination (increased levels).

PK/PD: Half-life: ~7-15 hours. Absorption: 7-32%. Metabolism: Hepatic via cytochrome P450 3A4. Elimination: Primarily feces.

Common adverse events: Alopecia, transplant diabetes, and hypomagnesemia thought to be greater incidence than cyclosporine. Renal insufficiency, hypertension, and other cosmetic side effects are slightly reduced. Ventricular hypertrophy and transaminitis rare.

Administration:
- Compounded suspension of 0.5 mg/mL.
- Capsules: 0.5 mg, 1 mg, 5 mg.

Other: Food does not alter extent of absorption. If attempting sublingual dosing, reduce dose by 30-50%.

Index

A
Aberrant right subclavian artery 218
Absent pulmonary valve syndrome 144–149
  anesthetic considerations 148
  surgical repair 148–149
Activated clotting time (ACT) 26–28
Acute respiratory distress syndrome (ARDS) 404
Admission to the intensive care unit 385
  admission checklist *386*
room setup *386*
Amiodarone 501
Amlodipine 498
Amniocentesis 369
Analgesia 388–402
Anesthesia for congenital heart disease 382–384
Animal therapy 433
Anomalous aortic origin of a coronary artery. See Coronary anomalies, congenital: anomalous aortic origin of a coronary artery
Anomalous left coronary artery from the pulmonary artery 224–232
  anesthetic considerations 226–227
  surgical repair 228–230
    coronary reimplantation *228*, 228–229
    Takeuchi repair 229, *230*
Anomalous pulmonary venous return
  partial. See Partial anomalous pulmonary venous return
  total. See Total anomalous pulmonary venous return
Antegrade cerebral perfusion 30, 204, 206, 214
Anticoagulation 421–427
  cardiopulmonary bypass. See Cardiopulmonary bypass: anticoagulation
  extracorporeal membrane oxygenation. See Extracorporeal membrane oxygenation: anticoagulation
  medication changes with major surgery 427
  medications *423*
  monitoring *425*
  prosthetic valves *422*
  single-ventricle prophylaxis 421
  ventricular assist devices 424
Antithrombin 504
Antithymocyte globulin 507
Aortic arch advancement 153, *186*, 191–192, *192*
Aortic coarctation. See Coarctation, aortic
Aortic root replacement 256
Aortic stenosis, subvalvar. See Subaortic stenosis
Aortic stenosis, supravalvar. See Supravalvar aortic stenosis
Aortic stenosis, valvar 163–170
  catheter-based intervention 166–167
  genetic evaluation *365*

Aortic uncrossing procedure 220
Aortic valve repair 167–168, *168*
Aortic valve replacement *168*, 168–169, 256
Aortopathy panel *368*. See also Genetic evaluation: aortopathy panel
Aortopulmonary window 209–216, *211*
  anesthetic considerations 212–213
  surgical repair 214
Arrhythmias 258–262
  atrioventricular block
    first-degree 259
    second-degree 259
    third-degree 259, 480–481
  junctional rhythm 258
  pacemaker-mediated tachycardia 310
  sick-sinus syndrome. See Arrhythmias: sinus node dysfunction
  sinus node dysfunction 258
  sinus tachycardia 258
  supraventricular 260–261, 311, 474–476
    algorithm for management *475*
    atrial ectopic tachycardia 261, 474
    atrial fibrillation 261
    atrial flutter 261, 474
    atrioventricular nodal reentrant tachycardia 260, 474
    atrioventricular reentrant tachycardia 260, 474
    intra-atrial reentrant tachycardia 300, 311, 353
    junctional ectopic tachycardia 261, 477–479
    multifocal atrial tachycardia 261
    premature atrial contraction 260
  ventricular 261–262
    premature ventricular contraction 261
    ventricular fibrillation 262, 264
    ventricular tachycardia 261, 263, 264
    torsades de pointes 262, 263
Arterial switch operation 97, *99*, *102*, 100–103
Arterial tortuosity syndrome 344, 350
Art therapy 433
Aspirin 504. See also Anticoagulation
Atenolol 501
Atrial septal defect 42–47
  catheter-based intervention 44–46
  coronary sinus 42
  primum 42
  secundum 42
  sinus venosus 42
  surgical repair 46–47
Atrial switch. See Double-switch operation; See Senning operation; See Senning/Rastelli operation
Atrioventricular canal. See Atrioventricular septal defect
Atrioventricular septal defect 80–87
  balanced 80
  complete 80, *83*, *84*
    anesthetic considerations 83–85

511

surgical repair 85–86
genetic evaluation *366*
partial 80, *84*
    anesthetic considerations 82
    surgical repair 85
    Rastelli classification 80
transitional 80
    anesthetic considerations 82
    surgical repair 85
unbalanced 80
Azathioprine 507

B
Balloon atrial septostomy 97, 137
Barth syndrome *370*
Beighton score 344
Bicuspid aortic valve 163
    genetic evaluation *365*
Bilevel positive airway pressure (BiPAP) 406–407
Bivalirudin 504–505. See also Anticoagulation
Blalock-Taussig-Thomas shunt, modified 89, *93*, 127, 137, 138, 282–284, 287, 292
    for Ebstein anomaly 159, 161, 162
    for tricuspid atresia 152
Bland-White-Garland syndrome. See Anomalous left coronary artery from the pulmonary artery
Bleeding, postoperative 482
Body surface area 26
Borderline left heart. See Left-heart hypoplasia
Bortezomib 507
Brain imaging 376, *377*
Breast milk 417
Brugada syndrome 263, 264–265

C
Calcium
    hypercalcemia 412
    hypocalcemia 411–412
Captopril 498
Cardiac catheterization
    angiography 18
    diagnostic 15–19
Cardiac Developmental Outcomes Program. See Neurodevelopmental outcomes
Cardiac magnetic resonance (CMR). See Magnetic resonance imaging (MRI)
Cardiomyopathy
    arrhythmogenic right-ventricular 248
    dilated 244, 245–246
    genetic testing 369–371, *370*
    hypertrophic 246–247
    noncompaction, left ventricular 247
    restrictive 247–248
    tachycardia-induced 246
Cardioplegia. See Myocardial protection

Cardiopulmonary arrest 469–473
    cardiopulmonary resuscitation. See Cardiopulmonary resuscitation
    management after arrest 473
    management algorithm *470*
    postcardiac-arrest syndrome 473
    sudden. See Sudden cardiac arrest
Cardiopulmonary bypass 26–31
    anticoagulation 26–27
    pH-Stat 29–30
    prime 26
    weaning 31
Cardiopulmonary resuscitation 472. See also Extracorporeal membrane oxygenation: ECMO-CPR
Carvedilol 501
Catecholaminergic polymorphic ventricular tachycardia 264
Central line 442–446
    insertion checklist *443*
Central line-associated bloodstream infection (CLABSI) 442
    prevention *443*, 445
Chaplain 434–437
CHARGE syndrome
    genetic evaluation *368*
Chest tube 450–456
Child life 432–433
Chorionic villus sampling 369
Chromosomal microarray 291, 363, *365–366*, *368*, 369
Chylothorax 419, 483–485
    algorithm for diagnosis and management *484*
    chemical pleurodesis 484–485, *485*
Circumflex aortic arch 219
Clonidine 498
Clopidogrel 505
Coarctation, aortic 181–196
    anesthetic considerations 190
    arch-watch protocol 190
    catheter-based intervention 192–193
        balloon angioplasty 192
        bare-metal stenting 192–193
        covered stents 193
    genetic evaluation *365*
    management algorithm *184*
    surgical repair 190–192. See also Aortic arch advancement; See also Extended end-to-end anastomosis; See also Sliding arch aortoplasty
        interposition graft placement *187*
        patch aortoplasty *187*
Complete atrioventricular block. See Arrhythmias: atrioventricular block: third-degree
Computerized tomography (CT) 12–13, 14

Cone operation. See Ebstein anomaly: surgical intervention: cone operation
Congenitally corrected transposition of the great arteries 105–114
  morphological variants 105, *106*
  surgical repair 109–114
    classic repair *108–109*, 109–110
    double-switch operation. See Double-switch operation
    Fontan operation. See Fontan: for congenitally corrected transposition
    Hemi-Mustard/Rastelli operation. See Hemi-Mustard/Rastelli operation
    left-ventricular retraining *108–109*, 112–113
    Senning/Rastelli operation. See Senning/Rastelli operation
Connective-tissue disorders 344–351
Continuous positive airway pressure (CPAP) 406
Coronary anomalies, congenital 233–243
  anomalous aortic origin of a coronary artery 233–243, *234*
    algorithm for diagnosis and management *235*
    surgical repair 239–240, *240*, *241*
      coronary translocation 240–239
      neoostium creation 240
      pulmonary artery translocation 240
      unroofing 239
    topographic map *237*
  intraseptal coronary 236
    surgical repair 241
  myocardial bridge 236
    surgical repair 241
Coronary artery aneurysm. See Kawasaki disease
Coumadin 426
Cyclosporine 507–508

D
Damus-Kaye-Stansel anastomosis 153, 205, 292
Deep hypothermic circulatory arrest 30, 206
Defibrillator 308–312
Delirium 398–402
  assessment 399–402
  pathway 399–402, *400–401*
Dialysis
  on extracorporeal membrane oxygenation support 329
  peritoneal. See Peritoneal dialysis
DiGeorge syndrome 88, 124, 128, 144, 148, 189, 209, *212*, 215, 216, 217, *378*, 411, 468
  genetic evaluation *368*
Digoxin 502
Discharge education 430–431
Double-outlet right ventricle 115–123
  anesthetic considerations 119–120
  classification 115, *116*, *118*
  genetic evaluation *365*
  surgical intervention 120–121
  Taussig-Bing anomaly. See Taussig-Bing anomaly
Double-switch operation *108–109*, 110–113, 113
Down syndrome. See Trisomy 21
Drugs 498–510
D-transposition of the great arteries. See Transposition of the great arteries
Ductal stent 127, 137, 138, 282–288, 292
  for Ebstein anomaly 159, 162
  for tricuspid atresia 152
Dysphagia lusoria 219

E
Ebstein anomaly 155–162
  anesthetic considerations 160
  surgical intervention 160–161
    cone operation 161
    Starnes procedure 159, 161, 162
    tricuspid valve repair 161, 162
    tricuspid valve replacement 161
Echocardiography
  fetal 8
  transesophageal 20–25
  transthoracic 11, 12–13
Ehlers-Danlos syndromes 344
  classical 347
  genetic evaluation *368*
  hypermobile 348
  vascular-type 347–348
Eisenmenger syndrome 71, 210
Elastin mutation 180, *365*, *368*. See also Williams syndrome
Electrolytes 409–413
Enalapril 498–499
Enalaprilat 499
Endocarditis 249–257
  acute 250
  subacute 250
  surgical intervention 256
End-of-life discussions 435–437
Enoxaparin 505
Epsilon-aminocaproic acid 428, *429*
Esmolol 502
Extended end-to-end anastomosis *185*, 191
Extracorporeal membrane oxygenation 245, 261, *285*, 322–332
  anticoagulation 330, 422–424
  for arrhythmias 479
  atrial septal defect creation 331–332
  cannulation 329–330
    venoarterial 322–323
    venovenous 327
  ECMO-CPR 325–326, *471*, *472*
  Impella. See Ventricular assist device: Impella
  mechanical ventilation while on ECMO 325, 405

sedation 330–331
venoarterial 322–326
  for sepsis 325–326
  weaning 326
venovenous 326–328
  recirculation 327–328
  weaning 328
Extubation 405–406

F

Feeding intolerance algorithm *416*
Feeding protocol for high-risk patients *415*
Feeding tube 462–463
Fetal aortic valvuloplasty 198
Fetal cardiology 9
Fetal circulation 7
Fetal intervention 8, 10
Fick principle 18
Flecainide 502
FLNA-related periventricular nodular heterotopia 351
Fluids 408–409
Fluoresecent in-situ hybridization (FISH) 364, *365, 368*, 369
Fontan *293*, 298–300, 343
  adults 352–358
  anesthetic considerations 354
  arrhythmias 353
  complications 352–353
  for congenitally corrected transposition 114
  failure 353–354
  fenestration 298, 354
  long-term follow-up 300–301
  mechanical support. See Ventricular assist device: for Fontan patients
  for pulmonary atresia with intact ventricular septum 139–143
  revision 355–357
  transplantation. See Transplant, heart: for Fontan patients
Fractional flow reserve 238, 273, 275

G

Gastrostomy 419
Genetic evaluation 363–371
  aortopathy panel 344
  by lesion *365*
  by suspected diagnosis *368*
Glenn, bidirectional 152, 153, *293*, 295–298, 343
  for Ebstein anomaly 161
  pulsatile 297, 343
Grief 434–437

H

HeartMate II *316*
Hemi-Mustard/Rastelli operation 110, *112*, 113
Hemostasis 428–429

Heparin 505–506. See also Anticoagulation
Heritable thoracic aortic disease 350–351. See also Genetic evaluation: aortopathy panel
Heterotaxy syndrome 341–343
  genetic evaluation *366*
High-flow nasal cannula 406
High-frequency oscillatory ventilation 404–405
Holter *378*
Holt-Oram syndrome
  genetic evaluation *368*
Hydralazine 499
Hypoplastic aortic arch. See Coarctation, aortic
Hypoplastic left-heart complex. See Hypoplastic left heart syndrome; See Left-heart hypoplasia
Hypoplastic left heart syndrome 201–208
  anesthetic considerations 204–205
  comfort care 207
  genetic evaluation *365*
  hybrid procedure 207
  transplantation 207. See also Transplant, heart

I

Imaging 11–14
Immune globulin 508
Implantable cardioverter defibrillator. See Defibrillator
Innominate artery syndrome 217
Intercoronary pillar 233
INTERMACS profiles *315*
Interrupted aortic arch 181–196
  classification 181
  genetic evaluation *365*
Interstage period 294–295
Intra-atrial reentrant tachycardia. See Arrhythmias: supraventricular: intra-atrial reentrant tachycardia
Intraseptal coronary. See Coronary anomalies, congenital: intraseptal coronary
Intravascular ultrasound 238
Intubation, endotracheal 440–441

J

Jacobsen syndrome 291
Junctional ectopic tachycardia. See Arrhythmias: supraventricular: junctional ectopic tachycardia

K

Karyotype 364, *365–366, 368*, 369
Kawasaki disease 267–276
  atypical. See Kawasaki disease: incomplete
  complete 267, *268*
  echocardiographic recommendations 270–272
  incomplete 267, *268*
  management
    cath-based intervention 275

complicated Kawasaki disease 269–270
  coronary bypass grafting 275
  uncomplicated Kawasaki disease 269
 shock syndrome 267–268
Kommerell diverticulum. See Vascular ring: right aortic arch with aberrant left subclavian artery
Konno operation, modified 174

L

Left-atrial line 447–449
Left-heart hypoplasia 197–200. See also Hypoplastic left heart syndrome
  anatomical patterns 197–198
  surgical considerations 199–200
    intracardiac exploration 199
Lidocaine 502–503
Lisinopril 499–500
Loeys-Dietz syndromes 344, 349–350
  genetic evaluation *368*
Long-QT syndrome 263
Low cardiac output syndrome 466–468
L-transposition of the great arteries. See Congenitally corrected transposition of the great arteries

M

Magnesium 412–413
  hypermagnesemia 413
  hypomagnesemia 412
Magnetic resonance imaging (MRI) 11
Major aortopulmonary collaterals. See also Pulmonary atresia with ventricular septal defect
  unifocalization 128, 130–131
    postoperative management 132
Malrotation, intestinal 342
Marfan syndrome 344, 344–346
  genetic evaluation *366*, *368*
  Marfan syndrome systemic score 344, *345*
Mechanical ventilation 403–405
Mee shunt 127, 128, 130, 282
Metoprolol 503
Milrinone 500
Mitral valve repair 256
Mitral valve replacement 256
Modified Blalock-Taussig-Thomas shunt. See Blalock-Taussig-Thomas shunt, modified
Multiplex ligation probe-dependent analysis (MLPA) 364
Music therapy 432–433
Mycophenolate 508
Myocardial bridge. See Coronary anomalies, congenital: myocardial bridge
Myocardial protection 26–31

Myocarditis 244–245

N

Near-infrared spectroscopy (NIRS) 30, 204, 206, 292, *377*, 461
Neurodevelopmental outcomes 361–362, *377*
Next-generation sequencing panels 366–367
Nicardipine 500
Nikaidoh procedure 121
Nitroprusside 500
Noninvasive mechanical ventilation 406–407
Non-invasive prenatal testing (NIPT) 369
Noonan syndrome *370*
  genetic evaluation *365*, 366, *368*
Norwood procedure *203*, 205–206, 292, 292–293
  Blalock-Taussig-Thomas shunt, modified 204, 205, 206, 207, 293
  Brawn modification 206, 293
  Lamberti modification 293
  Sano modification 205, 206, 207, 293
Nutrition 414–420
  nutritional needs *414*

O

Occupational therapy algorithm *418*
Oscillator. See High-frequency oscillatory ventilation
Overhaul, right ventricle. See Pulmonary atresia with intact ventricular septum: overhaul, right ventricle
Oxygenation index 326
Oxygen consumption 18
Oxygen delivery 327
Oxygen-extraction ratio 466
Oxygen-saturation index 326

P

Pacemaker 308–312
  nomenclature *310*
Palliative arterial switch 153, 154, 294
Parenteral nutrition guidelines *417*
Partial anomalous pulmonary venous return 48–55
  scimitar syndrome *51*, *52*, *53*, 54–55
  surgical repair 53–54
    two-patch repair 54
    Warden procedure 54
Patent ductus arteriosus 34–41
  anesthetic considerations 38–39
  catheter-based intervention 39
  ibuprofen treatment 37
  indomethacin treatment 37
  postligation cardiac syndrome 41
  stent. See Ductal stent
  surgical intervention 39–41
Patent foramen ovale 42
Pericardial effusion 277, 278, 279, 494–495

515

Pericarditis 277–280
　autoimmune 279
　bacterial 278, 279
　constrictive 280
　idiopathic 278, 279
　malignant 279
Peripherally inserted central catheter (PICC) 444
Peritoneal dialysis 457–460
P/F ratio 326
Pleural effusion 492–493
Pneumothorax 486–488
　tension 486
Postcardiotomy syndrome 46, 279, 494–495
Postcoarctectomy syndrome 194
Postligation cardiac syndrome. See Patent ductus arteriosus: postligation cardiac syndrome
Potassium 409–410
　hyperkalemia 409–410
　hypokalemia 409
Prednisolone 509
Prednisone 509
Preoperative evaluation 376–381
Propranolol 503
Protein-losing enteropathy 280, 353, 354
Pulmonary artery band 291–292
　for tricuspid atresia 152, 153
Pulmonary artery sling 217, *218*
Pulmonary atresia with intact ventricular septum 133–140
　1.5-ventricle repair 139–140
　biventricular repair 139–140
　Fontan circulation 139–143
　management algorithm *135, 141*
　overhaul, right ventricle 139–140
　right-ventricle-dependent coronary circulation 134, 136, 136–140, 137–140, 138
　right-ventricular decompression 138–140
Pulmonary atresia with ventricular septal defect 124–132. See also Major aortopulmonary collaterals
　anesthetic considerations 128–129
　catheter-based intervention 129
　diagnostic cardiac catheterization 125
　management strategy 126–128
　surgical intervention 129–132
　　aortopulmonary shunts 130. See also Mee shunt
　　Rastelli procedure 131–132. See also Rastelli procedure
　　unifocalization 130–131
Pulmonary hypertension 489–491
Pulmonary stenosis 140–143
　balloon valvuloplasty 141–142
　surgical intervention 142–143
　tetralogy of Fallot. See Tetralogy of Fallot
Pulmonary valve replacement 302–307
　indications 302
　surgical *303*, 305–307
　transcatheter 303–305
Pulmonary vascular resistance 19
Pulmonary vein stenosis 64–70
　catheter-based intervention 66–69
　surgical intervention 69–70

Q
Qp:Qs 18, 19

R
Rastelli procedure 121, 127, 131–132
Réparation à l'etage ventriculaire (REV) procedure 121
Right-ventricular outflow tract obstruction 133–143
Rituximab 509
Ross-Konno operation 169, 174
Ross operation 168, 170, 256
RotaFlow 315
ROTEM 330, 383, *425, 426*, 427, 428, 429, 482

S
Scimitar syndrome. See Partial anomalous pulmonary venous return: scimitar syndrome
Sedation 388–402
　clinical pathways 389–396
　FLACC scale 388, *389*
　Sedation Targeted Assessment and Review (STAR) 388
　State Behavioral Scale 388, *390*
　tolerance 396–402
　weaning 396–402
　withdrawal 396–402
　Withdrawal Assessment Tool 396–402, *397, 399, 400*
Segmental anatomy of the heart 2–6
Senning operation 110, *111*
Senning/Rastelli operation *108–109*, 110
Shone complex. See Left-heart hypoplasia
Shunts, aortopulmonary 282–288
　Blalock-Taussig-Thomas shunt, classic 282
　Blalock-Taussig-Thomas shunt, modified. See Blalock-Taussig-Thomas shunt, modified
　Mee shunt. See Mee shunt
　Potts shunt 282
　Waterston-Cooley shunt 282
Sickle-cell disease or trait *378*
Simulation 359–360
Single-gene sequencing 364
Single-ventricle palliation 289–301
　anticoagulation prophylaxis 421
Sirolimus 509
Sliding arch aortoplasty *187*
Sodium 410–411

hypernatremia 411
hyponatremia 410–411
Sotalol 503–504
Staphylococcus aureus infection prevention protocol *379*
Starnes procedure. See Ebstein anomaly: surgical intervention: Starnes procedure
Subaortic stenosis 171–175
  surgical repair 173–174
Sudden cardiac arrest 233, 235–236
  workup 265–266
Supravalvar aortic stenosis 176–180
  genetic evaluation *365*
  surgical repair 178
    Doty patch aortoplasty *178*, 178–179
Supraventricular tachycardia. See Arrhythmias: supraventricular
SynCardia total artificial heart *316*, 317
Systemic vascular resistance 19

T

Tacrolimus 509–510
Tamponade, cardiac 277, 278, 279
Taussig-Bing anomaly 102, 115, *117*, 118
  surgical intervention 121
Tetralogy of Fallot 88–94
  anesthetic considerations 90
  genetic evaluation *365*
  surgical repair 90–93
Thermodilution 17
Thrombosis
  arterial 424
  venous 424–425
Total anomalous pulmonary venous return 56–64
  anesthetic considerations 61–62
  cardiac 56, *60*
  in heterotaxy 341
  infracardiac 56, *58*, *59*
  mixed 56
  supracardiac 56
  surgical repair 62
Total artificial heart. See SynCardia total artificial heart
Tranexamic acid 428
Transcranial Doppler 30, 204, 206
Transitional circulation 7
Transition medicine 372–374
Transplant, heart 333–340
  anesthetic considerations *336*, 336–337
  contraindications 333, *334*
  evaluation of donor 335
  evaluation of recipient 333–334
  for Fontan patients 354, 357–358
  in hypoplastic left heart syndrome 207
  immunosuppression *338*, 338–340, 339–340
  indications 333
  rejection 338, 340
  status for listing 335
  surgical technique 335–336
  surveillance 337–338
Transposition of the great arteries 95–104
  anatomical variants 96
  anesthetic considerations 98–100
  congenitally corrected. See Congenitally corrected transposition of the great arteries
  coronary patterns 98
  left-ventricular retraining 100
  physiology 95, *96*
  surgical repair 100–103. See also Arterial switch operation
Tricuspid atresia 150–154
  classification 150
  management algorithm *153*
  surgical considerations 152–154
Trisomy 13 291
  genetic evaluation *368*
Trisomy 18 291
  genetic evaluation *368*
Trisomy 21 81, 83, 87, 190, 217, *378*
  genetic evaluation *366*, *368*
Truncus arteriosus 209–216
  anesthetic considerations 212–213
  classification 209, *210*
  genetic evaluation *365*
  surgical repair 214
Turner syndrome 291
  genetic evaluation *368*

U

Ultrafiltration 31, 329
Unifocalization. See Major aortopulmonary collaterals: unifocalization

V

VACTERL association 88, 209
Vascular ring 217–223
  anesthetic considerations 220–222
  double aortic arch 217, *218*
    surgical repair 219
  right aortic arch with aberrant left subclavian artery 217, *218*
    surgical repair 219, *221*
Ventilator-associated pneumonia
  prevention 405
Ventricular assist device 245, 246, 313–321
  anticoagulation 424
  Berlin EXCOR 315, *316*
  device selection *314*, 315–317, *316*
  driveline care 320–321
  for Fontan patients 357
  HeartWare HVAD 315, *316*
  Impella 315, *316*, 323, 331

   patient selection 313–315
   postoperative management 317–320
   surgical implantation 317
Ventricular septal defect 71–79
   catheter-based intervention 75–77
   doubly committed juxta-arterial 71, *72*
   inlet 71, *72*
   muscular 71, *72, 76, 77*
   perimembranous 71, *72, 76*
   supracristal. See Ventricular septal defect: doubly committed juxta-arterial
   surgical repair 78
Vertebral-artery tortuosity index 345, 346
von Willebrand syndrome, acquired 428

W

Warfarin 506–507. See also Anticoagulation
Whole-exome sequencing 291, 364–366, *368*
Williams syndrome 176, 177, 178
   anesthetic considerations 177–178
   genetic evaluation *368*
Withdrawal of life sustaining therapies 435
Wolff-Parkinson-White syndrome 105, 156, 474

Abbreviations

2D: 2-dimensional
3D: 3-dimensional
ABG: Arterial blood gas
ACT: Activated clotting time
AHA: American Heart Association
AS: Aortic stenosis
AI: Aortic insufficiency
ALT: Alanine aminotransferase
ARDS: Acute respiratory distress syndrome
ASA: American Society of Anesthesiologists
ASD: Atrial septal defect
AST: Aspartate transaminase
AV: Atrioventricular
BP: Blood pressure
Bpm: Beats per minute
BSA: Body surface area
BUN: Blood urea nitrogen
BVH: Biventricular hypertrophy
CBC: Complete blood count
CHD: Congenital heart disease
CHF: Congestive heart failure
CHS: Congenital heart surgery
CICU: Cardiac intensive care unit
CNS: Central nervous system
CO$_2$: Carbon dioxide
CPAP: Continuous positive airway pressure
CPB: Cardiopulmonary bypass
CPR: Cardiopulmonary resuscitation
CRNA: Certified registered nurse anesthesist
CT: Computed tomography
CTA: Computed tomography angiography
CV: Cardiovascular
CVP: Central venous pressure
CVOR: Cardiovascular operating room
CXR: Chest X-ray
DNA: Deoxyribonucleic acid
EACTS: European Association for Cardio-Thoracic Surgery
ECLS: Extracorporeal life support
ECG: Electrocardiogram
ECMO: Extracorporeal membrane oxygenation
eCrCl: Estimated creatinine clearance
ENT: Ears, nose, and throat (otolaryngology)
ETCO$_2$: End-tidal carbon dioxide
ETT: Endotracheal tube
FDA: Food and Drug Administration
FFP: Fresh frozen plasma
FiO2: Inspiratory fraction of oxygen
GERD: Gastroesophageal reflux disease
GI: Gastrointestinal
HFNC: High-flow nasal cannula
hpf: High-power field
ICU: Intensive care unit
IJ: Internal jugular
iNO: Inspired nitric oxide
INR: International normalized ratio
INTERMACS: Interagency Registry for Mechanically Assisted Circulatory Support
IV: Intravenous
IVC: Inferior vena cava
IR: Interventional radiology
JET: Junctional ectopic tachycardia
LA: Left atrium

LAD: Left anterior descending
LAP: Left atrial pressure
LCOS: Low cardiac output syndrome
LFT: Liver function test
LV: Left ventricle
LVH: Left ventricular hypertrophy
LVOT: Left ventricular outflow tract
MAP: Mean arterial pressure
MR: Mitral regurgitation
MRI: Magnetic resonance imaging
NICU: Neonatal Intensive Care Unit
NIRS: Near infrared spectroscopy
NP: Nurse practitioner
NPO: Nil per os (nothing by mouth)
NS: Normal saline
OR: Operating room
OT: Occupational therapy
PA: Pulmonary artery
PaCO$_2$: Arterial partial pressure of carbon dioxide
PaO$_2$: Arterial partial pressure of oxygen
PCA: Patient-controlled analgesia
PCR: Polymerase chain reaction
PDA: Patent ductus arteriosus
PediMACS: Pediatric Interagency Registry for Mechanically Assisted Circulatory Support
PEEP: Peak end-expiratory pressure
PFO: Patent foramen ovale
PGE: Prostaglandin E
PI: Pulmonary insufficiency
PICC: Peripherally inserted central catheter
PICU: Pediatric Intensive Care Unit
PIP: Peak inspiratory pressure
PK/PD: Pharmacokinetics / Pharmacodynamics
PO: Per os (by mouth)

PRBC: Packed red blood cells
PT: Physical therapy / Prothrombin time
PTT: Partial thromboplastin time
PVR: Pulmonary vascular resistance
Qp:Qs: Ratio of pulmonary flow to systemic flow
RA: Right atrium
ROTEM: Rotational thromboelastography
rSO$_2$: Regional oxygen saturation
RSV: Respiratory syncytial virus
RV: Right ventricle
RVH: Right ventricular hypertrophy
RVOT: Right ventricular outflow tract
SaO$_2$: Oxygen saturation
SvO$_2$: Mixed-venous oxygen saturation
SIMV-VC: Synchronized intermittent mandatory ventilation / volume control
SVC: Superior vena cava
SVR: Systemic vascular resistance
STS: Society of Thoracic Surgeons
TCH: Texas Children's Hospital
TEE: Transesophageal echocardiogram
TPN: Total parenteral nutrition
TR: Tricuspid regurgitation
TTE: Transthoracic echocardiogram
UAC: Umbilical arterial catheter
US: United States
UVC: Umbilical venous catheter
VAD: Ventricular assist device
VBG: Venous blood gas
VSD: Ventricular septal defect
Vt: Tidal volume
WBC: White blood cells

Lightning Source UK Ltd.
Milton Keynes UK
UKHW020700230222
399112UK00001B/7